Risk of Arrhythmia and Sudden Death

To my parents

Risk of Arrhythmia and Sudden Death

Edited by
Marek Malik
Professor of Cardiac Electrophysiology
St George's Hospital Medical School, London, UK

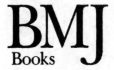

©BMJ Books 2001
BMJ Books is an imprint of the BMJ Publishing Group

First published in 2001
by BMJ Books, BMA House, Tavistock Square,
London WC1H 9JR

www.bmjbooks.com

British Library Cataloguing in Publication Data
A catalogue record for this book is available from the British Library

ISBN 0-7279-1581-9

Typeset by Phoenix Photosetting, Chatham, Kent
Printed and bound by Creative Print and Design Ltd

Contents

Part III: Clinical studies of risk assessment

Part IV: Antiarrhythmic trials

Contributors

Steen Z Abildstrom
Department of Cardiology, Gentofte University Hospital, Copenhagen, Denmark

James J Bailey
Center for Information Technology, National Institutes of Health, Bethesda, Maryland, USA

Velislav Batchvarov
Department of Cardiological Sciences, St George's Hospital Medical School, London, UK

Antoni Bayés de Luna
Departamento de Cardiología, Hospital de la Santa Creu i Sant Pau, Barcelona, Spain

Toni Bayés-Genis
Fellow, Mayo Clinic, Rochester, Minnesota, USA

Annalisa Bertoldi
Department of Cardiology, S. Chiara Hospital, Trento, Italy

Daniel M Bloomfield
Assistant Professor of Medicine, Division of Cardiology, College of Physicians and Surgeons, Columbia University, USA

Mark L Brown
Staff Scientist, Tachyarrhythmia Research Department, Atrial Fibrillation Research Group, Medtronic, Minneapolis, Minnesota, USA

Rory Childers
Professor of Medicine, Section of Cardiology, University of Chicago Medical Centre, Chicago, USA

Timothy R Church
Division of Environmental and Occupational Health, School of Public Health, University of Minnesota, Minneapolis, Minnesota, USA

Richard J Cohen
Whitaker Professor, Harvard University–Massachusetts Institute of Technology, Division of Health Sciences and Technology, Massachusetts, USA

Andrea Colella
Istituto di Clinica Medica e Cardiologia, Università di Firenze, Florence, Italy

Xavier Copie
Department of Cardiology, Broussais Hospital, Paris, France

Alessandro Costoli
Istituto di Clinica Medica e Cardiologia, Università di Firenze, Florence, Italy

Philippe Coumel
Hôpital Lariboisière, Paris, France

Harry JGM Crijns
Department of Cardiology, Thoraxcenter, University Hospital Groningen, Groningen, The Netherlands

Michael Cusack
Clinical Research Fellow, Department of Cardiology, Rayne Institute, St Thomas' Hospital, London, UK

Joseph T Dell'Orfano
Department of Medicine, Division of Cardiology, The State University of New York at Stony Brook, Stony Brook, New York, USA

Roberto Elosua
Unidad de Lípidos y Epidemiología Cardiovascular, Instituto Municipal de Investigación Médica, Barcelona, Spain

Fredrick Fernando
Sports Science Institute, Italian National Olympic Committee, Rome, Italy

Francesco Furlanello
S. Raffaele Scientific Institute, Milan-Rome, Italy

Amedeo Galassi
Arrhythmia and Electrophysiological Center, S Donato Institute, Milan, Italy

Gian Franco Gensini
Istituto di Clinica Medica e Cardiologia, Università di Firenze, Florence, Italy

Louis Guize
Department of Cardiology, Broussais Hospital, Paris, France

Josep Guindo
Departmento di Cardiologia, Hospital de la Santa Creui i Sant Pau, Barcelona, Spain

Harry Hemingway
Senior Lecturer in Epidemiology, International Centre for Health and Society, Department of Epidemiology and Public Health, University College London Medical School, London; Director of Research and Development, Department of Research and Development, Kensington & Chelsea and Westminster Health Authority, London, UK

Morrison Hodges
Minneapolis Heart Institute Foundation, Minnesota, USA

Stefan H Hohnloser
Department of Medicine, Division of Cardiology, J.W. Goethe University, Frankfurt, Germany

Katerina Hnatkova
Department of Cardiological Sciences, St George's Hospital Medical School, London, UK

Michiel J Janse
Cardiovascular Research, Academic Medical Center, Amsterdam, The Netherlands

Josef Kautzner
Department of Cardiology, Institute for Clinical and Experimental Medicine, Prague, Czech Republic

Robert E Kleiger
Professor of Medicine, Washington University School of Medicine; Medical Director of Washington University School of Medicine HRV Laboratory, St Louis, USA

Lars Køber
Department of Cardiology, Gentofte University Hospital, Copenhagen, Denmark

Piotr Kulakowski
Department of Cardiology, Postgraduate Medical School, Grochowski Hospital, Warsaw, Poland

Patrick Lam
Beth Israel Medical Center, New York, USA

Maria Teresa La Rovere
Fondazione "Salvatore Maugeri", IRCCS, Divisione di Cardiologia, Centro Medico Montescano, Pavia, Italy

Thomas Lavergne
Department of Cardiology, Broussais Hospital, Paris, France

Jean-Yves Le Heuzey
Department of Cardiology, Broussais Hospital, Paris, France

Steven Lindsay
Consultant Cardiologist, Bradford Royal Infirmary, Bradford, UK

Federico Lombardi
Cardiologia, Dipartimento di Medicina, Chirurgia e Odontoiatria Ospedale S Paolo, Università degli Studi di Milano, Milan, Italy

Pierre Maison Blanche
Hôpital Lariboisière, Paris, France

Marek Malik
Professor of Cardiac Electrophysiology, Department of Cardiological Sciences, St George's Hospital Medical School, London, UK

Antonio Martinez-Rubio
Departamento de Cardiología, Hospital de la Santa Creu i Sant Pau, Barcelona, Spain

Branco Mautner
President, International Society for Holter and Non-Invasive Electrocardiology; Academic Vice-Chancellor, Favaloro University, Belgrano, Buenos Aires, Argentina

William J McKenna
Professor of Cardiac Medicine, Department of Cardiological Sciences, St George's Hospital Medical School, London, UK

Antonio Michelucci
Istituto di Clinica Medica e Cardiologia, Università di Firenze, Florence, Italy

Andrea Mortara
Fondazione "Salvatore Maugeri", IRCCS, Divisione di
Cardiologia, Centro Medico Montescano, Pavia, Italy

Arthur J Moss
Professor of Medicine (Cardiology), Director, Heart
Research Follow-up Program, University of Rochester
Medical Center, Rochester, New York, USA

Gerald V Naccarelli
Chief, Division of Cardiology, MS Hershey Medical Center
of the Pennsylvania State University, Hershey,
Pennsylvania, USA

Jim Nolan
Consultant Cardiologist, Cardiothoracic Centre, North
Staffordshire Hospital, Stoke on Trent, UK

Luigi Padeletti
Istituto di Clinica Medica e Cardiologia, Università di
Firenze, Florence, Italy

Paolo Pieragnoli
Istituto di Clinica Medica e Cardiologia, Università di
Firenze, Florence, Italy

Gian Domenico Pinna
Servizio di Bioingegneria, Fondazione "Salvatore
Maugeri", IRCCS, Centro Medico Montescano, Pavia,
Italy

Olivier Piot
Department of Cardiology, Broussais Hospital, Paris,
France

Maria Cristina Porciani
Istituto di Clinica Medica e Cardiologia, Università di
Firenze, Florence, Italy

Simon Redwood
Senior Lecturer / Honorary Consultant Cardiologist,
Department of Cardiology, Rayne Institute, St Thomas'
Hospital, London, UK

Georg Schmidt
Deutsches Herzzentrum und Medizinische Klinik der
Technischen Universität München, Munich, Germany

Peter J Schwartz
Professor and Chairman, Department of Cardiology,
Policlinico S Matteo, IRCCS and University of Pavia, Italy

Paul Schweitzer
Beth Israel Medical Center, New York, USA

Phyllis K Stein
Research Assistant Professor of Medicine, Washington
University School of Medicine; Director of Washington
University School of Medicine HRV Laboratory, St Louis,
USA

Shlomo Stern
Emeritus Professor of Medicine, Hebrew University, and
the Bikur Cholim Hospital, Jerusalem, Israel

Peter Sutton
Departments of Cardiology, UCL Hospitals and Hatter
Institute, University College Hospital, London, UK

Peter Taggart
Departments of Cardiology, UCL Hospitals and Hatter
Institute, University College Hospital, London, UK

Christian Torp-Pedersen
Department of Cardiology, Gentofte University Hospital,
Copenhagen, Denmark

Isabelle C Van Gelder
Department of Cardiology, Thoraxcenter, University
Hospital Groningen, Groningen, The Netherlands

Xavier Viñolas
Departamento de Cardiología, Hospital de la Santa Creu i
Sant Pau, Barcelona, Spain

Johan EP Waktare
Cardiological Sciences, St George's Hospital Medical
School, London UK

Yee Guan Yap
Specialist Registrar in Cardiology, Department of
Cardiological Sciences, St George's Hospital Medical
School, London, UK

Gang Yi
Department of Cardiological Sciences, St George's
Hospital Medical School, London, UK

Preface

In the developed world, the cost of medical care is rapidly rising and practically every clinical, pharmacological or technological breakthrough brings not only an improved quality of life and prolonged patient survival but also a significant burden on healthcare providers irrespective of whether they are privately organised or government controlled. Despite the differences in the economies and healthcare arrangements of the Western world countries, the discussions about the ever rising cost of medical care are everywhere similarly heated. Clearly, there are no easy solutions since removing a potentially life-saving treatment from any human being is not ethical. At the same time, no country of the world is so wealthy that it could afford the best available treatment and care for all its citizens. Cardiology is no exception to this trend. For instance, studies that have confirmed the efficacy and appropriateness of the prophylactic use of implantable defibrillators are examples of findings that have both clinical and financial implications. Still, compared to comprehensive safety nets and resuscitation programs designed to save patients only after they have suffered from malignant ventricular arrhythmias, prophylactic use of implantable defibrillators is most likely a cost-saving option.

In general, prophylactic medicine is one of the most effective ways of reducing the overall costs of medical care while, at the same time, maintaining adequate quality of life and improving the survival of the overall population. It is therefore not surprising that prophylactic methods are presently receiving substantial attention from both clinical community and healthcare providers. The advances in prophylactic medicine are clearly dependent on improved risk markers and advanced risk stratification approaches. Again, cardiology is no exception. Cardiac risk stratification is presently being investigated not only to identify patients who might benefit from more cost-effective modes of prophylactic treatment but also, even more importantly, to save patients who would otherwise succumb to cardiac death and sudden cardiac death in particular.

For all these reasons, I was very pleased when I was offered the opportunity of editing this book on risk stratification of arrhythmias and sudden cardiac death. Indeed, some of the principles and methodologies of arrhythmia risk stratification are rather complex and, in some cases, perhaps not fully appreciated and understood by clinical cardiologists and electrophysiologists. In order to offer a comprehensive coverage of the field, I have divided the contents of the book into four sections. The first part contains chapters dealing with the general principles of risk stratification, explaining the individual facets of methodology and technology and summarising the goals of arrhythmic risk stratification studies. The second part is devoted to a detailed description of individual investigation techniques aimed at identification of patients at high risk of arrhythmia or sudden death. The third part describes the present experience with applying the risk stratification technologies and tests to patients of different clinically defined groups. Finally, the two chapters of the final part summarise the presently conducted clinical trials utilising the risk stratification techniques.

As with every multi-authored book, I faced the usual editoral dilemma of finding the proper balance between having the book compact with cross-references within individual chapters and having the chapters suited for separate reading. Eventually, I felt that with a book of this size aimed at providing a source of standard references, each chapter should contain a standard coverage of its subject. Hence, I am happy to recommend the reader to select chapters corresponding to his/her particular needs and interest. Needless to say, reading the book in its entirety offers much more comprehensive learning of the whole field.

Without the kind positive response of the authors of the individual chapters, this book would have never been written. I truly appreciate the efforts of the individual contributors and am very grateful for their kind help. My deep thanks also go to my secretary, Mrs Melanie Monteiro, who carefully organised the editorial office of this book and who helped me in many other ways. I am grateful to the publisher for their useful suggestions, significant technical help, and kind flexibility. My apologies go to my wife and children since far too frequently I have devoted the time that I should have spent with them to the editing of this text.

Marek Malik

Abbreviations

AECG	ambulatory electrocardiography	**NPV**	negative predictive value
AF/AT	atrial fibrillation/atrial tachycardia	**NSVT**	non-sustained ventricular tachycardia
APC	atrial premature contraction	**PCA**	principal component analysis
AT	attributable risk	**pNN50**	percentage of normal to normal RR intervals that differ ≥50 ms from the preceding interval
BRS	baroreflex sensitivity		
CHF	congestive heart failure		
DAD	delayed after-depolarisations	**PPV**	positive predictive value
EAD	early after-depolarisations	**PSVT**	paroxysmal supraventricular tachycardia
ECG	electrocardiograph	**rMSSD**	root mean square of successive differences of normal to normal RR intervals
EGM	electrogram		
ERP	effective refractory period	**ROC**	receiver-operating characteristic
FRP	functional refractory period	**SACT**	sinoatrial conduction time
HCM	hypertrophic cardiomyopathy	**SDNN**	standard deviation of normal to normal RR intervals
HF	high frequency		
HRV	heart rate variability	**SDNNIDX**	SDNN index
ICD	cardioverter/defibrillator	**SNRT**	sinus node recovery time
ILR	implantable loop recorder	**TO**	turbulence onset
LF	low frequency	**TP**	total power
LVEF	left ventricular ejection fraction	**ULF**	ultralow frequency
LVH	left ventricular hypertrophy	**VA**	ventricular arrhythmias
MAPs	monophasic action potentials	**VPC**	ventricular premature contraction
MI	myocardial infarction	**VT**	ventricular tachycardia

Part I

Problem and methodology

1 Clinical goals of risk stratification

Roberto Elosua, Josep Guindo, Xavier Viñolas, Antonio Martinez-Rubio, Toni Bayés-Genis and Antoni Bayés de Luna

The clinical goals of risk stratification of sudden death (SD) are to identify subjects who are at high risk and, eventually, to reduce the incidence of SD. We will focus in this chapter on aspects related to epidemiological and clinical issues to stratify risk of SD. We consider SD as a syndrome that may be associated with different diseases and situations. The term "sudden death" has been used in different ways by epidemiologists, clinicians, forensic pathologists, etc. Clinically, the term is used for deaths due to natural causes that occur within 1 hour of the onset of symptoms in a person with or without pre-existing heart disease, but in whom the time and mode of death are unexpected. In approximately one-third of cases the death is instantaneous, without symptoms or coinciding only during a few seconds with the presence of symptoms. If the patient is found dead, death is considered to be "sudden" if the subject was seen alive and well in the preceding 24 hours.[1]

In this chapter we shall discuss the need for identification of high-risk populations for malignant arrhythmias and sudden death. It is especially important to emphasise the paradox that the highest-risk subgroups (cardiac arrest survivors or patients with an ejection fraction <30%) account for a small proportion of SD events in a population. We emphasise how different is the clinical approach for risk stratification in the general population and in patients with already clear evidence of heart diseases, for example in post-myocardial infarction patients.

Clinical epidemiological aspects

Sudden death usually appears in the presence of clinical or silent heart disease.[2,3] Ischaemic heart disease (IHD) is by far the most common associated situation found in patients presenting with sudden cardiac death (SCD) (Box 1.1). Nevertheless, other heart diseases may present with SCD, especially in the presence of heart failure and/or left ventricular hypertrophy.[4,5] In some cases, there are only isolated electrophysiological abnormalities (WPW, long QT syndrome, Brugada syndrome, etc.)[6–8] or congenital defects of coronary arteries.[9] In a few cases (≅3%), there is no evidence of associated heart disease, probably because, with the current technology used, we are unable to define or demonstrate some undetectable, minor abnormalities. Such cases, now named "idiopathic SCD", will be fewer in the future.[10]

Box 1.1 Principal causes of sudden cardiac death
- Ischaemic heart disease
- Cardiomyopathies
  - idiopathic dilated cardiomyopathy – heart failure
  - hypertrophic cardiomyopathy
  - arrhythmogenic right ventricular dysplasia
- Valvular heart disease
  - aortic stenosis
  - mitral valve prolapse
- Electrophysiologic abnormalities
  - pre-excitation syndromes
  - long QT syndrome
  - conduction system abnormalities
  - Brugada syndrome
- Congenital cardiac abnormalities
- Sudden death without apparent structural heart disease

SCD is considered to be of ischaemic origin if it appears during an acute ischaemic event or in the presence of severe IHD. From a pathological point of view, SCD is considered ischaemic when stenosis of at least 75% of the area of the lumen of one coronary artery is found. Intraluminal or intra-intimal thrombi may or may not be present.[11] Severe coronary atherosclerosis may exist whether or not there are clinical symptoms (acute myocardial infarction or angina) before SCD.[12]

We will comment on the following epidemiological aspects related to SCD:

- the size of denominator pools in different population subgroups that determine the ability to identify potential victims within population subgroups of various sizes;[13]
- the time dependence of risk, which expresses risk as non-linear function of time after a conditioning clinical event;[13,14]

● the importance of the different risk factors and environment in the appearance of SCD.[1-3]

Population subgroups and sudden cardiac death

According to Myerburg,[13] if we consider all cases of SCD occurring in the USA, the overall incidence is in the range of 1–2/1000 population per year (0.1–0.2%). This large population base contains both those victims where SCD occurs as a first cardiac event, in which the possibility to predict sudden death is very limited (i.e. the general population), and those victims whose deaths may be predicted with greater accuracy because they come from higher risk subgroups (i.e. survivors of sudden cardiac death) (Fig. 1.1). Because of the size of the denominator, any intervention designed for the general population must be applied to more than 99% of population who will not have an event during the course of a year. These numbers limit the nature of a broad-based intervention and encourage the identification of specific higher-risk clinical subgroups. Nevertheless, with increasing specificity of subgroups, the absolute number of potential victims who can be identified decreases. Figure 1.1 expresses the incidence (percent per year) of SCD among various subgroups.

In clinical epidemiology it is very important to consider two different levels of risk: attributable risk versus relative risk.[15,16] Relative risk (RR) is the ratio of the incidence of an event, SCD in this case, in persons with and without a risk factor; whereas, attributable risk (AR) refers to the proportion of the incidence of an event that can be explained by the presence of the risk factor.[1]

By moving from the total adult population to a subgroup with higher risk there may be a more than 10-fold increase in the incidence of events annually, an important RR increase. As shown in Fig. 1.1, there is a progressive increase in the incidence of SCD as one moves from the general population to subgroups having had a prior coronary event and to those with low ejection fractions and heart failure, and to survivors of out-of-hospital cardiac arrest, and to those experiencing ventricular tachycardia or fibrillation (VT/VF) during the convalescent phase after myocardial infarction. However, the corresponding absolute number of deaths becomes progressively smaller as the subgroups become more focused, an important AR decrease. Thus, in these selected subgroups although the RR is higher the AR is lower.

Clinical application of new technologies and procedures appears to have had a favourable impact on the highest risk subgroups. Progress measured in terms of prevention of large numbers of sudden cardiac deaths in the general population, however, will be limited until it is possible to identify more easily higher risk individuals in the general population. At the moment it is impossible to know which patients in the general population present vulnerable plaques. Thus, the only way to prevent SCD in this population is to fight against classical cardiovascular risk factors (smoking, hypertension, lipid disorders).

Time dependence of risk

Furukawa and Myeburg[13,14] have also emphasised that risk of SCD does not appear to be linear as a function of time after a change in cardiovascular status. Survival curves after major cardiovascular events (cardiac arrest survivors, post-myocardial infarction patients, patients with recent onset of heart failure, etc.), which identify populations at high risk for both sudden and total cardiac death, generally demonstrate that the most dangerous period occurs during the first 6–18 months after the index event. By 24 months, the slope of a survival curve is not very different from one describing a similar population that has remained free of an interposed major cardiovascular event. Thus, there is a time dependence of risk after a major event, which stresses the importance of the most intensive intervention in the early period. The higher risk subgroup, as happens in survivors of cardiac arrest, has not only a different overall mortality rate but also a different pattern of attrition as a function of time. In Fig. 1.2 the actuarial analysis of recurrences among a population of 101 cardiac arrest survivors with IHD is shown. The risk is high in the first 6 months (11.2%) and then falls to 3.3% in the next

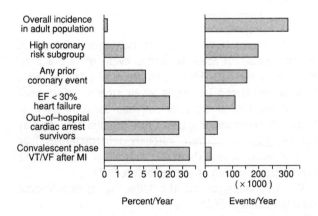

Figure 1.1 Bar graphs showing the relation between incidence and total numbers of sudden cardiac deaths in overall and population subgroups. The numbers are calculated for the US population. (Adapted form reference 13.) (Abbreviations: EF = ejection fraction; MI = myocardial infarction; VF = ventricular fibrillation; VT = ventricular tachycardia.)

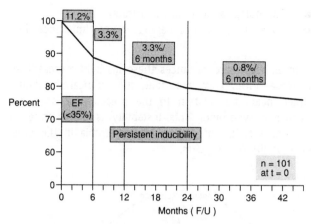

Figure 1.2 Time dependence of rate of recurrences among survivors of cardiac arrest. Actuarial analysis or recurrences among a population of 101 cardiac arrest survivors with coronary heart disease. Risk was higher in the first 6 months and then fell to 3.3% for the next three 6-month periods. After 24 months, the rate fell to 0.8% for each 6-month period thereafter. The most powerful predictor of death was a low ejection fraction (EF) during the 6 first months and persistent inducibility during programmed stimulation afterwards. (Adapted from reference 14.)

three 6-month blocks thereafter. Low ejection fraction is the most powerful predictor of death during the first 6 months, subsequently, persistent inducibility during programmed stimulation is the most powerful predictor of death.[13,14] In a study of a post-myocardial infarction population, Moss *et al.*[8] pointed out that 50% of the deaths that occur during the 48 months after myocardial infarction occur within the first 6 months. Therefore, the use of time as a dimension for measuring risk is extremely important.

Risk factors and the environment

The incidence of SCD varies considerably from country to country with relation to the prevalence of IHD. Since IHD is characteristic of industrialised societies and its ageing population, the prevalence of SCD is greater in the western countries than in the rest of the world. According to the World Health Organization,[17] the incidence of SCD in industrialised areas varies between 19 and 159 per 100 000 inhabitants per year among men between the ages of 35 and 64.

In the USA and other industrialised countries, the incidence of SCD is decreasing parallel to the overall decrease in IHD mortality.[18] This decrease has been attributed to a decrease in the incidence of IHD and to a lower fatality related to an improved medical therapy and a more effec-

tive system for resuscitating victims of out-of-hospital cardiac arrest. In spite of this, the incidence of SCD remains high and is still a major challenge confronting contemporary cardiology. On the other hand, the global burden of cardiovascular diseases including IHD and consequently of SCD is increasing in developing countries. Thus, we have to extend our preventive campaigns world-wide.

A number of studies have shown that SCD displays a prominent circadian pattern, with a primary peak occurring between 7 and 11 am.[19] In the Framingham Study,[20] the risk of SCD is approximately 70% greater from 7 to 9 am than during the rest of the day. A circadian variation of SCD, similar to that of the occurrence of non-fatal myocardial infarction and episodes of myocardial ischaemia, was observed.

Although the incidence of SCD parallels the incidence of IHD, which increases with age, the proportion of those who die suddenly is higher in younger patients. This differential effect of age may be due to older patients having more advanced coronary heart disease, and therefore the incidence of death due to heart failure is greater.

SCD is more common in males than in females by a ratio of 3 to 1. This is due to the lower prevalence of IHD in premenopausal women. Females attain a comparable incidence of SCD 20 years older than men. However, more females than males die suddenly without clinical evidence of IHD. Since the frequency of SCD is much higher in postmenopausal women compared to premenopausal women of the same age, it is likely that a hormonal factor influences the result.

Multivariate logistic analysis in the Framingham Study,[21] including all coronary risk factors, indicates that, in males, age, systolic blood pressure, cigarette smoking, and relative bodyweight are all independently related to the incidence of sudden death. In females, aside from age, only hypercholesterolaemia and vital capacity are associated independently with an increased risk of sudden death. Using these parameters, there is a wide variation in the risk of sudden death. Forty-two percent of sudden deaths in males and 53% in females occur in onetenth of the population in the top decile of multivariate risk.

It is important to conceptualise sudden cardiac death as a manifestation of IHD occurring as a consequence of a variety of risk factors and living habits. Small changes in blood pressure, cholesterol levels, and cigarette smoking pattern may not be of great importance if they are isolated, but they can interact to increase the risk of SCD.

Genetic factors are also important in less common causes of SCD, such as in the congenital long QT syndrome,[22] hypertrophic cardiomyopathy,[23] arrhythmogenic right ventricle dysplasia, or Brugada syndrome,[24] etc. Parental sudden death has been also identified as a risk factor for SCD.[25]

Pathophysiology of sudden cardiac death

Ischaemic heart disease

Most cases of SCD occur in patients with IHD. In these patients the chain of events leading to SCD may occur in two ways:

- an acute ischaemic syndrome (AIS), especially acute myocardial infarction (AMI), or
- a primary arrhythmic event (PAE) (Fig. 1.3).

It is practically impossible to predict the appearance of acute ischaemic syndrome (acute MI) when this is the first manifestation of the disease without previous heralding symptoms. This would only be possible if we could detect, easily and non-invasively, not only the presence of coronary atherosclerosis, but especially the existence of vulnerable plaques. Such plaques are at high risk of rupture or thrombosis.[26-28] From a pathological point of view, plaques are considered vulnerable when they have large lipid cores occupying more than 40% of the overall plaque volume, thin and inflamed fibrous caps separating the cores from the arterial lumen, a high density of macrophages, and a low density of smooth-muscle cells in the caps.[26]

On the other hand, the danger of a primary arrhythmic event often occurs in post-MI patients. In these cases, the danger of an acute ischaemic syndrome (severe and persistent ischaemia, usually appearing as acute myocardial infarction) is not the only cause of the vulnerability of the myocardium to SCD, although some degree of residual or transient ischaemia may be present. The most important markers that express this arrhythmic risk type of vulnerability are:

- clinical/ECG

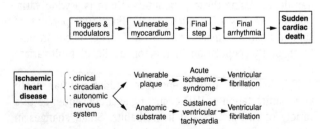

Figure 1.3 The chain of events that leads to final arrhythmia and sudden cardiac death. Some triggers and/or modulators acting in a vulnerable myocardium lead to the final step and final arrhythmia. The triggers and modulators may be similar in the two ways but the vulnerable myocardium is different: vulnerable plaque in the case of acute ischaemic syndrome leading to a ventricular fibrillation and anatomic substrate leading to a sustained ventricular tachycardia and ventricular fibrillation.

- morphological (anatomic substrate), and
- related to autonomic nervous system imbalance (Fig. 1.4).

In all these circumstances these markers represent an increase, often very important, in electrical instability, which bears no relation to the presence of an acute ischaemic syndrome. This instability is a substrate to develop a malignant ventricular arrhythmia in the presence of different triggers.

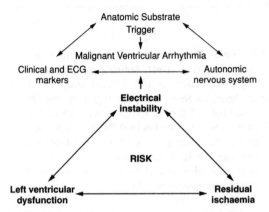

Figure 1.4 The triangle of risk in post-myocardial infarction patients with satellite triangle in the angle of electrical instability with different markers of bad outcome for a primary arrhythmic event.

The comparative role of acute ischaemic syndrome versus primary arrhythmic event in the presentation of SCD: a 50% responsibility

As we stated at the beginning of this article (Fig. 1.1), the population pool of SD represents an overall incidence of 1–2/1000 per year. This large population base include victims of SCD as a first manifestation of disease; in the majority of patients with first MI, in whom SCD is related to acute ischaemic syndrome (severe and persistent ischaemia), the danger of SCD is very difficult to predict. In this group there are also included a small number of cases of hypertrophic cardiomyopathy, primary ventricular fibrillation, etc. This group represents 40–60% of SCD cases. On the other hand, the remaining cases of SCD may be predicted with greater accuracy because they are included in higher-risk subgroups. The majority of these patients present IHD, but often the cause of the presentation of the final event is not an acute ischaemic syndrome, although some transient ischaemia may be present. There is considerable evidence[29,30] that, in patients with implanted defibrillator, thus in patients at a higher risk to present SCD, the cause of death is, in the majority of cases, a primary arrhythmic event and not an ischaemic-thrombotic acute syndrome. Henry et al.[29] demonstrated that in patients with implantable cardioverter–defibrillator (ICD) appropriate shocks for ECG-verified ventricular tachyarrhythmias were only very rarely (<3% of cases) preceded or followed by signs of acute myocardial infarction. Thereby supporting the idea that, in patients at higher risk of SCD, this is usually due to a primary arrhythmic event. On the other hand, Mont et al.[30] demonstrated that, in patients who have survived VF as the sole documented arrhythmia at the time of resuscitation and are currently receiving ICD therapy, VT is by far the most common ventricular arrhythmia recorded in device-incorporated electrograms during follow-up. This adds further support to the consideration that the primary cause of VF was a sustained VT not triggered by an acute ischaemic syndrome.

On the whole we may consider that acute ischaemic syndrome with thrombosis accounts for approximately 40–50% of cases of SCD. There are several arguments to support this. Clinically, the incidence of symptoms suggestive of ischaemia in cases of SCD is between 30 and 50%.[1,2] Furthermore, in our survey of patients who died while wearing a Holter device,[31] evidence of ischaemia detected by Holter monitoring was around 30%. From an angiographic point of view, Spaulding demonstrated[32] that the presence of acute coronary artery occlusion in a coronariography performed immediately in survivors of out-of-hospital cardiac arrest was 48%. Lastly, from a pathological point of view the frequency of active lessions varies greatly (from 13% to 95%)[11,12,33,34] depending on the type of patients studied (ambulatory versus CCU patients, methodological differences, etc.). Burke et al.[33] recently demonstrated that, in patients with IHD and presenting with a SCD, acute thrombosis was present in 52% of cases.

As a conclusion, it seems clear that in approximately 50% of cases SCD is explained by acute ischaemic syndrome and in the other 50% of cases by a primary arrhythmic event.

In other associated diseases

The chain of events leading to SCD in cases of other associated diseases flows a similar step-by-step approach. In Fig. 1.5 we may see this chain of events in hypertrophic cardiomyopathy, heart failure, Wolff–Parkinson–White (WPW) and congenital long QT syndrome.

Clinical goals

The clinical goals are to prevent the appearance of the disease if possible, and when the disease exists to avoid progression from silent to clinical, and when it has already been diagnosed to decrease the incidence of new events and complications. We will comment on some aspects focusing on IHD but also consider this problem in other situations.

In case of ischaemic heart disease

To detect the presence of ischaemic heart disease and especially of vulnerable plaque before the clinical appearance of the disease

At present, as previously described, the presence of vulnerable plaque by non-invasive methods cannot be investi-

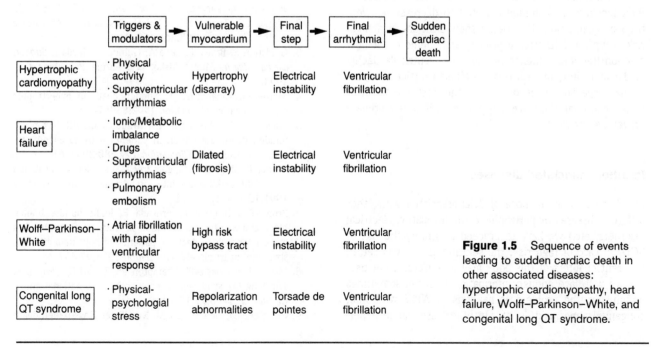

	Triggers & modulators	Vulnerable myocardium	Final step	Final arrhythmia	Sudden cardiac death
Hypertrophic cardiomyopathy	· Physical activity · Supraventricular arrhythmias	Hypertrophy (disarray)	Electrical instability	Ventricular fibrillation	
Heart failure	· Ionic/Metabolic imbalance · Drugs · Supraventricular arrhythmias · Pulmonary embolism	Dilated (fibrosis)	Electrical instability	Ventricular fibrillation	
Wolff–Parkinson–White	· Atrial fibrillation with rapid ventricular response	High risk bypass tract	Electrical instability	Ventricular fibrillation	
Congenital long QT syndrome	· Physical-psychologial stress	Repolarization abnormalities	Torsade de pointes	Ventricular fibrillation	

Figure 1.5 Sequence of events leading to sudden cardiac death in other associated diseases: hypertrophic cardiomyopathy, heart failure, Wolff–Parkinson–White, and congenital long QT syndrome.

gated. There is some evidence that magnetic resonance may be useful in the future.[35] What is possible is to suspect the presence of coronary atherosclerosis by special computed scanner and when some non-invasive ECG tests are very pathological (e.g. exercise testing). The sensitivity and specificity are also very high if this pathological non-invasive test is positive in patients with many risk factors or evidence of atherosclerotic disease in other locations. In this high-risk subgroup of asymptomatic patients, it may be necessary to perform other tests, even in some cases coronariography to rule out IHD, and if possible, to identify vulnerable plaques with more sophisticated techniques.[36]

Preventive campaigns are very important because, if we treat hypertension, decrease level of lipid disorders and smoking, we will decrease the incidence of IHD. If IHD is present, we can slow atherosclerosis progression or stabilise vulnerable plaques and consequently decrease the incidence of SCD. Nevertheless, there are still 20–30% of cases in which IHD is present in the absence of classical risk factors. Thus it is also very important to identify genetic aspects or other non-conventional risk factors that increase the risk of IHD.

To avoid recurrences of ischaemic syndrome and the presentation of primary arrhythmic event

When IHD is already established, our goal is to fight against the factors that are related to a negative outcome: residual ischaemia, left ventricular dysfunction, and electrical instability (Fig. 1.4). Therefore to decrease SCD we have to proceed with medical treatment or revascularisation procedures to decrease or, if possible, abolish residual ischaemia, and to give the best treatment (beta-blockers, ACE inhibitors, etc.) to decrease left ventricular dysfunction. If patients show markers of a high-risk group for SCD from a primary arrhythmic event (low ejection fraction, evidence of substrate, ventricular tachycardia in Holter, or previous sustained ventricular tachycardia, especially if it occurs in the first month after myocardial infarction), we may advise an ICD as a primary preventive measure.

In other associated diseases

In other cases, as in those of SCD associated with other different diseases (hypertrophic cardiomyopathy, electrical disorders, etc.) we have to proceed to stratify the risk of SCD. In case of high risk, the solution as you will see in different chapters of this book may be different, but usually we will have enough information to solve, sometimes definitively, the problem as happens in WPW syndrome, congenital abnormalities, etc. In other cases, as in hyper-

trophic cardiomyopathy, dilated cardyomyopathy, congenital long QT syndrome, or idiopathic ventricular fibrillation, the only solution at the present time in high-risk groups may be an ICD.

Conclusion

In the majority of cases the approach to reduce the number of SD victims has been based on secondary prevention among patients who have survived potentially fatal arrhythmias, or those who are identified as being at extraordinarily high risk because of a recent major cardiovascular event or specific clinical risk factors. Nevertheless, this approach does not emphasise that a large number of fatalities occur as a primary event. In patients with high risk of SCD, as in those who have already presented with out-of-hospital cardiac arrest, the most optimistic figures available for 1-year survival are in the range of 25–30%. In these cases an ICD implant is mandatory. However, primary prevention of cardiac arrest should have a much greater impact on overall outcome, but at the moment it is practically impossible to identify individual patients at high risk from amongst large population pools who usually do not present with markers of any real danger of SCD. Therefore we have to increase our ability to detect candidates of SCD in the global population if we want to fight efficaciously for SCD prevention in the future.

References

1. De Vreede-Swagemakers JJ, Gorgels AP, Dubois-Arbouw WI *et al.* Out-of-hospital cardiac arrest in the 1990s: a population-based study in the Maastrich area on incidence, characteristcs and survival. *J Am Coll Cardiol* 1997;**30**:1500–5.
2. Hinkle LE, Thaler HT. Clinical classification of cardiac deaths. *Circulation* 1982;**65**:457–4.
3. Goldstein S, Bayés de Luna A, Guindo Soldevila J. *Sudden cardiac death*. Mount Kisko, NY: Futura Publishing Co., 1994.
4. Maron BJ, Fananapazir L. Sudden death in hypertrophic cardiomyopathy. *Circulation* 1992;**85**:I57–63.
5. Stevenson WG, Stevenson LW, Middlekauff HR, Saxon LA. Sudden death prevention in patients with advanced ventricular dysfunction. *Circulation* 1993;**88**:2953–61.
6. Torner P, Brugada P, Smeets J *et al.* Ventricular fibrillation in Wolff–Parkinson–White syndrome. *Eur Heart J* 1991;**12**:144–50.
7. Brugada J, Brugada R, Brugada P. Right bundle branch block and ST-segment elevation in leads V1 through V3: a marker for sudden death in patients without demonstrable structural heart disease. *Circulation* 1998;**97**:457–60.
8. Moss AJ, Schwartz PJ, Crampton RS, Locati E, Carleen E. The long QT syndrome: a prospective international study. *Circulation* 1985;**71**:17–21.
9. Cheitlin MD, De Castro CM, McAllister HA. Sudden death

as a complication of anomalous left coronary origin from the anterior sinus of Valsalva: a not minor congenital anomaly. *Circulation* 1974;**50**:780.

10. Priori SG, Borggrefe M, Camm AJ, *et al.* Unexplained cardiac arrest. The need for a prospective registry. *Eur Heart J* 1992;**13**:1445–7.

11. Davies MJ, Thomas A. Thrombosis and acute coronary artery lesions in sudden cardiac ischemic death. *New Engl J Med* 1984;**310**:1137–40.

12. Warners CA, Roberts WC. Sudden coronary death: relation of amount and distribution of coronary narrowing at necropsy to previous symptoms of myocardial ischemia, left ventricular scarring and heart weight. *Am J Cardiol* 1984;**54**:65–73.

13. Myerburg RJ, Kessler KM, Castellanos A. Sudden cardiac death: structure, function, and time-dependence of risk. *Circulation* 1992;**85**(Suppl. I):I2–I10.

14. Furukawa T, Rozanski JJ, Nogami A, Moroe K, Gosselin AJ, Lister JW. Time-dependence risk of and predictors for cardiac arrest recurrence in survivors of out-of-hospital cardiac arrest with chronic coronary artery disease. *Circulation* 1989;**80**:599–608.

15. Nieto FJ, Peruga A. Riesgo atribuible: sus formas, usos e interpretación. *Gaceta San* 1990;**18**:112–17.

16. Greenland S, Rothman KJ. Measures of effect and measures of association. In: Rothman KJ and Greenland S eds. *Modern epidemiology.* Philadelphia: Lippincott-Raven Publishers, 1998, pp. 47–66

17. World Health Organization. Technical Report 726. *Sudden cardiac death.* Basel: WHO, 1985, pp. 3–26.

18. Feinleib M. The magnitude and nature of decrease in coronary heart disease mortality. *Am J Cardiol* 1984;**54**:2C–6C.

19. Muller JE, Ludmer PL, Willich SN *et al.* Circadian variation in the frequency of sudden cardiac death. *Circulation* 1987;**75**:131–8.

20. Willich SN, Levy D, Rocco MB, Tofler GH, Stone PH, Muller JE. Circadian variation in the incidence of sudden cardiac death in the Framingham Heart Study population. *Am J Cardiol* 1987;**60**:801–6.

21. Kannel WB, Schatzkin S. Sudden death: lessons from subsets in population studies. *J Am Coll Cardiol* 1985;**5**:141B–9B.

22. Zareba W, Moss AJ,Schwartz PJ *et al.* Influence of genotype on the clinical course of the long-QT syndrome. International Long-QT Syndrome Registry Research Group. *New Engl J Med* 1998;**339**:960–5.

23. McKenna WJ, Coccolo F, Elliot PM. Genes and disease expression in hypertrophic cardiomyopathy. *Lancet* 1998;**352**:1162–3.

24. Gussak I, Antzelevitch C, Bjerregaard P, Towbin JA, Chaitman BR. The Brugada syndrome: clinical, electrophysiologic and genetic aspects. *J Am Coll Cardiol* 1999;**33**:5–15.

25. Jouven X, Desnos M, Guerot C, Ducimetiere P. Predicting sudden death in the population: the Paris Prospective Study I. *Circulation* 1999;**99**:1978–83.

26. Davies MJ. The composition of coronary artery plaques. *New Engl J Med* 1997;**336**:1312–14.

27. Mann JM, Davies MJ. Vulnerable plaque. Relation of characteristics to degree of stenosis in human coronary arteries. *Circulation* 1996;**84**:928–31.

28. Gronholdt ML, Dalager-Pedersen S, Falk E. Coronary atherosclerosis: determinants of plaque rupture. *Eur Heart J* 1998;**19**(Suppl. C):C24–C29.

29. Henry PD, Pacifico A. Sudden cardiac death: still more questions than answers. *G Ital Cardiol* 1997;**27**:1319–24.

30. Mont L, Valentino M, Sambola A, Matas M, Aguinaga L, Brugada J. Arrhythmia recurrence in patients with a healed myocardial infarction who received an implantable defibrillator: analysis according to the clinical presentation. *J Am Coll Cardiol* 1999;**34**:351–7.

31. Bayés de Luna A, Coumel P, Leclercq JF. Ambulatory sudden cardiac death: mechanism of fatal arrhythmia on the basis of data from 157 cases. *Am Heart J* 1989;**117**:151–9.

32. Spaulding CM, Joly LM, Rosenberg A *et al.* Immediate coronary angiography in survivors of out-of-hospital cardiac arrest. *New Engl J Med* 1997;**336**:1629–33.

33. Burke AP, Farb A, Malcom GT, Liang YH, Smialek J, Virmani R. Coronary risk factors and plaque morphology in men with coronary disease who died suddenly. *New Engl J Med* 1997;**336**:1276–82.

34. Farb A, Tang AL, Burke AP, Sessums L, Liang Y, Virmani R. Sudden coronary death. Frequency of active coronary lesions, inactive coronary lesions, and myocardial infarction. *Circulation* 1995;**92**:1701–9.

35. Toussaint JF, LaMuraglia GM, Southern JF, Fuster V, Kantor HL. Magnetic resonance images lipid, fibrous, calcified, hemorrhagic and thrombotic components of human atherosclerosis in vivo. *Circulation* 1996;**94**:932–8.

36. Feld S, Ganim M, Carell ES *et al.* Comparison of angioscopy, intravascular ultrasound imaging and quantitative coronary angiography in predicting clinical outcome after coronary intervention in high-risk patients. *J Am Coll Cardiol* 1996;**28**:97–105.

2 Definition of arrhythmic risk

Steen Z Abildstrom, Christian Torp-Pedersen, and Lars Køber

Defining arrhythmic risk is the art of classifying clinical events, most often death, as being primarily caused by or not caused by a cardiac arrhythmia. In rare occasions this may be straightforward, but in most cases the amount of data available is modest and the classifications are presumptuous. Some classifications wisely take some distance to the goal of assuming arrhythmia, by using the concept of sudden death, but even this is presumptuous in many cases. The classifications all rely on the fact that sudden unexpected death can be classified as arrhythmic in many of those cases where documentation of the cardiac rhythm is available at the time of death or syncope. This is particularly true in the general population where there is ample documentation that unexpected (circulatory) collapse often is caused by ventricular fibrillation or ventricular tachycardia. However, classification is not focused in the general population, but in groups of heart disease patients where the risk of death is high and where specific interventions can be attempted to prevent certain causes of death. Death is in general related to a cardiac arrhythmia, eventually asystole, and the classifications must in some way try to identify those cases where a cardiac arrhythmia was likely to have been the primary event. This may in general be highly problematic in patients who already have a cardiac disease and where any event can be regarded as secondary to the disease and not completely unexpected. Primary arrhythmic cause becomes a more uncertain term relating to the circumstances immediately prior to death. The uncertainty has naturally generated numerous definitions and to some degree each group of investigators have in their dissatisfaction tried to improve classifications in the hope of being more accurate.

In the following we will summarise how arrhythmic risk has been defined. We will make no claim of presenting a completely exhaustive list of all definitions used, but will instead try to outline the circumstances where the definitions have been implied, the amount of data the investigators required, and the extent to which the classifications have been validated.

Sudden death

Sudden death (SD) is the more common and more modest of classifications, the name including the uncertainty of the classification. Often, but not always, SD has a time factor included, and death is classified as sudden when the time between death and new symptoms is below a certain figure. The time base for a definition of SD in relation to new symptoms has varied considerably from 24 hours to immediate, with a clear trend over the years toward using 1 hour or less as the limit. Before considering the time course of the terminal event, deaths with a documented non-cardiac or non-cardiovascular reason, or where the underlying reason is obscure, should be separated from the cardiac or cardiovascular deaths. In populations with manifest heart disease, this may have only little impact on the final result since most of the mortality is due to cardiac or cardiovascular reasons, but in the general population the results may be influenced.

In the mid-1960s Kuller using a time limit of 24 hours found that the leading finding in sudden unexpected death among 20–39-year-olds was alcoholism and fatty liver.[1] In a 1970 report from the World Health Organization Scientific Group, SD was referred to, but it was considered premature to define it.[2] SD was conceived as a very general concept describing unexpected cardiovascular death. The report describes other World Health Organization studies, where a time-based definition of SD is a death occurring within 6 hours from the onset of new symptoms. Nine years later in a report from WHO concerning the nomenclature for primary cardiac arrest, a definition of SD was "purposely omitted"; it stated that "The definition used should be operational."[3] Several studies evaluating the prognostic value of different non-invasive measures of arrhythmogenicity as a predictor of SD following myocardial infarction have set the time limit to 1 hour, giving the first indications that SD in some cases is arrhythmic. In order to understand the mechanism of SD, Goldstein in 1982 suggested that only witnessed deaths should be considered and a time limit of 1 hour used.[4] Roberts gave a restricted suggestion in an editorial in *The American Journal of Cardiology*.[5] Here SD was defined as death, which is non-violent, instantaneous, and occurring within a few minutes of an abrupt change in previous clinical state. The concept was specifically suggested to omit inclusion of patients dying during sleep or found dead. This concept is currently most often described as instantaneous, witnessed death. An even more rigid definition would require an autopsy ruling out a non-cardiac reason but, given the falling numbers of autopsies, the sensitivity would be very poor.

The place of death has been highlighted as an easy variable to record giving an indication whether death was both sudden and unexpected.[6] Death during hospitalisation is in most cases non-sudden and even when a terminal arrhythmia is documented it is, in many cases, secondary to the cause that brought the patient to the hospital, for instance myocardial infarction (MI) or worsening heart failure. However, patients suffering an out-of-hospital collapse may be brought to the hospital before they are declared dead and patients dying out-of-hospital may do so because they wish a peaceful end to a long illness. Place of death should be viewed in a broader context. Consider a case where a patient is entered in a post-MI study during hospitalisation for the index-infarction and dies still in-hospital. Such a death could be sudden but is likely to be secondary to the MI and can hardly be classified as both sudden and unexpected, unless the patient was about to be discharged. When deaths are classified in such studies, mortality should be divided into death during index-hospitalisation and death following discharge.

Patients dying in coma following a cardiac arrest are usually classified as SD even if some authors have required death to be declared within a certain time limit (for example 24 hours).[7]

The reason that SD is an appropriate entity is the anticipation that this in many cases represents arrhythmic death. At least the proportion of SDs being arrhythmic is larger than the proportion of non-SDs being arrhythmic, but this relation is highly dependable on the population studied. Hinkle and Thaler[8] found indeed that SD may not be arrhythmic, and arrhythmic death may not be sudden. Using data from a monitoring study in high-risk patients in New York they found that all 37 deaths occurring within 5 minutes could be classified as arrhythmic. Sixteen of 20 deaths occurring between 5 minutes and 1 hour were also classified as arrhythmic leading to 93% SDs (<1 h) being arrhythmic. However 29 of 84 deaths (35%) occurring later than 1 hour were also classified as arrhythmic suggesting an underestimation of the actual number of arrhythmic deaths when the classification based solely on the time from debut of symptoms till death was used. In the AIRE study all deaths among randomised patients were classified by both a time-based and a more descriptive algorithm.[7] Cleland *et al.* found that, even if 50% of the cardiovascular deaths were sudden, only approximately 50% of the SDs in this particular group of patients were arrhythmic.[9] However, proof of arrhythmic death was common in none of the definitions used in AIRE, and the different classifications used serve to illustrate that

different definitions of sudden or arrhythmic death may result in large differences in the result of classifications.

Although instantaneous witnessed death can have many causes aside from arrhythmias, the important relation between witnessed instantaneous death and arrhythmic death has been highlighted by the Seattle resuscitation studies. In one of their reports[10] ventricular fibrillation was recorded in 75% of patients with sudden witnessed collapse. When people attempt to extrapolate from such results to the groups of patients where prophylactic treatment of arrhythmias could be attempted, difficulties arise. The Seattle studies and similar studies in the general population indicate that instantaneous observed death is very likely to be preventable arrhythmic death; this is not necessarily the case in the populations of patients with heart failure and severe left ventricular dysfunction, where the risk of dying is sufficiently grave to warrant prophylactic intervention.

Arrhythmic death

Arrhythmic death will often be the focus of interest when SD is studied. An attempt to improve classification was provided by Hinkle and Thaler in 1982.[8] This work is important since it appears to be the first attempt to provide a surrogate endpoint for arrhythmic death, with data used that are more likely to be available than ECGs at the time of death. They proposed a clinical definition of arrhythmic death as "abrupt loss of consciousness and disappearance of pulse without prior collapse of the circulation". They examined four general methods of classifying cardiac deaths. One classification was made based on "the condition of the circulation immediately before death" (Box 2.1), and was considered to be the most useful. Other classifications examined were "classification in relation to clinical evidence of acute ischaemic heart disease at the time of death", "classification by the duration of the terminal acute illness", and classification by "location of the death". When a classification by state of the circulation at the time of death was found most useful, this is an assumption, since the truth is not known. This definition has had a major impact on later definitions and on the framework that classification committees have worked in. If the Hinkle and Thaler surrogate classification is correct, then SD within 1 hour used as synonym with arrhythmic death underestimates the occurrence of arrhythmic death.

Death classification in the Cardiac Arrhythmia Suppression Trial (CAST) as developed in the pilot study[11] was specifically designed to detect arrhythmic deaths possibly preventable by antiarrhythmic drugs. A surrogate definition of arrhythmic death/cardiac arrest was similar to the Hinkle/Thaler classification defined as "the abrupt spontaneous cessation of respiration and blood circulation

---

Box 2.1   Hinkle and Thaler classification of death

- Arrhythmic death (abrupt loss of consciousness and disappearance of pulse without prior collapse of the circulation)

  1. Not preceded by impairment of circulation
     Witnessed directly
     Not witnessed directly
  2. Preceded by chronic congestive heart failure – not disabling
     Witnessed directly
     Not witnessed directly
  3. Preceded by chronic congestive heart failure – disabling
     Witnessed directly
     Not witnessed directly

- Deaths in circulatory failure (gradual circulatory failure and collapse of circulation before disappearance of pulse)

  1. Primarily caused by failure of peripheral circulation
     Witnessed directly
     Not witnessed directly
  2. Primarily caused by myocardial failure
     Witnessed directly
     Not witnessed directly

- Deaths not classifiable

(pulse) and loss of consciousness in the absence of other progressive severe medical conditions likely to cause death". Documented arrhythmic death/cardiac arrest was considered present if ventricular tachycardia or fibrillation was recorded within 10 minutes of clinical death. Other cases were classified as "presumed arrhythmic". In evaluation of "other progressive medical conditions likely to cause death" in the definition of arrhythmic death, the event committee only classified death as arrhythmic if the patient would probably have survived at least 4 months had the arrhythmia not occurred. The resemblance to the Hinkle/Thaler criteria has in many cases led to the term "modified Hinkle/Thaler criteria" when the criteria used in CAST are being referred to.

In the CAST pilot study[12] the relation between SD (within 60 minutes of new symptoms) and arrhythmic death (documented or presumed) was studied. Of 29 cases of SD, nine were classified as non-arrhythmic death, and of 16 patients with non-SD three were classified as arrhythmic. This result differs from the classification by Hinkle and Thaler as described above, mainly because a significant proportion of SD was not classified as arrhythmic. It may be important that the populations studied were different, but a more likely cause of the discrepancy is that the CAST criteria of arrhythmic death require a clinician to assume that the patient would have been able to live for 4 months, had the arrhythmia not occurred. Nevertheless, there is overall agreement between the CAST criteria and the Hinkle/Thaler criteria, that SD within 1 hour of new symptoms is a reasonable marker for arrhythmic death as illustrated in Table 2.1 where the numbers of death giving the sensitivity and specificity are listed.

In a report from 1996 Narang *et al.*[7] demonstrated beyond doubt the heterogeneity among classifications used for deaths in chronic heart failure patients. They recommended that SD should not be time based, but rather should be death not attributable to terminal pump failure, stroke, or non-cardiac cause of death. The so-called ACME criteria take several factors into consideration:

- **a**ctivity or place of death
- **c**ause of death
- **m**ode of death, and
- **e**vents associated with death.

This new set of criteria has been developed for the Acute Infarction Ramipril Efficacy (AIRE) study and, as mentioned, a rather poor association between sudden and arrhythmic death was observed in this particular patient population.

Table 2.1   Sensitivity and specificity between sudden death (SD) and arrhythmic death (AD) in Hinkle and Thaler, and CAST Pilot Study, where AD is "the truth"

Hinkle & Thaler

AD	SD Yes	No	Total
Yes	53(93%)	29	82(65%)
No	4	55	59
Total	57	84	141

CAST Pilot Study

AD	SD Yes	No	Total
Yes	20(69%)	3	23(87%)
No	9	13	22
Total	29	16	45

Recently Epstein *et al.*[13] has published a classification of death for use in antiarrhythmic trials. This classification was particularly designed for trials of devices. It classifies death as cardiac (arrhythmic/non-arrhythmic/unknown), non-cardiac, and unknown. The temporal course is also included as sudden (<1 h), non-sudden, and unknown. Furthermore, a suggestion for the tabulation of documentation, operative relation, and system relation is suggested. Wisely, it does not incorporate device memory readouts in evaluation of devices because of the bias this may introduce. This suggestion mainly serves to suggest a uniform tabulation of certain data. Clearly the classification should now be modified to include also a classification as described by Hinkle and Thaler.

Arrhythmic events

In order to boost the number of endpoints investigators have tried to combine arrhythmic death and non-lethal ventricular arrhythmic events. This will be particularly obvious in implantable cardioverter defibrillator (ICD) settings. The problem is to define clearly when an arrhythmic event is potentially lethal. If just the number of shocks without electrogram (EGM) is used, documentation is inadequate. In the Coronary Artery Bypass Graft (CABG)-Patch trial, there was huge discrepancy between number of shocks in the ICD group and mortality in the control-group.[14] By the end of 4 years of follow-up, 70% of the ICD patients had received a shock, but the absolute arrhythmic death rate in the control group was 6.2%.[15] This relation has probably improved as ICD technology has developed better algorithms detecting truly ventricular arrhythmias. Even when EGM documentation is available, some kind of clinical manifestation of the arrhythmia should be warranted. Syncope in a patient with an arrhythmic disposition may by default be interpreted as an arrhythmia but in the general population this is invalid.

Use of classifications in studies

Over the years the different classifications have been applied to a number of patient populations and subsets of the general population. Table 2.2 lists some of the major randomised interventional studies that have tried to subdivide mortality into sudden or arrhythmic death versus non-sudden or non-arrhythmic death. The aim of the table is to show the heterogeneity, since the actual numbers are highly biased by the differences in patient subgroup, patient selection and follow-up, and randomisation procedures. In some cases we now know that applying the intervention actually increased the risk of dying, especially sudden or arrhythmic death, making the picture even more complex.

Of major importance, the classification of Hinkle and Thaler was used in MADIT.[16] Since this trial demonstrated an overall mortality benefit, it provides a unique opportunity to examine whether a clinical classification of arrhythmic death is likely to be preventable arrhythmic death. In this study there were 13 arrhythmic deaths in the conventional therapy group and three in the defibrillator group. There were 13 non-arrhythmic deaths in the conventional therapy group and seven in the defibrillator group. This important result provides the first indication that arrhythmic death by this classification does indeed relate to preventable arrhythmic death. It also provides some indication that the classification (or the classifiers) may underestimate preventable arrhythmic death since cardiac non-arrhythmic death was also reduced.

ICD trials are very interesting since an ICD can only treat arrhythmias efficiently and are only rarely pro-arrhythmic or induce non-arrhythmic death. In the Antiarrhythmics versus Implantable Defibrillators (AVID) study, the Canadian Implantable Defibrillator Study (CIDS), and the Cardiac Arrest Study Hamburg (CASH) study, the impact of ICD versus amiodarone was a 50% reduction in arrhythmic death and no influence on non-arrhythmic death.[17] These three trials all used the modified Hinkle/Thaler criteria being somewhat like the CAST criteria. This gives a notion that classification of deaths is indeed possible and meaningful at least in a patient population having suffered and survived a cardiac arrest.

Evaluation of classifications

When current definitions of surrogate arrhythmic death to describe modes of death are used in trials, they can easily be defended as "best available". The definitions become more problematic when they are used to search for populations where a high risk of arrhythmic death could warrant an interventional study. Using CAST criteria for defining arrhythmic death in a post-MI population, Hartikainen *et al.*[18] demonstrated that heart rate variability was highly efficient in predicting arrhythmic death in patients with preserved ejection fraction, and that low ejection fraction was efficient in predicting non-arrhythmic death in patients with preserved heart rate variability. In such an evaluation there is a risk of a circular argument. For death to be classified as arrhythmic by the CAST criteria it is required that the patient could be assumed to survive for a further 4 months if arrhythmic death had not occurred. If the ejection fraction is very low, this could be the reason for assuming that the patient would not survive 4 months, and thus death would be classified as non-arrhythmic. Thus, the low ejection fraction could *per se* be the reason that the patient was classified as having non-arrhythmic death.

Table 2.2 Major randomised interventional studies

Study	Subgroup of patients	Year	Intervention studied	Follow-up	No. deaths/ no. of participants	Classification used	No. sudden or arrhythmic deaths
CONSENSUS 1[23]	CHF	1987	ACE-I	1 d–20 m	118/253	<1h	28
CONSENSUS 2[24]	Post-MI & CHF	1992	ACE-I	41–180 d	598/6090	<1h	174
VHEFT 1[25]	CHF, 18–75 y, men	1986	ACE-I	6 m–5.7 y	211/642	Instantaneous	124
VHEFT 2[25]	CHF, 18–75 y, men	1991	ACE-I	6 m–5.7 y	285/804	Instantaneous	104
VHEFT 3[26]	CHF, men	1997	ca-blocker	4–39 m	60/650	"Sudden"	16
SOLVD Treatment[27]	CHF, <80 y	1991	ACE-I	22–55 m	962/2569	"Arrhythmic", no HF	218
SOLVD Prevention[28]	EF <35%, no HF	1992	ACE-I	14–62 m	647/4228	"Arrhythmic", no HF	203
SAVE[29]	EF <40%, no HF	1992	ACE-I	14–62 m	503/2231	"Sudden", unexpected	137
PRAISE[30]	CHF	1998	ca-blocker		413/1153	Hinkle & Thaler	185
Packer[31]	CHF	1996	carvedilol	6 m	53/1094	"Sudden"	29
BHAT[32]	Post-MI, 30–69 y	1982	beta-blocker	25.1 m	326/3837	<1 h	153
Julian[33]	Post-MI, 30–69 y	1982	sotalol	12 m	116/1456	<1 h	39
EIS[34]	Post-MI, 35–69 y	1984	beta-blocker	12 m	102/1741	Instantaneous	49
Singh[35]	CHF, EF <40%, PVCs	1995	amiodarone	45 m	274/674	"Sudden"	139
MIS[36]	Post-MI	1977	beta-blocker		126/3053	<2 h	86
AMIS[37]	Post-MI	1980	aspirin	3 y	464/4524	<1 h	106
Olsson[38]	Post-MI	1992	beta-blocker		411/5474	<2 h	166
Norwegian Multicenter[39]	Post-MI, 20–75 y	1981	beta-blocker	>12 m	250/1884	<24 h (instantaneous)	142(49)
MERIT-HF[40]	CHF, EF <40%	1999	beta-blocker		362/3991	<1 h	211
AIRE[9]	Post-MI & CHF	1997	ACE-I	15 m	392/2006	ACME	210
TRACE[41]	Post-MI, EF <35%	1995	ACE-I	24–50 m	673/1749	<1 h	238
CAST[42]	Post-MI	1989	class-I AAD	1 y	81/1498	CAST	53
SWORD[43]	Post-MI & EF <40%	1996	d-sotalol	148 d	126/3121	CAST	88
BASIS[44]	Post-MI & PVCs, <71 y	1990	amiodarone	1 y	30/312	<1 h	22
Ceremuzynski[45]	Post-MI & non-bb, <75 y	1992	amiodarone	1 y	54/613	<1 h	30
CIBIS I[46]	CHF, EF <40%	1994	beta-blocker	1.9 y	120/641	<1 h	45
CIBIS II[47]	CHF, EF <40%	1999	beta-blocker	1.3 y	384/2647	<1 h	131
MADIT[16]	Post-MI, EF <36%, nsvt	1996	ICD	27 m	54/196	Hinkle & Thaler	16
RALES[48]	CHF	1999	spiron	24 m	670/1663	<1 h	192
CABG-Patch[15]	Post-CABG, EF <36%, SAECG	1999	ICD	32 m	198/900	Hinkle & Thaler	43
EMIAT[49]	Post-MI & EF <40%	1997	amiodarone	21 m	205/1486	"Arrhythmic"	83
CAMIAT[50]	Post-MI & PVCs	1997	amiodarone	1.8 y	125/1202	CAST	57

Abbreviations: ACE-I = ACE-inhibitor; ca-blocker = calcium channel antagonist; CHF = congestive heart failure; d = days; EF = ejection fraction; h = hour; HF = clinical heart failure; m = months; nsvt = non-sustained ventricular tachycardia; Post-MI = following myocardial infarction; PVC = premature ventricular complex; SAECG = signal averaged ECG; spiron = spironolactone.

Perhaps a time-based definition for SD should also be studied in such studies, although it would be no guarantee, since the criterion of unexpectedness could include similar risk of a circular reasoning. Knowledge of a very low ejection fraction could raise the probability that death was not considered unexpected.

Fig. 2.1 shows the decision process of a CAST-like classification. This slightly simplified flowchart demonstrates that lack of data will increase the likelihood of death being classified by default as presumed arrhythmic. In descriptions of evaluations, it is never forgotten that the members of the event committees are experts, whereas the fact that autopsies are rare and few data are available in many cases is passed lightly.

An exact description of the handling of cases, where the amount of data is so poor or contradictory that classifi-

cation is truly random, is important since differences in these procedures may lead to different results. The lack of information may make it impossible to decide whether the

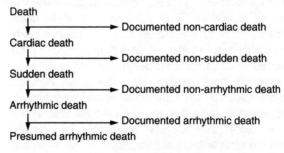

Figure 2.1 The decision process of a CAST-like classification.

death was due to a cardiac or cardiovascular reason or not, and, more commonly, whether a cardiac or cardiovascular death was sudden or non-sudden, arrhythmic or non-arrhythmic. Some investigators have classified deaths as non-sudden until proven sudden; others have only included the cases where the exact time course is known but most often the procedures are not described. In arrhythmic death the trend is opposite, since lack of data in many cases leads to the event being classified as arrhythmic but Hinkle and Thaler gave an important option of choosing "death not classifiable".

If the concept of SD is going to be used in the foreseeable future, it must in each case be defined whether the concept is used as a (relatively) strict time-based definition or whether more descriptive modes of death are included in the concept. Particular attention must be paid to the description of the handling of unobserved death. Some classifications have requested that the time from when the patient was last seen should be used. Most classifications state that suddenness should be classified by a "detailed review of the circumstances of death". Most likely, circumstances where the patient appears to have died instantaneously or has peacefully died during sleep are classified as sudden.

Validation of classifications

The basic problems inherent in any classification of arrhythmic death are related to validation of classifications and the quality of available data. Currently we have large-scale validation from the Seattle studies of cardiac arrest in the community that sudden, observed collapse in society is often preventable arrhythmic death. With MADIT, AVID, CIDS, and CASH we have small-scale evidence that death classified as arrhythmic by the Hinkle/Thaler or CAST criteria is also to a large extent preventable.

There are major problems with the quality of available data. In many studies autopsy reports are only available in a few percent of cases and, even in studies where specific efforts have been made, autopsy reports are only available in a minority of the cases. Because of the many difficulties of practical classification, committees are used to perform the classification. Usually, cases are classified by at least two members and various mechanisms of reaching consensus are used in cases of discrepancies. In a recent investigation of patients in different ICD studies, Pratt *et al.*[19] studied the inaccuracies of evaluation. With the use of CAST criteria, committee consensus was reached in classifying a 2% rate of arrhythmic death. Nearly twice as many, 3.6% was classified as SD by at least one committee member. In addition, the opinion of the committee was not in agreement with that of the investigator in 40% of the cases. Uncertainty of interpretation of the data is not

specific to this study, and it demonstrates that evaluation of such data is either difficult or truly uncertain.

It was anticipated that trials of implantable defibrillators would provide further insight because device memory might provide insight in many cases. Unfortunately, many devices are buried with the patient and in other cases the memory is filled with noise that obscures tracing at the time of death. Even when readable EGM-storage is available, Pratt[19] has reported that only in about half of what we conceive as arrhythmic death could it be confirmed by the recording. At the same time only looking at the terminal EGM led to erroneous classification of a pulmonary embolism as arrhythmic death. This shows that documenting an arrhythmia in the final phase of dying does not necessarily make the death arrhythmic. These recordings should probably be viewed in connection with the general circumstances of the terminal event.

Grubman[20] and Pires[21] have reported some data from patients dying with SD despite having an ICD. The electrograms showed that in most cases SD in these patients was not related to arrhythmia and that none of the SDs was due to ICD malfunction. These data cannot be used to comment on the relation between sudden and arrhythmic death, since these patients are highly selected and since the events, where the ICD did actually treat a potentially lethal arrhythmia, were not in the analysis. However, it is comforting to know that ICD malfunction is rare even in patients dying SD.

Future perspectives

Mortality studies of medical therapies and devices to treat or prevent arrhythmias must include a classification of mode of death. Current classifications have a major drawback in that the quality of data is not apparent from the tabulation. Even the finest committee can be forced to default classification in the majority of cases, if data are sparse resulting in an overreporting of arrhythmic death. For this reason, we would recommend that future tabulation of arrhythmic deaths include a tabulation to indicate the certainty of available data as shown in Box 2.2. Also the exact handling of cases where data are insufficient (death during sleep, unwitnessed death etc.) should be apparent from the report.

No study has yet provided sufficient data in their report to allow the reader to classify deaths by such strict criteria. Use of committees and/or tabulation of the committee conclusions cannot replace a presentation of the available data. It is to be hoped that investigators and editors will require that a breakdown as suggested or similar is included in future reports of death classifications.

Apart death being classified as arrhythmic or non-arrhythmic, it is of major interest to subclassify, in order

Box 2.2 Classification of arrhythmic death by certainty of data

- Documented arrhythmic death
  - Instantaneous death (<5 min of new symptoms) with documented VF or VT within 10 minutes of death
  - Number of patients with autopsy documenting absence of non-cardiac death should be recorded
- Arrhythmic death by exclusion
  - Observed instantaneous death or circumstances compatible with instantaneous death where history does not indicate severe disease incompatible with continued life for some time
  - Number of patients with autopsy documenting absence of non-cardiac death should be recorded
- Arrhythmic death by default
  - Abrupt loss of consciousness and disappearance of pulse without prior collapse of the circulation but no further data

to examine groups where the outcome of therapy might be different. The Hinkle/Thaler classification suggests one important classification based on the general severity of disease. It could also be of major interest to examine whether ischaemia is present at the time of arrhythmia, since arrhythmias provoked by ischaemia could very well have a different outcome than those unrelated to acute ischaemia. Hinkle and Thaler provide one suggestion for such a classification simply by pooling clinical information as to whether the patient in immediate relation to the arrhythmia had ischaemia or acute MI. The value of such a subclassification is currently unknown, but should be attempted.

Since all current evaluations of mode of death rely on unproved assumptions, no classification has yet the potential to be used as a primary endpoint in a trial. In accordance with this, recommendations for evaluation of ICDs should use total mortality as an endpoint.[22]

Given all the uncertainties of classification, proof of arrhythmic death can only be achieved by proving that prevention or treatment of arrhythmia saves life. Such proof has been established in the general population by the Seattle studies, and with MADIT, AVID, CIDS, and CASH we have emerging evidence of proof in at least part of the high-risk population. However, with the CABG-Patch study,[14] we also have an indication that the situation is more complex in high-risk patients. At this time a number of studies are being initiated, randomising wider groups of patients to receive a cardioverter defibrillator or standard treatment. The success or failure of these studies will provide critical insight. We can further hope that technical problems with devices as well as their prices will fall fur-

ther in order to allow true wide-scale intervention studies. These studies could very well resolve the uncertainties of classification of high-risk patients, yet perhaps obviate the need for future classification. In the meantime we must live with the uncertainties and hope that reports in the coming years will present their results in such a way that the uncertainties of each study are clearly presented.

References

1. Kuller L, Lilienfeld A, Fisher R. Sudden and unexpected deaths in young adults. An epidemiological study. *JAMA* 1966;**198**:248–52.
2. World Health Organization Scientific Group. The pathological diagnosis of acute ischemic heart disease. *Wld Hlth Org Techn Rep Serv* 1970;5–27.
3. Rapaport, E. Nomenclature and criteria for diagnosis of ischemic heart disease. *Circulation* 1979;**59**:607–8.
4. Goldstein S. The necessity of a uniform definition of sudden coronary death: witnessed death within 1 hour of the onset of acute symptoms. *Am Heart J* 1982;**103**:156–9.
5. Roberts WC. Sudden cardiac death: definitions and causes. *Am J Cardiol* 1986;**57**:1410–13.
6. Goldstein S, Friedman L, Hutchinson R *et al*. Timing, mechanism and clinical setting of witnessed deaths in post-myocardial infarction patients. *J Am Coll Cardiol* 1984;**3**:1111–17.
7. Narang R, Cleland JG, Erhardt L *et al*. Mode of death in chronic heart failure. A request and proposition for more accurate classification. *Eur Heart J* 1996;**17**:1390–403.
8. Hinkle LE J, Thaler HT. Clinical classification of cardiac deaths. *Circulation* 1982;**65**:457–64.
9. Cleland JG, Erhardt L, Murray G, Hall AS, Ball SG. Effect of ramipril on morbidity and mode of death among survivors of acute myocardial infarction with clinical evidence of heart failure. A report from the AIRE Study Investigators. *Eur Heart J* 1997;**18**:41–51.
10. Greene HL. Sudden arrhythmic cardiac death – mechanisms, resuscitation and classification: the Seattle perspective. *Am J Cardiol* 1990;**65**:4B–12B.
11. Greene HL, Richardson DW, Barker AH *et al*. Classification of deaths after myocardial infarction as arrhythmic or non-arrhythmic (the Cardiac Arrhythmia Pilot Study). *Am J Cardiol* 1989;**63**:1–6.
12. CAPS. Effects of encainide, flecainide, imipramine and moricizine on ventricular arrhythmias during the year after acute myocardial infarction: the CAPS. The Cardiac Arrhythmia Pilot Study (CAPS) Investigators. *Am J Cardiol* 1988;**61**:501–9.
13. Epstein AE, Carlson MD, Fogoros RN, Higgins SL, Venditti FJ J. Classification of death in antiarrhythmia trials. *J Am Coll Cardiol* 1996;**27**:433–42.
14. Bigger JTJ. Prophylactic use of implanted cardiac defibrillators in patients at high risk for ventricular arrhythmias after coronary-artery bypass graft surgery. Coronary Artery Bypass Graft (CABG) Patch Trial Investigators. *New Engl J Med* 1997;**337**:1569–75.

15. Bigger JTJ, Whang W, Rottman JN *et al.* Mechanisms of death in the CABG Patch trial: a randomized trial of implantable cardiac defibrillator prophylaxis in patients at high risk of death after coronary artery bypass graft surgery. *Circulation* 1999;**99**:1416–21.

16. Moss AJ, Hall WJ, Cannom DS *et al.* Improved survival with an implanted defibrillator in patients with coronary disease at high risk for ventricular arrhythmia. Multicenter Automatic Defibrillator Implantation Trial Investigators. *New Engl J Med* 1996;**335**:1933–40.

17. Connolly, S. J. *An overview of the CIDS, AVID, CASH, and Meta-Analysis.* Oral presentation, NASPE, 1999.

18. Hartikainen JE, Malik M, Staunton A, Poloniecki J, Camm AJ. Distinction between arrhythmic and non-arrhythmic death after acute myocardial infarction based on heart rate variability, signal-averaged electrocardiogram, ventricular arrhythmias and left ventricular ejection fraction. *J Am Coll Cardiol* 1996;**28**:296–304.

19. Pratt CM, Greenway PS, Schoenfeld MH, Hibben ML, Reiffel JA. Exploration of the precision of classifying sudden cardiac death. Implications for the interpretation of clinical trials. *Circulation* 1996;**93**:519–24.

20. Grubman EM, Pavri BB, Shipman T, Britton N, Kocovic DZ. Cardiac death and stored electrograms in patients with third-generation implantable cardioverter–defibrillators. *J Am Coll Cardiol* 1998;**32**:1056–62.

21. Pires LA, Lehmann MH, Steinman RT, Baga JJ, Schuger CD. SD in implantable cardioverter–defibrillator recipients: clinical context, arrhythmic events and device responses. *J Am Coll Cardiol* 1999;**33**:24–32.

22. Guidelines. Guidelines for Clinical Intracardiac Electrophysiological and Catheter Ablation Procedures. A report of the American College of Cardiology/American Heart Association Task Force on practice guidelines. (Committee on Clinical Intracardiac Electrophysiologic and Catheter Ablation Procedures). Developed in collaboration with the North American Society of Pacing and Electrophysiology. *Circulation* 1995;**92**:673–91.

23. Swedberg K, Kjekshus J. Effects of enalapril on mortality in severe congestive heart failure: results of the Cooperative North Scandinavian Enalapril Survival Study (CONSENSUS). *Am J Cardiol* 1988;**62**:60A–66A.

24. Swedberg K, Held P, Kjekshus J, Rasmussen K, Ryden L, Wedel H. Effects of the early administration of enalapril on mortality in patients with acute myocardial infarction. Results of the Cooperative New Scandinavian Enalapril Survival Study II (CONSENSUS II). *New Engl J Med* 1992;**327**:678–84.

25. Goldman S, Johnson G, Cohn JN, Cintron G, Smith R, Francis G. Mechanism of death in heart failure. The Vasodilator-Heart Failure Trials. The V-HeFT VA Cooperative Studies Group. *Circulation* 1993;**87**:VI24–VI31.

26. Cohn JN, Ziesche S, Smith R, *et al.* Effect of the calcium antagonist felodipine as supplementary vasodilator therapy in patients with chronic heart failure treated with enalapril: V-HeFT III. Vasodilator-Heart Failure Trial (V-HeFT) Study Group. *Circulation* 1997;**96**:856–63.

27. SOLVD-t. Effect of enalapril on survival in patients with reduced left ventricular ejection fractions and congestive heart failure. The SOLVD Investigators. *New Engl J Med* 1991;**325**:293–302.

28. SOLVD-p. Effect of enalapril on mortality and the development of heart failure in asymptomatic patients with reduced left ventricular ejection fractions. The SOLVD Investigators. *New Engl J Med* 1992;**327**:685–91.

29. Pfeffer MA, Braunwald E, Moye LA *et al.* Effect of captopril on mortality and morbidity in patients with left ventricular dysfunction after myocardial infarction. Results of the survival and ventricular enlargement trial. The SAVE Investigators. *New Engl J Med* 1992;**327**:669–77.

30. O'Connor CM, Carson PE, Miller AB *et al.* Effect of amlodipine on mode of death among patients with advanced heart failure in the PRAISE trial. Prospective Randomized Amlodipine Survival Evaluation. *Am J Cardiol* 1998;**82**:881–7.

31. Packer M, Bristow MR, Cohn JN *et al.* The effect of carvedilol on morbidity and mortality in patients with chronic heart failure. U.S. Carvedilol Heart Failure Study Group. *New Engl J Med* 1996;**334**:1349–55.

32. BHAT. A randomized trial of propranolol in patients with acute myocardial infarction. I. Mortality results. *JAMA* 1982;**247**:1707–14.

33. Julian DG, Prescott RJ, Jackson FS, Szekely P. Controlled trial of sotalol for one year after myocardial infarction. *Lancet* 1982;**1**:1142–7.

34. EIS. European Infarction Study (E.I.S.). A secondary prevention study with slow release oxprenolol after myocardial infarction: morbidity and mortality. *Eur Heart J* 1984;**5**:189–202.

35. Singh SN, Fletcher RD, Fisher SG *et al.* Amiodarone in patients with congestive heart failure and asymptomatic ventricular arrhythmia. Survival Trial of Antiarrhythmic Therapy in Congestive Heart Failure. *New Engl J Med* 1995;**333**:77–82.

36. MIS. Reduction in mortality after myocardial infarction with long-term beta-adrenoceptor blockade. Multicentre international study: supplementary report. *BMJ* 1977;**2**:419–21.

37. AMIS. The aspirin myocardial infarction study: final results. The Aspirin Myocardial Infarction Study research group. *Circulation* 1980;**62**:V79–V84.

38. Olsson G, Wikstrand J, Warnold I *et al.* Metoprolol-induced reduction in postinfarction mortality: pooled results from five double-blind randomized trials. *Eur Heart J* 1992;**13**:28–32.

39. Norwegian Multicenter Study Group. Timolol-induced reduction in mortality and reinfarction in patients surviving acute myocardial infarction. *New Engl J Med* 1981;**304**:801–7.

40. MERIT. Effect of metoprolol CR/XL in chronic heart failure: Metoprolol CR/XL Randomised Intervention Trial in Congestive Heart Failure (MERIT-HF). *Lancet* 1999;**353**:2001–7.

41. Kober L, Torp PC, Carlsen JE *et al.* A clinical trial of the angiotensin-converting-enzyme inhibitor trandolapril in patients with left ventricular dysfunction after myocardial infarction. Trandolapril Cardiac Evaluation (TRACE) Study Group. *New Engl J Med* 1995;**333**:1670–6.

42. Echt DS, Liebson PR, Mitchell LB *et al*. Mortality and morbidity in patients receiving encainide, flecainide, or placebo. The Cardiac Arrhythmia Suppression Trial. *N Engl J Med* 1991;**324**:781–8.
43. Waldo AL, Camm AJ, deRuyter H *et al*. Effect of d-sotalol on mortality in patients with left ventricular dysfunction after recent and remote myocardial infarction. The SWORD Investigators. Survival With Oral d-Sotalol. *Lancet* 1996;**348**:7–12.
44. Burkart F, Pfisterer M, Kiowski W, Follath F, Burckhardt D. Effect of antiarrhythmic therapy on mortality in survivors of myocardial infarction with asymptomatic complex ventricular arrhythmias: Basel Antiarrhythmic Study of Infarct Survival (BASIS). *J Am Coll Cardiol* 1990;**16**:1711–18.
45. Ceremuzynski L, Kleczar E, Krzeminska-Pakula M *et al*. Effect of amiodarone on mortality after myocardial infarction: a double-blind, placebo-controlled, pilot study. *J Am Coll Cardiol* 1992;**20**:1056–62.
46. CIBIS. A randomized trial of beta-blockade in heart failure. The Cardiac Insufficiency Bisoprolol Study (CIBIS). CIBIS Investigators and Committees. *Circulation* 1994;**90**:1765–73.
47. CIBIS. The Cardiac Insufficiency Bisoprolol Study II (CIBIS-II): a randomised trial. *Lancet* 1999;**353**:9–13.
48. Pitt B, Zannad F, Remme WJ *et al*. The effect of spironolactone on morbidity and mortality in patients with severe heart failure. Randomized Aldactone Evaluation Study Investigators. *New Engl J Med* 1999;**341**:709–17.
49. Julian DG, Camm AJ, Frangin G *et al*. Randomised trial of effect of amiodarone on mortality in patients with left-ventricular dysfunction after recent myocardial infarction: EMIAT. European Myocardial Infarct Amiodarone Trial Investigators. *Lancet* 1997;**349**:667–74.
50. Cairns JA, Connolly SJ, Roberts R, Gent M. Randomised trial of outcome after myocardial infarction in patients with frequent or repetitive ventricular premature depolarisations: CAMIAT. Canadian Amiodarone Myocardial Infarction Arrhythmia Trial Investigators. *Lancet* 1997;**349**:675–82.

3 Statistical methods for risk-stratification studies

Timothy R Church

Background

Scope of this chapter

Patients recovering from or afflicted with severe illness face many potential complications that cloud their future and make the choice of treatments difficult. This is particularly true of sudden cardiac death syndrome,[1] chronic congestive heart failure,[2] and myocardial infarction.[3] A common concern among these conditions is predicting whether the patient will experience sudden tachyarrhythmic death.[4] Although many clinical and electrocardiographic factors have been identified that have some degree of association with the chances that an individual will experience a life-threatening tachyarrhythmia, much work still needs to be done, and the appropriate design and execution of clinical studies is a necessary foundation on which this work must be built. The following material attempts to outline the biostatistical (that is, inferential) requirements for identifying and validating risk stratification and its use in selecting and validating the appropriate therapy for different risk strata. In addition, although the appropriate use of statistical methods that address the needs of risk-stratification studies can be no more than outlined in a single chapter such as this, such methods are described, reasons for their selection given, and helpful references are cited for the interested reader to learn more details regarding their implementation, including the underlying assumptions, computational considerations, and pitfalls.

Definitions

Risk stratification

Usually, risk stratification is the process of assigning individuals to homogeneous groups based on assessed risk in order to differentiate treatment efficacy or to predict common outcomes.[5] Those groups with high risk can be given more aggressive prevention or monitoring and those with lower risk can be spared treatment. Ideally, risk assess-

ment would separate perfectly those individuals who will have an event from those who will not, but currently no more than a probabilistic association between the risk variables and the events can be expected. For the purpose of this discussion, we will expand the definition of risk stratification to refer to the assignment of an individual probability or risk of sudden cardiac death.

Other activities resemble risk stratification, in that they attempt to categorise individuals based upon a set of factors associated with a condition of interest. These activities include mass screening, diagnosis, identification of risk factors, and prognostic staging (for example, in cancer). Mass screening[6] identifies asymptomatic individuals undergoing diagnosis of an underlying disease. Diagnosis[7] identifies precisely (or rules out) an underlying disease, but does not necessarily dictate a particular therapy (for example, one may not exist, or the therapeutic decision may require additional indications). Like screening, identification of risk factors[8] assigns to (usually) asymptomatic individuals a probability of developing disease, but, as opposed to screening, diagnosis or risk stratification, before any diagnosable disease is present for the purpose of preventing the development of disease. Prognostic staging,[9] which focuses on the extent of disease progression (as in staging cancer) rather than specific mechanisms of further morbidity, is perhaps the closest to risk stratification; it is also used to predict outcomes and tailor therapies. Although in the following we will not focus on the similarities of these activities to risk stratification, their associated methods can guide the development of methods for risk stratification.

Terminology

In the following, measurement will refer to any assessment of a characteristic of a patient, whether it is numeric (for example, heart rate, age in years, number of occluded vessels, or QT_c) or categorical (for example, sex, race, New York Heart Association Class, or presence of mitral valve regurgitation). Any function of one or more measurements is also a measurement. Any measurement that may be associated with the probability of a patient experiencing SCD is a predictor; and specifying a cut-point for the predictor, so that patients are divided into two groups, one at high risk and one at low risk, creates a test.

Statistical considerations and methods

Prediction

Some claim that the main challenge in modern clinical medicine is to make predictions regarding the patient.[10] Risk stratification, in which the challenge is to employ statistical methods that can emphasise the most pertinent data and filter irrelevant information, fits this description exactly. However, both misuse of and failure to use appropriate methods can lead to either serious error or underuse of information. Whatever useful information is collected should be used optimally to predict sudden cardiac death. A number of pitfalls, well known in the biostatistical literature, can be identified in advance and, therefore, avoided by the careful investigator. These pitfalls are often overlooked as fine points, even by able and experienced researchers. Traditionally, statistical methods have focused on parameter estimation and hypothesis testing, as opposed to prediction, but in the last decade some attention has been paid to predictive probabilities.[11]

Some of the problems peculiar to prediction are overfitting, model misspecification, and variable selection. Although these are highly interrelated, a brief description of each separately is in order. Overfitting refers to the tendency of a predictive model to appear to be more accurate in the set of data on which it is developed (the learning sample) than can be expected in a new set of data. For example, if a population of CHD patients are measured at baseline and followed until a number of them experience SCD, and if a predictive model using multiple independent predictor variables is developed, the model will correctly predict a certain fraction of SCD and a certain fraction of those not experiencing SCD. However, both theory and empirical evidence dictates that these fractions will, on the average, be higher than the rates of accurate prediction in a new set of patients, even though they are drawn from the same general population.[12] This stems from the tendency of model fitting methods to overfit the model to the patients in the "learning sample", so that not only will the model adapt to the characteristics of the learning sample that are representative of the larger population, but it will also adapt to those characteristics peculiar to that particular sample. Thus, the investigator must be chary of being overly optimistic about a model extracted from a particular data set and use methods that minimise this optimistic tendency.

The second problem of model misspecification simply refers to the potential that a parametric model (for example, a multiple logistic model) does not truly represent the underlying relationship between the predictor variables and the probability of SCD. If the true relationship is log-normal, say, instead of logistic, then the prediction will be off, especially at the tails of the distribution. Another potential for misspecification comes when it is decided how the variables interact when they enter the model. Do the effects add, multiply, or exponentiate? Using models that are flexible enough to adapt to the form that best represents the underlying relation between the predictors and the probability of SCD can combat this error. On the other hand, unless care is taken, such flexible models can exacerbate the problem of overfitting by allowing the model to reflect even more closely the idiosyncrasies of the learning sample.

Finally, the problem of variable selection, i.e. deciding which potential predictor variables to include in the predictive model, involves elements of the other two problems, with the additional complication that in common statistical software there are many available methods of accomplishing selection, each with its own appropriate context, but rarely is it accompanied by good advice on when to use it. Many variables potentially predict SCD in cardiac patients, but only a few are likely to be helpful in combination. If too many are used, the problem of overfitting becomes acute; if enough variables are used, apparently perfect prediction in the learning sample will result, with absolutely no usefulness in a new sample. On the other hand, if too few are used and especially if the appropriate set is not used, valuable predictive power will be left on the table with no one benefiting.

Use of multiple predictors

When several univariate predictors are available, for example, heart-rate variability and late potentials, frequently their individual predictive values are compared and the "loser" discarded in favour of the winner. On the other hand, when multiple predictors are considered in combination, it is usually after the optimal cut-point has been determined for each predictor and the resulting tests combined. However, both head-to-head comparison and combining tests can grossly underuse the predictive power of the combined predictors, as can be illustrated with a previously published simplified example.[5]

Suppose, in a population with a low-risk group and a high-risk group, that Predictor 1 and Predictor 2 are under consideration for discriminating members of one group from members of the other. Fig. 3.1 shows the hypothetical distributions of Predictor 1 for the two risk groups and Fig. 3.2 shows those for Predictor 2. Predictor 1 by itself predicts SCD only moderately well, but Predictor 2 is practically useless by itself. Casual observation would lead

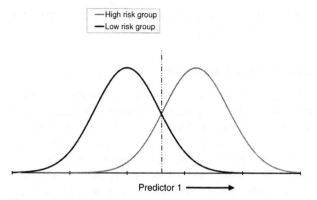

Figure 3.1 Distribution of hypothetical Predictor 1 for high-risk and low-risk groups, showing moderate discrimination.

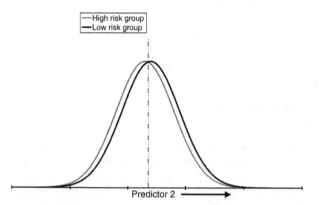

Figure 3.2 Distribution of hypothetical Predictor 2 for high-risk and low-risk groups, showing little discrimination.

to the conclusion that Predictor 2 should be discarded, and only Predictor 1 used to evaluate a patient's risk based on the vertical line separating the two groups. However, suppose the predictors are correlated, and the correlation coefficient (Pearson's r) = 0.80. Fig. 3.3 represents the joint distributions of Predictor 1 and Predictor 2 for each risk group by two ellipses, which enclose about 95% of each group. The reader can imagine them as enclosing the base of two peaks that represent where the majority of individuals in the two groups are located by their values of Predictor 1 and Predictor 2. Determining optimal cut-points for each predictor to create two tests and combining them would define the four quadrants (defined by the beaded horizontal and vertical lines) shown in the Fig. 3.3. It is easy to see that prediction would be less than optimal no matter how those quadrants are combined. On the other hand, an almost perfect separation of the low-risk group from the high-risk group is indicated by the diagonal dashed line. This line is based on a discriminant function.[12] Although this simplified example is based on idealised conditions, the general prin-

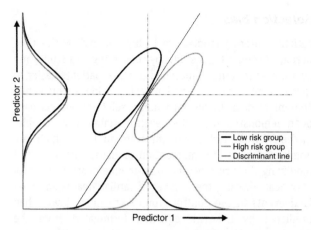

Figure 3.3 Joint distribution of Predictors 1 and 2 for high-risk and low-risk groups, showing high discrimination for linear combination.

ciple that poor to moderate predictors can be combined to produce an excellent prediction holds true in less ideal circumstances.

This example can be used to illustrate four underappreciated, but valuable points:

- Measurements with little apparent discriminating ability by themselves may be powerful predictors when combined with other predictors.
- High correlation with other predictors is not a good reason for discarding a predictor.
- Combining predictors can produce improved results over using tests based on individual predictors.
- Dichotomising predictors prior to combining them can weaken predictive power.

Censoring

Since SCD occurs over time, the most powerful way to examine its incidence is to analyse how long it takes for an SCD event to occur. However, not all individuals will experience an event during their follow-up period, a phenomenon called censoring. In addition, rarely are patients all followed for the same amount of time, so the researcher must either analyse the time to events or create a subset of patients all having a minimum amount of follow-up, and proceed to ignore all events past that point and all individuals with less follow-up. In the latter case, time-dependent effects may be missed and information lost. For example, measurement of initially low heart-rate variability may indicate increased risk of death immediately, but the risk may decrease for those surviving for a period of time. Estimates of risk must account for such time-dependence, and the basic appropriate survival models are the life-table[13] and Cox regression.[14]

Selection bias

Patients entering studies are highly selected by the time period they enroll in a study; by consenting to a study; and by study entry criteria intended to make patients easier to follow or to ensure the patient will provide a worthwhile amount of data. In several studies, selection effects have been demonstrated to affect even mortality. For example, in the Multiple Risk Factor Intervention Trial, which randomised subjects to intervention or usual care to see if modifying their risk factors could reduce death from coronary heart disease, the number of cardiac deaths and non-fatal events in the control group were much lower than predicted by the risk equation formulated from the Framingham Study and accounting for the explicit entry criteria.[15] Each successive eligibility screen reduced mortality relative to the predicted rate by 27, 40, and 50%, respectively. In the Minnesota Colon Cancer Control Study, the control group was 46% lower than the general population from which they were recruited.[16] Similar selection effects show up in other studies[17,18] and one group of investigators found selection to be common in prevention trials.[19]

Regression to the mean

If a predictor measurement fluctuates over time, even as the basic risk for the individual stays constant, a relatively high measurement of a predictor may more likely indicate a true value closer to the average, whereas a low measurement may be more likely to represent a higher value. This is a phenomenon known as "regression to the mean". For example, in hypertension, an individual blood pressure measurement may vary as much as 15 mmHg from time to time during the day,[20] but each individual measurement does not influence long-term risk; only the average about which the variation occurs is believed to be relevant. In a previous publication,[5] it has been shown that regression to the mean could result in an apparent drop of about 10 mmHg and, with a moderate sample size, this drop would appear to be a highly "statistically significant" result even if no treatment is applied.

By definition, risk stratification selects individuals with extreme values of inherently variable biological measurements, so regression to the mean invariably occurs. For example, if patients with a measured heart-rate variability (HRV) in the lowest quartile on a 24-h Holter recording are entered into a study, a comparison of the follow-up HRV to the baseline values will be biased; even the control group will show an artefactual increase in HRV. Further, if the relationship between HRV and outcome events is estimated from these biased baseline data, the actual number of events will be greater than the number of events predicted, if unbiased values are used for prediction. Care must be taken to avoid misinterpreting the comparison of risk-stratification scores when they are remeasured after selection.

Low structure methods

Although the development of optimal predictions using multiple predictors presents substantial technical challenges from a statistical point of view, there are a variety of approaches available. Discriminant analysis, a statistical tool closely related to logistic regression that optimally combines multiple variables to predict the status of individuals under certain assumptions, has been available for 30 years.[21] Because it is often difficult to verify those assumptions, one should use more recent "low-structure" methods, such as classification and regression trees,[22] generalised linear models,[23] generalised additive models,[24] neural networks,[25] and general smoothing techniques[26]; these require fewer assumptions and provide flexibility to account for more complex relations between predictors and the probability of an event.

Prior knowledge

The prediction equations that are developed must be updated as new information becomes available, either to refine predictions using existing predictors, or to incorporate new predictors. Bayesian methods not only provide a framework for previous information to be updated by new information, but also provide a coherent foundation for predictive inferences.[27] Such methods lend themselves to evidence-based medical practice.[28] The acceptability of Bayesian approaches in science is evidenced by the fact that their use in the literature has nearly doubled over the last 10 years, marking a turn in the practice of statistics.[29] Combining Bayesian methods with the low-structure methods described provides the solution to the problem of predicting sudden cardiac death from multiple predictors without precise physiologic theory to guide the specification of parametric statistical models. Cross-validation techniques can be used to assure that the selection of the prediction function is unbiased.[30,31] Confidence intervals can be created for prediction probabilities that adjust for missing data and still guarantee nominal coverage rates.[32,33] The Appendix to this chapter gives a hypothetical example of an estimated predictor function and its resulting positivity (the fraction of results that are positive) and positive predictivity.

Development of risk stratification

Setting out to risk-stratify a defined population (for example, all CHD patients), the investigator wishes to use clinical, laboratory, and electrocardiographic information to predict the chances that an individual will experience SCD within a certain time period (for example, 1 year). Once a stratification scheme is developed, a clinician will want to use the predictions from such a stratification scheme to determine the therapy that a patient will receive, i.e. watchful waiting, aggressive drug therapy, or implantation of a cardioverter/defibrillator. Naturally, the careful clinician will want to be reassured that the predictions are accurate. Thus, the two phases needed to develop a risk-stratification scheme are

- to develop a candidate scheme, and
- to validate the scheme.

Each of these phases requires separate specific steps. The development phase includes:

1. Identifying a target population.
2. Selecting candidate variables.
3. Collecting data on a representative sample of the population.
4. Developing a risk-stratification scheme with associated risk estimates.
5. Incorporating prior information.
6. Updating the risk estimates in the stratification scheme.

Target population

The target population must be one that is readily identified by history or some other symptom or sign, and in which we want to subcategorise the members by their risk of SCD. The population can be as narrowly defined as, for example, those with long-QT syndrome, or as broad as the population of the world. What is important is that it be well defined, so that the results can be analysed and generalised appropriately. For example, in a narrowly defined population like the long-QT example, which has a high underlying rate of SCD, more costly and invasive tests can be used to risk stratify, and, since the population is clearly defined, the applicability of the stratification to others with long-QT is fairly straightforward. For the population of the world, the rate of SCD is fairly low relative to the long-QT group, so less invasive and costly tests could be used, and, again because of the clear definition of the population, the generalisation would be straightforward as well. Once a suitable target population is identified, then a representative sample of that population must be selected to provide information about predictors and SCD rates.

Candidate variables

Note that the presence of long-QT syndrome, which defines the first population, might be used, in part, to risk-stratify the second population. Some underlying causal model should drive the decisions about what information to include in a risk-stratification scheme. Candidate variables can be

- demographic characteristics, such as age, sex, and race;
- clinical measurements, such as blood pressure, cardiac output, or prior history of MI, SCD, or bypass surgery;
- laboratory values, such as cholesterol fractions or triglyceride levels;
- electrocardiographic parameters, such as heart-rate variability, signal-averaged ECG, or QT interval.

What is important is that the chosen variables have some plausible association with SCD and that they be obtainable from members of the target population.

Although it is assumed that all of the candidate variables have some plausible connection with the chances of SCD, it will be useful in distinguishing between tests used in clinical decision-making and the underlying predictors that are used to form the test. In the following, the notion of a "predictor" will be distinguished from that of a "test", by defining a test to be any procedure that results in a binary decision such as "positive/negative", "rule in/rule out", "at risk/not at risk", and the like. Predictors, on the other hand, can be binary, polytomous (having multiple categories, either with some ordering or unordered), continuous, or any combination of these characteristics, as long as they contain information about the chances of SCD. To illustrate the difference, note that heart rate variability (HRV) expressed as a standard deviation is a continuous predictor of SCD but, by defining a critical value for HRV below which the patient is considered at high risk, creates a test. A second example is the number of VT episodes on 24-h Holter monitoring. As a predictor it takes on ordered categories 0, 1, 2, etc. but, if it is dichotomised by noting the presence or absence of VT, it creates a test.

Data collection

Data must be collected twice on the sample of the population to develop risk strata. First, baseline information, consisting of the value of each candidate predictor considered for risk stratification, must be collected on each individual at the beginning of the follow-up period. Collecting the results of tests, as will be illustrated, is inadequate, because some information could be lost in the collapsing of the candidate predictors. Although risk stratification can be performed when some data are missing for some individuals, minimising the number of missing values will maximise the usefulness of the risk stratification.

Next, the sample population must be followed for an adequate period of time for sufficient SCD events to be observed among them. Based on simulation studies, the size of the population and the period of follow-up need to produce a number of events roughly equal to 10 times the number of candidate predictors that will analysed.[34] For example, for 20 predictors, a minimum of 200 events is required. Thus, if the annual SCD rate for the target population is 1%, then a sample of 10 000 individuals followed for an average of 2 years or a sample of 20 000 followed for 1 year would be adequate to examine those 20 predictors.

Risk stratification

For many reasons, some pragmatic, some mistaken, SCD predictors have been used clinically as tests one at a time, or in informal combinations of two or three tests. Theoretically, a combination of all the predictors into a single "risk function" would optimally predict SCD. Such a risk function would provide for every conceivable combination of risk factors an estimated probability of SCD in the next period of time, say 1 or 5 years. This approach has not heretofore been used, however. Misunderstandings regarding the statistical constraints on the use of multiple predictors represent the mistaken reasons as to why this approach has not yet been undertaken (unpublished manuscript, M Hodges and TR Church "Identifying individual patients with coronary heart disease who are at risk of sudden cardiac death"). Non-parametric or low-structure methods outlined above provide a viable approach to optimal prediction.

Once a risk function has been estimated, the investigator will need to determine which prediction value (cutpoint) to use in deciding whether or not to implant an ICD. One way to evaluate a test for predicting SCD is to plot its sensitivity against its specificity on an X–Y coordinate system. A receiver-operating characteristic (ROC) curve results, and points along the curve represent all possible cut-points. In Fig. 3.4, two hypothetical tests are plotted. Each test predicts SCD within a specified period of time. It is easy to see that Test 2 is superior to Test 1: at any given specificity, Test 2 has a higher sensitivity. Although Test 2 is the obvious choice in this example, sometimes the ROC curves of the tests compared will not reveal a clear favourite. In such cases, the expected cost of mistakes at various cut-points can be used to compare tests and to set an optimal cut-point for the test chosen.

Risk function updates

As new information becomes available, the prediction equations that are developed must be updated either to

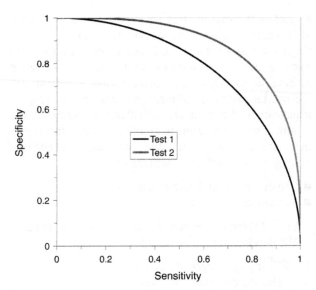

Figure 3.4 ROC curves for two hypothetical tests, showing the domination of Test 1 by Test 2.

refine predictions using existing predictors, or to incorporate new predictors. Bayesian methods not only provide a framework for previous information to be updated by new information, but provide a coherent foundation for predictive inferences.[27] Such methods lend themselves to evidence-based medical practice.[28] The acceptability of Bayesian approaches in science is further evidenced by the fact that their use in the literature has nearly doubled in the last 10 years, marking a turn in the practice of statistics.[29]

Validation of risk stratification

Once a candidate risk-stratification scheme is developed, the next phase is to validate the scheme prospectively on a population. It is tempting to assume that once the risk stratification has been developed applying it to the selected therapies is straightforward. In a situation where everything is known about the mechanisms of pathology and therapy, this assumption would be valid. Likewise, when the risk stratum under consideration is a subset of a population already shown to be effectively treated with the therapy, further validation also is not necessary. However, when risk stratification represents a new population in whom the therapy will be used, its application should be validated by first selecting individuals for therapy using the risk-stratification scheme, randomising the selected patients to either treatment or usual care, and then following both groups to determine whether the treatment is successful. In today's environment the treatment of choice for those with a high probability of SCD is the implantable cardioverter/defibrillator (ICD). Several clinical trials have proven the efficacy of this therapy over other therapies (AVID, CIDS, CASH, MUSTT, etc.). For the foregoing discussion, we shall assume that the therapy of choice in the high-risk group is the ICD.

The validation phase requires:

1. Selecting the therapy (ICD or medical care only) for each risk stratum.
2. Selecting and recruiting a population for testing.
3. Designing a trial to test those therapies in that population.
4. Measuring outcomes and assessing validity.

Selecting therapies

Clearly the problem of determining optimal therapy is complex, since combinations of ICD and medical therapy are commonly used to manage patients and, within each type of therapy, several options are available: for medical management several drug combinations are used and for ICD therapy, the determination of appropriate device settings is no small matter. Admittedly, it is a simplification of the clinical problem of determining optimal therapy to focus on deciding which individuals in the population have a great enough risk of SCD that an ICD is indicated, and which have low enough risk to be managed medically. However, as a first approximation the dichotomous decision of ICD versus medical management is reasonable. Unless there are solid data supporting a particular therapeutic approach (for example, dual-chamber pacing for ICD and amiodarone for medical management), determination of exact treatment decisions within the two broad categories might be left to the clinical judgment of the treating physician.

Selecting the population

If ICD versus medical management is to be studied, then the next step is to identify the population for whom the more aggressive treatment is justified. Studies[35,36] have shown that, in the first year after implantation, ICDs discharge appropriately in 25–45% of patients implanted under current indications. Assuming that a risk-stratification scheme yields an accurate estimate of the probability of SCD in the next year, it would seem reasonable to indicate those with a risk somewhere in excess of 25% over the next year. Again, this is an oversimplification, because under current indications the cumulative risk of appropriate discharge goes up as time passes, topping 90% after 5 years. However, as a starting point, this range is reasonable.

Designing the trial

Standard methods of trial design lend themselves to validating risk-stratification-based SCD prevention therapy. In multicentre trials, stratified randomisation with an overall sample size adequate to detect differences between treated and usual care groups is appropriate. An efficient design for validation of risk stratification for the purpose of assigning therapy involves a two-way 2×2 factorial design. This idea can be extended to multiple strata or treatments. Wu et al.[37] give a method for adjusting the sample size for the number of subjects expected to drop out of the study, cross-over to another treatment, or fail to comply with the assigned treatment. In any event, this design compares the treatment strategies across strata.

Measuring outcomes and assessing validity

Although an observational cohort study is used to develop the risk-stratification model, demonstrating the value of risk stratification and making preventive or therapeutic decisions based on it requires further study. Hypothetically, the risk-stratification model could identify increased risk, but therapy might have an equally large effect on the outcome events in all strata. Why? First, the relative reduction in mortality due to the therapy in the low-risk group might equal that in the high-risk group. Second, the therapy might not have any effect on the mortality in either group because it fails to address the appropriate mechanism or has large untoward effects. Hence the relative efficacy of the treatment in different strata must be examined.

The situation where two treatments, usual care and an implantable cardioverter–defibrillator, are being studied with two risk strata, high and low, is illustrated in Table 3.1, taken from Church.[5] The interesting results of the main comparisons, implantable cardioverter–defibrillator versus usual care and high versus low risk, and the stratum-specific comparisons, the implantable cardioverter–defibrillator versus usual care effect in the high-risk group and the same effect in the low-risk group are interpreted in Table 3.2, also taken from Church.[5] Other results may be difficult to interpret or represent conflicting outcomes.

Summary

Although common problems in predicting the occurrence of sudden cardiac death from clinical and electrocardiographic data can be identified, specifying a single solution to all them is impossible, because each situation is unique. However, the intent of this chapter is to indicate

Table 3.1   Groups in a two-by-two factorial design comparing treatments in two risk strata. Main treatment effect = (a + b) – (c + d). Main stratum effect = (a + c) – (b + d). Treatment effect in high risk = a – c. Treatment effect in low risk group = b – d. Equal treatment effects? = (a – c) – (b – d).

	High risk	Low risk
Implantable cardioverter–defibrillator	a	b
Usual care	c	d

general approaches that can be used to detect or circumvent the limitations of the datasets that are available. Enough information is given so that the reader educated in statistical inference can, through reviewing the cited literature, apply the ideas to a specific problem. It is not intended that the reader become a practitioner of statistics, instead the reader should become aware of the issues and collaborate with statistical colleagues when designing and analysing observational studies and clinical trials intended to develop or test risk-stratification schemes. In most circumstances, available multivariate methods allow the researcher to maximise the usefulness of information available, but for some purposes these methods must be modified.

Appendix

A hypothetical and simplistic example can be constructed to illustrate the concepts. Suppose that we collect data on 20 predictors from a large sample of symptomatic CHD patients. Label the variables representing the predictors $X_1,...,X_{20}$, and designate the vector of these variables **X**. Subsequently, we keep track of all SCDs among patients in the sample for 1 year, and use the values of **X** retrospectively to "predict" which patients were to experience SCD.

What would the predictor look like? It would first of all be a mathematical function of those variables. It could be called $f(x_1,...,x_{20})$, where x_i is a specific value of the variable X_i; denote the vector of specific values of **X** as **x**. The function would take on values between 0 and 1, estimating the probability of an event in the first year. The function can be estimated in any number of ways that allow a great deal of flexibility (generalised linear models, generalised additive models, generalised Cox models, smoothing splines, kernel smoothed models, artificial neural networks, classification and regression trees, etc.), or by using a combination of approaches, and cross-validating the result. If we assume a generalised linear model for the sake of illustration, the form of the predictive function is $f(\mathbf{X}'\beta)$, where **X** is a vector of the 20 values for an individual, β is a vector of regression coefficients, $\mathbf{X}'\beta = \beta_1 X_1 + ... + \beta_{20} X_{20}$, and f is an arbitrary smooth function. One could call $\mathbf{X}'\beta$ the risk score and $f(\mathbf{X}'\beta)$ the predictive function.

The predictive function could be graphed as the grey line in Fig. 3.5, with $\mathbf{X}'\beta$ on the horizontal axis and $f(\mathbf{X}'\beta)$ on the vertical axis. Although such a graph shows the probability that an individual with risk score $\mathbf{x}'\beta$ will have SCD in the next year (the positive predictive value), it does not indicate what fraction of individuals has a predic-

Table 3.2   Interpretation of results in a two-by-two study of treatment by risk stratum. See Table 3.1 legend for definitions of effects

Main treatment effect	Main stratum effect	Treatment in high risk group	Treatment in low risk group	Equal treatment effects?	Interpretation
Yes	Yes	Yes	No	–	Treatment is effective for one group, and stratification is effective in distinguishing the group in whom treatment is more effective
Yes	Yes	Yes	Yes	Yes	Treatment is effective, stratification is effective, but stratification is irrelevant to treatment efficacy or selection
Yes	Yes	Yes	Yes	No	Treatment is effective, stratification is effective, and stratification is relevant to treatment efficacy, but not to selection
Yes	No	Yes	Yes	–	Treatment is effective, stratification is not, so treatment should be applied to everyone
No	Yes	No	No	–	Treatment is ineffective, stratification is effective in predicting higher event rate
No	No	No	No	–	Neither treatment nor stratification is effective

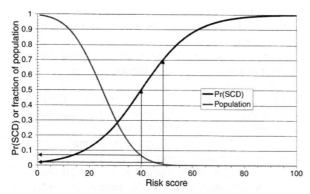

Figure 3.5 A hypothetical prediction function as a score plotted on the horizontal axis against the probability of an event, and against the proportion of the population with a score at least that high on the vertical axis. The vertical and horizontal arrows indicate two potential cut-points. Note that at a cut-point of 40, the probability of an event is 0.5, but the fraction of the population above this cut-point is about 6%. At a cut-point of 48, the probability of an event is 0.7, but only about 2% of the population would be positive.

tor value of $\mathbf{x}'\beta$. Multiplying the fraction (or prevalence) of individuals with a risk score of $\mathbf{x}'\beta$, designated p($\mathbf{x}'\beta$), by the predictive function at $\mathbf{x}'\beta$, i.e. p($\mathbf{x}'\beta$)f($\mathbf{x}'\beta$), predicts the incidence of SCDs in the next year for individuals with that risk score. A hypothetical curve for the fraction of the population having a risk score of at least $\mathbf{x}'\beta$ (call that fraction P($\mathbf{x}'\beta$)) is given by the black line in Fig. 3.5; p($\mathbf{x}'\beta$) is the slope or first derivative of this function. Integrating (essentially summing) over all such terms gives the total incidence of SCD in the next year.

Once data are collected from a large cohort of symptomatic CHD patients without prior events, and those experiencing SCD in the following year identified, the unknown parameters β and the unknown function f($\cdot$) can be estimated from the data. The estimates can be denoted $\hat{f}(\cdot)$ and $\hat{\beta}$. By substituting these estimates for the true values, estimated probabilities can be computed and calibrated for any given $\mathbf{x}$ using cross-validation techniques. Likewise, p($\mathbf{x}'\beta$) can be estimated by dividing the number of individuals with the risk score $\mathbf{x}'\hat{\beta}$ by the total population to get p*($\mathbf{x}'\hat{\beta}$). Confidence intervals for these estimates can be made using the bootstrap procedure.[38]

Creating a test requires selecting a cut-point value, c, for $\mathbf{X}'\hat{\beta}$. Those with a risk score above c would be "positive" and ICD implantation for them would be justified. For those with a score below c, ICD implantation would not be justified. By integrating the terms p*($\mathbf{x}'\hat{\beta}$)$\hat{f}$($\mathbf{x}'\hat{\beta}$) for all $\mathbf{x}'\hat{\beta}>c$, we get the estimated incidence of SCD in the next year among all patients with a positive result. The sensitivity of the test is equal to this incidence divided by the incidence in the total population of asymptomatic

CHD patients. The value of c is selected by trading off the "cost" of a false-positive result with that of a false-negative result to optimise the value of the test. Some subjectivity is involved in determining the acceptable number of false negative errors for each false positive error. However, some combination of the cost and pain of ICD implantation and the risk of dying of SCD must be evaluated in order to determine an optimal value of c.

References

1. Hallstrom A, Cobb L, Yu B. Influence of comorbidity on the outcome of patients treated for out-of hospital ventricular fibrillation. *Circulation* 1996;**93**:2019–22.
2. Ortiz J, Ghefter CGM, Silva CES, Sabbatini RME. 1-year mortality prognosis in heart failure: a neural network approach based on echocardiographic data. *J Am Coll Cardiol* 1995;**26**:1586–93.
3. Gomez-Marin O, Folsom A, Kottke T *et al.* Improvement in long-term survival among patients hospitalized after acute myocardial infarction, 1970 to 1980: The Minnesota Heart Survey. *New Engl J Med* 1987;**316**:1353–9.
4. Demirovic J, Myerburg R. Epidemiology of sudden cardiac death: An overview. *Prog Cardiovasc Dis* 1994;**37**:39–48.
5. Church TR. Risk assessment and risk stratification in sudden cardiac death – a biostatisticians view. *Pace-Pacing Clin Electrophysiol* 1997;**20**:2520–32.
6. Morrison A. *Screening in chronic disease.* New York, NY: Oxford University Press, 1985, pp. 42–47.
7. Lusted L. *Introduction to medical decision making.* Springfield, IL: CC Thomas, 1968.
8. Henderson M. Validity of screening. *Cancer,* 1976;**37**: 573–81.
9. Greenberg E, Baron J, Dain B *et al.*, Cancer staging may have different meanings in academic and community hospitals. *J Clin Epidemiol* 1991;**44**:505–12.
10. Feinstein AR. An additional basic science for clinical medicine: I. The constraining fundamental paradigms. *Ann Intern Med* 1983;**99**:393–7.
11. Geisser S. *Predictive inference: an introduction.* New York: Chapman & Hall, 1993.
12. Lachenbruch P. *Discriminant analysis.* New York, NY: Hafner Press, 1975.
13. Cutler SJ, Ederer F. Maximum utilization of the life table method in analyzing survival. *J Chron Dis* 1958;**8**:699–73.
14. Cox DR. Regression models and life tables. *J Royal Statist Soc B* 1972;**34**:187–200.
15. Neuwirth R. *Considerations in the estimation of the event rate in the control group for intervention trials.* Plan B Paper, in Division of Biostatistics, School of Public Health. Mineapolis: University of Minnesota, 1990.
16. Church TR, Ederer F, Mandel JS, Watt GD, Geisser MS. Estimating the duration of ongoing prevention trials. *Am J Epidemiol* 1993;**137**:797–810.
17. Wilhelmsen L, Ljungberg S, Wedel H *et al.*, A comparison between participants and non-participants in a primary prevention trial. *J Chron Dis* 1976;**29**:331–9.

18. Cairns J, Cohen L, Colton T *et al.* Issues in the early termination of the aspirin component of the Physicians' Health Study. *Ann Epidemiol* 1991;**1**:395–405.

19. Ederer F, Church TR, Mandel JS. Sample sizes for prevention trials have been too small. *Am J Epidemiol* 1993;**137**:787–96.

20. Hughes MD, Pocock SJ. Within-subject diastolic blood pressure variability: implications for risk assessment and screening. *J Clin Epidemiol* 1992;**45**:985–98.

21. Spiegelhalter DJ. Probabilistic prediction in patient management and clinical trials. *Stat Med*, 1986;**5**:421–33.

22. Breiman L, FJ, Olshen RA, Stone CJ. *Classification and regression trees*. Belmont, CA: Wadsworth, 1984.

23. McCullagh P, Nelder J. *Generalized linear models,* 2nd edn. London: Chapman & Hall, 1989.

24. Hastie T, Tibshirani R. *Generalized additive models*. London: Chapman & Hall, 1990.

25. Warner B, Misra M. Understanding neural networks as statistical tools. *Am Statistician* 1996;**50**:284–93.

26. Cleveland W, Robust, locally weighted regression and smoothing scatterplots. *J Am Stat Ass* 1979;**74**:829–36.

27. Davidoff F. Standing statistics right side up. *Ann Intern Med* 1999;**130**:1019–21.

28. Goodman S. Toward evidence-based medical statistics. 2:The Bayes' factor. *Ann Intern Med* 1999;**130**:1005–13.

29. Malakoff D. Bayes offers a 'new' way to make sense of numbers. *Science* 1999;**286**:1460–4.

30. Tanner M, Wong W. Data-based non-parametric estimation of the hazard function with applications to model diagnostics and exploratory analysis. *J Am Stat Ass* 1984;**79**:174–82.

31. Efron B. Estimating the error rate of a prediction rule: improvements on cross-validation. *J Am Stat Ass* 1983;**78**:316–31.

32. Robins JM, Ritov Y. Toward a curse of dimensionality appropriate (coda) asymptotic theory for semi-parametric models. *Stat Med* 1997;**16**:285–319.

33. Schemper M, Heinze G. Probability imputation revisited for prognostic factor studies. *Stat Med* 1997;**16**:73–80.

34. Peduzzi P, Concato J, Kemper E, Holford TR, Feinstein AR. A simulation study of the number of events per variable in logistic regression analysis. *J Clin Epidemiol* 1996;**49**:1373–9.

35. Moss AJ, Cannom DS, Daubert JP *et al.* Improved survival with an implanted defibrillator in patients with coronary disease at high risk for ventricular arrhythmia. *New Engl J Med* 1996;**335**:1933–40.

36. AVID Investigators. A comparison of antiarrhythmic-drug therapy with implantable defibrillators in patients resuscitated from near-fatal ventricular arrhythmias. *New Engl J Med* 1997;**337**:1576–83.

37. Wu M, Fisher M, DeMets D. Sample sizes for long term medical trial with time dependent dropout and event rates. *Control Clin Trials* 1980;**1**:109–21.

38. Efron B, Tibshirani RJ. *An Introduction to the Bootstrap*. New York: Chapman & Hall, 1993, p. 436.

4 Step-wise risk-stratification strategies

Stefan H Hohnloser

Prognosis of patients with ventricular arrhythmias is largely dependent on the underlying structural heart disease. The presence and severity of heart disease is the most important independent factor determining morbidity and mortality in that population. It is the purpose of this chapter to discuss step-wise risk-stratification strategies that could serve as a basis for the design of prospective interventional studies aiming at a reduction in arrhythmic events in patients prone to sudden cardiac death. Since the majority of studies dealing with the issue of risk stratification has been conducted in patients with ischaemic heart disease – and in particular in those with a recent myocardial infarction – we will mainly focus on this patient population. Accordingly, it appears appropriate to review the recent developments in postinfarction survival over time, the sensitivity and predictive value of various risk-assessment methods, and potential strategies of how the arrhythmogenic risk can be maximised by combining various risk stratifiers.

Mortality after myocardial infarction

The last two decades have observed a substantial improvement in survival of patients with acute myocardial infarction. In-hospital mortality has decreased from around 16% in the late seventies and early eighties to 8–10% in the

early nineties as recently documented in a prospective population-based survey.[1] For example, in-hospital mortality from congestive heart failure associated with acute myocardial infarction has been found to be significantly reduced over the last two decades.[2] The main reason for this reduction in mortality is the more widespread use of and adherence to contemporary therapeutic modalities, such as thrombolysis, administration of aspirin and beta-blockers.[1] The survival of patients discharged alive from hospital after myocardial infarction has also been considerably improved. As demonstrated in Table 4.1, the 1-year total mortality rate of patients discharged alive from hospital ranges between 3 and 11%.[1,3–7] However, it is important to note that total mortality appears to be also dependent on how the patient population under observation was selected. Uniformly, mortality rates reported from prospective controlled studies are significantly lower compared to those derived from more unselected consecutive series of patients; this is due to the strict adherence to exclusion criteria within controlled trials resulting in exclusion of patients at particularly high risk, such as older patients, patients with recurrent myocardial infarction, myocardial infarction after coronary artery bypass grafting, or ineligibility to thrombolysis. Given these considerations, it appears decisive that recommendations for risk stratification of patients after myocardial infarction are derived from observations of unselected patient cohorts.

Table 4.1 Mortality after myocardial infarction

Study	Year	Patient characteristics	Number of patients	12 months' mortality (%)
GISSI II[3]	1993	Only thrombolysed patients	10 219	3.5[a]
Aguirre *et al.* (TIMI II)[4]	1995	Only thrombolysed patients	2634	3.4–4.4[b]
SMILE[5]	1995	Anterior MI, no thrombolysis	1556	6.5
ISIS 4[6]	1995	Suspected acute MI	58 050	7.7
Feuvre *et al.*[1]	1996	Geographically determined unselected population	831	11.3
Copie *et al.*[7]	1996	Unselected post-MI patients	579	6.0
Frankfurt post-MI survey	1998	Unselected post-MI patients	439	2.5

[a]6 months' mortality; [b]4.4% = non-Q wave mortality; MI = myocardial infarction.

Despite these favourable trends in total postinfarction mortality, sudden arrhythmogenic death continues to represent a clinical challenge. Death from ventricular tachyarrhythmias is responsible for approximately 40–50% of all fatalities in the postinfarction population. It is of paramount importance to realise that the majority of all arrhythmogenic deaths occur during the first 12 months after the index infarct. For example, as shown in Fig. 4.1, the experience from the Frankfurt postinfarction survey, comprising 439 consecutive infarct survivors who were followed for an average of 42 ± 25 months, demonstrates that the vast majority of arrhythmic events occurs during the first year, particularly in patients with impaired left ventricular function. Accordingly, primary prevention of sudden death after myocardial infarction remains a valuable clinical goal, which has as yet not been achieved. Trials evaluating various antiarrhythmic drugs have failed to demonstrate a reduction in overall mortality in infarct survivors receiving preventive pharmacological therapy, with the one exception of beta-blocker therapy.[8–10] At present, the implantable cardioverter–defibrillator (ICD) is the most effective treatment for prevention of arrhythmogenic death both for primary and secondary prevention.[11,12] However, owing to the invasive nature of this therapy and its related costs, it will never be possible to fit all infarct survivors with such a device. Therefore, one of the biggest challenges in today's cardiology is represented by the need to risk-stratify patients surviving an acute myocardial infarction in order to select those patients who will benefit most from ICD therapy.

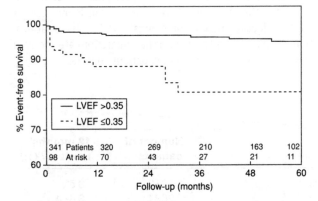

Figure 4.1 Survival free of sudden cardiac death, resuscitated ventricular fibrillation, and ventricular tachycardia during a mean follow-up period of 42 months in 439 consecutive survivors of acute myocardial infarction. Note that the majority of arrhythmic events occurred during the first year after the index infarct, particularly in patients with impaired left ventricular function.

Endpoints for future trials in survivors of myocardial infarction

An important consideration concerns the precise cause of death of patients surviving an acute myocardial infarction, particularly when risk stratification should result in therapeutic measures to decrease arrhythmogenic death. As discussed elsewhere, it is often very difficult to define retrospectively the precise cause of death of a patient enrolled in a controlled trial, particularly when suspected sudden arrhythmogenic death is concerned.[13] This problem becomes even more evident when population-based survey data are considered. The best estimate derived from numerous investigations is that arrhythmogenic death accounts for approximately 40–50% of total mortality in the first year after myocardial with a significant decrease over the next 12–24 months.[14] This time dependence of risk within the higher-risk patient groups limits the opportunity for effective intervention strategies to the early periods after the conditioning cardiovascular events.

There has been considerably dispute about the various study endpoints that should be elected to assess therapeutic interventions aiming at a reduction in sudden death in a defined patient population. Specifically, there is no general consensus as to whether in such trials total mortality should be considered as the primary study endpoint or whether other endpoints, such as sudden death mortality or appropriate interventions from an implantable cardioverter–defibrillator, would be more appropriate. The recent trend, however, is to use total mortality as opposed to total cardiovascular fatalities or death caused by more specific mechanisms, such as arrhythmias, myocardial infarction, or heart failure.[15] There are two major limitations of using arrhythmic death as the primary outcome measure of prospective trials:

- One relates to the already mentioned difficulties in accurate classification of death.[13]
- The other has been referred to as competing risks,[14] in which risks of multiple mechanisms of death may coexist and "compete" for causation of the terminal event.

Both of these reasons clearly favour the use of total mortality as the preferred measure of mortality outcome. Secondary stratification by cause of death is prudent and should be pursued in such trials.

Epidemiological impact of risk stratification

Risk stratification after myocardial infarction, which should ideally be performed prior to discharge of the patient from the initial hospitalisation, aims at two goals: to identify patients at very low risk of subsequent arrhythmic events, and, conversely, to select individuals at high risk of such events. In the first case, the risk stratifier used needs to show a high negative predictive value (usually much greater than 90% given the relatively low event rates of 5–10%). If one attempts to predict adverse events, the statistical criteria of an ideal test for risk stratification need to be tailored according to the therapeutic avenue that is envisaged. For instance, in trials evaluating the efficacy of the implantable defibrillator for primary prevention of sudden death, a costly and potentially complicated therapy, the test to identify eligible patients should have a high positive predictive accuracy. This would avoid exposure of many unnecessary patients to the intervention. Obviously, the test also needs to have a reasonable sensitivity. If, on the other hand, the proposed intervention is cheap and relatively safe (i.e. beta-blocker therapy) a test with a high sensitivity is mandatory. The positive predictive value may be lower in this circumstance since it is not a matter of concern if some patients receive unnecessary therapy. If these requirements are not fulfilled, the test or the combination of tests used will be too specific to impact on the epidemiological problem of sudden death simply because these tests will yield positive findings only in an insignificant tiny minority of the postinfarction population.

The first step towards this goal requires knowledge of the total number of sudden deaths within a specific patient population expressed as a fraction of total mortality within this group. For example, in a series of studies in patients with congestive heart failure, Kjekshus demonstrated that in studies in which the mean functional class was between I and II, the overall death rate was relatively low, but 67% of deaths were sudden.[16] In contrast, among studies with a mean functional class of IV, there was a high total mortality, but the fraction of sudden deaths was only 29%. Thus, for an intervention specific for the problem of sudden death, it is important not only to identify infarct survivors at high risk of death but also to predict the most likely mode of death, i.e. arrhythmic or non-arrhythmic death. Such a distinction would influence treatment strategy. Patients with a high propensity for arrhythmic death may benefit from preventive antiarrhythmic interventions, whereas such treatment may provide no advantage or even increase the risk of mortality in patients more likely to die from non-arrhythmic death. Accordingly, the various risk stratifiers currently in clinical use need to be examined towards their ability not only to predict total mortality but also with respect to their potential to predict specific causes of death.

A second prerequisite of risk stratification concerns the fact that the methods used must be available not only in specialised referral centres, but rather in the majority of all hospitals that are taking care of patients with acute myocardial infarction. For this reason, invasive procedures are much less likely to gain widespread popularity simply because they are only available at tertiary referral centres. As indicated above, the risk for arrhythmogenic death after myocardial infarction appears to be highest during the first 12 months following the index infarction. Accordingly, risk assessment should be commenced at the time patients are discharged from the hospital.

With these considerations in mind, it appears possible to design a step-wise risk-stratification strategy that can be tested in prospective well-controlled trials. If the expectations are fulfilled in such trials, this risk-stratification algorithm could subsequently been implemented in the routine assessment of patients surviving acute myocardial infarction.

Design of prospective interventional trials based on risk stratification

For the design of prospective studies, clinical data are needed which include prospectively recorded indices of various risk markers together with a sufficiently long follow-up period during which enough prespecified events occur.[17] Based on such data, a concept of a new trial can be modelled according to several important considerations. These include among others:

- the statistical association of the risk factors with the follow-up events;
- the statistical characteristics for individual and combined risk stratifier;
- an estimation of the expected mortality reduction within the high-risk group by an individual intervention.

The statistical aspects of this procedure have been recently detailed elsewhere.[17]

Step 1. Determination of left ventricular function

In patients with structural heart disease in general, left ventricular function has been demonstrated beyond doubt to be a decisive determinant of cardiac and overall mortality. For example, in a recent meta-analysis of 13 randomised controlled trials of prophylactic amiodarone therapy in patients with recent myocardial infarction or congestive heart failure, the strongest univariate predictor of risk of arrhythmic or sudden death was symptomatic heart failure.[18] In patients recovering from a recent acute myocardial infarction, numerous studies, both before and after the widespread use of thrombolysis, have convincingly demonstrated that depressed left ventricular function in postinfarction patients is associated with an increased mortality risk.[19–22] Unfortunately, the positive predictive value of left ventricular ejection fraction (LVEF) for arrhythmic events was found to be low. In addition, several investigators have shown that its predictive power was better for cardiac mortality than for arrhythmic events.[23,24] This is particularly relevant for patients with an ejection fraction in the range of 0.20–0.40. In patients with an LVEF of <15–20%, the vast majority of deaths are due to pump failure.[16] If one aims to identify patients at high risk, particularly for arrhythmic death, in order to subject these individuals to prophylactic antiarrhythmic therapy, infarct survivors with extensive myocardial damage resulting in an LVEF of <15–20% should probably be excluded from such intervention trials.[25] However, this issue is controversially discussed since the implantable defibrillator has been shown in secondary prevention trials to be significantly more effective in patients with depressed as compared to patients with better preserved left ventricular function.[12,26] Accordingly, left ventricular function alone appears to be not accurate enough for identifying patients at particularly high risk for arrhythmic events or sudden death,[23,24,27,28] but, on the other hand, it represents the strongest predictor of total cardiac mortality. Generally speaking, therefore, determination of left ventricular function should be the initial step in assessment of risk of sudden cardiac death in patients with structural heart disease and in particular in survivors of acute myocardial infarction.

Step 2. Maximising arrhythmogenic risk

As discussed above, the prerequisite for an interventional trial aiming to prevent specifically sudden cardiac death is to identify infarct survivors being at highest risk for arrhythmias. Research efforts over the last decade have therefore focused on finding ideal clinical markers which are non-invasive and highly correlated with arrhythmia-related sudden cardiac death. The majority of risk stratifiers evaluated for this purpose are based on electrocardiographic methods or on measurements of cardiac autonomic tone (Box 4.1). These methods are extensively discussed in subsequent chapters of this book. As a general rule, however, most of these various risk stratifiers have been demonstrated to have relatively low positive predictive values. Accordingly, several of these factors are analysed in combination in an attempt to increase the positive predictive accuracy to a more reasonable value.

A classical example of such a stepwise risk-stratification strategy was pursued by the MADIT (Multicenter Automatic Defibrillator Implantation Trial) investigators.[11] They sought to risk-stratify coronary patients with a remote myocardial infarction who presented with two risk markers:

Box 4.1 Methods for assessment of arrhythmogenic risk after myocardial infarction

- Clinical assessment
- Assessment of left ventricular function
- Resting ECG
  - heart rate
  - QRS duration, intraventricular conduction disturbances
  - QT duration
  - QT interval dispersion
- Signal-averaged ECG
- T-wave alternans
- Holter monitoring
  - frequency of ventricular premature beats
  - non-sustained ventricular tachycardia
  - heart rate variability
  - heart rate turbulence
  - QT interval/T wave dynamicity
- Baroreflex sensitivity
- Programmed ventricular stimulation

- reduced left ventricular ejection fraction (LVEF) (<0.36), and
- asymptomatic non-sustained ventricular tachycardia on Holter monitoring.

To further enhance arrhythmogenic risk, these patients were then subjected to programmed ventricular stimulation and, if inducible ventricular tachycardia or fibrillation was found that could not be suppressed by intravenous procainamide, these patients were randomised to defibrillator implantation or to conventional therapy.[11] This strategy identified a group of coronary patients in which implantation of a defibrillator turned out to improve prognosis to a substantial extent. Although the study does not provide information on how many patients had to be screened in order to complete the trial,[11] some have estimated that only 1 or 2% of all survivors of acute myocardial infarction fall in that category.[29] These patients would account for, at best, 5–10% of all postinfarction deaths.

At least two other prospective studies have evaluated the potential advantage of combining non-invasive risk-stratification methods with the invasive technique of programmed ventricular stimulation. Both studies differed from the MADIT trial in as much as infarct survivors were subjected to risk stratification early after the index infarct. However, in both studies, no specific therapeutic interventions were based on the results of risk stratification. Pedretti and associates[30] studied 303 survivors of myocardial infarction in a two-step protocol with assessment of various non-invasive risk stratifiers (LVEF <0.40, Holter-documented spontaneous ventricular ectopy including non-sustained VT, late potentials on signal-averaged ECG, heart rate variability, and mean heart rate) followed by programmed ventricular stimulation in individuals with more than two positive non-invasive risk stratifiers. In 47 patients, two or more non-invasive risk stratifiers were found to be present which resulted in a positive predictive value of 30% with a sensitivity of 87%.[30] Of these 47 patients, 20 were inducible into sustained monomorphic VT on programmed ventricular stimulation, which yielded a positive predictive value of 65% at a reasonable sensitivity of 81%. The authors correctly concluded from their observations that the combined use of non-invasive methods and programmed ventricular stimulation selected a group of infarct survivors with an arrhythmic event rate of 65% during the observation period. They argued that these patients could be selected for preventive implantation of an ICD. In the second study, Andresen and coworkers followed a similar study protocol.[31] From a series of 657 infarct survivors, 304 (46%) were selected who had either an abnormal Holter recording prior to discharge (defined as the presence of ≥ 20 VPBs/h, ≥ 10 ventricular pairs, or non-sustained VT) or an LVEF ≤ 0.40. The investigators performed programmed ventricular stimulation (PVS) in 146 out of these 304 patients, which yielded abnormal responses in 22. During a follow-up period of 37 months, the incidence of arrhythmic events was 18% in patients with an abnormal programmed ventricular stimulation result, compared to only 4% with a unremarkable PVERPVS ($P = 0.034$). Of note, however, the positive predictive value of programmed ventricular stimulation was only 18%, which is in marked contrast to the results obtained by Pedretti *et al.*[30] Clearly, this discrepancy is partially explained by methodological problems, such as the relatively low percentage of patients subjected to programmed ventricular stimulation in the study of Andresen *et al.*[31] or different stimulation protocols used. Moreover, differences in patient characteristics between both studies are apparent; for instance, the rate of thrombolysis and/or acute mechanical revascularisation was higher in the Andresen study compared with that of Pedretti.[30] In the latter investigation, antiarrhythmic drugs were more often used than in the former one and the rationale to use these agents was not apparent. Since programmed ventricular stimulation is often regarded as one of the most specific methods to assess arrhythmogenic risk in patients with structural heart disease, the combined use of non-invasive risk assessment as the first step to select patients followed by the second one, application of programmed ventricular stimulation may seem attractive. However, there is no general consensus as to the question whether such an approach can substantially increase the positive predictive accuracy of the entire risk-stratification strategy. Moreover, and probably most importantly, the invasive nature of programmed ventricular stimulation and its associated risks and costs seem unlikely to introduce this approach into widespread clinical routine. Accordingly,

some experts in the field of risk stratification have clearly stated that this technique is impractical for identifying patients at high risk for arrhythmia or sudden cardiac death after myocardial infarction.[25]

With these limitations of invasive risk-stratification methods in mind, numerous studies have tried to enrich arrhythmogenic risk in a given patient population by applying entirely non-invasive risk-stratification algorithms. One of the best examples for such a combined approach is the use of heart rate variability together with other non-invasive risk-stratification methods. In this case, the positive predictive accuracy of heart rate variability can be improved over a clinically important range of sensitivities (25–75%) for cardiac mortality and arrhythmic events.[32,33] Such improvements of positive predictive accuracy have been reported for combinations of heart rate variability with mean heart rate, LVEF, frequency of ventricular premature beats, and clinical assessment.[34] However, it has to be emphasised that it is unknown at present which other risk stratifiers are the most practical and most feasible to be combined with heart rate variability for multivariate risk stratification.

The largest prospectively designed post-myocardial infarction risk-stratification study is the ATRAMI (Autonomic Tonus and Reflexes After Myocardial Infarction) trial.[35] This multinational multicentre study enrolled 1284 survivors of acute myocardial infarction who were treated according to contemporary therapeutic guidelines with 63% of patients undergoing thrombolysis. Besides left ventricular function, heart rate variability, baroreflex sensitivity, spontaneous ectopy, and signal-averaged ECG were applied as risk stratifiers. Patients were followed for an average of 21 months during which time 49 prespecified endpoint events were observed. Low values of heart rate variability or baroreflex sensitivity carried a significant multivariate risk of cardiac mortality (3.2 and 2.8, respectively). When both values were below the cut-offs, the 2-year mortality was 17% compared with 2% when both were well preserved ($P < 0.0001$). A similar increase in risk could be established by step-wise risk stratification using the association of low heart rate variability or baroreflex sensitivity with depressed left ventricular function (LVEF < 0.36): the relative risk increased to 6.7 and 8.7 with this combined approach.[35]

In a similar study from our own institution, we could confirm these observations. In a series of 325 consecutive infarct survivors, a variety of currently available non-invasive risk stratifiers were assessed and patients were followed for 30 months.[36] In that study, we evaluated the predictive power of these risk stratifiers for cardiac mortality and in a second step for arrhythmic events only. Particularly for the secondary endpoint of arrhythmic events, the predictive accuracy was highest for heart rate variability and left ventricular function; however, when each stratifier was analysed separately, the positive predictive accuracy was low. Only when both predictors were combined, was a significant improvement in risk prediction achieved.

Therefore, the conclusion can be drawn from these investigations that the step-wise risk-stratification strategy using reduced left ventricular function and low values of autonomic markers are useful to identify a subgroup of postinfarction patients at truly high risk of preventable death. Actually, the predictive power of this risk-stratification algorithm appears to be comparable to that incorporating invasive programmed ventricular stimulation, but offers the clinical advantage of an entirely non-invasive procedure.

Step-wise risk assessment: an approach for prospective interventional trials

Currently, several prospective randomised intervention trials aiming at primary prevention of sudden death after acute myocardial infarction are being pursued based on a step-wise stratification strategy. The one which is most advanced is the so-called ALIVE trial (AzimiLide post-Infarct surVival Evaluation).[37] This study follows an innovative design to examine the potential of azimilide, a new antiarrhythmic agent, for improving survival after acute myocardial infarction in patients at high risk of sudden cardiac death. The trial proposes to target a selected group of infarct survivors at high risk for arrhythmic events. Accordingly, patients will be eligible for ALIVE if they have had an acute infarct within the previous 6–21 days, have a left ventricular ejection fraction between 0.15 and 0.35 (determined by any method), and have no contraindications for class III antiarrhythmic agents. To enrich arrhythmogenic risk, patients are being enrolled until a total of 2150 patients with a depressed heart rate variability (defined as an index of ≤20 U) have been enrolled. Heart rate variability is assessed from a 18–24-h Holter recording, which is started immediately after randomisation of the patient. This second step of risk stratification is hoped to be sufficient to select the targeted population with a high arrhythmic event rate. Patients will randomly receive placebo, 75 mg azimilide daily, or 100 mg daily. The primary endpoint based on an intent-to-treat analysis is all-cause mortality. The trial is designed based on the assumption that the 1-year all-cause mortality rate in this patient population will be 15% in the placebo group and that azimilide will decrease the mortality rate by ≥ 45%.[37] In addition, a number of secondary study endpoints will be evaluated. Azimilide or placebo medication is administered after patients have already been optimised on conventional therapy including aspirin, beta-blockers, ACE inhibitors, and statins where appropri-

ate. A second trial, which uses a very similar design with a two-step stratification strategy, is the DINAMIT study (Defibrillators In Acute Myocardial Infarction). To be enrolled in this study, postinfarction patients have to exhibit a left ventricular ejection fraction <0.36 and a depressed heart rate variability (SDNN <71 ms) and/or an increased average 24-h heart rate (mean RR <751 ms). Eligible patients will be randomised to optimal pharmacological therapy alone or to additional prophylactic defibrillator implantation.

Undoubtedly, both of these and perhaps additional other prospective trials will help to assess the efficacy of primary preventive therapy to reduce arrhythmic mortality after myocardial infarction using various treatment modalities. However, it is equally important to realise that these trials are the first to test the hypothesis that a step-wise risk-stratification strategy actually is able to select the targeted patient population after myocardial infarction which will benefit most from such preventive therapy.

References

1. Le Feuvre CA, Connolly SJ, Cairns JA, Gent M, Roberts RS. Comparison of mortality from acute myocardial infarction between 1979 and 1992 in a geographically defined stable population. *Am J Cardiol* 1996;**78**:1345–9.
2. Spencer FA, Meyer TE, Goldberg RJ et al. Twenty year trends (1975–1995) in the incidence, in-hospital and long-term death rates associated with heart failure complicating acute myocardial infarction. *J Am Coll Cardiol* 1999;**34**:1378–87.
3. Volpi A, De Vita C, Franzosi MG et al. Determinants of 6-month mortality in survivors of myocardial infarction after thrombolysis. results from the GISSI-2 data base. *Circulation* 1993;**88**:416–29.
4. Aguirre FV, Younis LT, Chaitman BR et al. Early and 1-year clinical outcome of patients evolving non-Q wave versus Q wave myocardial infarction after thrombolysis. *Circulation* 1995;**91**:2541–8.
5. Ambrosioni E, Borghi C, Magnani B for the Survival of Myocardial Infarction Long-Term Evaluation (SMILE) Study Investigators. The effect of the angiotensin-converting-enzyme inhibitor zofenobril on mortality and morbidity after anterior myocardial infarction. *New Engl J Med* 1995;**332**:80–5.
6. ISIS-4 Collaborative group. ISIS-4: A randomized factorial trial assessing early oral captopril, oral mononitrate, and intravenous magnesium sulphate in 58 050 patients with suspected acute myocardial infarction. *Lancet* 1995;**345**:669–85.
7. Copie X, Hnatkova K, Staunton A, Fei L, Camm AJ, Malik M. Predictive power of increased heart rate versus depressed left ventricular ejection fraction and heart rate variability for risk stratification after myocardial infarction.

Results of a 2-year follow-up study. *J Am Coll Cardiol* 1996;**27**:270–6.

8. Julian DG, Camm AJ, Frangin G *et al.* and the European Myocardial Infarct Trial Investigators. Randomised trial of effect of amiodarone on mortality in patients with left-ventricular dysfunction after recent myocardial infarction: EMIAT. *Lancet* 1997;**439**:667–74.

9. Cairns JA, Connolly SJ, Roberts R, Gent M. Randomised trial of outcome after myocardial infarction in patients with frequent or repetitive ventricular depolarizations: CAMIAT. *Lancet* 1997;**349**:675–82.

10. Hjalmarson A. Effects of beta blockade on sudden cardiac death during acute myocardial infarction and the postinfarction period. *Am J Cardiol* 1997;**80**:35J–39J.

11. Moss AJ, Hall WJ, Cannom DS *et al.* for the Multicenter Automatic Defibrillator Implantation Trial Investigators. Improved survival with an implanted defibrillator in patients with coronary disease at high risk for ventricular arrhythmias. *New Engl J Med* 1996;**335**:1933–40.

12. The Antiarrhythmics Versus Implantable Defibrillators (AVID) Investigators. A comparison of antiarrhythmic-drug therapy with implantable defibrillators in patients resuscitated from near-fatal ventricular arrhythmias. *New Engl J Med* 1997;**337**:1576–83.

13. Pratt CM, Greenway PS, Schoenfeld MH, Hibben ML, Reiffel JA. Exploration of the precision of classifying sudden cardiac death. Implications from the interpretation of clinical trials. *Circulation* 1996;**93**:519–24.

14. Myerburg RJ, Kessler M, Castellanos A. Sudden cardiac death: Epidemiology, transient risk, and intervention assessment. *Ann Intern Med* 1993;**119**:1187–97.

15. Myerburg RJ, Mitrani R, Interian A, Castellanos A. Interpretation of outcomes of antiarrhythmic clinical trials. Design features and population impact. *Circulation* 1998;**97**:1514–21.

16. Kjekshus J. Arrhythmias and mortality in congestive heart failure. *Am J Cardiol* 1990;**65**:421–8.

17. Malik M. Analysis of clinical follow-up databases: risk stratification studies and prospective trial design. *PACE* 1997;**20**:2533–44.

18. Amiodarone Trials Meta-Analysis Investigators. Effect of prophylactic amiodarone on mortality after acute myocardial infarction and in congestive heart failure: meta-analysis of individual data from 6500 patients in randomized trials. *Lancet* 1997;**350**:1417–24.

19. Bigger JT Jr, Fleiss JL, Kleiger R, Miller JP, Rolnitzky LM and the Multicenter Post-Infarction Research Group. The relationships among ventricular arrhythmias, left ventricular dysfunction, and mortality in the 2 years after myocardial infarction. *Circulation* 1984;**69**:250–8.

20. Kleiger RE, Miller JP, Bigger JT Jr, Moss AJ and the Multicenter Post-Infarction Research Group. Decreased heart rate variability and its association with increased mortality after acute myocardial infarction. *Am J Cardiol* 1987;**59**:256–62.

21. Hohnloser SH, Franck P, Klingenheben T, Zabel M, Just H. Open infarct artery, late potentials, and other prognostic factors in patients after acute myocardial infarction in the thrombolytic era. *Circulation* 1994;**90**:1747–56.

22. Copie X, Hnatkova K, Staunton A, Fei L, Camm AJ, Malik M. Predictive power of increased heart rate versus depressed left ventricular ejection fraction and heart rate variability for risk stratification after myocardial infarction. Results of a 2-year follow-up study. *J Am Coll Cardiol* 1996;**27**:270–6.

23. Richards D, Byth K, Ross D, Uther J. What is the best predictor of spontaneous ventricular tachycardia and sudden death after myocardial infarction? *Circulation* 1991;**83**:756–63.

24. Odemuyiwa O, Malik M, Farrell T, Bashir Y, Poloniecki J, Camm AJ. Comparison of the predictive characteristics of heart rate variability index and left ventricular ejection fraction for all-cause mortality, arrhythmic events, and sudden death after myocardial infarction. *Am J Cardiol* 1991;**68**:434–9.

25. Pratt CM, Waldo AL, Camm AJ. Can antiarrhythmic drugs survive survival trials? *Am J Cardiol* 1998;**81**(6A):24D–34D.

26. Connolly SJ, Gent M, Roberts RS *et al.* Canadian implantable defibrillator study (CIDS): a randomized trial of the implantable cardioverter defibrillator against amiodarone. *Circulation* 2000;**106**:1297–302.

27. Hartikainen JEK, Malik M, Staunton A *et al.* Distinction between arrhythmic and non-arrhythmic death after acute myocardial infarction based on heart rate variability, signal-averaged electrocardiogram, ventricular arrhythmias and left ventricular ejection fraction. *J Am Coll Cardiol* 1996;**28**:296–304.

28. Hohnloser S H, Klingenheben T, Zabel M. Identification of patients after myocardial infarction at risk of life-threatening arrhythmias. *Eur Heart J* 1999;**1**(Suppl. C):C11–C20.

29. Wilber DJ, Kall JG, Kopp DE. What can we expect from prophylactic implantable defibrillators? *Am J Cardiol* 1997;**80**(5B):20F–27F.

30. Pedretti R, Etro MD, Laporta A, Braga SS, Caru B. Prediction of late arrhythmic events after acute myocardial infarction from combined use of non-invasive prognostic variables and inducibility of sustained monomorphic ventricular tachycardia. *Am J Cardiol* 1993;**71**:1131–41.

31. Andresen D, Steinbeck G, Brüggemann T *et al.* Risk stratification following myocardial infarction in the thrombolytic era. A two-step strategy using non-invasive and invasive methods. *J Am Coll Cardiol* 1999;**33**:131–8.

32. Task Force of The European Society of Cardiology and the North American Society for Pacing and Electrophysiology. Heart rate variability: standards of measurement, physiological interpretation, and clinical use. *Circulation* 1996;**93**:1043–65.

33. Hohnloser S H, Klingenheben T, Zabel M, Li Y-G. Heart rate variability used as an arrhythmia risk stratifier after myocardial infarction. *PACE* 1997;**20**(Pt II):2594–601.

34. Camm AJ, Fei L. Risk stratification following myocardial infarction. In: Malik M, Camm AJ eds. *Heart rate variability*. Armonk, NY: Futura Publishing Co. Inc., 1995:369–92.

35. La Rovere MT, Bigger JT Jr, Marcus FI, Mortara A, Schwartz PJ for the ATRAMI Investigators. Baroreflex sensitivity and heart-rate variability in prediction of total car-

diac mortality after myocardial infarction. *Lancet* 1998;**351**:478–84.

36. Hohnloser S H, Klingenheben T, Zabel M, Schoepperl MD, Mauss O. Prevalence, characteristics, and prognostic value during long-term follow-up of non-sustained ventricular

tachycardia after myocardial infarction in the thrombolytic era. *J Am Coll Cardiol* 1999;**33**:1895–902.

37. Camm AJ, Karam R, Pratt CM. The azimilide post-infarction survival evaluation (ALIVE) trial. *Am J Cardiol* 1998;**81**(6A):35D–39D.

5 Risk-stratification studies for prospective trial design

Marek Malik

The appropriateness and efficacy of every novel treatment should be validated and tested in a prospective study. However, reasonable design of new prospective studies has to use detailed retrospective evaluations of clinical data. Experience shows that the goals of prospective trials based on traditional beliefs and consensus assumptions are far less frequently fulfilled than the goals of prospective studies, the design of which was retrospectively modelled within existing data sets. Indeed, the hypothetical concepts derived only from speculations about the contemporary state-of-the-art knowledge might be easily misleading and, in the past, many such concepts were used in proposals of new prospective studies, although data were available, which, if properly analysed, would clearly show that the new proposal is unrealistic.

Modelling a proposal of a new prospective study in an existing data set is, of course, based on the assumption that the nature and character of data accumulated in the past will be repeated in the future. Whilst this is rarely the case, a retrospective modelling test is certainly much more accurate than a hypothetical consideration.

Sample of clinical data

In order to demonstrate the individual concepts and data analytical approaches, this chapter will use follow-up data accumulated in the database of the Post-Infarction Research Survey of St George's Hospital. The examples will use a population of 644 patients (mean age 56.5 ± 8.9 years, 131 women) who suffered from acute myocardial infarction and survived until hospital discharge.[1,2] For all these patients, complete data were available for a 3-year follow-up, during which 74 patients died. Of these, 62 deaths were classified as cardiac and 41 as sudden cardiac (i.e. within 1 hour of the onset of new symptoms or during sleep). In addition, 22 patients suffered from sustained symptomatic ventricular tachycardia. Based on these data, an arrhythmic death was defined as "sudden cardiac death without new signs of myocardial ischaemia or progressive heart failure" or as a cardiac death in a patient with a history of sustained symptomatic

ventricular tachycardia after the index infarction. Using this definition, 44 deaths were considered as cardiac arrhythmic, 19 deaths as cardiac non-arrhythmic, and 11 deaths as non-cardiac. While this distinction between arrhythmic and non-arrhythmic deaths certainly has its limitations,[3] it is probably reasonable in statistical terms.[4]

All patients had left ventricular ejection fraction (LVEF) assessed either by angiography or by a radionuclide MUGA scan. A nominal 24-h Holter recording was obtained from each patient and all these recordings had at least 18 hours of analysable data. The mean RR interval duration was obtained by averaging all sinus rhythm RR intervals, and the heart rate variability (HRV) was measured by the HRV triangular index method and expressed in technical units corresponding to the 128 Hz sampling bins.

The examples presented in this text consider a model of an antiarrhythmia treatment in patients surviving acute myocardial infarction and selected according to these risk predictors. Although some practically relevant conclusions might be drawn from the examples, the chapter is mainly concerned with the methodology of data analytical techniques.

Risk assessment and trial design

Thus, having this data set available, we would like to propose a new prospective trial aiming at testing a certain treatment option designed to reduce arrhythmia mortality in patients surviving acute myocardial infarction. Naturally, because of a rather low incidence of arrhythmia as well as total mortality (6.8% and 11.5% in the first 3 years, respectively), the new treatment option cannot be applied to all patients. Instead, we would like to select a high-risk group for this purpose, using LVEF, 24-h mean heart rate, or HRV as risk stratifiers.

The appropriate plan for testing the new idea with existing data is to carry out the following steps:

- The data of the risk factors need to be investigated in terms of their distribution in the whole population and their statistical association with follow-up events.

- The stratification characteristics (i.e. sensitivity, specificity, etc.) need to be evaluated for the individual risk factors and, if appropriate, for their multivariate combinations.
- The stratification characteristics have to be converted into estimates of the mortality reduction that can be expected within the high-risk group and need to be projected into optimum trial design in terms of number of patients, screening cost, etc.

Statistical descriptors

Review of data

Fig. 5.1 shows scatter diagrams of the risk factors in the existing population. Displays of this kind are particularly useful if you are dealing with risk factors quantified numerically with many different possible values (for instance with values of LVEF rather than of NYHA class, which is also expressed numerically but has only four possible values). In the graphs of Fig. 5.1, note that, although the values of LVEF are measured on a discrete scale (the results of the LVEF are only integers), there are no clear preferential values. If we were dealing with manual readings of some measurements, say calliper and ruler-based measurement of total QRS duration in EKG recorded with a paper speed of 25 mm/s, preferential values of 80 and 120 ms might be too numerous invalidating the whole data set.

Further, note in Fig. 5.1 that, while arrhythmic mortality is truly associated with low HRV values, the association with low LVEF is rather modest.[5] It can also be seen that the values of risk factors in patients with follow-up events do not create two or more distinct populations, as might be the case with some biochemical data. This has an implication for optimising the dichotomy limits (i.e. thresholds of risk factors differentiating between high-risk and low-risk cases). In cases of separate populations of risk factors in event-positive patients, step-wise rather than continuous adjustment of the dichotomy limits is needed.

Cumulative distributions of risk factor values enable us to assess the correspondence of different dichotomy limits to the percentages of the complete population. In the data discussed here, criteria of LVEF $\leq$40%, mean RR $\leq$750 ms, and HVR index $\leq$20 units are all satisfied in approximately 30% of the complete population (naturally, the groups of patients satisfying individual criteria are different). More strict criteria of LVEF $\leq$30%, mean RR $\leq$600 ms, and HRV index $\leq$15 units are satisfied in only approximately 16, 4, and 12% of the complete population, respectively.

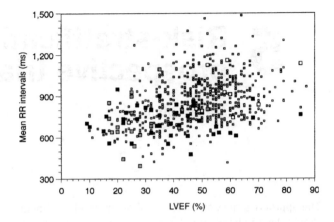

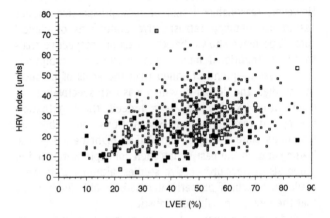

Figure 5.1 Scatter diagram of the data used in the examples. Large open, large shaded, and large full squares correspond to patients who, during a follow-up of 3 years, suffered from non-cardiac, cardiac non-arrhythmic, and cardiac arrhythmic deaths, respectively.

Statistical testing

Table 5.1 shows the statistical differences in risk factors of patients who did and did not survive first 3-year follow-up and of patients who did and did not suffer from cardiac arrhythmic death. In both these groups of comparisons, the differences are highly significant. This confirms the visual observations regarding the association of risk factors with follow-up events. However, for a design of a risk-stratification strategy, statistical comparisons of this kind are of little help. In particular, no conclusion can be drawn from statistical comparisons in respect of the optimum dichotomy limits of individual risk factors.

Moreover, the relationship between statistical differences of the means and the practical performance of risk stratification (i.e. selection of a high-risk group) is rather complex. Although in many cases a strongly significant difference between the means leads to a powerful selection of high-risk group, this relationship is not absolute. Some

Table 5.1 Statistical differences in risk predictors between survivors and non-survivors

Risk predictor	3-year all-cause mortality		*P*
	Survivors N = 570	Non-survivors N = 74	
Left ventricular ejection fraction (%)	48.3 ± 14.2	38.7 ± 16.9	1×10^{-5}
Mean RR interval (ms)	870 ± 165	750 ± 150	6×10^{-9}
Heart rate variability index (units)	28.2 ± 10.2	21.1 ± 11.9	4×10^{-6}
	3-year arrhythmic mortality		
	Survivors N = 600	Non-survivors N = 44	
Left ventricular ejection fraction (%)	47.8 ± 14.5	38.9 ± 16.3	1×10^{-4}
Mean RR interval (ms)	866 ± 167	724 ± 109	5×10^{-8}
Heart rate variability index (units)	28.1 ± 10.5	18.1 ± 9.4	2×10^{-8}

Values of individual risk predictors are shown as mean ± SD, standard two-sample t-test assuming unequal variances was used for comparisons.

risk factors with a strongly significant difference between the means of positive and negative patients perform rather poorly when a high-risk group is selected (e.g. the depressed LVEF used in predicting arrhythmia mortality – see below). If the distribution of the data of the risk factor is very non-normal, a practically useful risk stratification is possible, even if the means of the positive and negative patients do not significantly differ.

Descriptors

Statistical tests related to dichotomy limits of risk factors are also possible. Each dichotomy limit divides the complete population into two groups, namely patients with the risk factor lower and higher than the dichotomy. The incidence of mortality levels in these two groups can be compared using a suitable categorical test, such as χ^2 test or Fisher exact test. Figure 5.2 shows the results of such tests performed for different dichotomy limits of individual risk factors. To compare the results of these tests for different risk factors, the dichotomies used can be converted into the proportion of the complete population using the data of the cumulative distributions of risk factor values. As discussed in the following sections, the proportions of the population corresponding to dichotomy limits of the risk factors can only be used as a very approximate guide. Practical suggestions of specific stratification strategies should not be based on this type of statistical analysis.

Different dichotomy limits of a risk factor can also be used to express the relative risk, i.e. the proportion between the mortalities among patients with the risk factor lower and higher than the given dichotomy. Again, the dichotomy limits can be converted into percentages of the complete population. Unfortunately, when the dichotomy limit is moved from very abnormal to less abnormal values, both the mortality among patients with the risk factor lower and higher than the dichotomy decreases while their proportion may not change much. Consequently, within a broad range of risk factor values, the relative risk is frequently almost independent of the precise dichotomy. This, of course, means that the assessment of relative risk is not helpful in the design of a risk-stratification strategy.

Actually, relative risk analysis is only helpful in risk-stratification studies when the performance is compared of the same or different risk factors recorded in different populations with different event rate.

Characteristics of the power of risk stratification

Sensitivity and specificity

The division of a population between patients with and without a risk factor is most frequently described in terms of sensitivity and specificity.

Every criterion distinguishing high and low-risk patients, such as a dichotomy limit of a risk-predicting variable (say, 40% of LVEF), divides the complete population into test positive (e.g. LVEF ≤40%) and test negative (e.g. LVEF >40%) patients. At the same time, the com-

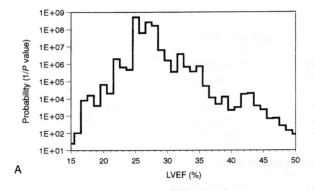

A

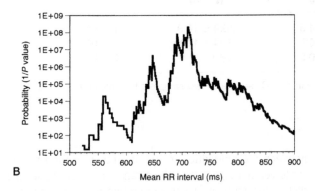

B

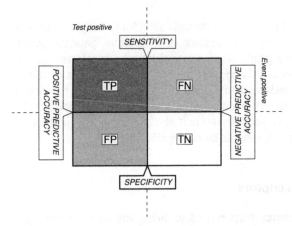

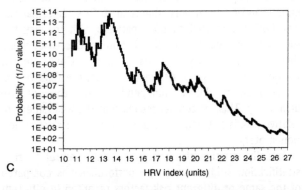

C

Figure 5.2 Association of risk factors with 3-year all-cause mortality. Panels A, B, and C: for each dichotomy limit of the corresponding risk factor, the graphs shows the reciprocal *P* value of the χ^2 test evaluating the hypotheses that the cases of mortality are differently frequent in patients with the risk factor below/equal and above the dichotomy.

- *true negative* are those without clinical events and with a negative test;
- *false positive* are those without a clinical event but with a positive test, and
- *false negative* are those with a clinical event but with a negative test.

As shown schematically in Fig.5.3, *sensitivity* is the proportion of true positive among event-positive patients, and *specificity* is the proportion of true negative among event-negative patients. Hence, the values of sensitivity and specificity show how many event-positive and event-negative patients are correctly classified as such by the classification test under consideration. *Positive predictive accuracy* is the proportion of true positive among test-positive patients (how many high-risk patients selected by the test really had an event) and *negative predictive accuracy* is the proportion of true negative among test-negative patients (how many low-risk patients selected by the text really had been event free).

Figure 5.3 Schematic representation of distinctions of true-positive (TP), true-negative (TN), false-positive (FP), and false-negative (FN) patients. See the text for details.

Every dichotomy limit of a risk factor measured on a numerical scale defines a different classification criterion and is therefore associated with different values of sensitivity and specificity. These values may be plotted for different values of dichotomy limits and the resulting graph of both sensitivity and specificity values has a typical X-shaped form. As the dichotomy limit is moved from very abnormal towards the more normal values, the sensitivity increases (more and more event-positive patients are classified as test-positive) and the specificity decreases (more and more patients without an event are classified as test-positive). Similar to the graphical representation of the statistical parameters, the dichotomy limits of individual risk factors can be converted into proportions of the

plete population is divided into patients with and without clinical events or categories (e.g. death within a certain follow-up period). The combination of the criterion with clinical events leads to the division of the complete population into four mutually exclusive groups:

- *true positive* are those with the clinical event and a positive test;

investigated population. Then, the sensitivity and specificity graphs derived from different risk factors can easily be compared (Fig. 5.4).

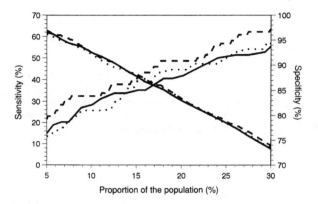

Figure 5.4 Sensitivity and specificity associated with different dichotomies of individual risk factors. The dichotomies were converted into proportions of the complete population; full line = LVEF; dotted line = mean RR interval; dashed line = HRV index.

Positive predictive accuracy

To some extent, the values of sensitivity and specificity are independent of the incidence of clinical events in the total population. Having representative samples of patients with and without clinical events is sufficient to assess sensitivity and specificity. The values of sensitivity and specificity do not principally change by increasing or decreasing the number of patients with and without events. On the contrary, the values of positive and negative predictive accuracy depend on the true incidence of events in the complete population, and a consecutive population of patients (or, at least, a population representative of a consecutive population) is needed to assess their values. Adding more patients with events into the investigated population increases, in principle, positive predictive accuracy and decreases negative predictive accuracy, while adding more patients without events decreases positive and increases negative predictive accuracy, respectively. To avoid an artificial bias introduced by mixing arbitrarily some event positive and some event negative patients, the true real incidence of events has to be maintained within the investigated data set.

It is easy to see that the values of positive predictive accuracy equal the event rate in the high-risk population selected by the given test. As certain positive predictive accuracy is associated with every dichotomy limit of a risk factor, a graph can be constructed showing the event rate in a population of patients having the risk factor lower (or higher) than the given dichotomy. Again, it is practical to

convert the dichotomy limits of individual risk factors into proportions of the complete population. An example of such graphs is shown in Fig. 5.5. For instance, panel A of Fig. 5.5 shows a 3-year mortality of 25% among the quintile (20%) of the complete population with lowest values of LVEF. (These patients were approximately those with LVEF <35%.)

In cases of classified events, the graphs of event rate can easily be modified to show proportions of individual event categories. Panels A, B and C in Fig. 5.5 distinguish different mortality modes. It can easily be seen that the increase of total mortality with depressed LVEF is mainly due to the increase of non-arrhythmic deaths, whilst the increase of total mortality with depressed HRV is predominantly caused by an increased incidence of arrhythmic events.

Receiver operator and positive predictive curves

Any value of sensitivity can be achieved with any risk factor just by selecting a correct dichotomy. (By changing the dichotomy, the group of true positive patients can be made to grow one, by one event-positive patient.) Thus quoting the value of sensitivity without the corresponding value of specificity is completely meaningless. The dependency between sensitivity and specificity can be assessed from graphs such as those in Fig. 5.4. However, it is also possible to plot specificity directly as a function of sensitivity. Such an interdependency is termed *receiver operator characteristic*.

Since the pairs of sensitivity and specificity do not reflect the incidence of events (see previous section), it is frequently more useful to plot positive predictive accuracy against sensitivity and negative predictive accuracy against specificity. These graphs are called *positive* and *negative predictive characteristics* (Fig. 5.6).

By relating the specificity and positive predictive characteristics to sensitivity rather than to a dichotomy limit of a risk factor, the characteristics can be used to describe the power of multivariate risk stratification in which two or more risk factors are combined. In principle, there are two ways of combining risk factors. Either, independent dichotomies of individual factors can be combined,[6] or a linear combination of two or more factors can be used.[7] Examples of multivariate positive predictive characteristics are shown in Fig. 5.7. The graphs are not informative in respect of the individual dichotomies or combinations but, for instance, the top panel in Fig. 5.7 shows that when dichotomies of all three risk factors (i.e. LVEF, mean RR interval, and HRV) are combined, a positive predictive accuracy of approximately 50% can be achieved for predicting 3-year mortality at a sensitivity level of 40%. In other words, the graph indicates that a risk-stratification

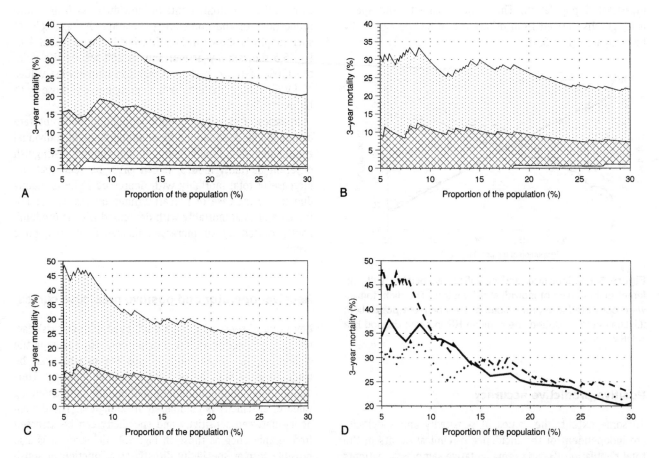

Figure 5.5 Positive predictive accuracy (= 3-year mortality) associated with different dichotomies of individual risk factors. The dichotomies were converted into proportions of the complete population. In panels A, B, and C, different modes of 3-year mortality are distinguished: open area at the bottom of the panels = non-cardiac mortality; cross-hatched area = cardiac non-arrhythmic mortality; dotted area = cardiac arrhythmic mortality. In panel D, the total mortalities of individual risk factors are compared. Panel A and full line in panel D = LVEF. Panel B and dotted line in panel D = mean RR interval. Panel C and dashed line in panel D = HRV index.

strategy exists that combines all three factors and that selects a test positive group with a 3-year mortality of 50%, which included 40% of all patients who died during the 3-year follow-up.

Statistical comparisons of positive predictive curves

Different positive predictive characteristics can be statistically compared at different levels of sensitivity. When characteristics derived from different and mutually independent populations are compared, the comparison is simple, as a binomial test can be used.

A more elaborate approach is needed to compare positive predictive characteristics constructed for different risk factors applied to the same population. The easiest is to employ a standard sign test to compare misclassifications of both

strategies. Such a comparison is performed in steps corresponding to individual sensitivity values. For each level of sensitivity, corresponding dichotomy limits of both risk factors are found defining test-positive groups with this sensitivity (multivariate characteristics are compared in the same way, relevant combinations of dichotomies rather than individual dichotomies are established). These dichotomy limits define two different stratification strategies, each of which leads to the division of the complete population into test-positive and test-negative patients. The patients for whom both strategies disagree (i.e. patients test-positive in one test and test-negative in the other) are identified. These patients are further divided into those classified correctly (i.e. as test-positive if event-positive, and as test-negative if event-negative) by one strategy and those classified correctly by the other strategy. Finally, the proportions of the numbers of patients in these two groups can be compared statistically, for instance by the sign test (Fig. 5.8).

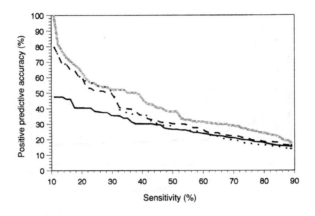

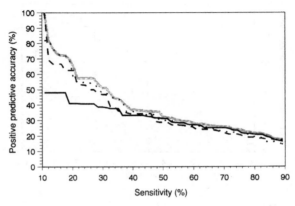

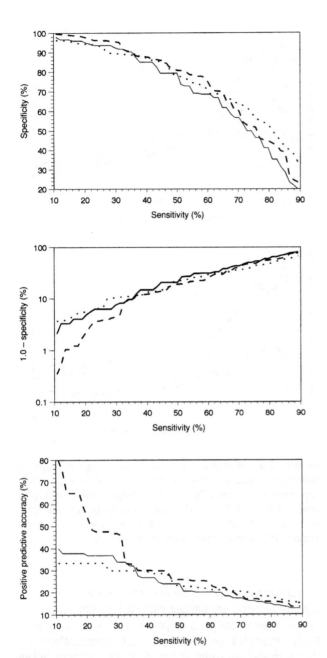

Figure 5.7 Multivariate positive predictive characteristics for prediction of 3-year all-cause mortality. Top panel: characteristics computed with independent dichotomies of individual risk factors; bottom panel: characteristics computed with linear combinations of individual risk factors (see the text for details). Full black line = LVEF + mean RR interval; dotted line = LVEF + HRV index; dashed line = mean RR interval + HRV index; bold grey line = combination of all three risk factors.

Figure 5.6 Receiver-operator characteristics (top and middle panel) and positive predictive characteristics (bottom panel) for the prediction of 3-year all-cause mortality; full line = LVEF; dotted line = mean RR interval; dashed line = HRV index.

Trial design

Models of mortality

Ideally, graphs such as those presented in Fig. 5.5 should be used in computations assessing the sample sizes of the new trial. However, the unsmoothed nature of such graphs makes them unsuited for this purpose.

The principal trend of these graphs may be obtained by approximating them with mathematically defined functions. Figure 5.9 shows negatively exponential approximation of graphs presented in Fig. 5.5 as well as corresponding graphs showing the incidence of arrhythmic rather than all-cause mortality in stratified populations.

Trial parameters

The mathematically defined functions used for graph approximation in Fig. 5.9 can be used to postulate not only the all-cause mortality for individual stratification strategies but also the proportion of arrhythmic and non-arrhythmic mortality in different high-risk groups.

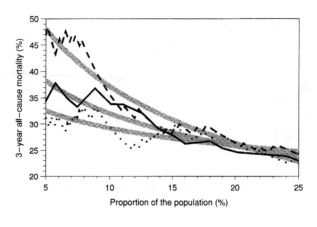

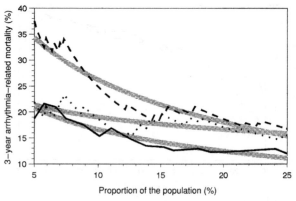

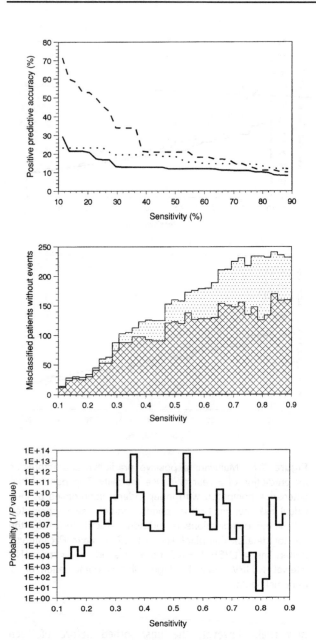

Figure 5.9 Mortality levels corresponding to different dichotomy limits of individual risk factors (see Figure 5.7) and their mathematically defined interpolations (bold grey lines). Top panel: 3-year all-cause mortality; bottom panel: 3-year cardiac arrhythmic mortality; full line = LVEF; dotted line = mean RR interval; dashed line = HRV index.

Figure 5.8 Example of statistical comparisons of positive predictive characteristics. Top panel: positive predictive characteristics for prediction of 3-year cardiac arrhythmic mortality; full line = LVEF; dotted line = mean RR interval; dashed line = HRV index. Middle panel: for dichotomy limits corresponding to individual levels of sensitivity, the disagreement between HRV index and LVEF is shown (see the text for details): cross-hatched area = HRV index correct and LVEF incorrect; dotted area = LVEF correct and HRV index incorrect. Bottom panel: the proportions of disagreement between LVEF and HRV index is tested by the sign test (repeated for each sensitivity level).

Assuming a certain reduction of arrhythmic mortality with a new treatment option, the graphs of mortality can be combined with the appropriate statistical formula expressing the power of the new trial, to show how many high-risk patients are needed with each stratification strategy to achieve, say a study power of β = 80% (at α = 0.05). Examples of results of such computations are shown in the top panel of Fig. 5.10. For instance, when tuning the dichotomy limit of HRV to select only 5% of all postinfarction patients and expecting 40% reduction of 3-year arrhythmic mortality in the on-treatment group, approximately 200 patients will be needed in each arm of the new trial to guarantee its power of β = 80% (at α = 0.05) to show a significant reduction of all-cause mortality in the on-treatment group. Returning to the graphs in Fig. 5.9, we shall see that selecting 5% of patients with the lowest HRV leads to a 3-year all-cause mortality of 48% of which 34.5% are arrhythmic deaths. Assuming 40% reduction of arrhythmic deaths reduces 3-year all-cause mortality to 34.2%. Indeed, a simple power estimate shows that 201 patients in each limb are needed to show an event difference of 48% versus 34.2% at β = 80% and α = 0.05.

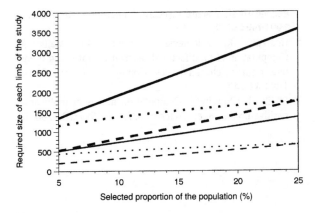

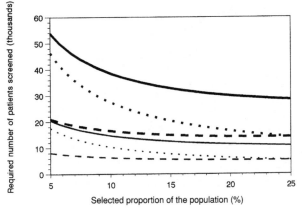

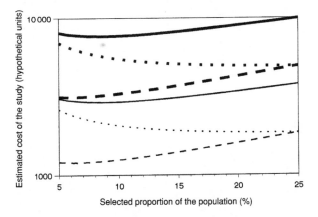

Figure 5.10 Characteristics of a new trial design (see the text for details). Top panel: required size of each limb of the study (β = 80%, α = 0.05) for different dichotomies of the individual risk factors (converted into proportions of the complete population). Middle panel: required number of patients screened. Bottom panel: hypothetical cost of the study assuming 1/20 proportion between screening and enrolment cost. Fine lines = expected 40% reduction of arrhythmic mortality; bold lines = expected 25% reduction of arrhythmic mortality; full line = LVEF, dotted line = mean RR interval, dashed line = HRV index.

Whilst tuning the dichotomies of risk stratifiers to select a very small proportion of all postinfarction patients

(and to achieve a high placebo mortality) leads to the smallest sizes of the new study, the number of patients to be screened needs to be considered. Graphs of the top panel of Fig. 5.10 can easily be converted into predictions of the numbers of patients to be screened (Fig. 5.10, middle panel). For instance, if 200+200 patients represent 5% of the total screened population, 8000 patients are needed to select them.

Various other descriptors can be derived from these estimates. For instance, the bottom panel of Fig. 5.10 shows estimates of the total trial cost assuming that enrolment of one patient is 20 times more costly than screening one patient. It can be clearly seen that the financial optimum, in terms of the proportion between screened and enrolled patients (horizontal axis) is very different for different risk predictors.

Conclusion

The data analytical possibilities presented in this text constitute only the core of methods used for researching clinical follow-up databases and modelling new trial proposals. For instance, confidence intervals need to be introduced for individual risk-stratification characteristics used in studies of this kind.

Some of the steps demonstrated in this text are rather complex, especially when applied to multivariate risk-stratification approaches, in which different combinations of dichotomies or different algebraic combinations of risk factors have to be considered. Despite this complexity, these data analytical procedures should be considered when a new prospective study is being designed, aimed at prophylactic reduction of clinical events. Without detailed analyses of existing data, we cannot be certain that a new concept of a prospective trial reflects the true pathophysiologic reality and not only our optimistic assumptions.

References

1. Cripps TR, Malik M, Farrell TG, Camm AJ. Prognostic value of reduced heart rate variability after myocardial infarction: clinical evaluation of a new analysis method. *Brit Heart J* 1991;**65**:14–19.
2. Copie X, Hnatkova K, Staunton A, Fei L, Camm AJ, Malik M. Comparison of the predictive power of increased heart rate with that of depressed left ventricular ejection fraction and heart rate variability for risk stratification after myocardial infarction: results of a 2-year follow-up study. *J Am Coll Cardiol* 1996;**27**:270–6.
3. Gottlieb SS. Dead is dead – artificial definitions are no substitute. *Lancet* 1997;**349**:662–3.
4. Hartikainen JEK, Malik M, Staunton A, Poloniecki J, Camm AJ. Distinction between arrhythmic and non-arrhythmic

death after acute myocardial infarction based on heart rate variability, signal-averaged electrocardiogram, ventricular arrhythmias and left ventricular ejection fraction. *J Am Coll Cardiol* 1996;**28**:296–304.

5. Odemuyiwa O, Malik M, Farrell T, Bashir Y, Poloniecki J, Camm AJ. A comparison of the predictive characteristics of heart rate variability index and left ventricular ejection fraction for all-cause mortality, arrhythmic events and sud-

den death after acute myocardial infarction. *Am J Cardiol* 1991;**68**:434–9.

6. Hnatkova K, Poloniecki J, Camm AJ, Malik M. Computation of multifactorial receiver operator and predictive accuracy characteristics. *Comput Meth Prog Biomed* 1994;**42**:147–56.

7. Malik M, Church TR. Computation modes of multivariate positive predictive characteristics. *PACE* 1997;**20**:1708–13.

Part II

Techniques of risk assessment

6 Basic clinical assessment

Branco Mautner

I never manage arrhythmias but patients with arrhythmias.

It is surprising that most books on general medicine, clinical cardiology, or even specialised ones, when dealing with arrhythmias, do not mention the clinical aspects, but point directly to the ECG and other non-invasive or invasive studies, both for diagnosis and risk stratification.

In common clinical practice, the first contact between the physician and his patient should be through verbal communication followed by clinical examination, i.e. performing a clinical history. Sometimes the patient is consulting because of one or more symptoms evidently related or caused by an arrhythmia. In other cases, after an arrhythmia is suspected or found, the patient is referred to a cardiologist or for an ECG. This takes some time, during which the patient may be at risk. Thus, it is commonsense and good clinical practice to perform an initial clinical assessment of the patient in this first approach. Even in such extreme situations as sudden death episodes, a quick basic clinical evaluation of the situation preceding CPR or ECG monitoring is unavoidable.

When arrhythmias are being assessed clinically, remember that there are two ways in which they can affect human beings: by altering their quality of life or by reducing their survival. Quality of life will be mostly altered by the existence of symptoms, whilst danger of increased mortality will be indicated by the coexistence of structural heart disease, diseases of other parts of the body, and by the functional status of the patient; gender and age participating factors in both situations.

Age and gender

The first thing that a physician will note when approaching a patient is age and sex. We should differentiate between "normal", "healthy", and "asymptomatic" people, since often arrhythmias are present without symptoms and in otherwise healthy subjects. We would like to call "normal" people those without arrhythmias, "healthy" those with asymptomatic arrhythmias that do not increase the risk of death, present in normal hearts and without any evidence of other pathologic entities. On the other hand a subject can be sick, in high risk for sudden death and still asymptomatic, in which case we would not call him normal or healthy.

There does not seem to be an important difference in symptoms frequency between gender at any age. The presence of arrhythmias in the embryo in the first trimester of pregnancy seems to be a predictor of pregnancy loss.[1] A low birthweight (<2500 g) predicts an increased tendency towards arrhythmias in early childhood, the OR being 14.6; children of 1–15 years of age with supraventricular arrhythmias from the presence of accessory pathways were more often born with low birthweight than normal ones.[2]

In healthy children arrhythmias are rare, although isolated premature ventricular beats are present in up to 20% of ambulatory monitoring studies.[3] Pre-excitation syndrome was found in 0.04% of the total population since childhood and no significant variation with age was detected, being around 60% in males and 40% in women.[4]

Supraventricular tachyarrhythmias are more frequent in young people. They are usually felt as palpitations, with or without dizziness and syncope episodes. Remember that often palpitation, shortness of breath, and chest discomfort are present without evidence of arrhythmias, these being due to psychological distress such as panic disorders.

Asymptomatic ectopic atrial tachycardia is not an uncommon finding in young males, having been found in 0.34% of 3556 asymptomatic males of 17–21 years of age[5] and in 0.46% of 3700 symptomatic (mostly palpitations) arrhythmia hospital patients of a mean age of 26 years.

Among young people, specially when they are engaged in competitive sports, sudden cardiac death owing to ventricular fibrillation is a distressing outcome that is extremely rare in well-trained professionals under medical supervision, occurring more frequently in a sporting population with a lesser degree of training and medical care;[6] generally the structural disease has an underlying hyperthrophic cardiomyopathy,[7-8] an anomalous coronary arteries origin, or arrhythmogenic right ventricular cardiomyopathy,[9] although it may be related only to an impact to the chest.[10]

Although some woman complain of more arrhythmia-related symptoms during menstruation, difference in arrhythmia frequency has not been detected.[11] There seems to be an increased incidence of arrhythmias during normal pregnancy that consist mostly in atrial and ventricular premature beats,[12] but during Holter monitoring arrhythmias were found in only 10% of symptomatic episodes.

Premature beats, either supraventricular or ventricular, are felt as isolated palpitations. They can produce anxiety in the patient. Supraventricular premature beats are common at any age, whilst ventricular ones are more common in adulthood and older people.

As in other cardiac situations, arrhythmias of functional origin are more frequent in women, although mitral valve prolapse, rheumatic valve disease, myocardiopathies, and other structural heart alterations can produce them. In adult males the most common cause is ischaemic heart disease, although all other causes, including psychological stress, are possible.

Atrial fibrillation (AF) is relatively rare in the first two decades of life. When present in the fetus or neonates, it is almost always related to an accessory AV pathway, and in adolescents to hyperthyroidism.[13] In a survey made in 43 hospitals in Argentina[14] of 1003 patients with AF, mean age was 65.8 years (ranging from 6 to 100 years), (54% men and 46% woman). Most frequent symptoms were: palpitations (44%), dyspnoea (44%), anginal pain (19%), and less often syncope, dizziness, and asthenia. Only 2% of the patients were asymptomatic. Prevalence of AF increases with age: 3.1% cases in men and 1.9% in women aged 55–64 years; 6.2% in men and 4.8% in women over 65 years of age, and rising to 38.0% in man and 31.4% in women age 85–94.[15–16] There is an annual increase in stroke associated with AF with age, from 1.5% for those aged 50–59 years to 23.5% for those aged 80–89 years.[17] The presence of AF has a risk of all-cause mortality ranging from an adjusted relative risk of 1.3 to an unadjusted relative risk of 2.6.[18] Recently a follow-up over 40 years from the Framingham Heart Study of subjects aged 55–94 years was made:[19] the OR for death when AF was present was 1.5 (95% CI 1.2–1.8) for men and 1.9 (95% CI 1.5–2.2) for women, when adjusted for age, hypertension, smoking, diabetes, left ventricular hypertrophy, myocardial infarction, congestive heart failure, valvular heart disease, stroke, and transient ischaemic attack. The risk of mortality did not significantly vary by age, but it did by sex, diminishing female survival more than men's, the age-adjusted OR for death being 2.4 for men and 3.5 for women.

During monitoring 383 asymptomatic middle-aged men over 6 hours, at least one premature beat during the study[20] was found in over 90%, more than one supraventricular premature beat present in 6.4%, paired supraventricular beats in 17.7%, more than one premature ventricular beat in 8.8%, ventricular premature contractions (VPC) in two or more foci in 23.1%, paired ventricular premature beats in 15.9%, paroxysmal ventricular tachycardia in 3.2%, and intraventricular block in 7.7% of the subjects studied. Age was an important independent predictor of increased presence of ventricular premature beats and ventricular tachycardia in Holter data from more than 17 000 post-myocardial infarction patients analysed from the CAST Registry,[21] while there were no significant differences in any arrhythmia present among both sexes in 49 250 post-MI patients.[22]

Exercise-induced supraventricular arrhythmias increase mostly with advancing age[23] and male gender.

After 40 years of age ventricular tachyarrhythmias caused by ischaemic heart disease are the most frequent cause of sudden cardiac death. The same changes, but less dramatic in outcome, can be felt like palpitations with or without chest pain and shortness of breath.

In elderly subjects over 65 years of age without other clinical signs of heart disease, conduction disturbances were present in 33.6% of cases, and a statistically significant increase in the presence of first-degree AV block was found in the group of very old (over 80 years). In these very old patients, premature beats and tachycardias were found in 96% of cases, most of them (89%) being supraventricular.[24] In another recent and large study[25] (5201 adults aged >65 years, with 1512 ambulatory ECG controls), ventricular arrhythmias were present in 16% of woman and 28% of man ($P = 0.0001$ for gender difference); supraventricular arrhythmias were present in 56% of woman and 57% of man ($P = $ NS for gender difference); bradycardia and conduction blocks were present in 1.9% of woman and 5.6% of man ($P = 0.0001$ for gender difference). Although most of these patients were asymptomatic, the production of cerebral symptoms caused by disturbed cerebral autoregulation of blood pressure is not unusual, nor is an insufficient adaptation of the circulation to the decreased cardiac output caused by the rhythm alteration.[26]

Symptoms

The physician will ask the patient the reason for consultation, thus taking careful notice of symptoms and signs. Arrhythmias may pass unnoticed because many individuals do not perceive abnormal rhythms. Others will feel an exaggerated heart activity, although the rhythm is regular and frequency normal, and refer to it as palpitations. Bradyarrhythmias are felt usually as dizziness, followed or not by Stokes–Adams episodes.

Any of the following symptoms and signs can be associated with cardiac arrhythmias, although often none of them is present[27]:

- palpitations
- intermittent dyspnoea
- intermittent chest discomfort or pain
- intermittent dizziness
- complaints of unsteadiness, blurred or distal vision, or altered auditory perception
- weakness
- confusion
- faintness without loss of consciousness (near-syncope)
- syncope
- polyuria related to attacks of tachycardia (urina spastica)
- unexplained traumatic accidents.

In a study[28] of 762 patients with symptoms suggesting arrhythmias, in whom a structured history was taken by a general practitioner and a transtelephonic ECG was performed to assess the value of symptoms in diagnosing arrhythmias in general practice, arrhythmias were found in 28.3% of cases, this being 8.8% clinically relevant. Collapse and dyspnoea had both a positive predictive value (OR 1.9 and 1.4, respectively), palpitations had a negative one; neither angina, nor fatigue, nor other symptoms supported the diagnosis of arrhythmia.

Because palpitations were the most frequent symptom reported by patients suspected of having an arrhythmia and syncope the most dramatic one, we will only expand on those.

Palpitations

In normal conditions heart beat is not perceived except during physical or mental stress.

Many extracardiological disturbances such as fever, hyperthyroidism, chronic anaemia, increased sympathetic tone or serum cathecolamines level, and arteriovenous shunts provoke the increased perception of the heart beat that is called palpitation. From 125 patients evaluated with Holter monitoring because of palpitations,[29] only one-third of them had significant cardiac arrhythmias. From the remaining two-thirds, 29% had a psychiatric disorder and 83% of these had major depression or panic disorders, but is noteworthy that this did not result in referral or psychiatric treatment in most cases.

They occur also in abnormal hearts, mainly hypertropic or dilated, and in aortic insufficiency. In these cases, sinus rhythm is present and palpitations are perceived as regular precordial strikes.

Isolated irregular beats are generally due to premature beats, either supraventricular or ventricular, and most commonly what the patient perceives as the postextrasystolic pause.

Fast regular beats are called *tachycardias*, and when they are very fast and still asymptomatic they are probably of supraventricular origin, whilst the presence of dizziness or syncope usually means a ventricular origin. The presence of very fast irregular beats generally indicates that atrial fibrillation is present.

Very slow regular beats identify extreme *bradycardia*, often from high-degree AV block.

In a study of 352 patients referred for ambulatory ECG monitoring,[30] the reason for the study was in 42.6% chest pain, in 31% palpitations, in 13.9% unexpected dyspnoea, and in 12.5% syncope or dizziness. Of this population less than 50% of the patients complained during monitoring of the symptom for which they were referred.

Syncope

"An attack of syncope and convulsions resulting from extreme slowing of the arterial pulse" was the original description by Stokes of the Adams–Stokes syndrome, but it has been long known that episodes[31] of syncope, although more commonly caused by conduction defects that produce a ventricular rate below 36 beats per minute, are caused not only by bradyarrhythmias but also by rapid ventricular rates. ECGs taken during Stokes–Adams attacks showed episodes of ventricular arrest lasting 5 seconds or more in 90% of patients and torsade de pointes-type ventricular tachycardia in the remaining 10%.[32]

Symptoms and examination led to the cause of syncope in 222 of 497 patients enrolled in a recent study,[33] but they were not useful in risk-stratifying patients, the underlying cardiac disease being the only predictor for 1-year mortality.

Syncope is a serious event in patients with structural heart disease. In a study[34] of 491 patients with advanced heart failure referred for pretransplant evaluation, 12% had a history of syncope, 35% attributable to ventricular tachycardia. The risk for sudden death in patients with syncope in this group was 45% at 1 year.

Other intervening factors

Genetical and congenital alterations

Some forms of arrhythmias are recognised to be of genetic origin, being discovered when an adequate family history has been taken. This is the case of long Q-T syndrome –

one of the inborn alterations produced by a single genetic alteration,[35] arrhythmogenic right ventricular cardiomyopathy/dysplasia,[36] Naxos disease,[37] etc. Others, like the Wolff–Parkinson–White syndrome[38] that is present in 0.1–0.3% of the general population, are congenital defects that seem to have a familiar occurrence.[39]

Race and place of origin

In some cases there is a race prevalence, such as in Brugada syndrome, more frequent in Thai males.[40] In other cases, the place from where the patient comes is crucial, as for example with Chagasic cardiomyopathy, one of the most arrhythmogenic types of structural heart disease, in Latin American natives.[41,42]

Obesity

In obese young people who have suffered sudden death, significant pathological findings in the conduction system have been reported.[43]

Pro-arrhythmic drug effect

Medication taken by the patient should be investigated, since there are many drugs that have a pro-arrhythmic effect, among them most antiarrhythmic drugs.[44] Older age increases the susceptibility to adverse cardiac events of antiarrhythmic therapy,[45] including pro-arrhythmia.

Psychosocial factors

There is increasing evidence that anxiety, depression, anger, mental stress, and personality are triggers of acute cardiac events and at the same time increase the risk of long-term adverse cardiac events in post-MI patients, especially when silent ischaemia,[46] decreased LVEF,[47] or autonomic nervous system imbalance[48] are present. This has been linked with ventricular malignant arrhythmias and sudden cardiac arrhythmic death. It is therefore of the outmost importance that the physician explores and considers the psychosocial situation of the arrhythmic patient.

Functional assessment

Atrial fibrillation is common in patients with heart failure, occurring in 15–30% of patients during the evolution of the disease, and present in 31% of cases in a recent population-based study;[49] it is considered as the primary aetiological factor of heart failure in 5% of the cases. The assessment of left ventricular systolic function when AF is present is not reliable, especially when ventricular rate is fast. Often, returning to sinus rhythm after cardioversion normalises an impaired left ventricular function. In an analysis of SOLVD Trials,[50] patients with AF, when compared with those in sinus rhythm, had greater all-cause mortality (34% versus 23%, $P <0.001$) and death attributed to pump failure (16.7% versus 9.4%, $P <0.001$). After other variables had been adjusted, AF was associated to an increase in all-cause mortality (RR 1.34, 95% CI 1.12–1.62; $P = 0.002$) and pump failure death (RR 1.42; 85% CI 1.09–1.85; $P = 0.01$), but not to sudden death (RR 1.13; 95% CI 0.75–1.71; $P = 0.55$). Independent variables associated with increased risk of death included, amongst others: age, with a 10% increased risk for every 5 years increase in age, and decline in left ventricular ejection fraction (LVEF), 45% increased risk for every 10% decrease in the latter.

In the older population, the prevalence of ventricular arrhythmias was 15% in women and 26% in men with normal LVEF, and 26% in women and 43% in man with abnormal LVEF.[51]

There are numerous studies that convincingly show that depressed left ventricular function in post-MI patients increases the mortality risk, LVEF <35% being the most powerful predictor of total mortality in the first year after a MI.[52] Patients with LVEF <12–15% die mostly from pump failure, whilst those with an LEVF between 15 and 35% suffer more often from sudden arrhythmic death.

The combination of depressed heart rate variability, frequent ventricular ectopic beats, and low LVEF is a powerful predictor of non-arrhythmic death in post-MI patients,[53] whereas arrhythmic death in patients with the same pathology was best predicted by depressed heart rate variability and runs of ventricular tachycardia. In the group of 96 patients followed over 2 years, 33% of those who suffered an arrhythmic death had premature ventricular beats and 30% runs of ventricular tachycardia, in contrast to 14.5% of premature ventricular beats and 12.3% of runs of ventricular tachycardia present in survivors ($P <0.001$ in both).

Functional classification of the New York Heart Association

Since this is one of the most used clinical classifications of functional capacity,[54] it is important to relate it to arrhythmic risk stratification.

In AF, NYHA class III/IV increases the risk for all-death mortality relative to class I/II to 74%.[13]

Asymptomatic ventricular arrhythmias are common in

patients with chronic heart failure and related to their functional class. In 102 patients with heart failure,[55] rare premature ventricular beats (<100/24 h) were observed in 21.6%, moderately frequent (101–1000/24 h) in 30.4%, and frequent ones (>1000/24 h) in 48%. When gender was male, age was older than 60 years or a low LVEF was present, there was a significant greater incidence in premature ventricular beats. Contrary to what would have been expected, no statistically significant differences (Table 6.1) were present in relation to the NYHA functional class classification.

On the contrary, in the same study, LVEF is related to the prevalence of asymptomatic ventricular arrhythmias (Table 6.2). Low LVEF predicts[56] inducible sustained ventricular tachycardia on electrophysiological study, and 1-year mortality increases with worsening of NYHA functional class and LVEF.

Sudden death episodes are originated by arrhythmias, 80% of them being monomorphic/polymorphic ventricular tachycardia or primary ventricular fibrillation, and 20% bradyarrhythmias.[57] Assuming that this is also true in heart failure patients, the relationship between NYHA functional class, total annual death, and arrhythmic (sudden) death[58] would be as shown in Table 6.3.

In post-MI patients with heart failure it was found[59] that, when the mean NYHA functional class was I–II, the overall death rate was low and 67% of these deaths were sudden, whereas, with a NYHA functional class IV, sudden death rate was 29% but with a high total mortality. In another study of patients with heart failure due to ischaemic cardiomyopathy, LVEF had a strong relation to the presence of ventricular premature beats (r = 0.54).[60]

Ischaemic heart disease

AF develops in 21% of acute myocardial infarction (AMI) patients, decreasing from 15% in days 1–2, to 13% in days 3–4, and 10% from day 5.[61] Patients with AMI/AF are older, with left ventricular dysfunction and the presence of congestive heart failure being significantly higher than in patients with AMI but without AF. The same applies for paroxysmal atrial fibrillation.[62] Mortality in a recent study[63] of 517 acute MI was 30.6% when AF was present versus 16.7% when absent, with a relative risk of 1.83%.

Bigger *et al.*[64] in a classical study have shown that the presence of even a few premature ventricular beats is linked to increased mortality in post-MI patients.

An analysis[65] of 1067 post-MI patients found that mortality was higher in females, the presence of ventricular tachycardia being significantly higher in deceased women than in men.

Sinus bradycardia occurs in 40% of patients in the first hours of AMI;[66] 13% of inferior infarcts develop complete heart block, producing a two- to three-fold increase of mortality, and it is well known that, even if properly treated, the latter is highly ominous in the setting of anterior AMI.

Killip and Kimball classifications

Clinical evaluation is still important in post-MI risk stratification and the Killip and Kimball classification[67] is a traditional way of doing it. When related to atrial fibrillation in AMI, Killip and Kimball peak class was one of the main predictors of outcome.

Table 6.1 Asymptomatic ventricular arrhythmias related to NYHA classification

Functional class	Total PVCs/24 h (%)	>1000 PVCs/24 h (%)	>25 repetitive PVCs/24 h (%)	With VT events (%)
NYHA II	49	49	45	43
NYHA III	51	51	55	57

No statistically significant difference between any value.
(Adapted from reference 55.)

Table 6.2 Asymptomatic ventricular arrhythmias related to left ventricular ejection fraction

LVEF (%)	>1000 PVCs/24 h (%)	>25 repetitive PVCs/24 h (%)	With VT events (%)
>30	27	19	22
<30	73	81	76

(Adapted from reference 55.)

Table 6.3 Relation between NYHA functional class, total death, and arrhythmic (sudden) death

NYHA class	Annual death (%)	Sudden death (%)
II	5–15	50–80
III	20–50	30–50
IV	30–70	5–30

(Adapted from reference 58.)

Table 6.4   Post-MI risk stratification by Killip and Kimball classification

Class Killip and Kimball	Women		Men	
	Cardiac death (N = 13) (%)	No cardiac death (N = 95) (%)	Cardiac death (N = 28) (%)	No cardiac death (N = 320) (%)
I	15	87	50	80
II	31	10	21	14
III	39	3	14	5
IV	15	0	14	1

(Adapted from reference 68.)

Results of a 3-year follow-up of 456 myocardial infarction patients,[68] who were risk-stratified by the Killip and Kimball classification and separated by gender, is presented in Table 6.4 showing, as one would have expected, an increase in Killip class parallel to increased cardiac mortality, with no differences between women and men.

References

1. Vaccaro H, Amor F, Leyton M, Sepulveda W. Arrhythmias in early pregnancy: a predictor of first trimester pregnancy loss. *Ultrasound Obstet Gynecol* 1998;**12**:248–51.

2. Kelmanson IA, Adrianov AV, Zolotukhina TA. Low birth weight and risk of cardiac arrhythmias in children. *J Cardiovasc Risk* 1998;**5**:47–51.

3. Southall DP, Johnston F, Shinebourne EA. 24 hour electrocardiographic study of heart rate and rhythm patterns in a population of healthy children. *Br Heart J* 1981;**45**:281–6.

4. Scherf D, Cohen J. *The atrioventricular node and selected cardiac arrhythmias*. New York: Grune & Stratton Inc., 1964, pp. 372–447.

5. Poutiainen AM, Koistinen MJ, Airaksinen EJ *et al.* Prevalence and natural course of ectopic atrial tachycardia. *Eur Heart J* 1999;**20**:694–700.

6. Furlanello F, Bettini R, Cozzi F *et al.* Ventricular arrhythmias and sudden death in athletes. In: Greenberg HM, Kulbertus HE, Moss AJ, Schwartz PJ eds. *Clinical aspects of life-threatening arrhythmias. Ann NY Acad Sci* 1984;**427**:253–79.

7. Maron BJ, Shirani J, Ploiac LC, Mathenge R, Roberts, WC, Mueller FO. Sudden death in young competitive athletes: clinical, demographic, and pathological profiles. *JAMA*1996;**276**:199–204.

8. Corrado D, Basso C, Schiavon M, Thiene G. Screening for hypertrophic cardiomyopathy in young athletes. *New Engl J Med* 1998;**339**:364–9.

9. McKenna WJ, Thiene G, Nava A *et al*, on behalf of the Working Group of Myocardial and Pericardial Disease of the European Society of Cardiology and of the Scientific Council on Cardiomyopathies of the International Society and Federation of Cardiology, supported by the Schooepfer Association. Diagnosis of arrhythmogenic right ventricular dysplasia/cardiomyopathy. *Br Heart J* 1994;**71**:215–18.

10. Marob BJ, Poliac LC, Kaplan JA, Mueller FO. Blunt impact to the chest leading to sudden death from cardiac arrest during sport activities. *New Engl J Med* 1995;**333**:337–42.

11. Fuenmayor AJ, Araujo X, Fuenmayor AM. Cardiac arrhythmias during two different stages of the menstrual cycle. *Int J Cardiol* 1998;**63**:267–70.

12. Shotan A, Ostrzega E, Mehra A, Johnosn JV, Elkayam U. Incidence of arrhythmias in normal pregnancy and relation to palpitations, dizziness and syncope. *Am J Cardiol* 1997;**79**:1061–4.

13. Prystowsky EN, Benson DW, Fuster V *et al*. Management of patients with atrial fibrillation. A statement for healthcare professionals from the Subcommittee on Electrocardiography and Electrophysiology, American Heart Association. *Circulation*, 1996;**93**:1262–77.

14. CONAREC, Oral presentation, Argentine Congress of Cardiology, Buenos Aires, 1995.

15. Benjamin EJ, Levy D, Vaziri SM, D'Agostino RB, Belanger AJ, Wolf PA. Independent risk factors for atrial fibrillation in a population-based cohort: the Framingham Heart Study. *JAMA* 1994;**427**:840–4.

16. Furnerg CD, Psaty BM, Manolio TA *et al*. Prevalence of atrial fibrillation in elderly subjects (The Cardiovascular Health Study). *Am J Cardiol* 1994;**74**:236–41.

17. Wolf PA, Abbott RD, Kannel WB. Atrial fibrillation as an independent risk factor for stroke: the Framingham Study. *Stroke*, 1991;**22**:983–8.

18. Krahn AD, Manfreda J, Tate RB, Mathewson FA, Cuddy TE. The natural history of atrial fibrillation: incidence, risk factors, and prognosis in the Manitoba follow-up study. *Am J Med* 1995;**98**:476–84.

19. Benjamin EJ, Wolf PA, D'Agostino RB, Silbershatz H, Kannel WB, Levy D. Impact of atrial fibrillation on the risk of death: The Framingham Heart Study. *Circulation* 1998;**98**:946–52.

20. Bellet S. *Clinical disorders of the heart beat*, 3rd edn. Philadelphia: Lea & Febiger, 1971:120–1.

21. Josephson RA, Papa LA, Brooks MM, Morris M, Akiyama T, Greene HL. Effect of age on postmyocardial infarction ventricular arrhythmias (Holter Registry data from CAST I and

CAST II). Cardiovascular Arrhythmias Suppression Trials. *Am J Cardiol* 1995;**76**:710–13.

22. Kostis JB, Wilson AC, O'Dowd K *et al*, for the MIDAS Study Group. Sex differences in the management and long-term outcome of acute myocardial infarction. A statewide study. *Circulation* 1994;**90**:1715–30.

23. O'Connor FC, Mayuga R, Arrington CT, Fleg JL. Do echocardiographic changes explain the age-associated increase in exercise-induced supraventricular arrhythmias? *Aging (Milano)* 1997;**9**:120–6.

24. Tomaszewski A, Prasal M, Dabrowski P, Markiewicz M. Arrhythmias in patients after 80 years of age. *Wiad-Lek* 1993;**46**:881–4.

25. Manolio TA, Furberg CD, Rautaharju PM *et al*. Cardiac arrhythmias on 24–hours ambulatory electrocardiophy in older women and men: The Cardiovascular Health Study. *J Am Coll Cardiol* 1994;**23**:916–25.

26. Lang E. Significance of arrhythmias in advanced age. *Ther Umsch* 1991;**48**:322–8.

27. Chamberlain DA, Kulbertus H, Mogensen L, Schlepper M. Cardiac arrhythmias in the active population-management recommendations. In: Chamberlain DA, Kulbertus H, Mogensen L, Schlepper M eds. *Cardiac arrhythmias in the active population-prevalence, significance and management.* Mölndal, Sweden: AB Hässle, 1980, pp. 142–3.

28. Zwietering PJ, Knottnerus JA, Rinkens PELM, Klejne MAWJ, Gongels APM. Arrhythmias in general practice: diagnostic value of patients characteristics, medical history and symptoms. *Fam Pract*, 1998;**15**:343–53.

29. Barsky AJ, Delamater BA, Clancy SA, Antman EM, Ahern DK. Somatized psychiatric disorder presenting as palpitations. *Arch Int Med* 1996;**156**:1102–8.

30. Krasnov AZ, Bloomfield DK. The relationship between subjective symptomatology and objective findings from ambulatory ECG monitoring studies in a large unselected population. In: Stern S ed. *Ambulatory ECG monitoring.* Chicago: Year Book Medical Publishers Inc., 1978, pp. 149–69.

31. Watanabe Y, Dreifus LS. *Cardiac arrhythmias.* New York: Grune & Stratton Inc., 1977, pp. 320–38.

32. Sandae E, Sigurd B. *Arrhythmia – A guide to clinical electrocardiology.* Bingen: Publ Partners Verlag GmbH, 1991, pp.262–70.

33. Oh JH, Hanusa BH, Kapoor WN. Do symptoms predict cardiac arrhythmias and mortality in patients with syncope? *Arch Intern Med* 1999;**159**:375–80.

34. Stevenson WG, Stevenson LW, Middlekauff HR, Saxon LA. Sudden death prevention in patients with advanced ventricular dysfunction. *Circulation* 1993;**88**:2953–61.

35. Priori SG, Barhanin J, Hauer NRW *et al*. Genetic and molecular basis of cardiac arrhythmias: impact on clinical management. Part III. *Circulation* 1999;**99**:674–81.

36. Danieli JA, Nava A, Rampazzo A. A first insight into molecular genetics. In: Nava A, Rossi L, Thiene G eds. *Arrhythmogenic right ventricular cardiomyopathy/dysplasia.* Amsterdam: Elsevier, 1997, pp.166–73.

37. Coonar AS, Prrotonotarios N, Tsatsopoulou A *et al*. Gene for Arrhythmogenic Right ventricular cardiomyopathy with nonepidermolytic palmoplantar keratoderma and woolly hair (Naxos disease) maps to 17q21. *Circulation* 1998;**97**: 2049–58.

38. Gallagher JJ, Pritchett ELC, Sealy WC. The preexcitation syndromes. *Progr Cardiovasc Dis* 1978;**20**:285–327.

39. Vidaillet HJ, Presley JC, Henke E, Harrel FE, German LD. Familial occurrence of accessory atrioventricular pathways preexcitation syndrome. *New Engl J Med* 1987;**317**:65–9.

40. Alings M, Wilde A. "Brugada" syndrome. Clinical data and suggested pathophysiological mechanism. *Circulation* 1999;**99**:666–73.

41. Mautner B. Arrhythmias and abnormalities of cardiac conduction in Chagas disease. *Rev Latina Cardiol* 1992;**11**:8–12.

42. Milei J, Mautner B, Storino R, Sánchez JA. Does Chagas disease exist as an undiagnosed form of cardiomyopathy in the United States? *Am Heart J* 1992;**123**:1732.

43. Bharati S, Lev M. Cardiac conduction system involvement in sudden death of obese young people. *Am Heart J* 1995;**129**:273–81.

44. Goldstein RE, Tibbits PA, Oetgen WJ. Proarrhythmic effects of antiarrhythmic drugs. In: Greenberg HM, Kulbertus HE, Moss AJ, Schwarts PJ eds. *Ann NY Acad Sci* 1984;**427**:94–100.

45. Akiyama T, Pawitan Y, Cmpbell WB *et al*. Effects of advancing age on the efficacy and side effects of antiarrhythmic drugs in post-myocardial infarction patients with ventricular arrhythmias. The CAST Investigators. *J Am Geriatr Soc* 1992;**40**:666–72.

46. Rozanski A, Bairey CN, Krantz DS *et al*. Mental stress and the induction of silent myocardial ischemia in patient with coronary artery disease. *New Engl J Med* 1988;**318**:1005–12.

47. Denollet J, Brutsaert DI. Personality, disease severity and risk of long-term cardiac events in patients with a decreased ejection fraction after myocardial infarction. *Circulation* 1998;**97**:167–73.

48. Schwarz PJ. The autonomic nervous system and sudden death. *Eur Heart J* 1998;**19**:F72–F80.

49. Cowie MR, Wood DA, Coats JS, *et al*. Incidence and aetiology of heart failure. A population-based study. *Eur Heart J* 1999;**20**:421–8.

50. Dries DL, Exner DV, Gersh BJ, Domansky MJ, Waclawiw MA, Stevenson LW. Atrial fibrillation is associated with an increased risk for mortality and heart failure progression in patients with asymptomatic and symptomatic left ventricular systolic dysfunction: a retrospective analysis of SOLVD trials. *J Am Coll Cardiol* 1998;**32**:695–703.

51. Prystowsky EN, Benson DW, Fuster V *et al*. Management of patients with atrial fibrillation. A statement for healthcare professionals from the Subcommittee on Electrocardiography and Electrophysiology, American Heart Association. *Circulation*, 1996;**93**:1262–77.

52. Hohnloser SH, Klingenheben T, Zabel M. Identification of patients after myocardial infarction at risk of life threatening arrhythmias. *Eur Heart J* 1999;**1**(Suppl. C):C11–C20.

53. Hartikainen JEK, Malik M, Staunton A, Poloniecki J, Camm AJ. Distinction between arrhythmic and nonarrhythmic death after acute myocardial infarction based on heart rate variability, signal-averaged electrocardiogram, ventricular

arrhythmias and left ventricular ejection fraction. *J Am Coll Cardiol* 1996;**28**:296–304.

54. The Criteria Committee of the New York Heart Association. *Nomenclature and criteria for diagnosis of disease of the heart and great vessels*. 9th edn. Boston: Little, Brown and Co., 1994.

55. Anastasiou-Nana MI, Menlowe RL, Mason JW, for the Western Enoximone Study Group. Quantification of prevalence of asymptomatic ventricular arrhythmias in patients with heart failure. *Ann Non-Invasive Electrocardiol* 1997;**2**:346–53.

56. Greene HL. Clinical significance and management of arrhythmias in the heart failure patient. *Clin Cardiol* 1992;**15**:I13–I21.

57. Bayes de Luna A, Coumel P, Leclerq JF. Ambulatory sudden cardiac death: mechanisms of production of fatal arrhythmia on the basis of data from 157 cases. *Am Heart J* 1989;**117**:151–9.

58. Uretsky, BF, Sheahan, RG. Primary prevention of sudden cardiac death in heart failure: will the solution be shocking? *J Am Coll Cardiol* 1997;**30**:1589–97.

59. Kjekshus J. Arrhythmias and mortality in congestive heart failure. *Am J Cardiol* 1990;**65**:421–8.

60. Min JY, Meissner A, Alexander H, El-Mokhtari NE, Simon R. Heterogeneity of noninvasive arrhythmic risk indicators in patients with ischemic cardiomyopathy. *J Electrocardiol* 1998;**31**:221–6.

61. Pedersen OD, Bagger H, Torp-Pedersen C, on behalf of the TRACE Study group. The occurrence and prognostic significance of atrial fibrillation-flutter following acute myocardial infarction. *Eur Heart J* 1998;**20**:748–54.

62. Eldar M, Canetti M, Rotstein Z *et al.* for the SPRINT and Thrombolysis Survey Group. Significance of paroxysmal atrial fibrillation complicating acute myocardial infarction in the thrombolytic era. *Circulation* 1998;**97**:965–70.

63. Madias JE, Patel DC, Singh D. Atrial fibrillation in acute myocardial infarction: a prospective study based on data from a consecutive series of patients admitted to the coronary care unit. *Clin Cardiol* 1996;**19**:180–6.

64. Bigger JT Jr, Fleiss JL, Kleiger R, Miller JP, Rolnitzky LM and the multicenter postinfarction research group. The relationship among ventricular arrhythmias, left ventricular dysfunction, and mortality in the 2 years after myocardial infarction. *Circulation* 1984;**69**:250–8.

65. Kenda MF, Turk J, Stare J, Rebolj M, Demsar J. Sudden and expected death after acute myocardial infarction. The impact of sex differences. *CARDIOnet J* 1998 (Abstract from International Congress New Frontiers in Arrhythmias, Marrileva, Italy).

66. Brezinski DA. Supraventricular arrhythmias and heart block in acute myocardial infarction. In: Califf RM, Mark DB, Wagner GS eds. *Acute coronary care*. St. Louis: Mosby-Year Book Inc., 1995, pp. 603–16.

67. Killip T, Kimball JT. Treatment of myocardial infarction in a coronary care unit. A two years experience with 250 patients. *Am J Cardiol* 1967;**20**:457–64.

68. Copie X, Knatkowa K, Frei L, Staunton A, Camm AJ, Malik M. Gender specificities in risk stratification after myocardial infarction. *Ann Non-Invasive Electrocardiol* 1997;**2**:59–68.

7 Left ventricular ejection fraction and wall motion score

Steen Z Abildstrom, Christian Torp-Pedersen and Lars Køber

The absolute risk in a patient with a particular disease is closely related to the possible benefit of treatment. The higher the risk the higher is the potential of benefit from treatment. Risk assessment technologies help clinicians to select the appropriate treatment for the appropriate patient. The likelihood of finding a patient with a high risk of arrhythmic death is greatest in a population of cardiac arrest survivors, but these patients constitute only a small fraction of the total population at risk. Arrhythmic death is frequent in patients with congestive heart failure or following a myocardial infarction, but the risk in the individual patient is lower than in a cardiac arrest survivor. In an unselected adult population the risk of arrhythmic death is approximately to be 2 per 1000 persons per year in western societies.[1] Overall, most cases of arrhythmic death occur in the general population because of the small number of high-risk patients compared to the vast size of the general population.[2]

In a population of patients surviving a myocardial infarction, left ventricular systolic function can be used for risk assessment. Left ventricular systolic function expressed as left ventricular ejection fraction or wall motion score is considered to be one of the most powerful predictors of mortality in infarct survivors. In contrast, estimation of left ventricular systolic function with the aim of predicting arrhythmic death in the normal population would probably be futile, as the likelihood of encountering people with reduced left ventricular function is very small. This illustrates that the different technologies used for risk assessment should be applied only in relevant populations. In this chapter we will focus on the value of assessing left ventricular systolic function in patients with heart disease, where the assessment is relevant, and compare this with other relevant technologies for risk assessment. All the studies we are able to cite use surrogate markers of arrhythmic death – sudden death or presumed arrhythmic death. This overview will not deal with the inherent problems of classification and use the terms given by the studies.

Left ventricular systolic function

A measure of left ventricular function should ideally combine information on the contractile function of the left ventricle, dilatation of the chamber as well as remodelling of the surviving myocardium. It should reflect the damage and the consequences imposed on the heart, but no method can to fully extent do this. All available methods for studying left ventricular systolic function are closely correlated. It is noteworthy that these methods have achieved their high status because they are useful risk markers, since their ability to predict exercise capacity or any other indicator of pump function is rather poor. Practically, left ventricular systolic function can be measured by a variety of techniques such as radionuclide cardiography, echocardiography, ventriculography and magnetic resonance imaging. Whether the systolic function is expressed as left ventricular ejection fraction (LVEF) or as an assessment of wall motion, as often used by echocardiography, is not important from a prognostic viewpoint. All of these methods can be used for risk assessment in patients following acute myocardial infarction.[3–9] Echocardiography has the advantage that it can be performed bedside in the very ill patient making it available for consecutive patients admitted to hospital. In addition, it contains information on hyperkinesia, left ventricular chamber size, regional wall motion differences, and valve diseases.

With the use of wall motion score index, an estimate of left ventricular systolic function can be obtained in more than 95% of patients. In brief, the left ventricle is divided into segments and each segment is scored according to its systolic function. Adding segments together and dividing with number of segments establishes a wall motion index (WMI).[10] We have used from 9 to 16 segments and a reversed scoring system compared to USA. By this reverse scoring system there is a linear correlation between LVEF and WMI, and WMI multiplied by 30 corresponds to an estimate of LVEF.[11]

Relation between LV systolic function and sudden death

Ventricular ectopy defined as a high number of premature ventricular beats and/or the presence of non-sustained ventricular tachycardia is found in patients with a wide range of left ventricular systolic dysfunction. These arrhythmias are predictors of mortality and appear to be independent of left ventricular systolic dysfunction.[12] Conversely, patients with congestive heart failure and/or left ventricular systolic dysfunction frequently have increased ventricular ectopy.[12,13] Studies have shown that stretch or myocardial fibrosis results in electrophysiological changes which predisposes to arrhythmias.[14–16] Progressive left ventricular dilatation following an AMI will result in a parallel increase in ventricular ectopy. However, patients with severely depressed systolic function demonstrate a great variation in prevalence of arrhythmias.[17] In addition to left ventricular systolic dysfunction, increasing left ventricular chamber size is a risk factor for arrhythmias.[17,18] Thus, studies of the association between left ventricular systolic dysfunction and arrhythmias indicate that left ventricular function is an indirect and unspecific markers of those mechanisms which predisposes to the presence of arrhythmias.

The Multicenter Post-Infarction Study Group evaluated the occurrence of sudden death over a period of 2 years.[19] The study population were patients discharged alive after a myocardial infarction and the overall risk of death was 17% over 4 years. As ejection fraction determined by radionuclide cardiography decreased, there was a corresponding increase in risk of arrhythmic death, as well as death from progressive heart failure.[19] This moderate relation between decreasing ejection fraction and increasing occurrence of sudden death or arrhythmic events has also been found in studies of more selected patients and with focus on other methods for predicting arrhythmic death.[12,20–24] Available evidence indicates that left ventricular systolic dysfunction is an efficient way to select patients with a high risk of total death, which is more or less equally distributed between arrhythmic death and death from heart failure. Thus left ventricular function is not an efficient way of selecting patients where the proportion of patients with arrhythmic death is high. In patients with preserved left ventricular function, the risk of any mode of death is low, and those with future events will not be identified by assessing left ventricular function.

Prediction of total mortality versus sudden death following an acute myocardial infarction

Following a myocardial infarction, 1-year mortality may be as high as 22–28% in the western societies including the USA for unselected, hospitalised patients, even after the implementation of revascularisation strategies.[25–28] These figures are often reported to be declining, but the sources used vary considerably. Data from studies investigating new concepts or where patients are part of a clinical trial will usually report a lower mortality than will epidemiological studies because of selection biases. Subjects in clinical trials have to consent and be able to take part in the scheduled follow-up programme. Similarly, patients with significant comorbidity are often excluded as are elderly patients. If a new technology for risk assessment is investigated, it may even be so complicated that it can only be applied to a minority of the patients.

It is most often reported that sudden death accounts for approximately 50% of all cardiovascular deaths following a myocardial infarction, and that these deaths are often the result of ventricular tachyarrhythmias.[19] This relation is based on unproven assumptions, and the uncertainty of classifying sudden death is highlighted by the finding of a 3-fold variation of sudden death in similar populations.[29–31] The relationship between tachyarrhythmic and bradyarrhythmic events is largely unknown. This relationship could differ according to the time period studied, but this is at present speculative, and tachyarrhythmias as well as bradyarrhythmias will often be categorised as sudden. In order to compare arrhythmic death from one study to another it is important to examine the prevalence in conjunction with total death. This may highlight differences between populations and offer an explanation of different results obtained in different studies.

Left ventricular systolic function has been used in several studies in order to identify patients with an increased mortality who might benefit from ACE-inhibition.[30,32,33] The inclusion of high-risk patients and the assumption that 50% of all cardiovascular death is arrhythmic has resulted in the use of reduced left ventricular systolic function for selection of patients presumed to be relevant for testing of antiarrhythmic drugs such as *d*-sotalol, amiodarone, and dofetilide.[34–36] There are no data to support or reject whether patients with reduced left ventricular systolic function die proportionately more from arrhythmic causes than patients with preserved left ventricular function. In the studies mentioned above patients were required to have an LVEF <40% (or 35%) and this resulted in populations where approximately 50% of all deaths were classified as sudden. Table 7.1 provides a list of studies where left ventricular function was used to predict all-cause mortality. The studies with exclusion criteria resulted in considerably lower mortality compared to the studies without any reported exclusion criteria. Mode of death is not available from these studies.

Non-sudden versus sudden death in patients with moderate to severe left ventricular systolic dysfunction

The potential value of left ventricular systolic function is to identify groups of heart patients where left ventricular

Table 7.1 Different studies assessing the prognostic information of left ventricular systolic function

Studies assessing left ventricular function	No.	Method	Total mortality	Excluded patients	Prognostic value of LV dysfunction on total mortality	Prediction of sudden or arrhythmic death
MPIG[19]	867	RNC[a]	9% (1–year)	≥70 years in-hospital death	RR 2.4 (LVEF ≤ 40%)	NA
Bigger[12]	766	RNC[a]	9% (1–year)	≥70 years in-hospital death	RR 3.5 (LVEF ≤ 30%)	NA
Kelly[5]	171	RNC	18.1% (15 months)	None	Sen: 84% Spe: 67% (LVEF <35%)	Sen: 90% Spe: 64%[b]
Kan[7]	345	E	20% (1–year)	None	Sen: 88% Spe: 86% RR 18 (WMS >10)	NA
Shah[9]	114	RNC	18% (1–year)	None	RR 9.0 (LVEF ≤ 30%)	NA
Ong[6]	222	RNC	11% (30–day)	Killip class 3 and 4	RR 6.6 (LVEF <30%)	NA
Trace[8]	6676	E	23% (1–year)	None	RR 4.9 (WMI, pr. unit)	NA

[a]Same patients; [b]only sudden death after hospital discharge; [c]cardiac mortality; [d]arrhythmic events

Abbreviations: AF = atrial fibrillation/flutter; BBB = bundle branch block; BRS = baroreflex sensitivity; CHF = congestive heart failure; DM = diabetes mellitus; E = echocardiography; NA = not available; RNC = radionuclide cardiography; RR = relative risk; Sen = sensitivity; Spe = specificity; V = ventriculography at catheterisation; WMI = wall motion index; WMS = wall motion score.

function varies, enabling subgroups to be defined with a particular high risk of either sudden or non-sudden death.

In the TRAndolapril Cardiac Evaluation (Trace) study, consecutive patients with AMI were screened by echocardiography for detection of moderate to severe left ventricular systolic dysfunction. The patients included in the study had a very high mortality, reflecting that they represent patients with left ventricular systolic dysfunction following an AMI, and also reflecting the effort of including representative patients in this study.[25] Patients enrolled in the study had a WMI ≤ 1.2 (corresponding to an ejection fraction ≤ 35%) and were prospectively separated into two groups according to WMI (Table 7.2).[25] Among the patients with a WMI <0.8 (corresponding roughly to an LVEF <0.25), 37 (20.7%) died suddenly, but of those who died (N = 115) this mode of death constituted 32.2%. Of patients with a higher WMI (estimated LVEF of 0.25–0.35), 201 (12.8%) died suddenly and, of those who died (N = 558), this constituted 36.0%. It appears that, in patients with moderate to severe left ventricular dysfunction, approximately one-third dies suddenly relatively independent of the severity of left ventricular dysfunction. Similarly, documented arrhythmic death (confirmed by an end-points committee and requiring ECG measurements) were seen in 7.3% of the patients with WMI<0.8, corresponding to 11.3% of those dying in that group during a

Table 7.2 Total, cardiovascular, sudden, and arrhythmic mortality in patients with moderate to severe left ventricular systolic dysfunction following an acute myocardial infarction

Events	WMI <0.8 N = 179	WMI 0.8–1.2 N = 1570
Documented arrhythmic death (%)	13 (7.3)	30 (1.9)
Sudden death (%)	37 (20.7)	201 (12.8)
Cardiovascular death (%)	91 (50.8)	423 (26.9)
Total death (%)	115 (64.3)	558 (35.6)

Abbreviation: WMI = Wall motion index.

follow-up of 2–4 years. For the other group with WMI from 0.8 to 1.2, the corresponding figures were 1.9% and 5.4%, respectively. Thus, documented arrhythmic death seems to be a little higher in the group with severe left ventricular dysfunction, but the requirement of documentation of the arrhythmia results in very few events.

Patients could also be divided into groups according to NYHA class and WMI (Table 7.3). All patients with WMI <0.4 died non-suddenly irrespective of NYHA class, and

Table 7.3 Sudden death (%) in relation to wall motion index and NYHA classification

NYHA classification	Wall motion index			
	<0.4	0.4–0.6	0.7–0.9	1.0–1.2
Class I	0 (0)	6 (7.2)	26 (31.3)	51 (61.5)
Class II	0 (0)	9 (9.5)	31 (32.6)	55 (57.9)
Class III	0 (0)	5 (20.0)	9 (36.0)	11 (44.0)
Class IV	0 (0)	0 (0)	9 (45.0)	11 (55.0)

Missing information of NYHA class in 15 patients.

among those with WMI from 0.4 to 0.6 and NYHA class IV, none died suddenly (Table 7.3).

Prediction of arrhythmic death in patients with congestive heart failure

Mode of death in a consecutive group of patients with congestive heart failure has never been reported. The difficulties with establishing a diagnosis of congestive heart failure in patients with normal left ventricular systolic function increases the likelihood that patients will differ from study to study and a different frequency of reported arrhythmic death will result. Some data exist in patients with congestive heart failure and reduced left ventricular systolic function from the Diamond (Dofetilide in patients with congestive heart failure and left ventricular dysfunction) Study.[37] A total of 1518 patients out of 2531 (60%) consecutive patients with congestive heart failure and left ventricular systolic dysfunction determined by echocardiography were included in the study. Owing to this selection, the results are difficult to extrapolate to other populations with congestive heart failure and left ventricular systolic dysfunction. Nevertheless, patients were definitely at high risk with a 2-year mortality of 40%. There were 628 deaths in the population and 307 were classified as arrhythmic (49%). Left ventricular systolic dysfunction was a powerful predictor of mortality when patients were divided according to the median WMI. Patients with severely reduced left ventricular function had a crude mortality of 46% (392 of 858 patients died), whilst the mortality in patients with moderately reduced left ventricular systolic function was 36% (336 of 660 died). Arrhythmic death was seen at similar frequency in the two strata of left ventricular systolic function (unpublished). Thus, left ventricular systolic function can select high-risk patients with congestive heart failure, and the Diamond Study implies that the mode of death is arrhythmic in approximately 50% of fatalities regardless of whether ejection fraction is below 25% (WMI <0.8) or between 26% and 35% (0.8≤WMI≤1.2). Analogous to the situation in the post-myocardial infarct situation is that severe left ventricular dysfunction identifies a group of patients with a very high risk of death, but the ratio between sudden and non-sudden death does not vary much. Such analyses do not exclude that an effective treatment of arrhythmias would have a very different impact in subgroups of left ventricular systolic function. It might be anticipated that patients with very severe left ventricular function would die from heart failure even if they were protected against arrhythmic death with devices or drugs.

Left ventricular systolic function in patients surviving ventricular arrhythmias

Several randomised studies have included patients following cardiac arrest for intervention but patients are highly selected and not representative of patients surviving cardiac arrest or rapid ventricular tachycardia. The best data originate from the registry to the antiarrhythmics versus implantable defibrillators (AVID) study.[38] Patients were included in the registry if they had a documented or symptomatic arrhythmic event. Left ventricular ejection fraction was registered and patients were followed for at least 2 years with respect to mortality. Survival according to type of arrhythmia and left ventricular systolic function is presented in Table 7.4. Left ventricular systolic function was a predictor of mortality in all types of arrhythmias except in patients with unexplained syncope. However, in these patients survival was better than in all of the other groups. In all other groups, left ventricular systolic function predicted future events. Accordingly, the benefit of ICD treatment seems to be more pronounced in patients with left ventricular dysfunction.

Comparison with other methods for risk assessment

In general, it would be preferable to use selection procedures that ensure a high proportion of arrhythmic death when the intervention to be tested is specific for certain orders of arrhythmias. In order to predict arrhythmic death many methods have been used:

- late potentials
- heart rate variability
- T wave alternans
- arrhythmias seen on Holter monitoring or during exercise testing

Table 7.4   Two-year survival rates by arrhythmia type and left ventricular ejection fraction (EF)

	No.	EF ≥0.35 (%)	No.	EF <0.35 (%)	No.	All (%)
VF	656	85.7	680	73.6	1399	79.7
VT with syncope	241	81.5	339	73.0	598	75.7
Non-syncopal VT with symptoms	419	84.7	624	78.6	1065	81.3
Haemodynamical stable VT	235	85.3	217	67.7	497	77.2
Transient/correctable VT/VF	167	86.1	88	70.8	270	80.6
Unexplained syncope	158	84.8	209	82.7	390	84.1

Abbreviations: VF = ventricular fibrillation; VT = ventricular tachycardia.
(Modified from ref. 38.)

- electrophysiological testing
- baroreflex sensitivity assessment.

The list is incomplete but, more importantly, each method has methodological problems when compared to other methods, including left ventricular dysfunction. The predictive power of heart rate variability with respect to arrhythmic death has been compared with other methods in patients following AMI in a very important study, showing that heart rate variability is superior to most other methods.[20] However, heart rate variability cannot be assessed in patients with atrial fibrillation and this important subgroup of high-risk patients were excluded from the comparisons, thus creating a bias in favour of heart rate variability. Similarly, T wave alternans requires an exercise test in order to obtain a heart rate of 100 beats per minute and exercise testing is often not performed in the very ill patients. Also, in some studies patients with diabetes are excluded,[21,22] whilst others have excluded patients not treated with thrombolysis or patients having bundle branch block.[39,40] Patients over 75 years of age are also often excluded.[12,20–24]

The prognostic importance of left ventricular systolic function in post-MI patients in these studies are shown in Table 7.5.[20,21,23,41] The populations studied differ and the relative importance of left ventricular systolic function in univariate analyses is less in the studies assessing other risk factors compared with studies primarily assessing left ventricular function (Table 7.5). As the complexity and number of tests increases, the number of patients where the tests are actually applied decreases. The problem is that many of the excluded patients in each study are high-risk patients. This important bias must be taken into account when the value of several methods are compared. Preferably, the outcome of consecutive patients should be reported whether or not they had all tests performed. Of all the different methods used for prediction of sudden death, none has been used in unselected patients following AMI. Assessment of left ventricular dysfunction has

been applied to representative patients and this is not a specific marker for arrhythmic events.[20,25] Our data suggest that patients with very reduced LVEF (WMI <0.4) could be restricted from treatment intended to reduce arrhythmic death. However, it does not seem justified to exclude patients with less severe left ventricular dysfunction from treatment unless there is suspicion that the treatment will be especially harmful in these patients. Conversely, using only left ventricular dysfunction to select patients for an antiarrhythmic treatment can only be supported if the treatment is not harmful.

In order to select a group of patients who would not die suddenly, we also included a grading of CHF by NYHA classification. Among the 62 patients who died and with NYHA class IV at time of randomisation, only one died suddenly if WMI was less than 0.8, in contrast to 19 deaths occurring suddenly in the patients with a WMI from 0.8 to 1.2 (Table 7.3). Thus, the combination of a severely depressed WMI and NYHA class IV seems to identify patients who will die from causes other than arrhythmias. In comparison, the study by Kelly showed that patients with in-hospital death owing to pump failure had an LVEF of 18%, whilst the remaining patients dying in-hospital had an LVEF of 44%.[5] Among all patients dying with NYHA class IV, 42 (67%) deaths were non-sudden. In the group of patients with a WMI from 0.8 to 1.2, 38% of the deaths were judged to be sudden and 62% to be nonsudden. This may be used as an argument for trying to prevent sudden death, even in patients with severe symptomatic CHF, if WMI is not less or equal to 0.7 (or LVEF <20%).

In clinical trials testing antiarrhythmic treatment, patients with severe CHF (NYHA class IV) are often excluded, which seems to be justified.[34,42] Others have tried to make algorithms in order to predict mechanism of cardiac death and found that by excluding patients with low LVEF (lowest 20th percentiles) they were able to identify a group of patients in whom 75% of deaths were arrhythmic, if a low heart rate variability was combined

Table 7.5 Studies assessing other risk factors as well as left ventricular function

	No.	Method	Total mortality	Excluded patients	Prognostic value of LV dysfunction on total mortality	Prediction of sudden or arrhythmic death
Farrell[20]	416	ET ECG, HRV, LP, RNC/V	11.3% (2 years)	≥70 years, non-SR, BBB, cancer, etc.	NA	RR: 3.7[c] (LVEF <40%)
Odemuyiwa[23]	385	RNC/V, HRV	11.4% (½ year)	≥70 years, non-SR, in-hospital death	Sen: 48% Spe: 78% (LVEF ≤ 40%)	Sen: 40% Spe: 73% (LVEF ≤ 40%)
Richards[44]	361	LP, EPS, ET ECG, RNC	9.4% (2 years)	>70 years, various drugs, CHF, ischaemia, early death	Sen: 75%[c] Spe: 76%[c] RR: 5.2[c] (LVEF <40%)	Sen: 71%[d] Spe: 74% RR: 4.8 (LVEF <40%)
Pedretti[45]	305	E, HRV, EPS, LP	2% (15 months)	>70 years, BBB, AF, CHF, early death	NA	Sen: 79% Spe: 85% RR: 16[d] (LVEF <40%)
Hartikainen[21]	575	HRV, LP, RNC/V	9.6% (2 years)	>70 years, BBB, DM, AF, PM	NA	RR: 3.0[c] (LVEF = 40%)
ATRAMI[41]	1284	E/RNC/V, HRV, BRS	5.1% (21 months)	>80 years, AF, CHF at discharge	NA	RR: 3.9–4.7 (Cardiac death + CA) (LVEF ≤ 0.35)

[a]Same patients; [b]only sudden death after hospital discharge; [c]cardiac mortality; [d]arrhythmic events.
Abbreviations: AF = atrial fibrillation/flutter; BBB = bundle branch block; BRS = baroreflex sensitivity; CD = non-fatal cardiac arrest; CHF = congestive heart failure; DM = diabetes; E = echocardiography; EPS = electrophysiological testing; ET ECG = exercise testing; HRV = heart rate variability; LP = late potentials; NA = not available; RNC = radionuclide cardiography; RR = relative risk; Sen = sensitivity; Spe = specificity; V = ventriculography at catheterisation.

with long filtered QRS duration or ventricular arrhythmias.[21] This study by Hartikainen followed 575 survivors of an AMI but included only cardiac deaths in their comparative analyses. The cardiac mortality after 2 years was only 8.2%, and the total mortality was as low as 9.6% making comparison to other patient groups with a higher mortality difficult. The algorithm was made retrospectively and there is a need for a prospective trial including patients by an algorithm combining different methods. Also, it seems to be important to include all patients with the disease who wished to be studied, since it previously has been shown that extrapolating results from one part of a population to the remaining part is difficult.[25]

In the Autonomic Tone and Reflexes After Myocardial Infarction (ATRAMI) study, heart rate variability (measured as SDNN), baroreflex sensitivity, and LVEF were used alone or in combination in order to develop an algorithm for prediction of cardiac death in combination with non-fatal cardiac arrest.[41] This study indicates that there was only a borderline additional effect of heart rate variability or baroreflex sensitivity compared to the effect of clinical risk makers (age, heart failure class) and LVEF. In the Nordic Pilot Study the combination of reduced left ventricular systolic function was combined with reduced heart rate variability in order to find patients at high risk of arrhythmic death suitable for implantation of an intracardiac cardioverter defibrillator.[43] This pilot study showed that patients selected had a relatively low risk owing to high-risk patients not having both risk markers assessed. This was primarily due to difficulties in obtaining heart rate variability (atrial fibrillation, ventricular ectopy, tape quality, etc.).

Future perspective

As left ventricular systolic function declines, there is an increase in risk of death. The mode of death in subgroups defined by left ventricular function is more or less equally distributed between death from progressive heart failure and sudden death. Thus, left ventricular systolic dysfunction is an unspecific marker of high risk. This association seems to be independent of the ethiology of reduced left ventricular systolic dysfunction and independent of any initial presenting arrhythmia. Arrhythmic death or tachyarrhythmic events can be triggered by many factors. Left ventricular systolic dysfunction is one of the substrates on which other mechanisms can act. In contrast, several markers of autonomic dysfunction appear to identify patients where the risk of arrhythmic death is higher than the risk of death from heart failure. In order to identify a method that can select patients at a high risk of arrhythmic death, it would appear promising to combine the presence of moderate or severe reduced left ventricular systolic function with a marker of autonomic dysfunction.

Comparison between currently available studies is hampered by selection and exclusion, and reports should include information on those not included. This would make extrapolation to other patient groups more reliable. A perspective could be that all methods used for prediction of mode of death should at least include the following information:

- a definition of all screened patients;
- total mortality (1- or 2-year);
- arrhythmic/sudden death of all screened.

Combination with non-fatal events (e.g. non-fatal arrhythmias) can then be compared to these results. Left ventricular systolic function as well as baseline characteristics must be available for all patients, and multivariate analyses or stratified analyses need to be performed.

References

1. Kligfield P, Levy D, Devereaux RB, Savage DD. Arrhythmias and sudden death in mitral valve prolapse. *Am Heart J* 1987;**113**:1298–307.
2. Myerburg RJ, Mitrani R, Interian A, Castellanos A. Interpretation of outcomes of antiarrhythmic clinical trials. *Circulation* 1998;**97**:1514–21.
3. The Multicenter Postinfarction Research Group. Risk stratification and survival after myocardial infarction. *New Engl J Med* 1983;**309**:331–6.
4. Berning J, Steensgaard-Hansen F. Early estimation of risk by echocardiographic determination of wall motion index in an unselected population with acute myocardial infarction. *Am J Cardiol* 1990;**65**:567–76.
5. Kelly MJ, Thompson PL, Quinlan MF. Prognostic significance of left ventricular ejection fraction after acute myocardial infarction. A bedside radionuclide study. *Br Heart J* 1985;**53**:16–24.
6. Ong L, Green S, Reiser P, Morrison J. Early prediction of mortality in patients with acute myocardial infarction: A prospective study of clinical and radionuclide risk factors. *Am J Cardiol* 1986;**57**:33–8.
7. Kan G, Visser CA, Koolen JJ, Dunning AJ. Short and long term predictive value of admission wall motion score in acute myocardial infarction. A cross sectional echocardiographic study of 345 patients. *Br Heart J* 1986;**56**:422–7.
8. Køber L, Torp-Pedersen C, Carlsen J, Videbæk R, Egeblad H. An echocardiographic method for selecting high risk patients shortly after acute myocardial infarction for inclusion in multicentre studies (as used in the TRACE study). *Eur Heart J* 1994;**15**:1616–20.
9. Shah PK, Maddahi J, Staniloff HM *et al.* Variable spectrum and prognostic implications of left and right ventricular ejection fractions in patients with and without clinical heart failure after acute myocardial infarction. *Am J Cardiol* 1986;**58**:387–93.
10. Heger JJ, Weyman AE, Wann IS, Rogers EW, Dillon JC, Feigenbaum H. Cross-sectional echocardiographic analysis of the extent of left ventricular asynergy in acute myocardial infarction. *Circulation* 1980;**61**:1113–18.
11. Berning J, Rokkedal Nielsen J, Launbjerg J, Fogh J, Mickley H, Andersen PE. Rapid estimation of left ventricular ejection fraction in acute myocardial infarction by echocardiographic wall motion analysis. *Cardiology* 1992;**80**:257–66.
12. Bigger JT, Fleiss JL, Kleiger R, Miller JP, Rolnitzky LM and the Multicenter Post-infarction Research Group. The relationships among ventricular arrhythmias, left ventricular dysfunction, and mortality in the two years after myocardial infarction. *Circulation* 1984;**69**:250–8.
13. Uretz EF, Denes P, Ruggie N, Vasilomanolakis E, Messer JV. Relation of ventricular premature beats to underlying heart disease. *Am J Cardiol* 1984;**53**:774–80.
14. Taggert P, Sutton P, John R, Lab M, Swanton H. Monophasic action potential recordings during acute changes in ventricular loading induced by the Valsalva manoeuvre. *Br Heart J* 1992;**67**:221–9.
15. Dean JW, Lab MJ. Arrhythmia in heart failure: role of mechanically induced changes in the electrophysiology. *Lancet* 1989;**1**:1309–12.
16. Cranfield PF, Wit AL, Hoffman BF. Genesis of cardiac arrhythmias. *Circulation* 1973;**47**:190–5.
17. Koilpillai C, Quinones MA, Greenberg B *et al.* Relation of ventricular size and function to heart failure status and ventricular dysrhythmia in patients with severe left ventricular dysfunction. *Am J Cardiol* 1996;**77**:606–11.
18. Søgaard P, Gotzsche CO, Ravkilde J, Norgaard A, Thygesen K. Ventricular arrhythmias in the acute and chronic phase after acute myocardial infarction: effect of intervention with captopril. *Circulation* 1994;**90**:101–7.
19. Marcus FI, Cobb L, Edwards J *et al.* Mechanism of death and prevalence of myocardial ischaemic symptoms in the terminal event after acute myocardial infarction. *Am J Cardiol* 1988;**61**:8–15.
20. Farrell TG, Bashir Y, Cripps T, Malik M, Poloniecki J, Bennett D *et al.* Risk stratification for arrhythmic events in postinfarction patients based on heart rate variability, ambulatory electrocardiographic variables and the signal-averaged electrocardiogram. *J Am Cardiac Coll* 1991;**18**:687–97.
21. Hartikainen JEK, Malik M, Staunton A, Poloniecki J, Camm AJ. Distinction between arrhythmic and non-arrhythmic

deaths after acute myocardial infarction based on heart rate variability, signal-averaged electrocardiogram, ventricular arrhythmias and left ventricular ejection fraction. *J Am Cardiac Coll* 1996;**28**:296–304.

22. Farrell TG, Paul V, Cripps T *et al*. Baroreflex sensitivity and electrophysiological correlates in patients after acute myocardial infarction. *Circulation* 1991;**83**:945–52.

23. Odemuyiwa O, Malik M, Farrell TG, Bashir Y, Poloniecki J, Camm AJ. Comparison of the predictive characteristics of heart rate variability index and left ventricular ejection fraction for all-cause mortality, arrhythmic events and sudden death after acute myocardial infarction. *Am J Cardiol* 1991;**68**:434–9.

24. Bigger JT, Kleiger R, Fleiss JL *et al*. Components of heart rate variability measured during healing of acute myocardial infarction. *Am J Cardiol* 1988;**61**:208–15.

25. Køber L, Torp-Pedersen C. Clinical characteristics and mortality of patients screened for entry into the trandolapril cardiac evaluation (TRACE) study. *Am J Cardiol* 1995;**76**:1–5.

26. Stevenson R, Ranjadayalan K, Wilkinson P, Roberts R, Timmis A. Short and long term prognosis of acute myocardial infarction since introduction of thrombolysis. *BMJ* 1993;**307**:349–53.

27. McGovern PG, Pankow JS, Shahar E *et al*. Recents trends in acute coronary heart disease. Mortality, morbidity, medical care, and risk factors. *New Engl J Med* 1996;**334**:884–90.

28. Emanuelsson H, Karlson BW, Herlitz J. Characteristics and prognosis of patients with acute myocardial infarction in relation to occurrence of congestive heart failure. *Eur Heart J* 1994;**15**:761–8.

29. Pratt CM, Greenway PS, Schoenfeld MH, Hibben ML, Reiffel JA. Exploration of the precision of classifying sudden cardiac death. Implications for the interpretation of clinical trials. *Circulation* 1996;**93**:519–24.

30. The SOLVD investigators. Effect of enalapril on survival in patients with reduced left ventricular ejection fractions and congestive heart failure. *New Engl J Med* 1991;**325**:293–302.

31. Cohn JN, Archibald DG, Ziesche S *et al*. Effect of vasodilator therapy on mortality in chronic congestive heart failure: results of a Veterans Administration cooperative study. *New Engl J Med* 1986;**314**:1547–52.

32. Pfeffer MA, Braunwald E, Moyé LA *et al*. Effect of captopril on mortality and morbidity in patients with left ventricular dysfunction after myocardial infarction. Results of the Survival and Ventricular Enlargement trial. *New Engl J Med* 1992;**327**:669–77.

33. Køber L, Torp-Pedersen C, Carlsen J *et al*. A clinical trial of the angiotensin-converting-enzyme inhibitor trandolapril in patients with left ventricular dysfunction after myocardial infarction. *New Engl J Med* 1995;**333**:1670–6.

34. Waldo AL, Camm AJ, deRuyter H *et al*. Effect of d-sotalol on mortality in patients with left ventricular dysfunction after recent and remote myocardial infarction. The SWORD investigators. Survival With Oral d-Sotalol. *Lancet* 1996;**348**:7–12.

35. Julian DG, Camm AJ, Frangin G *et al*. Randomised trial of efect of amiodarone on mortality in patients with left-ventricular dysfunction after recent myocardial infarction: EMIAT. *Lancet* 1997;**349**:667–74.

36. The Diamond study group. Dofetilide in patients with left ventricular dysfunction and either heart failure or acute myocardial infarction: rationale, design, and patient characteristics of the DIAMOND studies. *Clin Cardiol* 1997;**20**:704–10.

37. Torp-Pedersen C, Møller M, Bloch-Thomsen PE *et al*. Dofetilide in patients with congestive heart failure and left ventricular dysfunction. *New Engl J Med* 1999;**341**:857–65.

38. Anderson JL, Hallstrom AP, Epstein AE *et al*. Design and result of the antiarrhythmics versus implantable defibrillators (AVID) registry. *Circulation* 1999;**99**:1692–9.

39. Vaishnav S, Stevenson R, Marchant B, Lagi K, Ranjadayalan K. Relation between heart rate variability early after acute myocardial infarction and long-term mortality. *Am J Cardiol* 1994;**73**:653–7.

40. Singh N, Mironov D, Armstrong PW, Ross AM, Langer A for the GUSTO ECG substudy investigators. Heart rate variability assessment early after acute myocardial infarction. Pathophysiological and prognostic correlates. *Circulation* 1996;**93**:1388–95.

41. La Rovere MT, Bigger JT, Flather MI, Mortara A, Schwartz PJ. Baroreflex sensitivity and heart-rate variability in prediction of total cardiac mortality after myocardial infarction. ATRAMI (Autonomic Tone and Reflexes After Myocardial Infarction) Investigators. *Lancet* 1998;**351**:478–84.

42. Moss AJ, Jackson HW, Cannom DS *et al*. Improved survival with an implanted defibrillator in patients with coronary disease at high risk for ventricular arrhythmia. *New Engl J Med* 1996;**335**:1933–40.

43. Thomsen PE, Huikuri H, Kober L, Linde C, Koistinen J, Ohm O *et al*. Lessons from the Nordic ICD pilot study. *Lancet* 1999;**353**:2130.

44. Richards DAB, Byth K, Ross DL, Uther JB. What is the best predictor of spontaneous ventricular tachycardia and sudden death after myocardial infarction? *Circulation* 1991;**83**:756–63.

45. Pedretti R, Etro MD, Laporta A, Braga SS, Caru B. Prediction of late arrhythmic events after acute myocardial infarction from combined use of non-invasive prognostic variables and inducibility of sustained monomorphic ventricular tachycardia. *Am J Cardiol* 1993;**71**:1131–41.

8 Risk assessment: the 12-lead electrocardiogram

Rory Childers

The power of the resting 12-lead electrocardiogram (ECG) to assess the risk of arrhythmia is double-tiered. A tracing with normal sinus rhythm may be the harbinger of an abnormal, even calamitous, arrhythmia. If the latter is already present, there may be features suggesting it is about to worsen, or conversely, revert to normal.

Quantity of ECG data: evolution of electrocardiograph devices

In the last four decades the average number of heart beats recorded in a routine 12-lead ECG has fallen from approximately 45–50, using a single channel device (55–60 with a lead II "rhythm strip"), to the current 11–13 in the 10-s computerised and digitised sheet (the companion multichannel rhythm strip looks at the same 11–13 beats). In a few centres a 20–30 second multichannel rhythm strip is recorded if the initial computer diagnosis is other than simple sinus rhythm, bradycardia, or tachycardia; storage and reimbursement problems have caused a decline in this desirable practice. These contractions have reduced the opportunities of observing changes in rhythm. While the 12-lead ECG, even with a rhythm strip, is not the chosen instrument for counting ectopy of any kind, a high frequency of such will obtrude on the data. However, predisposition to major arrhythmia is related not so much to ectopic count but to concomitant, or entirely separate, features. The illustrations here are formed from the full range of 12-lead ECG devices.

Risk of sudden cardiac death

Idiopathic ventricular fibrillation

Idiopathic ventricular fibrillation[1] accounts for 3–9% of those out-of-hospital deaths not involving coronary heart disease.[2] Most cases, including the catecholaminergic form in children,[3] show no special ECG features.[4] In a rare form of torsade de pointes, closely coupled ("short-coupled"),[5] ventricular premature contractions (VPCs) induce VF even in the absence of a prolonged QT (Fig. 8.1). The condition may be familial. It is not clear whether subjects who habitually show closely coupled VPCs and R-on-T without mishap are at similar risk (Fig. 8.2).

The idiopathic long QT syndromes (LQTS)

These carry the risk of SCD from torsade de pointes (TDP), and consist of six genetically separable entities each with a different "ionopathy".[6] LQT1 and LQT2 have reduced potassium currents, the result of defects in the genes *KVLQT1* (chromosome 11p15.5) and *HERG* (7q35–36) respectively. Reduction in the said current delays the completion of repolarisation. LQT3 results from a defect in *SCN5A* (3p21–24), which abnormally sustains the sodium inward current. Our sole knowledge of LQT4 is its locus on chromosome 4q25–27. LQT5 (21q22.1) involves the *minK* (or *KCNE1*) gene and is functionally symmetric to LQT1, each consisting of a subunit protein of the same potassium channel and current. The lengthening of the QT interval is due to a delayed phase 3 of the action potential in LQT1, 2, and 5; phase 2 is delayed in LQT3.

Clinical presentations of the LQT syndromes

These entities are differentiated by the presence or absence of congenital nerve deafness and by the mode of inheritance. The QT is habitually long but the magnitude of the prolongation can fluctuate markedly over hours or days. The presenting symptoms are either death, syncope, or convulsions; a similar sibling history is often obtainable. Syncope is due to ventricular tachycardia, generally TDP. The latter is almost certainly the actual event in most reported cases of "spontaneously arresting ventricular fibrillation".[7,8] If the latter lasts long enough, the resulting seizures may earn the child the false diagnosis of epilepsy. Syncopal attacks often appear in clusters that can be separated by months or years, appearing as early as the first

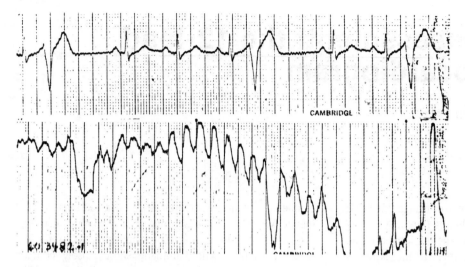

Figure 8.1 R-on-T inducing ventricular fibrillation. The 38-year-old patient was having his tongue pulled down to better visualise his sore throat at the time the lead II rhythm strip was being recorded. Short-coupled PVCs and a normal QT interval (and 12-lead ECG).

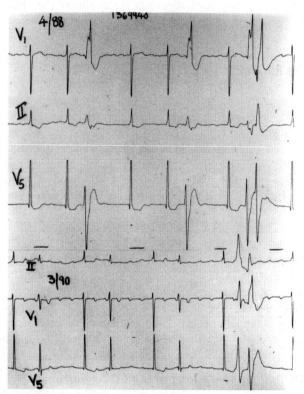

Figure 8.2 R-on-T ventricular ectopy, benign over a 2-year period. Whenever there are couplets, the second PVC climbs off the T wave nadir [or apex] of the first PVC.

month of life or as late as age 36 (median age is 3). The mortality can be as high as 78%.[9] These presentations are four in number:

- *Jervell and Lange-Nielsen syndrome*[10] (LQT1 and 5): children have neural deafness (with mutism); the inheritance is dominant for the long QT, but recessive for the deafness.

- *Romano–Ward syndrome*[11,12]: no deafness; transmission is via an autosomal dominant pattern (LQT1 through 5). Identification of the genetic defect is more reliable than the QTc in identifying carriers of the syndrome.[13]

- *Sporadic non-familial cases.*[14] Among these three presentations the second and third are commoner than the first, which constitutes only 5–6%.

- *Atypical forms*: These are seen later in life. They may have normal QTs, T waves, and U waves, at all times except immediately prior to torsades. Alternatively they get torsades when adrenergic stimulation is combined with type 1A drugs.[15]

LQT1 and 2 have a higher incidence of cardiac events than LQT3, but the latter is more lethal. Among all four groups the QTc is normal in only 6%. Among probands in the International LQTS Registry, 70% were female, 6% were deaf, 30% showed bradycardia <60 bpm, half had a QTc >0.5 s.[16]

ECG morphology in LQTS

With QT prolongation of any kind two elementary shapes may be encountered:

- the entire T wave is splayed or spread out, giving it a broad base, the ST starting its ascent immediately;
- the T wave is "moved bodily" to the right, the ST remaining isoelectric for a longer than usual interval.

In hypocalcaemia the T wave is of the latter kind but otherwise normal in shape and amplitude. Both types are seen in the LQTS patients; many show intermediate forms. The ECG often shows distorted and incongruous T wave shapes, which change over the minutes and hours. Their deformity can be gross enough to raise the question of artefact. In order to classify LQT morphology in general, and more specifically, to quantify the degree to which a given patient manifests either form, a series of basic measurements has been devised by specialists in the field. These are executed in leads II, aVF and V_5.[17] They include measurement parameters in the subunits of the traditional QT interval, each corrected according to Bazett's formula,[18] using the units suggested by Molnar *et al.*[19]:

- $QT_{onset-c}$ – the time from q to the departure of the commencing T wave from the isoelectric baseline ("time-to-start-of-T");
- the time-to-peak-of-T (whether positive or negative);
- the standard corrected QT_c, finishing either with the end of T, or with its caesura with a U wave;
- T wave duration;
- T amplitude in mV referential to the PR segment.

Linkage of long QT genotypes to a typical ST-T wave pattern

This was postulated in a multicentre blinded trial where investigators were asked to compare a group of unknown congenital LQT cases to 10 index ECG patterns, distilled from the above five measurements. These patterns were either typical or atypical for each of the first three genotypes. Among 265 carriers from 46 families (16 LQT1, 24 LQT2, and 6 LQT3), typical patterns were found in 75% of LQT1 and 2, and in half of the LQT3 carriers. Four non-specialist cardiologists sorted through the cases with correct predictions in 75–80% of the LQT1 and 2.[20] For example T wave duration was longest in the chromosome 11 genotype; the time-to-start-of-T was especially long in those patients with mutations of the sodium channel (SCN5A) on chromosome 3. In the latter instance, one finds a prolonged isoelectric ST segment, all of the voltage energy – whether positive, negative, or biphasic – being concentrated as a bizarre excrescence in the terminal portion of the QT interval.

Gender and the QT interval

There may or may not be a gender difference[21] in the QT_c, but the female interval alone expands with age.[22] Clarifying these issues, a recent study[23] split the QT into its component parts: time-to-peak-of-T (QT_p), and peak-to-end-of-T. In cohorts of normal males and normal females, the slope of RR intervals was plotted against each component measurement. The QT_p in women was significantly longer than in men; the T wave descent interval on the other hand, was longer in men than in women. In all subjects the first component was strongly responsive to change in RR interval, the second only weakly so. The slope of QT_p was steeper in females than in males and

increased its slope with age. There was no such age change in men. This difference becomes all the more remarkable when one remembers that the female QRS duration is less than that of the male, but also uniquely, shrinks a tad with age.[23]

Gender and congenital LQTS

In LQT1 families there are quite pronounced differences in event rates between the sexes at various age periods. Males were younger than females at the age of first event (mean age 8 versus 14), and had a higher event rate up to age 15. From 15 to 40 females had a higher event rate. There was no such gender–age disparity for carriers of the LQT2 and LQT3 genes.[24] Among all comers in congenital LQTS the female to male ratio is 7:3.

Other ECG features of congenital LQTS

Additional to the prolongation of repolarisation, and the often distinctive morphology of same, the other attendant ECG findings – used together with clinical and family history in a diagnostic scoring system – are T wave alternans, TDP, low heart rate for age, and notching of the T wave in at least 3 leads.[25]

Acquired LQT syndrome

Acquired LQT syndrome producing TDP is seen most commonly as a pro-arrhythmic consequence of quinidine,[26] procainamide,[27] or disopyramide[28] administration. The relevant serum levels of the drug need not be in the toxic range.[29] It is most likely to occur when the rate slows, after conversion of fibrillation to sinus rhythm, when electrolyte ion depletion is superadded, or when these factors freshly appear in combination. In half the cases the arrhythmia appears in the first four days of therapy; in the other half it develops weeks to years after commencement, generally by the intrusion of the aforesaid changes. The new development of ventricular bigemini, as a result of the introduction of a type 1A drug is a warning sign for torsade. Whilst combined electrolyte depletion is more often a cause of torsades, it can also be caused alone by hypokalaemia,[30] hypomagnesaemia,[31] and rarely by hypocalcaemia.[32] Other causative agents include oral,[33] or intravenous[34] amiodarone, bepridil,[35] sotalol,[36] intravenous erythromycin,[37] liquid protein diets,[38] chronic complete AV block with a bradycardic rhythm[39] (Fig. 8.3), the tricyclic, and tetracyclic antidepressants, the phenothiazines,[40] and the organophosphate insecticides.[41] There have been case reports of torsade with trimethoprim sulfamethoxazole,[42] pentamidine,[43] haloperidol,[44,45] and chloral hydrate.[46] Of recent interest has been the impact of the newer non-sedating antihistaminics terfenadine and astemizole. When TDP develops with the latter, such patients will often be found to have hepatic disease, or undergoing concomitant treatment with either macrolide antibiotics, such as erythromycin, or ketoconazole.[47] Erythromycin may impose its effect in part by increasing magnesium excretion and depleting this ion.[48] Other agents implicated in TDP are cited in recent reviews.[6] If no agent or electrolyte depletion can be identified, it should first be assumed that one is dealing with one of the congenital LQT syndromes in an adult.

Torsade de pointes[49] ("twisting of the points")

The visual impact of the QRS cadences in this form of ventricular tachycardia was likened by Smirk to a choreographic sequence: "cardiac ballet":[50] Like a row of dominoes each dancer bends her body down and up again forming graceful undulations. Electrocardiographically this very special type of ventricular tachycardia has the following features:

- The R-on-T phenomenon is seldom[51] observed with the first ventricular ectopic beat, but is overt with the subsequent complexes, each of which seemingly climbs out of the apex of the preceding T wave.
- The ventricular ectopic complexes show the following features:

1. The tachycardia is untidy looking and superficially reminiscent of the artefactual "V tacs" often recorded on monitor strips in ICUs. It is neither unifocal nor polymorphic. Each beat differs slightly from its neighbour in shape, size and crudity.
2. In the great majority of beats, the QRS duration cannot be measured. Neither the start of the QRS, nor the J point, nor the onset and offset of the T wave, can be clearly discerned. Each beat is a conjoined QRST, as opposed to a QRS-T. The only helpful localising feature of the T is its polarity, which opposes that of the QRS. The iso-electric line can only be defined by extrapolating from the TP interval of the last sinus cycle.

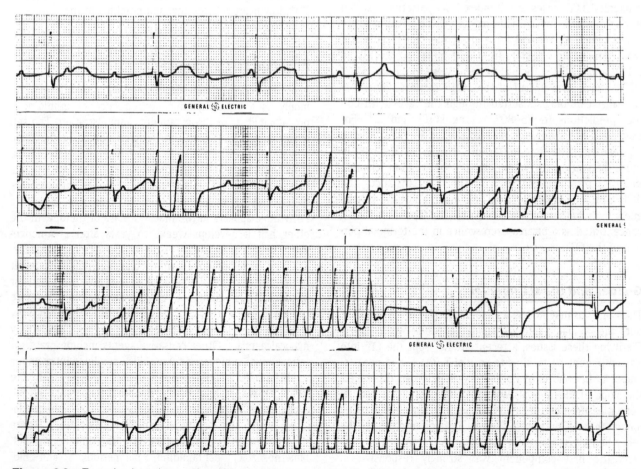

Figure 8.3 Torsade de pointes related to complete atrioventricular block and an idioventricular rate of 36 bpm. [NB The nadirs of the tachycardic QRS complexes are artefactually amputated by the ECG machine.]

3. The beats can be crudely grouped in repeating morphologic sequences, each constituting a single torsade of 5–22 beats. Most episodes consist of two to four torsades, the tachycardia thereafter spontaneously aborts, or becomes ventricular fibrillation.

4. The conjoined QRST beats show four basic shapes:

   (a) the rapid large voltage verticle scribble with a spike at both ends (any given spike may be notched);

   (b) a large amplitude beat with one spike and one rounded, squared or bifid opposing extremity; most beats are of this type;

   (c) a frankly curvaceous and sinusoidal complex, ressembling published examples of ventricular flutter;

   (d) small polyphasic complexes, in which the QRS and T are occasionally separable.

5. Each torsade shows, in consecutive beats, a gradual increase and then decrease in overall amplitude.

6. Companion to these shifting voltages are changes in shape and polarity: the complexes may appear to switch gradually from being *above* the putative baseline, to a negative disposition *below* it. This change often coincides with the moment when consecutive 4(b)-type beats showing positive R wave spikes or "points" yield to negative S wave spikes or *vice versa*. Thus the points or spikes "twist around the isoelectric line"[52] as described by Desertenne.[49] The positive and negative cadences are often bridged by two to five low amplitude 4(d)-type polyphasic complexes, and a slight decrement in rate. The amplitude may remain unchanged for up to 10 beats when sinusoidal beats 4(c) form a given torsade.

7. Although the torsade can be said to "repeat", the morphology is never precisely the same. The overall visual impression at a distance can suggest a taut vibrating guitar wire.

8. The rate of TDP ranges from 175–280 bpm and invariably fluctuates by as much as 15 bpm, the slower rates are seen with the 4(c) "sine wave" beats, the faster rates are seen with spike-containing complexes 4(a) or 4(b).

9. Variations from the foregoing description include a relatively abrupt change in amplitude (small to big rather than the converse), and instances where the cadence of ectopy is briefly chaotic.

Occasionally one will see a choreographically perfect torsade. Movement interference related to syncope is generally present, defiling the quality of the tracing. Thus there are very few standard 12-lead recordings of TDP. It is not rare for regular non-sustained monomorphic tachycardia to be found in adjacent strips. Single monitor strips may lack the above variations, and resemble monomorphic ventricular tachycardia. The differential diagnosis of TDP is from ventricular fibrillation and from artefact of the vertical-scribble type.

Retention of the name TDP

Because of the 10 or so alternative appellations given this arrhythmia in the literature, it has been argued that it should be replaced by the less specific "polymorphic ventricular tachycardia". But the original definition of TDP required not only the above morphologic description, but also a long QT interval. TDP should not be used in the absence of the latter. Failure to distinguish TDP from other forms of polymorphic VT may result in inappropriate treatment: for example with a type 1A agent.[52] The original conception of TDP has been reinforced by characterisation of the ECG structures recorded at the moment of initiation, or in the wake of its conversion to NSR.

Jackman's unified hypothesis

For all long QT syndromes: the triggering physiology of TDP is postulated to be of three types: pause-dependent, adrenergically-mediated, and other. (Cases of the latter are triggered by both or neither of these mechanisms.)[15] There are now modifications to the original hypothesis.

● *Pause-dependent torsades de pointes*. The triggering event in the common form of torsades is a pause, often induced by a PAC or ventricular premature contraction (VPC). The voltage of the T wave (Fig.8.4) or U wave of the subsequent (generally sinus) beat becomes unusually exaggerated. Off the descending limb of the enhanced T or U arises the first ventricular complex of the tachycardia; thus the first beat of torsades de pointes arises to the right of the vulnerable period. In a minority of cases, exclusively in the wake of the said pauses, the U wave appears for the first time. This U wave is probably an *early after-depolarisation* or EAD. (EADs are the hallmark of one type of *triggered automaticity* in which a hump or upward deflection emerges out of the action potential phase 3 descent before it reaches the baseline.) A freshly lengthened QT interval in this context is the collective expression at the body surface of EADs developing in a sufficiently large number of myocytes.[53]

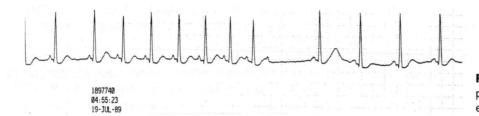

1897740
04:55:23
19-JUL-89

Figure 8.4 QT prolongation: pause-dependent T wave enhancement.

Jackman nomenclature

Because it is sometimes unclear whether the augmented wave is T or U, Jackman suggested calling the enhanced repolarisation hump UH.[15] In fact with a simultaneous 12-lead tracing, identification is not so difficult. Often both T and U are enhanced but optimally seen in different leads. As already stated, pause-dependent T or U enhancement does not presage the tachycardia, even though it appears to be a requisite for its advent. If an EAD reaches threshold, a VPC will appear. If this process becomes regenerative, each ectopic producing yet another threshold-attaining EAD, torsade de pointes is the result. Torsade is more likely to appear when QT prolongation is attended by some degree of ST depression, generally of rounded shape. The latter, like the above described adventitious U wave, may first appear shortly before the onset of the arrhythmia. The twisting pattern of torsade could reflect a recurrent migration across the ventricles, of those after-potentials which are earliest to be triggered.

Properties of the pause-dependent U wave

- Assuming a constant pause, the U amplitude varies directly with the prepause rate (Fig. 8.5).
- Assuming a constant prepause rate, the amplitude varies directly with the length of the preceding pause.
- The larger the torsade-provoking U wave, the greater the total of torsade beats (or the larger the number of torsades).
- In a given lead, the U may be enhanced at the expense of the T (Fig. 8.6) and *vice versa*.

- Augmentation of the U may prolong the Q-U, but does not directly lengthen or alter the Q-caesura or extrapolated QT interval.
- Pause-dependent augmentation of U often initiates a bigeminal-type rhythm, each supraventricular beat being followed by 1–4 VPCs; the greater the number of these sequential ectopy in each salvo of VT, the taller the subsequent U (see the first bullet above). Since the ectopy are followed by a pause the U enhancement is self-sustaining (as in the "Rule of Bigemini"). Short runs of VT are sometimes monomorphic; when the U becomes critically large, the full torsade de pointes emerges.
- The pause-induced appearance or augmentation of the U wave may be followed, in the absence of further pauses, by slow shrinkage of the wave over 2–3 beats, or by U wave alternation (especially if electrolyte depletion is present).

Adrenergically-induced TDP

When associated with the congenital, familial, or sporadic QT syndromes, the triggering factor is often some form of adrenergic stimulation: exercise (especially swimming), sudden unplanned exertion,[54] fright, anger, a loud noise,[55] abrupt awakening from sleep by an alarm clock, thunder, the telephone, or acute anxiety – triggered, for example, by bad news such as opening mail to find a large credit card bill. Exercise is particularly an inciting event in LQT1. Menstruation may encourage events. In some families in successive generations,[56] all events take place dur-

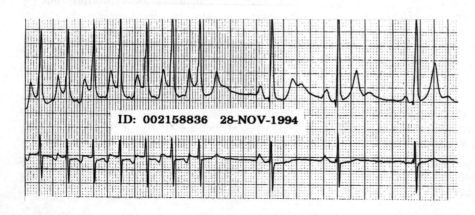

ID: 002158836 28-NOV-1994

Figure 8.5 Pause-related augmentation of the U wave. Termination of supraventricular tachycardia in presence of hypokalaemia. Augmentation enhanced by fast prepause rate.

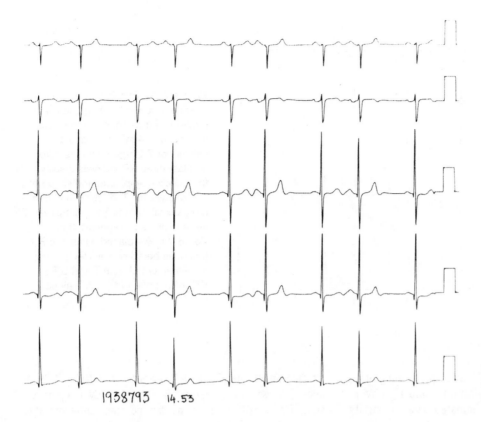

Figure 8.6 Pause-dependent U wave enhancement at the expense of T: 3/2 sinoatrial block.

1938793   14.53

ing sleep (especially in LQT3). The stimulus may be exclusive and specific in a given patient. On exercise, subjects with the Romano–Ward LQTS fail to shorten their QT appropriately with increments in heart rate;[57] instead of shrinking or remaining level (the two normal responses), the QT_c increases. The increase in the U wave can produce grotesque shapes and often makes its appearance minutes or seconds before the torsade. T or U wave alternans is very common. The separation of "adrenergic" and "pause-dependent" breaks down with many cases of congenital LQTS who reach adulthood. LQT3 is seldom stress-related. The presence of stress or even sinus acceleration does not deny the advent of a VPC inducing a pause-dependent event. Uncommonly a presumed acquired LQT is actually a congenital one unmasked by the drug. Most difficult of all are those cases of syncope where the QT is in the normal range and there is no family history. Repeated 12-lead tracings may eventually reveal the long QT; the presence of bifid or double-humped T waves in the frontal or left chest leads is also indicative, especially after adolescence. Finally, pause-dependent torsade can be unexplained or idiopathic.

Value of 12-lead ECG in prevention of TDP

Figure 8.7 shows a 12-lead tracing with all the warning features of possibly impending torsade de pointes. The recipe for the latter was very completely satisfied: a patient being treated for pneumonia with intravenous erythromycin had depletion of both potassium and calcium. The tracing permitted the service to be warned.

Simulation of these pause-dependent events

There are other time-related perturbations in repolarisation that may be confused with those discussed above; they have no relationship to TDP, and are three in number:[58]

- *Pause-dependent T wave inversion.* In this context, the QRS of non-aberrant PACs have a normal upright T wave, but in the postectopic sinus beat T is inverted. A simple sinus pause has the same result. If the pause is generated by a VPC, the polarity of the latter's QRS has no effect on the subsequent T inversion. If inversion of T is already present the pause will deepen it.

- *Post-VPC T wave change.* Here the directionality of T is anamnestic to that of the preceding abnormally depolarised QRS (as in "cardiac memory"[59]). Only in a lead where the ectopic QRS is powerfully positive will the subsequent sinus T wave be "enhanced"; other leads will show dispersion of the QRS-T wave axial angle, which is unchanged in true pause-related T-U enhancement.

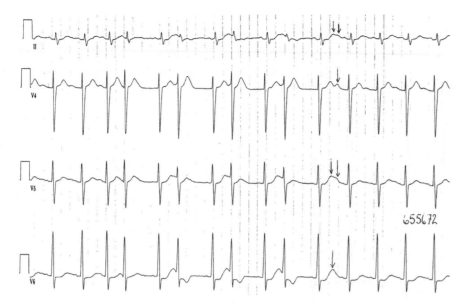

Figure 8.7 Possible prodromata to torsade de pointes. The patient was receiving intravenous erythromycin, had a K of 2.4 mEq/litre and a calcium of 7.1 mg/dl. The first two and last three RR intervals display the baseline amplitude and shape of T and U waves. The four PACs form a bigeminal rhythm. The post-pause T wave is grossly exaggerated in V5,V6. Arrows placed within the RR [unencumbered by any PAC] show enhancement of both T and U (II, V5), of U alone (V4), and T alone (V6).

● *Pseudo-enhancement of T or U.* Superpositioning of a strongly positive atrial repolarisation hump (T$_a$ wave) can occur when a pause is terminated by a low atrial (p inverted) escape, or by a junctional escape complex with a retrograde P. The T is enhanced in the first instance; in the second, the T is enhanced and a "U" wave appears, or is enhanced.

The QT$_c$ is not prolonged in any of the above three contexts; this alone distinguishes them from true pause-dependent T-U augmentation of the kind predisposing to TDP.

T wave alternans or ST-T alternans

This is either obvious or covert.[60,61] Either way, it has an association with ventricular fibrillation, tachycardia, or sudden cardiac death. Although most commonly seen in the classic congenital LQT syndromes, it is also seen during Prinzmetal's angina, coronary angioplasty,[62] acute myocardial infarction, catechol poisoning, and electrolyte imbalance, especially in the terminal hypocalcaemia and hypomagnesaemia of hepatic failure. In some instances, electrolyte depletion can cause selective U wave alternation, the U wave being also greatly enlarged. In Fig. 8.8 there is profound alternation of T wave polarity and QT interval. It may be observed that the deepness of alternate inversions is variable. A given patient can show great variation in the morphology of T alternans over a short period of time, ranging from similar Ts and QTs that simply alternate depth of inversion (Fig. 8.9a) to alternation of the QT and T shape (Fig. 8.9b). VPCs or fatal TDP will be initiated off a particularly deep inversion (Fig. 8.10). T alternans can be transiently initiated by an APC (Fig. 8.11). Slight pairing of sinus beats, or atrial bigemini of minimal prematurity are common with true alternans (Fig. 8.9b).

QRS widening in sinus rhythm without new BBB

If such a change is seen with an attack of angina (together with marked ST depression), one should suspect left main coronary stenosis or its three vessel equivalent (Fig. 8.12). This pattern of global ventricular ischaemia (also seen as a response to a stress test) is commonly followed by arrest, a malignant arrhythmia, or acute infarction during the subsequent 72 hours. The other major consideration with such widening is severe hyperkalaemia: a valuable but understressed sign of the latter is a companion widening of the P wave in lead II. The serum potassium under these circumstances is probably 7.0 mEq/litre or higher. Even more dangerous is the disappearance of P waves with such QRS widening, the result of atrial paralysis.

Prinzmetal's angina

This high-risk event is probably more common during sleep where it is said to coincide with REM.[63] It often fails to awake the patient. Ventricular ectopy frequently appears in the resolving phase, conceivably the outcome

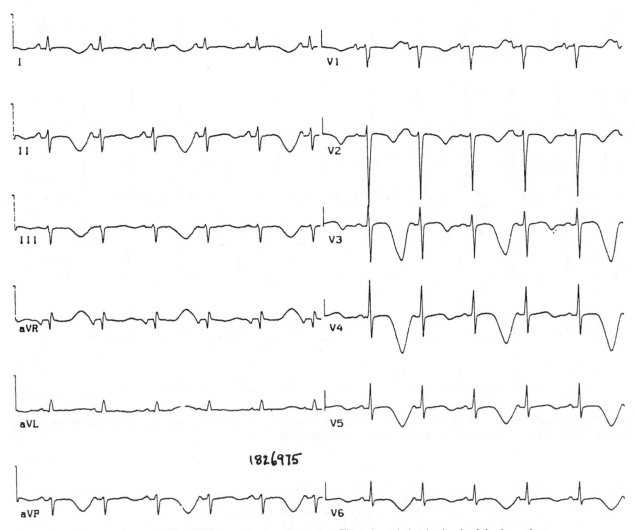

Figure 8.8 T wave alternans. The QT interval is also alternating. There is variation in depth of the inversion.

of "reperfusion".[64] Companion T wave alternans is an additional risk factor (Fig. 8.13). The attack can be notoriously brief. Incomplete RBBB is the most common complicating conduction disturbance, and may cause V_1 to be reminiscent of the pattern seen in the Brugada syndrome. The ST elevation may be severe in both planes. The greater the deviation the worse the risk. If unequal, the frontal is more likely to be worse than the horizontal plane. The axis of the ST segment can be anywhere; it is more likely to be concordant with the QRS in lead III when the latter is negative. As originally noted by Prinzmetal,[65] the R waves are invariably augmented in mid-precordial leads when these show marked ST elevation.[66] In follow-up, SCD occurred in 45% of Prinzmetal patients whose coronary spasm was accompanied by ectopy; the incidence was only 6% in those without the latter.[67] During spasm attacks AV dissociation may be transient. In Fig. 8.14 the coronary spasm clearly affected the

sA nodal structure reducing the sinus rate to a quarter of its prespasm rate of 71 over a short period of time.

Prediction of death in AMI at first presentation

Sinus tachycardia in the context of cardiogenic shock has surely the worst prognosis of all rhythm disturbances. Rare but more inevitably fatal is the presence of acute atrial infarction, which generally requires the associated presence of complete heart block to be visible (Fig. 8.15). In Fig. 8.16 acute inferior and atrial infarction is associated with sinoatrial Wenckebach sequences. Advanced AV nodal block as a complication of right coronary occlusion may cause the inferior MI to be concealed or cryptically evident, especially if an idioventricular rhythm fails to show any ST elevation (Fig. 8.17).

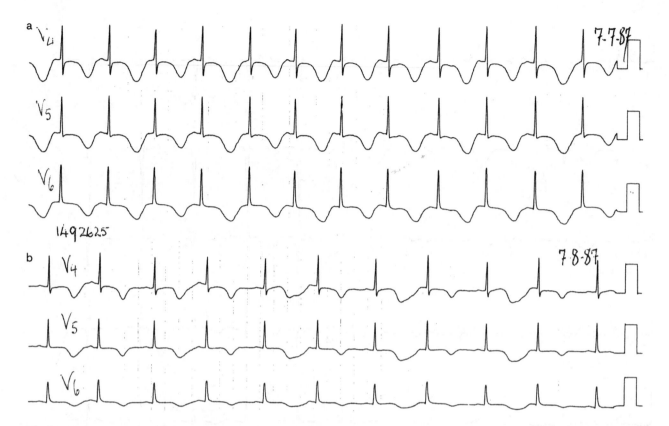

Figure 8.9 Variations of T wave alternans: Above: change is mainly in depth of T. Next day, the QT length shows marked alternation. Both tracings show a slight alternation in the sinus cycle length.

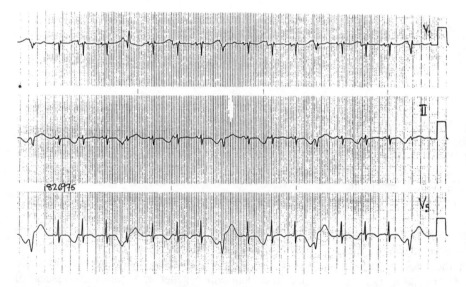

Figure 8.10 T wave alternans; the deeper of the inverted T waves generate PVCs.

Complete bundle branch block complicating acute MI

Of 1013 patients, this problem was seen in about 10%. Such cases are more commonly anterior MI in location, older, female, have a larger peak CK-MB, a higher Killip class, more frequent pericarditis, and get atrial flutter, fibrillation, AV block, and ventricular fibrillation more frequently. Mortality was greater in the BBB cohort than in those with normal IV conduction: in-hospital deaths 32 versus 10%; 3-year mortality 37 versus 18%.[68] When other IVCDs (including transient and alternating) were exam-

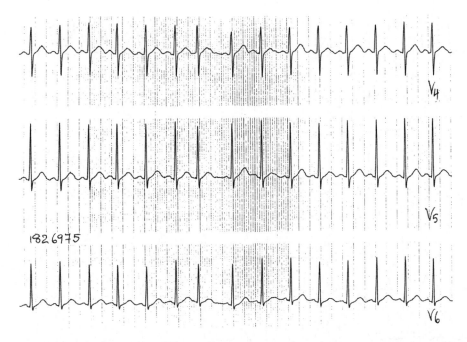

Figure 8.11 Temporary T wave alternans induced by a premature atrial beat.

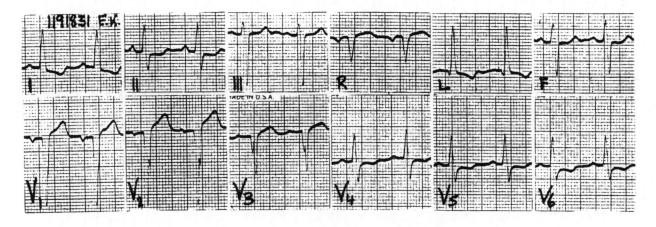

DURING CHEST PAIN (2 minutes later)

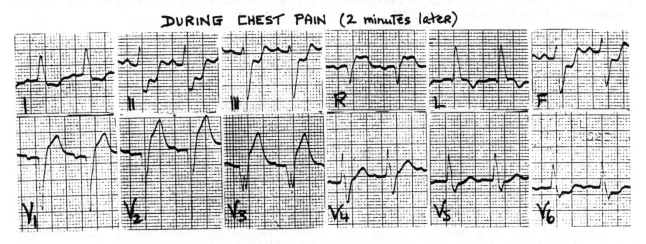

Figure 8.12 Global ventricular ischaemia: old ASMI. During pain the QRS became splayed out while preserving individual features of the baseline QRS, e.g. notching in V3. The patient was found to have left main coronary osteal stenosis.

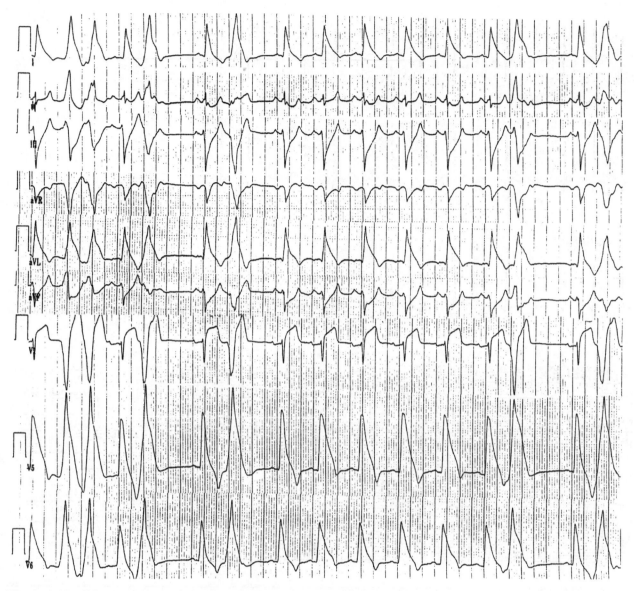

Figure 8.13 Prinzmetal's angina; the upright QRS resembles an action potential. T wave alternans is best seen in lead II. Ventricular ectopy follow the deeper T waves in V5.

ined using continuous seamless ECG monitoring after thrombolytic therapy, mortality was lower, except in those with persistent BBB.[69] Of those that get ventricular fibrillation during the first 30 days after acute MI, 47% have anterior MI complicated by BBB. Within the latter subset the incidence of SCD is 35%, and this danger persists for 6 weeks before it starts to abate.[70] Of those patients getting recurrent VF after acute MI, 9/10 have an associated AV or IV block problem.[71] The prognosis of acute MI complicated by IVCDs is more dependent on size of infarct than anything else.

Cardiac rupture

Death in the acute phase of infarction is not rarely due to cardiac rupture especially in elderly woman with hypertension. Recognition of the the actual event at the bedside is ECG-dependent: sinus rhythm continues in the complete absence of any pulse. Prediction by the ECG has been postulated by Oliva who states that the rapid restitution of the inverting T in Q wave leads, and its combination with ST elevation in a patient with pleurocardiac pain is a significant cluster of findings.[72]

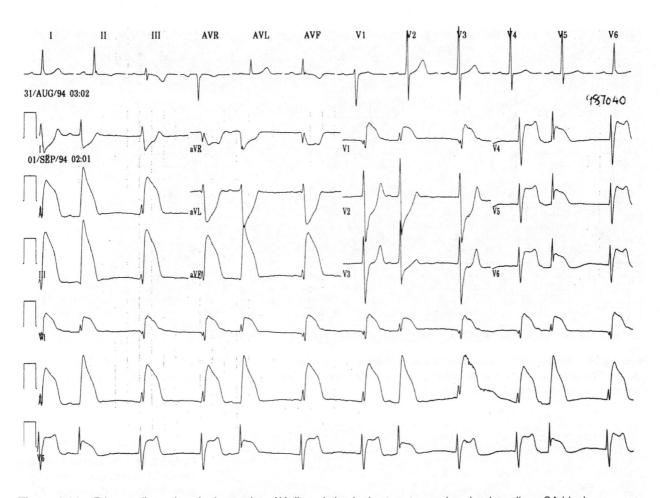

Figure 8.14 Prinzmetal's angina; the incomplete AV dissociation is due to extreme sinus bradycardia or SA block.

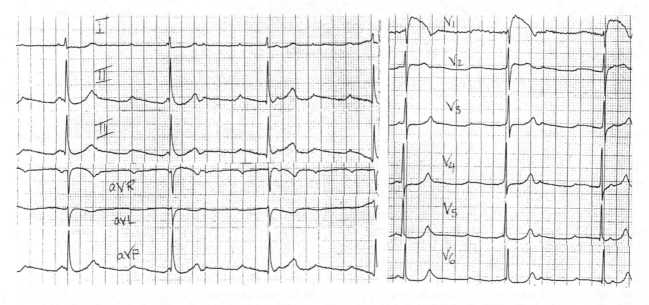

Figure 8.15 Fatal autopsy-proven atrial and right ventricular infarction: complete AV block with P waves showing elevation of the atrial ST segment or Ta wave. RV infarction suggested by the selectively elevated ST in V1.

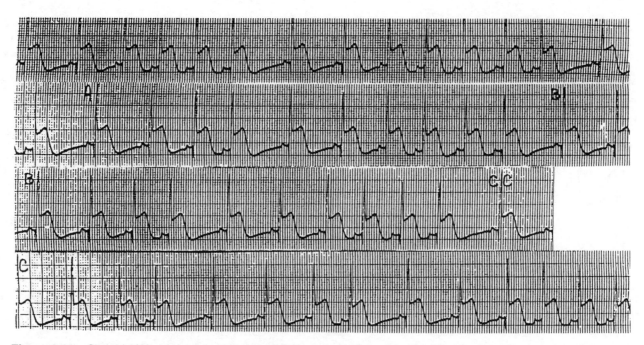

Figure 8.16 Sinoatrial Wenckebach in fatal acute inferior and atrial infarction. The PPs shorten progressively and terminate in a pause. The first cycle following the latter is always longer than the cycle preceding the pause. The PR segment is elevated suggesting acute atrial infarction (no autopsy).

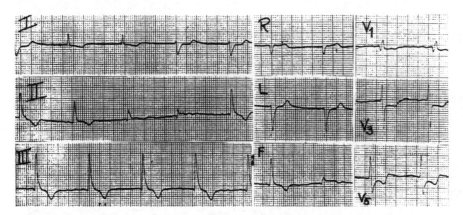

Figure 8.17 Presentation of acute inferior MI already complicated by atrial fibrillation and advanced AV nodal block. The ventricular rate is so slowed by ischaemic AV nodal block that much of the time there is idioventricular rhythm [lead III]. The diagnosis is revealed by the narrower capture-QRS complexes in leads II and aVF, which show Qs and ST elevation.

Post–MI: ST depression

The risk of a second MI, unstable angina, or cardiac death was examined in a 23-month follow-up of almost 1000 subjects who underwent Holter study, 12-lead ECG at rest, and exercise treadmill with thallium. In the landmark result, it was found that persistent non-glycoside ST depression in the 12-lead ECG was the only variable that predicted a serious risk. Non-predictive were the presence of Q waves, persistent ST elevation, a positive and "reversible" thallium scan, and the demonstration of silent ischaemia by Holter.[73] These findings were recently reinforced by examining the prognosis of patients presenting with ST depression and acute MI: mortality at 18 months was 10% worse in ST depression than ST elevation MI. These patients were older, received less thrombolytics, beta-blockade and ace inhibitor modelling.[74] Additional confirmation of the risk associated with ST depression was reported in a New Zealand cohort who found that overall survival with 1 mm, 2 mm, or 3 mm ST depression was 70, 56, and 48%, respectively.[75] Non-sustained ventricular tachycardia (including AIVR) was similarly examined for its predictive capacity for a second event: when seen in the first 7 days post–MI, it is non-predictive, but from day 8 to 28 the SCD incidence is 2.4 times that of post–MI subjects without the arrhythmia.[76,77] Ventricular vulnerability is greatly increased during acute myocardial infarction when the current required for R-on-T fibrillation with a pulse or shock may approach diastolic threshold.[78] For this reason the most imminent danger of fibrillation that an ECG can possibly exhibit is when a temporary pacemaker loses sensing and fires in the fixed rate mode in the context of acute myocardial infarction (Fig. 8.18). The presence of multiple ventricular responses fortifies the assumption of danger.

Statistical risks of common ECG abnormalities

In a 26-year follow-up, the Framingham Heart Study showed an increase in the likelihood of SCD using multi-

variate risk factors, which included ECG evidence for LVH (from any cause) and IVCD.[79] Hearts of SCD victims are heavier than those of subjects whose death is not sudden.[80] In the West of Scotland Coronary Prevention Study, minor 12-lead ECG abnormalities (Minnesota Codes 4-2, 4-3, 5-2, 5-3) in men at entry carried the highest risk of a cardiac event, exceeding such risk actors as smoking, reduced HDL, and hypertension.[81] Among 7735 British urban men of middle age followed over 8 years, three risk factors appeared to be specific for SCD, two of them electrocardiographic: heavy drinking, an elevated sinus rate, and ectopy or atrial fibrillation.[82] This contrasts with another study of the same population profile, which failed to show predictive features in the ECG unless the patient already had symptomatic coronary disease.[83]

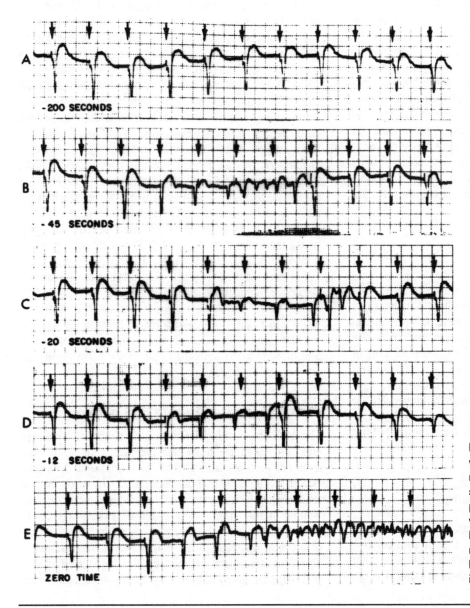

Figure 8.18 Fixed-rate mode of ventricular pacing in acute myocardial infarction. Lead II rhythm strip. The absence of sensing permits the stimulus to fall on the vulnerable zone of a spontaneous beats (sixth in strip B) causing multiple ventricular responses. In the bottom strip, this process terminates in ventricular fibrillation.

Mitral valve prolapse can be associated with SCD

The strongest predictors are syncope and abnormal ST-T waves in the inferior,[84,85] or inferolateral[86] leads. QT prolongation is not a required component There are no specific ECG markers in those cases where familial SCD and mitral prolapse coexist.[87]

Wolff–Parkinson–White (WPW) syndrome

WPW, by definition, warns of frequent arrhythmia. Sudden cardiac death in pre-excitation occurs when atrial fibrillation impulses, conducted down the accessory tract, induce ventricular fibrillation by an R-on-T occurrence. The hierarchy of tissue refractory periods (especially those of the AV node and trifascicular system) that normally confront an excessively early PAC are actually protecting the ventricle from an R-on-T. When impulses travel antegrade down an accessory tract these protective antifibrillatory hurdles are bypassed. Still not well explained is why patients with the WPW syndrome but without mitral, thyroid, hypertensive disease, or atrial enlargement are prone to atrial fibrillation. Neither the latter arrhythmia nor SCD can be predicted from the disposition of delta waves in the ECG. Ventricular fibrillation is more likely to occur when RR intervals during atrial fibrillation are as close as 250 ms.[6] Ventricular fibrillation has a strong situational frequency with the intravenous administration of digoxin in such cases.[88]

Hypertrophic cardiomyopathy

Hypertrophic cardiomyopathy of the obstructive type, when familial, carries a risk of death that is maximal under the age of 25.[89] A subset of these patients (probably less than 20%[90]) shows ECG features that invite the thought of risk or vulnerability: QS or Q wave patterns of frank anteroseptal, anterolateral, lateral, or inferolateral MI, or Q waves excessively deep and narrow in V_5–V_6.[91] The correlation of these features with sudden death or even with outflow obstruction is evidently zero. ECG evidence of LVH correlates with death from cardiac failure, but not to SCD.[92]

Idiopathic dilated cardiomyopathy

In patients with cardiac failure and an EF less than 20%, a single polymorphic ventricular triplet is strongly predictive of increased overall mortality, but not of SCD. The total ectopic count and the number of salvos of non-sustained ventricular tachycardia in a 22-h Holter tape did not refine this prediction.[93] LBBB,[94] and AV block of first or second degree[95] both predict early death.

The Brugada syndrome

First described in 1992[96] the ECG of these subjects shows an elevation of the ST segment in V_1/V_2 of a particular shape: the J point is elevated in V_1 or both leads to resemble an r prime from which the ST segment curves to a T inversion with a convex upward curvature.[97] When the latter pattern is seen in V_1, a "saddle-shaped" ST elevation may be seen in V_2: a horizontal segment with a negative dip near its mid-point. Evidence that the latter pattern is less arrhythmogenic is wanting. These morphologies are reminiscent of the J or Osborn wave of hypothermia (typified in V_4 or V_5) only in that termination of QRS, and start of ST (the J point) is not clearly defined.[98] The r prime in some subjects represents a true complete or incomplete RBBB with the equivalent features in aVR (rSr'), but in most cases V_5/V_6 lacks the fat s wave that goes with a true RBBB. Many subjects also show left anterior fascicular block. Subjects with this pattern are at risk from sudden cardiac death, which is probably more closely associated with the degree of right precordial ST elevation than with RBBB *per se*.[99] Surviving victims of ventricular tachycardia or fibrillation are all inducible by programmed stimulation. Their asymptomatic siblings may also be inducible, and should be regarded as at risk. The condition, often familial,[100] is more common in South Asia than in the USA or Europe.[101] It probably includes the majority of those young men who have suffered SCD or near-fatal arrest of a kind so familiar that it carries a special local name: *Lai Tai* ("died during sleep") in north-east Thailand,[102] *Bangungut* ("moaning and dying during sleep") in the Philippines,[103] and *Pokkuri* ("sudden unexpected nocturnal death") in Japan.[104] These syndromes became the focus of interest with the SCD of young migrant workers in Singapore[105] and Cambodian and other Asian immigrant refugees in the USA.[106]

Phasic change in Brugada ECG pattern

The ECG pattern can wax and wane, disappear with exercise or with simple heart rate increase; thus its absence does not exclude patients from this syndrome. The variation is in the ST elevation rather than any other component of the electrocardiographic complex. The waxing and waning of the latter is a true modal "switch" (as in Fig. 8.19). Prodromal to the arrest, some subjects may show a quantitative increase in the magnitude of ST elevation.[107] The Brugadas[96] have emphasised the absence of cardiac pathology in this syndrome, which they regard as a func-

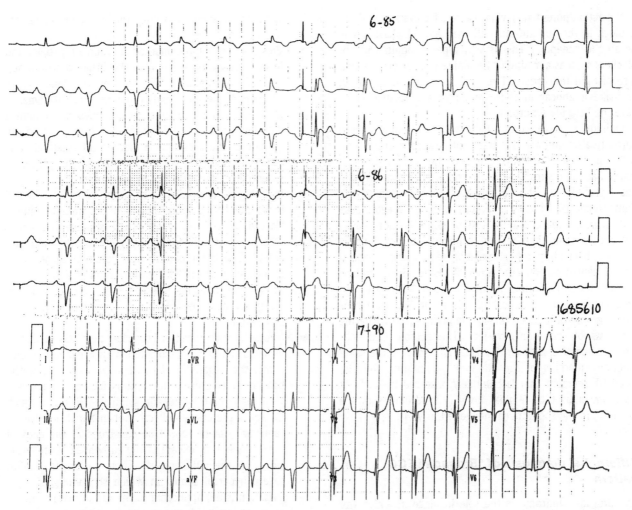

6-85

6-86

1685610

7-90

I aVR V1 V4
II aVL V2 V5
III aVF V3 V6

Figure 8.19 Brugada syndrome. Family history of SCD (father and brother < age 50). This woman suffered near-syncope at age 58; she had His bundle electrocardiography because of the bifascicular pattern. The HV was prolonged. She was aged 72 in the 1990 tracing, which shows the ST segment totally normalised in V1, V2. Died of Alzheimer's age 74.

tional electrophysiologic disorder. By way of contrast an identical ECG pattern was linked to right ventricular myopathy by groups in Padua[108] and Osaka,[109] but recent studies found this variant in only 11 out of the 174 subjects accumulated in the literature. The total represents those patients who were symptomatic, plus those of their relatives showing the specific Brugada ECG pattern.[110] This cohort showed a greater than 10:1 male/female ratio, and a 60% Asian origin; most subjects were in their 40s, with a wide age range. A fifth had a family history of VF, SCD, or syncope. Even in the absence of obvious or biopsied RV pathology, the frequency of a prolonged H-V time[111] suggests that the His–Purkinje system may be damaged or "dispersed".[112] Unlike the long QT syndrome, the R-R cycles prodromal to the syncopal event do not have pause-dependent or other structural features. The event is most likely to be nocturnal.

Cellular mechanisms in Brugada syndrome

Maintenance of an isoelectric ST segment is dependent on the absence of an voltage gradient between endocardial and epicardial myocytes. The latter normally exhibit a spike-and-dome shape in the action potential, the spike being the phase zero, the nadir between the latter, and the dome being phase 1. While the latter morphology is the mark of the transient outward current (I_{to}), the sodium current determines the voltage value at which this phase commences. The Brugada type right precordial ST elevation may arise if I_{to} is "unopposed" by, for example, loss or diminution of the calcium inward current (I_{ca}). This permits a gross exaggeration in the "depth" of the nadir, potentially reaching the baseline, with a resulting diminution or loss of the epicardial dome, and shortening of the action potential. A gradient thus appears during phase 2 of the action potentials giving rise to ST elevation. If there is block in the sodium current, the nadir of phase 1 will be all the "deeper". This is why type 1 sodium current blockers such as ajmaline or flecainide can restore the pattern of right precordial ST elevation if it has disappeared, or make it appear in those asymptomatic relatives who have the Brugada syndrome.[113]

Quinidine on the other hand while blocking sodium current, also inhibits the transient inward current, and will achieve the opposite effect. If the loss of dome is marked at some sites but not at others, re-entrant arrhythmia is facilitated. The confining of ST elevation to the right precordial leads is in accord with the greater ease with which, experimentally, loss of dome is more easily induced in right than in left ventricular myocardium.[114] Whereas beta-adrenergic stimulation reduces right precordial ST elevation, beta-adrenergic blockade, alpha-adrenergic and muscarinic stimulation enhance it.[107] In case 6 of probably the earliest report of this syndrome, treatment with metoprolol induced torsade de pointes; the triggering VPC was of the R-on-T variety. The ectopic QRS was strongly negative with an rS shape, and showed the same indefinite merging of the elevated J point into the elevated ST segment that is habitually observed in V_2.[115] At least one subset of familial Brugada syndrome shows a mutation in the sodium channel gene (*SCN5A*).[116]

Differential diagnosis of "Brugada" ECG pattern

The Brugada syndrome is the sole instance in which the threat of SCD is exhibited in the ECGs of individuals without structural heart disease, or long QT interval. It is vital that the very idiosyncratic and specific elements of this ECG morphology be considered, because each component ECG feature, taken in isolation, is commonly seen in the ECGs of individuals in no danger of losing their lives. Among the 10 electrode locations of the standard 12-lead ECG the V_1 and V_2 locations are intrinsically distinctive:

- They are the closest to the heart; in many subjects there is not even a slip of lung tissue between V_2 and the right ventricular epicardium.
- Aside from Einthoven's lead III, and aVL, V_1 is the only adult lead permitted to show positive or negative T waves.
- It can also show an initial Q wave, rather than an r, though this is less common before the age of 30.
- V_2 is the lead most likely to show R wave-coupled artefact in the early ST segment, possibly owing to right ventricular mechanical "thump".
- V_2 is the lead most likely to show both J point elevation and ST segment elevation[117] in entirely normal

subjects (maximum value for J point elevation: 330 mcV[118]).

- This feature is more marked in younger people, and in men (features common to the Brugada syndrome). Nor is the aforesaid ST elevation fundamentally a component piece of "early repolarisation": it demands no inferolateral components and does not diminish with heart rate. The J point in V_1/V_2 is quite often isoelectric in the presence of marked inferolateral early repolarisation, which, in the horizontal plane, is essentially, a post-transitional phenomenon.
- In 2.9% of the normal population[119] an rSr^1 is found in V_1 and or V_2, variously called "incomplete RBBB", "late depolarisation of the crista supraventricularis", "the rSr^1 pattern", "right ventricular basal conduction delay". The latter pattern is a common cause of an exaggeration of the ST elevation seen in V_2 (as if the r prime was hoisting the segment in question Fig. 8.20). In these tracings, the T wave is generally not inverted in V_2.
- In case 3 of the triad of Brugada-type ECGs published in 1953[120] but not associated with a dangerous outcome, the negativity of the T wave in V_2 below the baseline was present but minuscule, as is the case with many of the Brugada syndrome ECGs. In such instances the entire collective of maximal positive ST value or "J point" could be construed as the apex of the T wave – an exceptionally early apex – unusually close to the QRS onset. Such closeness typifies severe hypercalcaemia, in which shortening of repolarisation is not applicable to the QT interval so much as to the interval between onset of QRS and the apex of T in V_1 and or V_2 (Fig. 8.21). At cellular level the underlying causes of this pattern and that of the Brugada syndrome are not dissimilar.[121]
- Recently raised[122] is the possibility that right precordial ST elevation with the typical fat r prime and convex upward ST descent to a T inversion – identical to that of the Brugada syndrome – can be induced by a type 1C agent alone in a subject not otherwise at risk.
- Finally, acute right ventricular infarction can selectively elevate the ST in V_1, even without the usual companion evidence of acute inferior injury (see Fig. 8.15)

The aforementioned biphasic variation or dyad (from elevation of the J point, to its isoelectric restoration), are shown in Figs 8.19 and 8.22. The former female patient had suffered syncope 20 years before, had shown H-V prolongation during His bundle ECG (performed because of the presumption of bifascicular block:left anterior hemiblock plus incomplete RBBB), but was not subjected to "provocative" ventricular stimulation. She remained quite

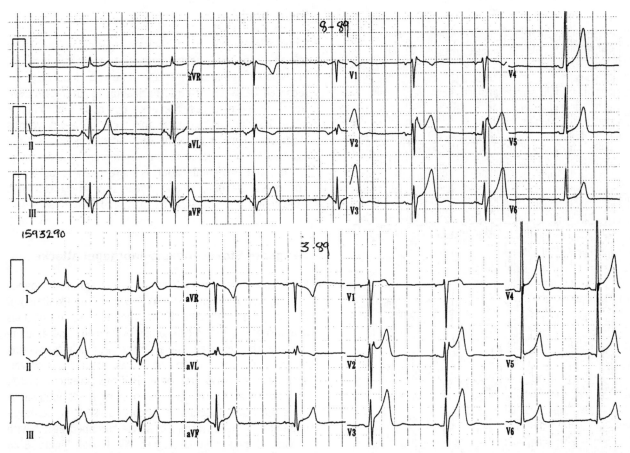

Figure 8.20 ST segment peculiarities with incomplete RBBB. Early repolarisation is present in inferolateral leads. ST elevations are marked in V2; variable definition of the J point.

active until she developed Alzheimer's dementia at the age of 73. The family history was positive for SCD. Figure 8.22 also comes from a woman in her 70s without either a family history or ventricular arrhythmia. She suffered atypical chest pain; angiography showed normal coronary arteries and ventricular function. The isoelectric restoration of the ST in V_1, V_2 in Fig. 8.22 is not of variable quantitative degree (as might be blamed on lead placement), but categoric and unequivocal. Conspicuous is how little change is seen in the other ten leads during the change in phase.

Arrhythmogenic right ventricular dysplasia or cardiomyopathy

This can share electrocardiographic features with the Brugada syndrome[108,109] but has a definite structural basis: the excessive infiltration of the right heart with fatty tissue (the left heart is eventually involved also). The ECG usually shows a widened QRS which is more overt in V_1 than in V_6. T is inverted in V_1–V_3. In 30% of cases there is

an epsilon wave, a very small depolarisation blip in the ST segment of V_2; it represents extreme delay of myocardial conduction within a small mass of right ventricular tissue. Ventricular tachycardia is common and can originate in one of three right ventricular sites.

Familial SCD with a euthermic Osborn wave

Familial SCD with a euthermic Osborn wave, but without any sign of cardiomyopathy, was reported in a Hispanic family. The ECG showed, in left ventricular precordial leads, the terminal slow wave that one would usually see in hypothermia. Neither complete or incomplete RBBB were present. The inferior leads, also left ventricular in shape (axis 55–70°) showed a tiny early dip in the ST segment, resembling a small retrograde P, or an epsilon wave: a small area of myocardium depolarised late. It corresponded with a late potential in the signal-averaged high resolution recording. Echo and complete catheterisation were normal. The abnormality in the ECG was completely eliminated by quinidine.[124]

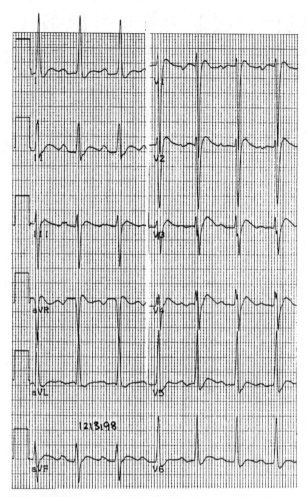

Figure 8.21 Peculiarities of repolarisation in V1, V2: there is no clear definition of the J point; the ST-T appears elevated. A case of severe hypercalcaemia (Ca^{2+}: 17.2 mg/dl).

Simulation of epsilon or ST segment depolarisation blips

Notoriously, V_2 is subject to R wave-coupled artefact of the ST blip type (Fig. 8.23). That these are not true late depolarisations is shown by their lack of reproducibility and the absence of any right ventricular dysplasia etc. in such subjects.

Risk of bradycardic death

Bradycardic SCD

Bradycardic SCD constitutes about 11% of all SCD. The ECG is only of prognostic value when it shows evidence of deterioration in the specialised nodes and fibres of the conduction system.

Sinus bradycardia

Sinus rates below 40, a constant shifting in successive tracings from atrial tachyarrhythmia to sinus or junctional bradycardia, prolonged escape intervals following the recorded cessation of atrial fibrillation or after cardioversion – all these suggest the sick sinus node syndrome, or more descriptively accurate: the tachycardia–bradycardia syndrome. A major cause of asystolic syncope, it is often associated with disease in the conduction system downstream, and this combination is more likely to be lethal. The respective one, 5- and 7-year survival figures for a large cohort were 85–92%, 62–65%, and 52%.[125]

Danger of Stokes–Adams–Morgagni attacks

Bifascicular block by itself has a 4% per annum incidence of complete or symptomatic AV block.[126] The likelihood of this event is increased if, in the absence of digitalis administration, the P-R becomes prolonged. The assumption that this represents delay in the residually conducting fascicle was correct in 66% of 40 cases studied. However, such delay was also present by H-V measurement in 30% of bifascicular blocks showing a normal PR interval. A more pressing prediction of syncopal asystole is the development in 12-lead tracings of single "dropped beats" with Mobitz II type second degree AV block. Figure 8.24 shows such an occurrence in every third beat. Type II second degree AV block most often develops in a substrate of fixed bifascicular block: Right bundle branch plus left anterior fascicular block commands 70–85% of this group, followed then by complete left bundle branch block, and RBBB plus posterior fascicular block. In the minority the tracing shows a narrow QRS. The lesion may be in the mainstem His bundle. In Figure 8.25 there is a normal 12-lead ECG (except for ectopic atrial rhythm). Two events are repeatedly seen: type II AV block and type II block in the left bundle branch. This tracing raises the possibility of a single lesion in the mainstem His bundle, which at times induces complete transverse blocking of the supraventricular impulse, and at other times imposes block predivisionally on only those fibres destined or "predestined" for the left bundle branch. Alternatively there are two distinct mainstem and left bundle lesions. In rare instances one records recurrent beat-by-beat degeneration into trifascicular block, the first beat of each cadence showing near normal IV conduction (Fig. 8.26).

Acute atrioventricular block: rhythm options

Either conduction resumes, an escape rhythm develops, or death ensues. The symptoms with the first two conditions

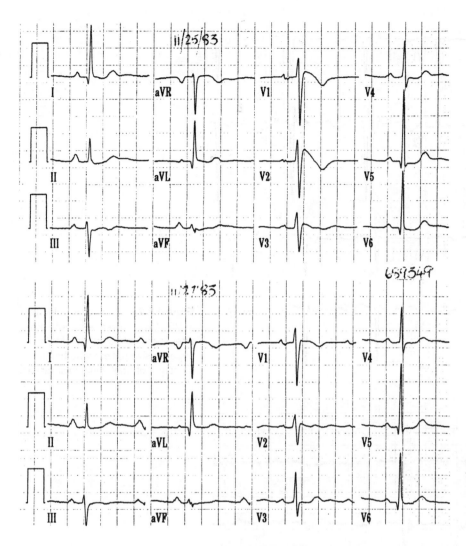

Figure 8.22 Brugada physiology. The bottom tracing shows that the normalisation phase exclusively changes V_1–V_3. The other leads remain identical.

depend on the duration of asystole, ranging from no symptoms to dizziness, to syncope, to anoxic convulsions. Restoration of the heart beat by either may not fully restore consciousness. The patient will remain deeply obtunded if the restored heart beat is excessively bradycardic. This can happen if resumed conduction is not 1/1 but, for example, high degree AV block (5/1, 4/1), or if the escape rhythm fails to "warm up" and continues at 20 bpm. Without an artificial pacemaker, the prognosis is dire in these situations.

Acute nodal versus infranodal block

Acute AV nodal block often shows companion sudden sinus slowing, the two events being due to a vagal surge (with or without evidence of carotid sinus hypersensitivity, which often shows a baseline P-R prolongation). The sinus rate is unchanged in infranodal block. The higher the level of block

the greater the number of potential subsidiary escape centres, and the faster the intrinsic escape rate ("the lower the slower"). When acute AV block is trifascicular, the escape rhythm is either idioventricular or, less commonly, fascicular, just distal to the final blocking lesion (generally in the posterior fascicle, the idio-QRS is unchanged from that of sinus rhythm). The time to the first escape is powerfully influenced by the sinus rate at the time of conduction failure: "the faster the rate, the longer the wait". Physiologically there is an actual moment of expectation with regard to the time to the first escape beat. Loss of pulse wave will induce a baroreceptor-mediated adrenergic reflex that will steepen the diastolic slope of sluggish latent idioventricular pacemakers. Figure 8.27 shows when such a sympathetic release causes the PP interval to shorten, at about 2.7 s into the arrest. If the escape rhythm fails to show "warm–up" and remains excessively slow, the patient will stay obtunded until artificially paced. Death in patients with these clinical substrates may be due to absence of either resumed con-

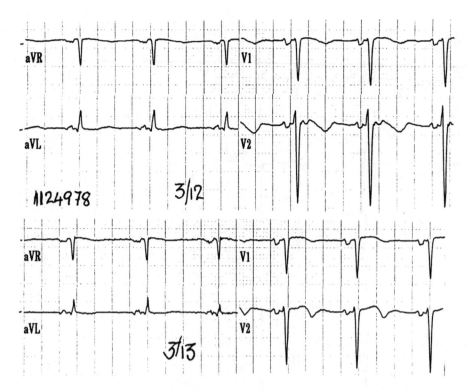

Figure 8.23 Pseudo-epsilon blip in V2. It was never seen before or after in multiple tracings of this hypertensive patient who had no evidence of right ventricular disease.

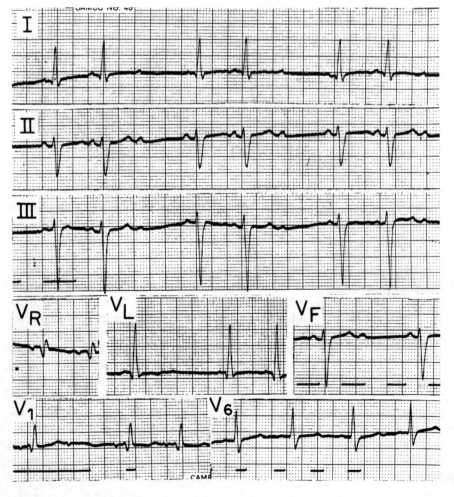

Figure 8.24 Trifascicular block: in a substrate tracing of RBBB and left anterior hemiblock there is 2nd-degree AV block with 3/2 Mobitz II sequences.

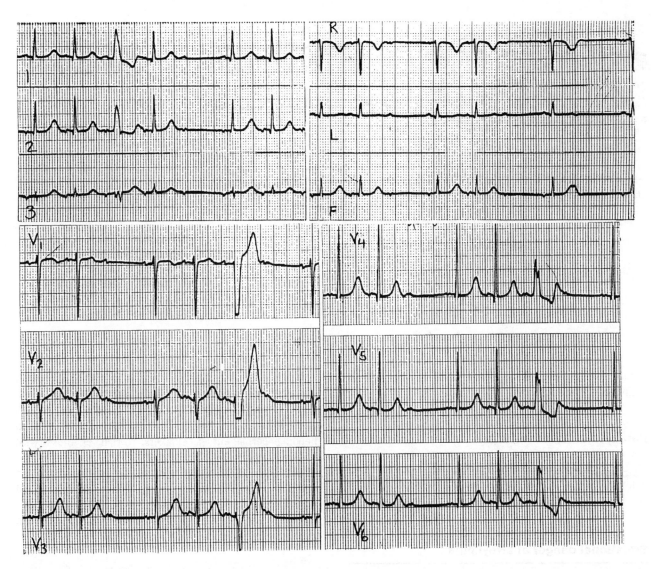

Figure 8.25 Presumption of either predivisional LBBB or two separate lesions. Many Mobitz II dropped QRS complexes suggesting main stem His bundle block. Also present: single Mobitz II phenomena in the LBB. A single lesion in the main His bundle may express itself as either "fully transverse" or "hemisectional", blocking only those fibres predestined for the LBB.

duction, or an escape beat. It should not be forgotten that many patients with bifascicular block get syncope from paroxysmal ventricular tachycardia, not complete heart block. It may be that mortality is more closely related to the severity of the underlying disease rather than the conduction deficit *per se*.

The postectopic catastrophe

AV block

Proposed by Langendorf, who showed it occurring in the wake of a blocked PAC,[127] this phenomenon is controversial. It has long been noted that Mobitz II AV block some-

times follows a VPC (see Fig. 8.27). Attempts to reproduce this phenomenon by intracavitary premature ventricular stimulation have been fruitless.[128] One is left with the possibility that the occurrence of the ectopic is merely coincidental, that AV block was going to occur at this time anyhow, or one is forced to seek a physiologic explanation. One candidate mechanism is bradycardia or phase 4-induced AV block, made possible by the postectopic pause (see bradycardia-related BBB).

Extinction of automaticity

Transient postectopic depression of sinus rate by a PAC is common. During unpaced complete heart block, idioven-

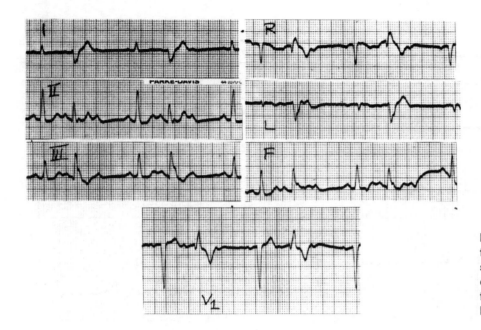

Figure 8.26 Beat-by-beat fascicular block. The sinus Ps shows consecutively: near-normal conduction, RBBB plus posterior fascicular block, and trifascicular block; PR unchanging.

tricular rhythm can similarly be depressed or even perhaps extinguished by a VPC.

Paroxysmal AV or exit block

AV block or asystole from exit block (Fig. 8.28) can suddenly occur without premature stimulation in both sinus and idiorhythms.[129]

Situational danger of arrhythmia

Situational AV block

Invasive or surgical procedures. Apart from the addition of a long PR interval to fixed bifascicular block, patients with the latter pattern are greatly at risk if a procedure threatens the controlateral conducting fascicle. The classic example is the passage of a Swann–Ganz or Cournand right heart catheter in the presence of complete LBBB. Less threatening is the passage of left ventricular cavity catheters in the presence of complete RBBB. Other situations are the development of acute pulmonary embolism in patients with LBBB. In such instances the embolism is announced by an asystolic arrest.

Surgical AV block: tetralogy of Fallot

Whilst RBBB follows correction of most VSDs and tetralogy of Fallot (as well as 80% of cardiac transplantations),

it is a benign complication. It may be due to the patch placement or resection of a right ventricular infundibulum. Temporary complete heart block is seen in up to 22% of patients in the first few hours, but only 2% end up needing permanent pacemakers.[130] Half of those with transient complete block retain a bifascicular pattern. About 1% of these patients have late asystole or SCD a decade or more following surgery. Congenitally corrected transposition of the great vessels has a unique predisposition to complete AV block both with and without surgical correction of the occasionally associated VSD.

Ventricular tachycardia after congenital heart surgery

This is rare under the age of 5 and is a more common cause of SCD than heart block. Both may occur without cardiac surgery. The leading malformations associated with SCD are tetralogy of Fallot, aortic stenosis, and Eisenmenger's physiology. Ventricular tachycardia is not seen in subjects who fail to show VPCs in follow-up 12-lead ECGs. Holter recordings do not refine or hone this simple observation. Of the 19% who do show VPCs in follow-up ECGs, the SCD mortality is 30%. Those who develop ventricular tachyarrhythmias or SCD often show an unusually widened QRS (>180 ms). Certain operative procedures for correction of congenital heat disease anomalies carry a higher than usual risk of complete AV block: the closure of very high VSDs is an example of same.

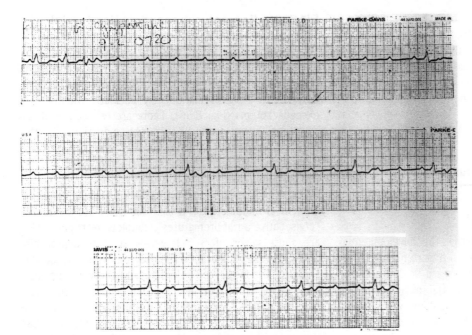

Figure 8.27 Stokes–Adams attack in presence of LBBB. Reflex increase in sinus rate is evident in the 4th "empty" PP interval about 2.7 seconds from the last QRS. The first escape falls 8 seconds after the latter. Note AV block starts after a PVC.

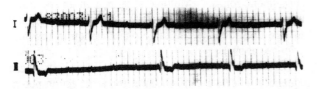

Figure 8.28 Complete heart block with idioventricular rhythm and type II single impulse exit block. (Reproduced with permission from Langendorf R, Pick A. Causes and mechanisms of ventricular asystole in advanced A-V block. In: Surawicz B, Pellegrino ED eds. *Sudden cardiac death.* New York: Grune & Stratton, 1964.)

Transposition: postoperative arrhythmias

After the "atrial switch" procedure of Mustard, these may show evidence of a "sick sinus node", the result of compromise of its blood supply. Late SCD after surgical correction of transposition may not be easy to explain. There is the suggestion that part of the problem may reside in the conduction system[131]: a pathologic reaction to the surgical procedure *per se*.

Risk of arrhythmia in Ebstein's anomaly

One-third of patients develop paroxysmal supraventricular arrhythmias, even without the commonly present accessory pathways. The latter may be multiple, unidirectional, and often intermittent. RBBB is seen in 75–95%. Neither complete heart block nor ventricular tachycardia are common. Once atrial fibrillation becomes chronic, death is

likely within 5 years,[132] a statistic that includes those subjects in whom ablation of tracts had not yet been performed. The longer the survival the wider the sinus P wave becomes, the result of right atrial stretch, which predicts eventual fibrillation or flutter.

Pharmacologic interventions with risk of AV block

Unique among these are the intravenous digitalisation of a patient with hypokalaemia or hypercalcaemia. These events are much less likely nowadays with measurable serum digoxin levels. The most common induction of AV block occurs when a patient, fully or excessively digitalised, is given intravenous calcium for some reason. It is particularly hazardous if the patient already has a raised serum calcium.

Situational asystole

Temporary pacemakers are sometimes required when a completed inferior MI is complicated by advanced AV nodal block. When the pacemaker is turned off to establish the status of the native rhythm, a long period of asystole may follow if the rhythm is idioventricular and the paced rate is not first reduced to a minimum ("the faster the rate, the longer the wait"). The same phenomenon is seen in the tachycardia–bradycardia syndrome when a paroxysm of atrial fibrillation finishes and there is no sinus or subsidiary escape of any kind. In this syndrome

(Fig. 8.29), a generalised disorder of automaticity, the sinus and ectopic atrial escape centres can be regarded as overdrive – suppressed by the atrial fibrillatory impulses – and the His–Purkinje centres suppressed by the rapid ventricular rate. The situation can sometimes be iatrogenically duplicated by cardioverting lone atrial fibrillation in the elderly.

Arrhythmia and decreased survival

Risk of atrial fibrillation

The Framingham Study[133] showed that the development of atrial fibrillation was associated with hypertension, congestive failure and rheumatic heart disease in that order. It nearly doubled the overall mortality, and made a cardiovascular death twice as likely. Similar outcome was noted in a large cohort of patients with coronary disease.[134] Quite apart from these named diseases, there is the more recently-ventilated but still fluid issues of fibrillation-related ventriculopathy,[135] and atriopathy,[136] the former owing to an habitually uncontrolled ventricular rate, the latter from the induction – by fibrillation *per se* – of atrial enlargement, with possibly a specific histopathology,[137] and "electric remodelling".[138]

Electocardiographic presentiments of atrial fibrillation and flutter

Flutter is intimately related to P wave width. Intra-atrial block is more closely associated with paroxysmal atrial flutter than atrial fibrillation,[139] particularly when P in II exceeds 160 ms (Fig. 8.30). There are two stages of risk of either flutter or fibrillation. The induction of either requires atrial premature beats, so there is a statistical risk related to the frequency of atrial ectopic impulse formation (significant with >10/min), but there is also a sign of impending atrial flutter or fibrillation. This is the development of *multiple atrial responses*. These are not merely "consecutive atrial prematures", couplets, or triplets. They are short salvos of 3–5 P waves at rates approaching 300 bpm (Fig. 8.31). Typically they follow a blocked PAC and, like the latter, fail to conduct to the ventricle, each of them entering and "dying within" the AV node; however deeply they traverse the latter, they leave a refractory wake that blocks the succeeding impulse, which repeats the process, creating primary, secondary, tertiary, etc. concealment zones.[140] Multiple atrial responses are examples of encroachment on the atrial vulnerable period, and thus are congruent to the same phenomonon in the ventricle (see above).

The shortness of the atrial cycle length in these sequences reflects a contraction of the atrial action poten-

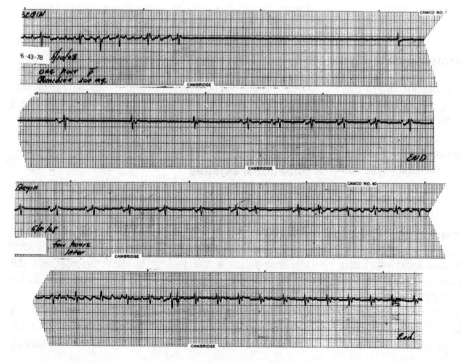

Figure 8.29 Prediction of asystolic syncope in the tachycardia-bradycardia syndrome. Spontaneous arrest of the paroxysmal atrial fibrillation is not followed by any prompt sinus, atrial, junctional, or ventricular escape. A junctional escape fires after a pause of 5.6 seconds. Sinus rhythm is slow to return. Hours later fibrillation returns, then junctional tachycardia with retrograde conduction.

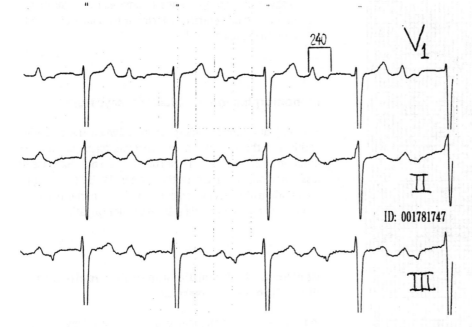

240

V_1

II

ID: 001781747

III.

Figure 8.30 Marked intra-atrial block recorded shortly before paroxysmal atrial flutter. The P wave duration was 240 ms.

tial duration and refractory period. It has been shown that maladaptation of refractorines to changes in rate is commonly present.[141] Multiple responses may be seen both before the onset and soon after the conversion of atrial fibrillation, particularly if the latter seems unlikely to hold.

Identifying the 12-lead characteristics of the provoking PAC

This has proven difficult. P wave shape and axis can be the same with multiple sites of origin. Morover, there is not as yet a typical or even recognisably common geographic site of origin for such a PAC, though recent studies have focused on extensions of atrial myocardium into the inserting pulmonary veins.[142]

Arrhythmia: signs of bad becoming worse or *vice versa*

Clandestine events in digitalis intoxication

When digitalis excess causes complete heart block at the AV nodal level in atrial fibrillation, the tracing not rarely looks like a simple junctional rhythm. Advanced glycoside excess often causes, selective to the upper cardiac chambers, an excessively low voltage, or even seeming absence, of atrial events, be they P waves, the F waves of flutter or the ff oscillations of fibrillation. This apparent banishment of ECG events is the result of high resistance or effective

"closure" of atrial gap junctions by the glycoside[143]: essentially a state of atrial paralysis may ensue. The unwary observer may assume that the absent P waves are "retrograde within the QRS". In such a fashion all three diagnoses may be missed: atrial fibrillation, complete AV nodal block, and digitalis poisoning.[144]

Severity of digitalis poisoning

While "PAT with block" is attributed to delayed afterdepolarisations in the atria, similarly triggered automaticity in the ventricle is more subtle – short of actual ventricular tachycardia. The fundamental feature is the foreshortened ventricular escape interval. It is induced to appear when the RR intervals shorten. Fig. 8.32 shows such an example.

Monomorphic right ventricular tachycardia: prognosis by QRS pattern

A pattern of LBBB defines the several tachycardias that originate in the right ventricle.

● If the baseline sinus rhythm ECG shows LBBB or a non-specific IVCD, and the rate of the tachycardia is very rapid (cycle length circa 280 ms), a bundle branch re-entrant mechanism should especially be considered if the underlying diagnosis is dilated cardiomyopathy. Ablation of the RBB in this context removes a major cause of SCD in this disease, since

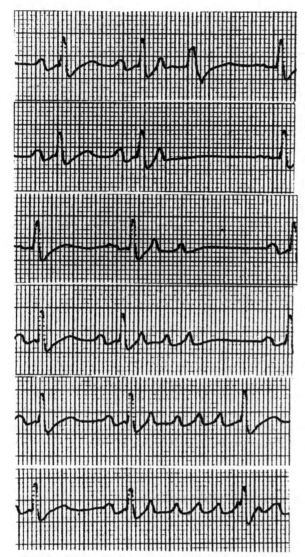

Figure 8.31 Harbinger of fibrillation/flutter. Selections from a lead II rhythm strip showing multiple atrial responses to a PAC (blocked in all but the top strip). A sustained arrhythmia is finally induced at bottom.

bundle branch re-entry constitutes 64% of all ventricular tachycardias seen with DCM.[145]

- If the patient is male, the baseline ECG shows T inversion in V_1–V_3, the QRS showing some QRS widening (0.11 s), with or without incomplete RBBB, right ventricular dysplasia should be considered; the tachycardia frontal axis may show axis deviation of either extreme.
- A normal heart, and excellent prognosis can be expected if the frontal axis is +90° to −180°, the QRS in aVL shows QS, and there are no qR or QR shapes anywhere. Exercise may be the trigger for such a

tachycardia. The presence in any lead of a qR or QR in a LBB-type ventricular tachycardia points directly to an ischaemic origin.[146]

Monomorphic left ventricular tachycardia

The only difference in morphology between the rare idiopathic and the very common ischaemic forms is the QRS duration: 125 +/− 9 versus 166 +/− 25 ms. Exercise is less commonly a trigger in the former. While the prognosis of idiopathic tachycardia is good, its perpetual form can result in a tachycardia-related cardiomyopathy.[147]

Ventricular tachycardia: impending ventricular fibrillation – or conversion?

Ventricular tachycardia may change in the following three ways:

- increase its rate
- decrease its rate
- widen its already widened QRS.

The significance of these changes depend very substantially on whether one is administering antiarrhythmic medication. The last two responses are common just prior to conversion with procain amide. Nor does the widening automatically signify overdosage. When sinus rhythm reappears, the QRS will probably be normal or "baseline": the widening with tachycardia simply a use-dependent change. Spontaneous acceleration and slowing are common preconversion changes, the first suggesting that the impulse within the re-entrant loop may be "catching up on itself", the second that conduction is decrementing within the loop. The most likely sign of impending ventricular fibrillation is a widening of the self-same QRS *in the absence of* treatment.

"Priming" of ventricular fibrillation

"Priming" of ventricular fibrillation during cardiopulmonary resuscitation is signified by larger fibrillatory waves with increased dV/dT; the latter reflects an improved rise time in the individuated myocyte action potentials. This promising change is achieved by epinephrine and the elimination of an acidemic milieu by adequate closed–chest massage oxygenation, and possibly also bicarbonate administration.

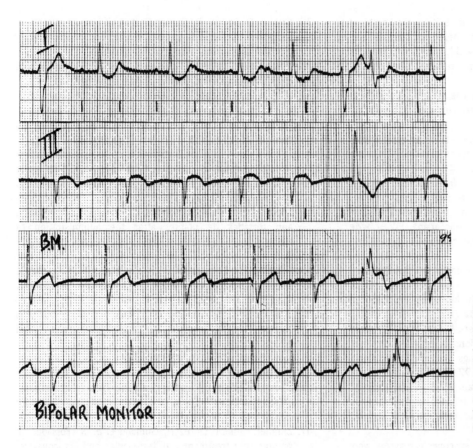

Figure 8.32 Advanced digitalis intoxication. Incomplete AV nodal block [vertical bars: P waves]. Ventricular ectopy with "foreshortened" escape intervals appear when RR intervals shorten (AV captures). Presumption of ventricular delayed after-depolarisations (DADs).

References

1. Viskin S, Belhassen B. Polymorphic ventricular tachy-arrhythmias in the absence of organic heart disease: Classification, differential diagnosis and implications for therapy: *Prog Cardiovasc Dis* 1998;**41**:17–34.

2. Viskin S, Lesh MD, Eldar M *et al*. Mode of onset of malignant ventricular arrhythmias in idiopathic ventricular fibrillation. *J Cardiovasc Electrophysiol* 1997;**8**:1115–1120.

3. Leenhardt A, Glaser E, Barguera M *et al*. Short-coupled variant of torsades de pointes. A new electrocardiographic entity in the spectrum of idiopathic ventricular tachy-arrhythmias. *Circulation* 1994;**89**:206–15.

4. Belhassen B, Shapira I, Shoshani D *et al*. Idiopathic ventricular fibrillation: Inducibility and beneficial effects of Class 1 antiarrhythmic agents. *Circulation* 1987;**75**:809–16.

5. Leenhardt A, Lucet V, Denjoy I *et al*. Catecholaminergic polymorphic ventricular tachycardia in children. A 2-year follow-up of 21 patients. *Circulation* 1995;**91**:1512–19.

6. Zipes DP, Wellens HJJ. Sudden cardiac death. *Circulation* 1998;**98**:2334–51.

7. Tye KH, Desser KB, Benchimol A. Survival following spontaneous ventricular flutter–fibrillation association with QT syndrome. *Arch Intern Med* 1980;**140**:255–6.

8. Schwartz SP, Orloff J, Fox C. Transient ventricular fibrillation. I. The prefibrillatory period during established auriculoventricular dissociation with a note on the phonocardiograms obtained at such times. *Am Heart J* 1949;**37**:21–9.

9. Schwartz PJ, Periti M, Malliani A. The long QT syndrome *Am Heart J* 1975;**89**:378–90.

10. Jervell A, Lange-Nielsen F Congenital deaf-mutism, functional heart disease with prolongation of the QT interval, and sudden death. *Am Heart J* 1957;**54**:59–68.

11. Romano C. Congenital cardiac arrhythmia. *Lancet* 1965;1:658–9.

12. Ward OC. The electrocardiographic abnormality in familial cardiac arrhythmia. *Ir J Med Sci* 1965;**6**:553–7.

13. Vincent GM, Timothy KW, Leppert M, Keating M. The spectre of symptoms and QT intervals in carriers of the gene for the long-QT syndrome. *New Engl J Med* 1992;**327**:846–52.

14. Coumel P, Leclercq JF, Lucet V. Possible mechanisms of the arrhythmias in the long QT syndrome. *Eur Heart J* 1985;**6**:115–29 (Suppl. D).

15. Jackman WM, Friday KJ, Anderson JL, Aliot EM, Clark M, Lazzara R. The long QT syndrome: a critical review, new clinical observations and a unifying hypothesis. *Prog Cardiovasc Dis* 1988;**31**:115–72.

16. Moss AJ, Schwartz PJ, Crampton RS *et al*. The long QT syndrome. Prospective longitudinal study of 328 families. *Circulation* 1991;**84**:1136–44.

17. Moss AJ, Zareba W, Benhorin J *et al*. ECG T–wave patterns in genetically distinct forms of the hereditary long QT syndrome. *Circulation* 1995;**92**:2929–34.

18. Bazett HC. An analysis of the time relations of electrocardiograms. *Heart* 1920;**7**:353–67.

19. Molnar J, Weiss JS, Rosenthal JE. The missing second: what is the correct unit for the Bazett corrected QT interval? *Am J Cardiol* 1995;**75**:537–8.

20. Zhang L, Timothy KW, Vincent GM *et al*. Can cardiologists predict long QT syndrome genotypes by ECG ST-T wave patterns? *PACE* 1999 (Suppl.);**22**:714.

21. Te–Chuan Chou. *Electrocardiography in clinical practice*. Philadelphia: WB Saunders, 1996, p. 14.

22. MacFarlane PW, Lawrie TDV. The normal electrocardiogram and vectocardiogram. In: MacFarlane PW, Lawrie TDV eds. *Comprehensive electrocardiology 1*. New York: Pergamon Press, 1989, p. 424.

23. Savelieva I, Camm AJ, Malik M. Gender-specific difference in QT interval components duration and relation to cardiac cycle length: why are women at higher risk of drug-induced torsade de pointes. *PACE* 1999;**22**:715.

24. Locati EH, Zareba W, Moss AJ *et al*. Age- and sex-related difference in clinical manifestations in patients with congenital long-QT syndrome: findings from the International LQTS Registry. *Circulation* 1998;**97**:2237–44.

25. Schwartz PJ, Locati EH, Napolitano C *et al*. The long QT syndrome. In: Zipes DP, Jalife J eds. *Cardiac electrophysiology. From cell to bedside*, 2nd edn. Philadelphia: WB Saunders, 1995, p. 804.

26. Selzer A, Wray HW. Quinidine syncope: paroxysmal ventricular fibrillation occurring during treatment of chronic atrial arrhythmias. *Circulation* 1964; **30**:17–26.

27. Strasberg B, Sclarovsky S, Erdberg A *et al*. Procainamide-induced polymorphous ventricular tachycardia. *Am J Cardiol* 1981;**47**:1309–14.

28. Robert EW, McMorrow M, Martin RP. Atypical ventricular tachycardia as a manifestation of disopyramide toxicity. *Am J Cardiol* 1978;**42**:1049.

29. Clark M, Lazzara R, Jackman WM. Torsades de pointes: serum drug levels and ECG warning signs. *Circulation* 1982;**66**:II–71(Abstr.).

30. Bens JL, Quiret JC, Lesbre JP. Torsades de pointes, une expression syncopale par hypokaliemie. *Coeur Med Intern* 1968;**1**:293.

31. Topol EJ, Lerman BB. Hypomagnesemic torsades de pointes *Am J Cardiol* 1983;**52**:1367–8.

32. Kahn MM, Logan KR, McComb JM *et al*. Management of recurrent ventricular tachyarrhythmias associated with QT prolongation. *Am J Cardiol* 1981;**47**:1301–8.

33. Jackman WM, Clark M, Friday KJ *et al*. Ventricular tachyarrhythmias in the long QT syndrome. *Med Clin North Am* 1984;**68**:1079–109.

34. Ostermaier R, vonEssen R. Amiodarone and torsade de pointes (letter). *Circulation* 1996;**94**:2316–18.

35. Manouvrier J, Sagot M, Caron C *et al*. Nine cases of torsades de pointes with bepridil administration. *Am Heart J* 1986;**111**:1005–7.

36. Kuck KH, Kunze KP, Roewer N *et al*. Sotalol-induced torsades de pointes. *Am Heart J* 1984;**107**:179–80.

37. Guelon D, Bedock B, Cartier C *et al*. QT prolongation and recurrent "torsades de pointes" during erythromycin lactobionate infusion *Am J Cardiol* 1986;**58**:666.

38. Singh BN, Gaarder TD, Kanegae T *et al*. Liquid protein diets and torsades de pointes. *JAMA* 1978;**240**:115–19.

39. Johansson BW. Adam–Stokes syndrome: A review and follow-up study of forty-two cases *Am J Cardiol* 1961;**8**:76–93.

40. Krikler DM, Curry PVL. Torsades de pointes, an atypical ventricular tachycardia. *Br Heart J* 1976;**38**:117–20.

41. Ludomirsky A, Klein HO, Sarelli P *et al*. QT prolongation and polymorphous ("torsades de pointes") ventricular arrhythmias associated with organophosphate poisoning. *Am J Cardiol* 1982;**49**:1654–8.

42. Lopez JA, Harold JG, Rosenthal MC *et al*. QT prolongation and torsades de pointes after the administration of trimethoprim–sulfamethoxazole. *Am J Cardiol* 1987;**59**: 376–7.

43. Wharton JM, Demopulos PA, Goldschlager N. Torsades de pointes during administration of pentamidine isethionate. *Am J Med* 1987;**83**:571–6.

44. Zee–cheng CHS, Mueller CE, Seifert CHF, Gibbs HR. Haloperidol and torsades de pointes. *Ann Intern Med* 1985;1**02**:18.

45. Kriwisky M, Perry GY, Tarchitsky D, Gutman Y, Kishon Y. Haloperidol-induced torsades de pointes. *Chest* 1990;**98**:2.

46. Young JB, Vandermolen LA, Pratt CM. Torsades de pointes: an unusual manifestation of chloral hydrate poisoning *Am Heart J* 1986;**112**:181–4.

47. Zimmermann M, Duruz H, Guinand O *et al*. Torsades de pointes after treatment with terfenadine and ketoconazole. *Eur Heart J* 1992;**13**:1002–3.

48. Martyn R, Somberg J, Kenn N. Proarrhythmia of non-antiarrhythmic drugs *Am Heart J* 1993;**126**:201–5.

49. Dessertenne F. La tachycardie ventriculaire a deux foyers opposés variables. *Arch Mal Coeur* 1966;**59**:263–72.

50. Smirk FH, Ng J. Cardiac ballet: repetition of complex electrocardiographic pattern. *Br Heart J* 1969;**31**:426–34.

51. Coumel P, LeClercq J-F, Lucet V. Possible mechanisms of the arrhythmias in the long QT syndrome. *Eur J Cardiol* 1985;**6**(Suppl. D):115–29.

52. Haverkamp W, Shenasa M, Borggrete M *et al*. Torsade de pointes. In: Zipes, DP, Jalife J eds. *Cardiac electrophysiology. From cell to bedside*, 2nd edn. Philadelphia, WB Saunders, 1995, Ch. 79.

53. Zipes DP. Cardiac electrophysiology: promises and contributions. *J Am Coll Cardiol* 1989;**13**:1329–52.

54. Phillips J, Ichinose H. Clinical and pathologic studies in the hereditary syndrome of a long QT syndrome, syncopal spells, and sudden death. *Chest* 1970;**58**:236–43.

55. Wellens HJJ, Vermeulen A, Durrer D. Ventricular fibrillation occurring on arousal from sleep by auditory stimuli. *Circulation* 1972;**46**:661–5.

56. Viersma JW, May JF, de Jongste MJL *et al*. Long QT syndrome and sudden death during sleep in one family. *Eur Heart J* 1988;**9**(Suppl. 1):45.

57. Vincent GM, Jaiswal D, Timothy KW. Effects of exercise on heart rate, QT, QTc and QT/QS2 in the Romano–Ward inherited long QT syndrome. *Am J Cardiol* 1991;**68**:498–503.

58. Childers RW. Time-related perturbations in repolarisation. *J Electrocardiol* 1995;**28**:124.

59. Rosenbaum MB, Blanco HH, Elizari MV, Lazzari JO, Davidenko JM. Electrotonic modulation of the T wave and cardiac memory. *Am J Cardiol* 1982;**50**:213–22.

60. Verrier RL, Nearing BD. T wave alternans as a harbinger of ischemia-induced sudden cardiac death. In: Zipes, DP, Jalife J eds. *Cardiac electrophysiology. From cell to bedside*, 2nd edn. Philadelphia, WB Saunders, 1995, Ch. 45.

61. Rosenbaum DS, He B, Cohen RJ. New approaches for evaluating cardiac electrical activity: repolarisation alternans and body surface Laplacian imaging. In: Zipes, DP, Jalife J eds. *Cardiac electrophysiology. From cell to bedside*, 2nd edn. Philadelphia, WB Saunders, Ch. 104.

62. Sochanski M, Feldman T, Chua KG et al. ST segment alternans during coronary angioplasty. *Catheter Cardiovasc Diag* 1992;**27**:45–8.

63. King MJ, Zir LM, Kaltman AJ et al. Variant angina associated with angiographically demonstrated coronary spasm and REM sleep. *Am J Med* Sci 1973;**265**:419–24.

64. Rihal CS, Gersh BJ. Role of acute myocardial ischemia in the pathogenesis of sudden cardiac death. In: Akhtar M, Myerburg RJ, Ruskin JN eds. *Sudden cardiac death*. Philadelphia: Williams & Wilkins, 1998, p. 302.

65. Rakita L, Borduas SL, Rothman S, Prinzmetal M. Studies on the mechanism of ventricular activity. XII. Early changes in the RS-T segment and QRS complex following acute coronary artery occlusions: Experimental study and clinical applications. *Am Heart J* 1954;**49**:351–8.

66. Childers RW. R wave amplitude in ischemia, injury, and infarction. *J Electrocardiol* 1997;**29**:171.

67. Miller DD, Waters DD, Szlachcic J et al. Clinical characteristics associated with sudden death in patients with variant angina. *Circulation* 1982;**66**:588–93.

68. Dubois C, Pierard LA, Smeets JP et al. Short and long-term prognostic importance of complete bundle branch block complicating acute myocardial infarction. *Clin Cardiol* 1988;**11**:292–6.

69. Newby KH, Pisano E, Krucoff MW et al. Incidence and clinical relevence of the occurrence of bundle-branch block in patients treated with thrombolytic therapy. *Circulation* 1996;**94**:2424–8.

70. Lie KI, Leim KL, Schuilenberg RM et al. Early identification of patients developing late in hospital ventricular fibrillation after discharge from the coronary care unit. *Am J Cardiol* 1978;**41**:674–80.

71. Myerburg RJ, Conde CA, Sung RJ et al. Clinical, electrophysiologic and hemodynamic profile of patients resuscitated from prehospital cardiac arrest. *Am J Med* 1980;**68**:568–74.

72. Oliva PB, Hammil SC, Edwards WD. Cardiac rupture, a clinically predictable complication of acute MI: report of 70 cases with clinicopathologic correlations. *J Am Coll Cardiol* 1993;**22**:720–6.

73. Moss AJ, Goldstein RE, Hall WJ et al. Detection and significance of myocardial ischemia in stable patients after recovery from an acute event. Multicenter Myocardial Ischemia Research Group. *JAMA* 1993;**269**:2379–85.

74. Sapsford RJ, Morrell C, Jackson B et al. Electrocardiograph at presentation for patients hospitalised with acute myocardial infarction – baseline characteristics and value in risk stratification. *Heart* 1999(Suppl. 1);**81**:26.

75. Hyde TA, Straznicky IT, French JK et al. Severity of ST depression predicts 8 year outcome in acute coronary syndromes. *Heart* 1999(Suppl. 1);**81**:36.

76. Campbell RW, Murray A, Julian DG. Ventricular arrhythmias in the first 12 hours of acute myocardial infarction: Natural history study. *Br Heart J* 1981;**46**:351–7.

77. Kleiger RE, Miller JP, Thanavaro S et al. Relationship between clinical features of acute myocardial infarction and ventricular runs two weeks to one year after infarction. *Circulation* 1981;**63**:64–9.

78. Axelrod PJ, Verrier RI, Lown BJ. Vulnerability to ventricular fibrillation during acute coronary arterial occlusion and release. *Am J Cardiol* 1975;**36**:776

79. Kannel WB, Schatzkin A. Sudden death: lessons from subsets in population studies. *J Am Coll Cardiol* 1985;**5**(Suppl.):141B–149B.

80. Friedman M, Manwaring JH, Rosenman RH et al. Instantaneous and sudden deaths: Clinical and pathological differentiation in coronary artery disease. *JAMA* 1973;**225**:1319–28.

81. West of Scotland Prevention Group. West of Scotland Coronary Prevention Study: Identification of high-risk groups and comparison with other cardiovascular intervention trials. *Lancet* 1996;**348**:1339–42.

82. Wannamethee G, Shaper AG, MacFarlane PW, Walker M. Risk factors for sudden cardiac death in middle-aged British men. *Circulation* 1995;**91**:1749–56.

83. Whincup PH, Wannamethee G, MacFarlane PW, Walker M, Shaper AG. Resting electrocardiogram and risk of coronary heart disease in middle-aged men. *J Cardiovasc Risk* 1995;**2**:533–43.

84. Bhutto ZR, Barron JT, Liebson PR et al. Electrocardiographic abnormalities in mitral valve prolapse. *Am J Cardiol* 1992;**70**:265–71.

85. Pocock WA, Bosman CK, Chesler E et al. Sudden death in primary mitral valve prolapse. *Am Heart J* 1984;**107**:378–83.

86. Campbell RWF, Godman MG, Fiddler GI et al. Ventricular arrhythmias in syndrome of balloon deformity of mitral valve: Definition of possible high risk group. *Br Heart J* 1976;**38**:1053–8.

87. Hauer RNW, Wilde AAM. Mitral valve prolapse. In: Zipes, DP, Jalife J eds. *Cardiac electrophysiology. From cell to bedside*, 2nd edn. Philadelphia, WB Saunders, 1995, Ch. 74.

88. Klein GJ, Bashore TM, Sellers TD et al. Ventricular fibrillation in the Wolff–Parkinson–White syndrome. *New Engl J Med* 1979;**301**:1080.

89. Maron BJ, Roberts WC, Epstein SE, et al. Sudden death in hypertrophic cardiomyopathy: A profile of 78 patients. *Circulation* 1982;**65**:1388–94.

90. Maron BJ, Wolfson JK, Ciro E et al. Relation of electrocardiographic abnormalities and pattern of left ventricular hypertrophy identified by 2-dimensional echocardiography in patients with hypertrophic cardiomyopathy. *Am J Cardiol* 1983;**51**:189.

91. Frank S, Braunwald E. Idiopathic hypertrophic subaortic

stenosis: Clinical analysis of 126 patients with emphasis on the natural history. *Circulation* 1968;**37**:759.

92. Ikeda H, Mali S, Yoshida N *et al*. Predictors of death from congestive heart failure in hypertophic cardiomyopathy. *Am J Cardiol* 1999;**83**:1280–3.

93. Doval HC, Nul DR, Grancelli HO *et al*. Non-sustained ventricular tachycardia in severe heart failure. Independent marker of increased mortality due to sudden death. *Circulation* 1996;**94**:3198– 203.

94. Olshausen KV, Stienen U, Schwartz F *et al*. Long term prognostic significance of ventricular arrhythmias in idiopathic dilated cardiomyopathy. *Am J Cardiol* 1988;**53**: 146–51.

95. Schoeller R, Andresen D, Buttner P *et al*. First or second degree atrioventricular block as a risk factor in idiopathic dilated cardiomyopathy.

96. Brugada P, Brugada J. Right bundle branch block, persistent ST segment elevation and sudden cardiac death: a distinct clinical and electrocardiographic syndrome. A multicentre report. *J Am Coll Cardiol* 1992;**20**:1391–6.

97. Bjerregaard P, GussakI, Antzelevitch C. The enigmatic ECG manifestation of Brugada syndrome. *J Cardiovasc Electrophysiol* 1998;**9**:109–11.

98. Harumi K, Chen CY. Miscellaneous electrocardiographic topics. In: MacFarlane PW, Lawrie TDV eds. *Comprehensive electrocardiology 1*. New York: Pergamon Press, 1989, p. 687.

99. Gussak I, Antzelevitch C, Bjerregaard P *et al*. The Brugada syndrome: Clinical, electrophysiologic and genetic aspects. *J Am Coll Cardiol* 1999;**33**:5–15.

100. Nademanee K. Sudden unexplained death syndrome in Southeast Asia. *Am J Cardiol* 1997;**79**:10–11.

101. Nademanee K, Veerakul G, Nimmmannit S *et al*. Arrhythmogenic marker for the sudden unexplained death syndrome in Thai men. *Circulation* 1997;**96**:2595–600.

102. Tungsanga K, Sriboonlue P. Sudden unexplained death syndrome in northeast Thailand. *Int J Epidemiol* 1993;**22**:81–7.

103. Aponte GE. The enigma of bangungut. *Ann Intern Med* 1960;**52**:1258–63.

104. Gotoh K. A histopathological study on the conduction system of the so-called 'pokkuri disease' (sudden unexplained cardiac death of unknown origin in Japan). *Jap Circ J* 1976;**40**:753–68.

105. Goh KT, Chao TC, Chew CH. Sudden nocturnal deaths among Thai construction workers in Singapore. *Lancet* 1990;**335**:1154.

106. CDC. Update: sudden unexplained death syndrome among southeast Asian refugees: United States *Mortal Morbid Week Rep* 1988;**37**:568–70.

107. Miyazaki T, Mitamura H, Miyoshi S *et al*. Autonomic and antiarrhythmic drug modulation of ST segment elevation in patients with Brugada syndrome. *J Am Coll Cardiol* 1996;**27**:1061–70.

108. Carrado D, Nava A, Buja G *et al*. Familial cardiomyopathy underlies syndrome of right bundle branch block, ST-segment elevation, and sudden death. *J Am Coll Cardiol* 1996;**27**:443–8.

109. Tada H, Aihara N, Ohe T *et al*. Arrhythmogenic right ventricular cardiomyopathy underlies the syndrome of right bundle branch block, ST-segment elevation, and sudden death. *Am J Cardiol* 1998;**81**:519–22.

110. Alings M, Wilde A. "Brugada" syndrome. Clinical data and suggested pathophysiological mechanism. *Circulation* 1999;**99**:666–73.

111. Shimada M, Miyazaki T, Miyoshi S *et al*. Sustained monomorphic ventricular tachycardia in patient with Brugada syndrome. *Jap Circ J* 1996;**60**:364–70.

112. Kirschner RH, Echner FAO, Baron RC. The cardiac pathology of sudden unexplained nocturnal death on southeast Asian refugees. *JAMA* 1986;**256**:2700–95.

113. Gussak I, Bjerregaard P, Greenwait T, Chaitman BR. Electrophysiological peculiarities of the ECG J wave: from hypothermia to Brugada syndrome In: Liebman J ed. *Electrocardiography '96: from the cell to the body surface*. Singapore: World Scientific Publishing Co. Pte. Ltd., 1996, p. 261–4.

114. Lukas A, Antzelevitch C. Differences in the electrophysiological response of canine ventricular epicardium and endocardium to ischemia: role of the transient outward current. *Circulation* 1993;**88**:2903–15.

115. Lemery R, Brugada P, Della Bella P. Ventricular fibrillation in six adults without overt heart disease. *J Am Coll Cardiol* 1989;**13**:911–16.

116. Chen Q, Kirsch GE, Zhand D, Brugada R *et al*. Genetic basis and molecular mechanism for idiopathic ventricular fibrillation. *Nature* 1998;**392**:293–6.

117. Edeiken J. Elevation of RS-T segment, apparent or real in right precordial leads as probable normal variant. *Am Heart J* 1954;**48**:331–9.

118. MacFarlane PW, Lawrie TDV. The normal electrocardiogram and vectorcardiogram. In: MacFarlane PW, Lawrie TDV eds. *Comprehensive electrocardiology*. New York: Pergamon Press, 1989, p. 445.

119. Hiss RG, Lamb LE. Electrocardiographic findings in 122 043 individuals. *Circulation* 1962;**25**:947–53.

120. Osher HL, Wolff L. Electrocardiographic pattern simulating acute myocardial injury. *Am J Med* Sci 1953;**226**:541–6.

121. DiDiego JM, Antzelevitch C. High (Ca^{2+}-induced electrical heterogeneity and extrasystolic activity in isolated canine ventricular epicardium: phase 2 reentry? *Circulation* 1994;**89**:1839–50.

122. Krishnan SC, Josephson ME. ST segment elevation induced by Class 1C antiarrhythmic agents: *J Cardiovasc Electrophysiol* 1998;**9**:1167–72

123. Fontaine G, Fontaliran F, Lascault P *et al*. Arrhythmogenic right ventricular dysplasia. 1964, Ch. 69.

124. Garg A, Finneran W, Feld G. Familial sudden cardiac death associated with a terminal QRS abnormality on surface 12-lead electrocardiogram in the index case. *J Cardiovasc Electrophysiol* 1998;**9**:642–7.

125. Sutton R, Kenny R-A. The natural history of sick sinus syndrome. *PACE* 1986;**9**:1110–14.

126. Langendorf R, Pick A. Atrioventricular block. type II (Mobitz) – its nature and clinical significance. *Circulation* 1968;**38**:819–21.

127. Langendorf R, Pick A. Causes and mechanisms of ventricular asystole in advanced A-V block. In: Surawicz B,

Pellegrino ED, eds. *Sudden cardiac death*. New York: Grune & Stratton, 1964, p. 103.

128. Rosen, M. Personal communication to the author circa 1977.

129. Rardon DP, Miles WM, Mitrani RD *et al*. Atrioventricular block and dissociation. In: Zipes, DP, Jalife J eds. *Cardiac electrophysiology. From cell to bedside*, 2nd edn. Philadelphia, WB Saunders, 1995, p. 939.

130. Natterson PD, Perloff JK, Klitzner TS *et al*. Electrophysiologic abnormalities: Unoperated occurrence and postoperative residua and sequelae. In: Perloff JK, Child JS eds. *Congenital heart disease in adults*. Philadelphia, WB Saunders, 1998, pp. 316–45.

131. Bharati S, Lev M. Role of the specialised conduction system abnormalities in sudden cardiac death. In: Akhtar M, Myerburg RJ, Ruskin JN eds. *Sudden cardiac death*. Philadelphia: Williams & Wilkins, 1998, p. 274–89.

132. Gentles TL, Calder AL, Clarkson PM *et al*. Predictors of long-term survival with Ebstein's anomaly of the tricuspid valve. *Am J Cardiol* 1992;**69**:377.

133. Kannel WB, Abbott RD, Savage DD *et al*. Epidemiologic features of chronic atrial fibrillation. The Framingham Study. *New Engl J Med* 1982;**306**:1018–22.

134. Cameron A, Schwartz MJ, Kronmal RA *et al*. Prevalence and significance of atrial fibrillation in coronary artery disease (CASS Registry). *Am J Cardiol* 1988;**61**:714–17.

135. Packer D, Bardy G, Worley S *et al*. Tachycardia induced cardiomyopathy: a reversible form of left ventricular dysfunction. *Am J Cardiol* 1986;**57**:563–70.

136. Langberg JJ. "Atrial fibrillopathy": Is atrial fibrillation really self-perpetuating? *J Cardiovasc Electrophysiol* 1999;**10**:1109–11.

137. Frustaci A, Chimente C, Bellocci F *et al*. Histologic substrate of atrial biopsies in patients with lone atrial fibrillation. *Circulation* 1997;**96**:1180–4.

138. Wijffels MCEF, Kirchof CJHJ, Dorland R *et al*. Atrial fibrillation begets atrial fibrillation. A study in awake chronically instrumented goats. *Circulation* 1995;**92**:1954–68.

139. Leier CV, Meacham JA, Schaal SF. Prologed atrial conduction: A major predisposing factor for the development of atrial flutter. *Circulation* 1979;**57**:213–16.

140. Childers R. The AV node: normal and abnormal physiology. *Prog Cardiovasc Dis* 1977;**19**:361–84.

141. Attuel P, Childers R, Cauchemez B *et al*. Failure in the rate adaptation of the atrial refractory period:Its relationship to vulnerability. *Int J Cardiology* 1982;**2**:179–97.

142. Haissaguerre M, Jais P, Shah DC *et al*. Spontaneous initiation of atrial fibrillation by ectopic beats originating in the pulmonary veins. *New Engl J Med* 1998;**339**:659–66.

143. Levi AJ, Dalton GR, Hancox JC *et al*. Role of intracellular sodium overload in the genesis of cardiac arrhythmias. *J Cardiovasc Electrophysiol* 1997;**8**:700–21.

144. Childers RW. New and neglected aspects of atrial depolarisation and repolarisation. *J Electrocardiol* 1998;**30**(Suppl.):44–52.

145. Tchou PPJ, Keim SG, Kinn R. Sudden death in patients with idiopathic dilated cardiomyopathy. In: Akhtar M, Myerburg RJ, Ruskin JN eds. *Sudden cardiac death*. Philadelphia: Williams & Wilkins, 1998, p. 155.

146. Wellens HJJ, Rodriguez L-M, Smeets JL. Ventricular tachycardia in structurally normal hearts. In: Zipes DP, Jalife J eds. *Cardiac electrophysiology. From cell to bedside*, 2nd edn. Philadelphia: WB Saunders, 1995, p. 939.

147. Toivonen L, Nieminen M. Persistent ventricular tachycardia resulting in left ventricular dilatation treated with verapamil. *Int J Cardiol* 1986;**13**:361–5.

9 Electrophysiological study for risk stratification of cardiac patients

Velislav Batchvarov

Two milestone innovations in the late 1960s gave birth to the intracardiac electrophysiological (EP) study of the heart: the introduction of direct catheter recording of the His bundle potential,[1] and the discovery of electrical stimulation for reproducible initiation and termination of supraventricular[2,3] and, later, of ventricular[4] tachycardias. In essence, this was the beginning of the modern era of clinical cardiac electrophysiology.

In the following decades EP study expanded beyond recognition the knowledge of all aspects of arrhythmias. The potential prognostic value of the new method was also realised soon after its advent. Atrial pacing, His-bundle recording and programmed electrical stimulation became the main tools for risk stratification of patients with bradyarrhythmias and tachyarrhythmias in the 1970s and 1980s.

However, in recent years the clinical use of EP study, both as a diagnostic tool as well as a risk stratifier, decreased. This was a result of changes in the general concepts of arrhythmia management, development of non-invasive electrophysiology, and realisation of its inherent limitations. Today patients with bradyarrhythmias undergo His bundle recording and atrial pacing much less frequently than 20 years ago. In patients with supraventricular tachycardias and tachyarrhythmias the EP study is almost always (planned as) an introduction to a same-session catheter ablation.

The role of EP study in the management of today's major arrhythmic problem, sustained ventricular arrhythmias in patients with heart disease, also decreased, reflecting changes in the understanding of this problem during the last decade. The response of the arrhythmia substrate to artificial electrical stimuli (arrhythmia inducibility) is still used to predict spontaneous arrhythmia occurrence or recurrence in certain patient groups,[5] largely because better predictors are still lacking. It is becoming clear, however, that suppression of arrhythmia inducibility by antiarrhythmic drugs is an unreliable predictor of outcome.[5] Similarly, 10 years ago the fruitlessness of suppression of ventricular premature beats by antiarrhythmic drugs was realised.[6]

Nevertheless, in certain clinical conditions, the EP study is still as indispensable for establishing a diagnosis and making a prognosis as it was 20 years ago. In the following text, an attempt has been made to summarise in brief the clinical use of EP study as a risk stratifier for major bradyarrhythmic and tachyarrhythmic events. Before that we shall outline briefly the basic elements of a standard diagnostic EP study, which are relevant to its role as a risk stratifier.

Basic elements of the electrophysiologic study

The general goals of EP study are:

- to establish diagnosis and reveal the mechanism of a suspected, undocumented, or unclear arrhythmia;
- to make prognosis about its recurrence, or about the occurrence of other related arrhythmias; and
- to guide or help its treatment.

Prognostically, EP studies are performed to estimate the risk of sudden cardiac death, either from asystole, or much more frequently, from ventricular tachyarrhythmias. This is achieved by endocardial recording of electrical potentials and by diagnostic electrostimulation of the heart. The techniques of recording and stimulation have changed little since the time of their introduction.

Recording of electrical potential

Potentials recorded directly from the endo-, myo-, or epicardium are denoted as "electrograms",[7] to be distinguished from those recorded from the body surface, or from other sites remote from the heart (e.g. subcutaneously implanted antiarrhythmic devices), generally referred to as "electrocardiograms". Generally, both unipolar and bipolar electrograms contain much more information about local electrical events than surface electrocardiograms.

The recording of monophasic action potentials (MAPs)[8–10] is presently the only clinical technique for recording indirectly (i.e. extracellularly) the transmembrane potential at and in the immediate vicinity of the recording site.[11] MAPs provide unique information mainly about the time course of repolarisation.[12] However, they are not recorded routinely during EP studies and their role for risk stratification is largely unproven.

Below are listed the basic conduction intervals, measured in sinus rhythm during a standard EP study. Their normal values are given in Table 9.1.

- The PA interval (from the beginning of the P wave in the surface lead in which it appears first to the beginning of the A wave in the H bundle electrogram) reflects *approximately* the time of intra-atrial conduction. The PA is of little clinical value and today is measured rarely, if ever.

- The AH interval (from the beginning of the atrial [A] deflection to the beginning of the H wave in the His bundle electrogram) represents *approximately* the conduction time through the AV node (Fig. 9.1). The AH interval is influenced by many factors, the two most important being the heart rate and the autonomic tone. Since these vary widely even within a single EP study, the AH interval also can vary widely and its value *per se* for assessment of the atrioventricular conduction is small.[13]

- The HV interval (from the beginning of the H deflection to the beginning of the QRS complex, in whichever surface lead it starts first, or, less frequently, to the beginning of the V deflection on the His bundle electrogram) represents the conduction time through the His–Purkinje system (somewhat erroneously referred to as the "intraventricular" conduction time) (Fig. 9.1). The HV interval is not changed by the heart rate and is insignificantly influenced by changes in the autonomic tone. It is stable within a single EP study and is sufficiently reproducible in consecutive studies in one and the same patient in the absence of factors that influence it (e.g. drugs).[13] In the presence of bundle branch or fascicular block, the duration of the HV interval is a measure of the con-

duction time through the remaining fascicle or bundle. The HV interval is the most important electrophysiological parameter for risk stratification of patients with intraventricular conduction disturbances.

- The H potential reflects the conduction through the His bundle. Its prolongation (especially when it is also notched or fragmented) or, more importantly, its splitting into ≥ 2 separate distinct deflections, signifies conduction disturbances within the His bundle, which are usually symptomatic and/or carry unfavourable prognosis for development of high-degree AV block.[14,15]

The H potential and the HV interval are of major importance not only in the assessment of the intraventricular conduction, but also in the analysis of supraventricular and ventricular tachyarrhythmias.

Additional intervals can also have prognostic value. For example, sometimes it is important to distinguish proximal right bundle branch block (at the level of main branch of the right bundle), from distal right bundle branch block (at the level of the moderator band) and from terminal right bundle branch block (in the distal conduction system of the right bundle). It can be achieved by analysis of the potentials of the right bundle (with the His bundle catheter), the right ventricular apex and the right ventricular outflow tract.[16]

The analysis of the morphology of the endocardial electrograms can provide information about local electrical phenomena, mainly local conduction disturbances. In addition to diagnostic and therapeutic information (e.g. localising key elements of the arrhythmia substrate as a target for catheter ablation), the morphology of endocardial electrograms may also contain some prognostic information,[17–19] but this is not yet established.

Diagnostic electrical stimulation of the heart

Diagnostic electrostimulation is used for two main purposes:

Table 9.1 Baseline conduction intervals during sinus rhythm (ms)

Author	PA	AH	H	HV
Narula	25–45 (37 ± 7)	50–120 (77 ± 16)	15–20	35–45 (40 ± 3)
Damato	25–45	60–140	10–15	30–55
Castellanos	20–50	50–120	–	25–55
Schuilenburg	–	85–150	–	35–55
Peuch	30–55	45–100	–	35–55
Bekheit	10–50	50–125	15–25	35–45
Rosen	9–45	54–130	–	31–55
Josephson	–	60–125	10–25	35–55
Ross and Mandel	20–45	60–125	–	35–55

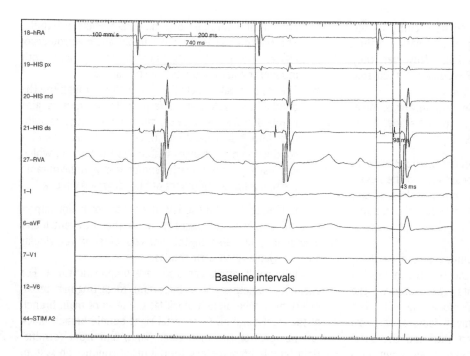

Figure 9.1 Basic conduction intervals during standard electrophysiological study. From top to bottom: recordings of the high lateral right atrium (hRA), proximal (HIS px), middle (HIS md) and distal (HIS ds) His bundle deflections, right ventricular apex (RVA), surface leads I, AVF, V₁, and V₆, and a channel displaying the stimulus artifacts during stimulation. Recording speed 100 mm/s. The AH interval is measured between the beginning of the A potential and the H potential in the distal His bundle electrogram and is equal to 98 ms. The HV interval is measured between the beginning of the H potential at the distal His bundle electrogram and the earliest beginning of the QRS in the surface ECG (in AVF) and is equal to 43 ms. The PA interval is not measured.

- to study the electrophysiological properties of the heart (automaticity, conduction, refractoriness);
- to induce tachyarrhythmias and study their mechanism and substrate.

Both the electrophysiological properties and the inducibility of tachyarrhythmias depend on the stimulation parameters (rate, duration, cycle length variation, synchronisation with the spontaneous heart rate, current strength, pulse duration, site of stimulation, application of drugs, and possibly others). Therefore diagnostic stimulation should always be performed according to a standardised protocol.

The basic assumption behind diagnostic stimulation is that, in general, the response of the heart to artificial electrical stimuli is practically the same as (and therefore can be used to predict) its reaction to naturally occurring impulses. Time has proven the validity of this assumption when the electrophysiological properties (automaticity, conduction, refractoriness) of separate cardiac structures are studied. However, it is more difficult and less reliable to predict the response of a substrate of tachyarrhythmia to the complexity of factors that comprise "natural electrical stimulation", from its response to diagnostic electrical stimulation.

Study of the electrophysiological properties of the heart

Automaticity. Normal automatic foci (sinus or subsidiary) are temporarily suppressed by electrical stimula-tion or by other foci with a rate higher than their spontaneous rate (overdrive suppression).[20,21] The degree of prolongation of the post-stimulation pause (the sinus node recovery time, SNRT) is assumed to reflect the degree of depression of the sinus node automaticity. SNRT is still the best and most widely used test for assessment of the sinus node function.[22,23] The upper normal limit of the SNRT is 1400–1600 ms.[24,25] Since the SNRT strongly depends on the resting sinus cycle length, different formulae for correction of the SNRT for the resting sinus cycle length have been proposed. The most frequently used formula for the "corrected" SNRT (CSNRT) is "CSNRT = SNRT − SCL", with upper normal values of 525–550 ms.[26,27]

The measurement of the sinoatrial conduction time (SACT) is part of the routine examination of the sinus node function, since prolonged SNRT, spontaneous sinus pauses, and sinus arrest may sometimes be due to sinoatrial block. SACT can be measured directly by recording the sinus node electrogram[28] or, much more frequently, indirectly by delivering atrial stimulus with a coupling interval sufficient to enter and depolarise (to "reset") the sinus node.[29,30] Upper normal values of around 150 ms for the SACT in one direction have been reported.[31] The refractoriness of the sinus node can also be determined by the extrastimulus technique and has been reported to have diagnostic value.[32]

Evaluation of conduction. The functional properties of the atrioventricular (AV) conduction system are assessed by the baseline conduction intervals, by its response to drugs and/or pharmacological interventions and by measurement of the refractory periods of its components.

The normal response of the AV conduction system to atrial pacing is gradual lengthening of the AH interval, as the pacing cycle length is decreased, until AV nodal conduction block of the Wenckebach type develops. The pacing cycle length at which AV nodal block Wenckebach type normally develops varies largely, depending mainly on age and autonomic tone, but in the majority of patients it is between 500 and 350 ms (i.e. pacing rate between 120 and 170 bpm).[13] The conduction through the His–Purkinje system is normally not affected by atrial pacing.[13]

The functional properties of the His–Purkinje system are assessed by the baseline HV interval and by its reaction to atrial pacing,[33] and to the intravenous application of antiarrhythmic drugs that affect it (e.g. ajmaline,[34,35] procainamide,[36] and disopyramide[37]).

Measurement of refractory periods. In clinical electrophysiology it is mainly the effective, the functional, and, to a lesser degree, the relative refractory periods that are measured.

The effective refractory period (ERP) of a structure is the longest interval between two impulses entering the structure, the second of which fails to propagate through it. In terms of stimulation, the ERP is the longest coupling interval of the premature impulse (S_1S_2) that is not propagated through the structure. The effective refractory periods are measured between the potentials of the nearest proximal structure, that can be recorded (e.g. between two atrial potentials [AA interval] for the ERP of the AV node, HH interval for the His–Purkinje system, etc.).

The functional refractory period (FRP) of a structure is the shortest interval between two consecutively conducted impulses entering the structure, regardless of the interval between them at entering. The FRP is measured between the potentials of the nearest distal structure, that can be recorded (e.g. HH intervals for the AV node, VV intervals for the His–Purkinje system, etc.). Obviously, the FRP of a structure limits the measurement of the ERP of the next structure; e.g. the ERP of the AV node cannot be determined if it is shorter than the FRP of the atrium.

Electrical stimulation for induction of tachyarrhythmias

Electrical stimulation for reproduction (i.e. initiation and termination) of tachyarrhythmias deals almost only with re-entry arrhythmias.

Automatic arrhythmias cannot be induced or terminated by spontaneous or artificial electrical stimuli. Their response to overdrive stimulation is either suppression during stimulation (overdrive suppression) with resumption after cessation of pacing, or no response. Unlike normal automatic foci, abnormal automatic foci are generally not suppressed by overdrive stimulation,[38] and can even be temporarily accelerated (overdrive acceleration).[39] The reproducible initiation and/or termination of sustained arrhythmia by electrical stimulation effectively exclude both normal and abnormal automaticity as an underlying mechanism.

Triggered activity can be regarded as a form of automaticity, as long as impulses are initiated within a cell or a group of cells.[40–42] However, unlike automatic rhythms, the initiation of a triggered rhythm depends on a pre-existing impulse (spontaneous or paced). Therefore, unlike automaticity and like re-entry, triggered activity can be initiated and terminated by timed electrical stimuli, although its initiation and termination are generally less reproducible than those of re-entry arrhythmias. The mode of initiation and termination and the response of a triggered arrhythmia to programmed stimulation also differ from those of re-entry arrhythmias and may help to differentiate the two mechanisms.

The overwhelming majority of all clinically significant tachyarrhythmias are due to re-entry, including the two most important, namely atrial fibrillation (of all cause) and sustained ventricular arrhythmias in patients with heart disease.

The heart is naturally protected against the occurrence of re-entry both by the high conduction velocity through the myocardium and the conduction system, as well as by the long refractory period of all cardiac structures (any one of the two is sufficient). Owing to the fast conduction and to the long refractoriness, the wave of excitation is normally extinguished long before any region of the myocardium regains excitability. Re-entry can occur when an impulse is conducted with sufficient delay (owing to slow conduction and/or to an obstacle that has to be circumvented), to allow tissues ahead of the impulse to recover excitability and be re-excited. If zones of altered electrophysiological properties (slow conduction, non-excitability, short refractoriness) are arranged functionally and anatomically in a suitable way, they can form a substrate for re-entry, within which the impulse can circulate, always finding an excitable tissue ahead of it.

Therefore re-entry can arise almost only on the basis of pre-existing substrate, usually created by some form of cardiac disease. Since conduction and refractoriness in the circuit change dynamically within the cardiac cycle, it is crucial that the impulse enters the circuit in a suitable moment to initiate or terminate re-entry. Therefore during electrical stimulation an impulse is introduced periodically, with gradual shortening of its coupling interval to the proceeding spontaneous or paced impulse. It is believed that, provided a substrate exists somewhere in the myocardium, at a critical moment the impulse will enter into it and initiate or terminate re-entry (Fig. 9.2).

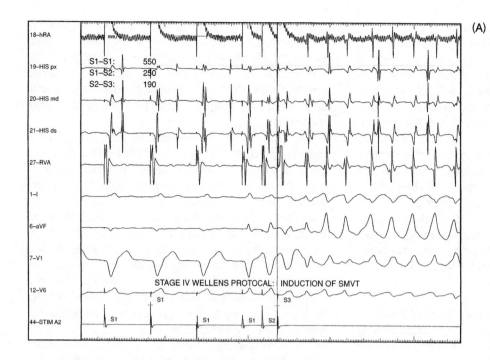

(A)

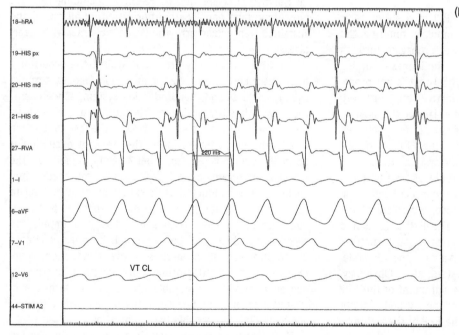

(B)

Figure 9.2 Induction and termination of sustained monomorphic ventricular tachycardia by programmed ventricular stimulation in a 46-year-old man with cardiac sarcoidosis and a history of sustained ventricular tachycardia for 10 years. The patient had been on antiarrhythmic therapy (sotalol 120 mg bd, disopyramide 300 mg bd) and had had no symptoms while on this therapy. The therapy was stopped 48 hours before the electrophysiological study. (A) Induction of sustained monomorphic ventricular tachycardia with programmed ventricular stimulation with drive cycle length $(S_1 - S_1)$ of 550 ms and two extrastimuli at a coupling intervals of $S_1 - S_2 = 250$ ms and $S_2 - S_3 = 190$ ms, respectively. The same intracardiac and surface leads are displayed as in Figure 9.1. (B) Intracardiac and surface ECG recording during the tachycardia. Cycle length of the tachycardia = 220 ms (273 bpm). The same intracardiac and surface leads as in Figure 9.2A.

The basic assumption behind electrical stimulation as a method of induction of re-entry arrhythmias is that failing to initiate the arrhythmia by delivering impulses at a wide range of coupling intervals implies that arrhythmia *on the basis of the existing substrate* is highly unlikely to occur spontaneously. There are many factors that limit the validity of this assumption and, consequently, the predictive value of programmed electrical stimulation.

Numerous attempts have been made to characterise the

arrhythmogenic substrate by the morphology of the endocardial electrograms. Findings, such as fractionation of paced electrograms in hypertrophic cardiomyopathy[17,18] or in primary ventricular fibrillation,[19] prolonged and multiphasic electrograms in patients with hypertrophic cardiomyopathy,[17,18] dispersion of repolarisation measured by MAPs[43] may have some prognostic value for the occurrence of ventricular arrhythmias, but it is still unknown.

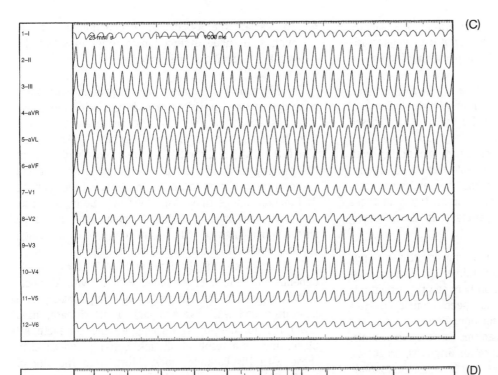

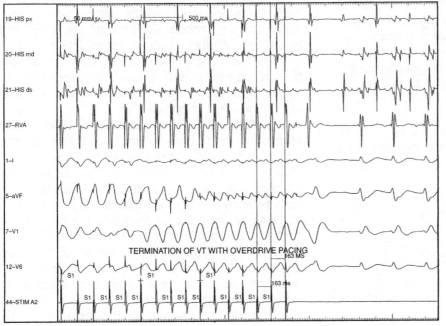

Figure 9.2 (C) Standard 12-lead ECG during the tachycardia. (D) Termination of the tachycardia with pacing from the right ventricular apex with a pacing rate faster than the tachycardia rate (overdrive pacing). The pacing cycle length is gradually shortened to 163 ms.

Risk stratification of patients with bradyarrhythmias

Some simple, yet often forgotten, truths about patients with bradyarrhythmias are worth remembering. Generally, the pathology of the conduction system tends to develop at more than one level. For example, AV block develops in patients with sinus node dysfunction with an annual rate of 0.6–1.8%,[45,46] high-degree AV block in patients with fascic-ular blocks in about one-half of all cases develops in the AV node,[47] etc. Generally speaking, bradyarrhythmias tend to co-exist with, or to predispose to, tachyarrhythmias. Therefore, in patients with bradyarrhythmias, symptoms often are (also) due to, and prognosis is often determined (mainly) by, concomitant tachyarrhythmias. Arrhythmias described as "functional" are usually assumed to be benign, while those described as "organic" are assumed to carry bad prognosis. Both assumptions are not necessarily right.

Figure 9.3 presents a simplified algorithm for a diagnostic work-up of a patient with inappropriate symptomatic bradycardia, not related to the application of drugs or another reversible cause.

The indications for permanent pacing in patients with bradyarrhythmias (owing to either sinus node dysfunction or conduction disturbances) are, for the most part, based on the history, physical examination, and non-invasive evaluation (standard ECG, ambulatory monitoring with Holter, event recorder or implantable devices for cardiac monitoring, exercise stress test, tilt-table, and other autonomic tests). The EP study has a limited role in these patients and is in indicated, generally, in the following cases[48]:

- in symptomatic patients in whom arrhythmia (sinus node dysfunction or His–Purkinje AV block) is suspected, but a causal relation between the arrhythmia and the symptoms has not been established after complete non-invasive evaluation;

- to determine the mechanisms of the arrhythmia, which may be of importance for diagnosis, prognosis, and therapy. Abnormalities may be due to autonomic dysfunction rather than intrinsic disease and respond to pharmacologic therapy instead of permanent pacing. Patients with sinus node dysfunction may also have carotid sinus hypersensitivity. Concealed atrial or junctional premature beats may be revealed as a cause for "pseudosinus node disease" or "pseudo-AV block;

- to find another cause, e.g. supraventricular or ventricular tachyarrhythmia, which may contribute to (or is the main cause of) symptoms;

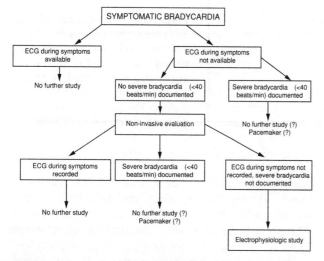

Figure 9.3 A simplified algorithm for diagnostic work-up of a patient with inappropriate symptomatic bradycardia, not related to the application of drugs or another reversible cause. See text for details.

- to evaluate the AV and VA conduction in patients with sinus node dysfunction in order to select the most appropriate pacing modality.

The EP study has a limited role in patients with sinus node dysfunction. In limited cases it may help to establish diagnosis and select patients who are likely to benefit from permanent pacing or other therapy.[48,49] When combined, the SNRT and the SACT have a sensitivity of about 65% and specificity of about 88%, with higher negative and low positive predictive value.[50] In patients with sinus node dysfunction, unlike those with AV block, permanent pacing, both ventricular and dual-chamber, have not been shown convincingly to reduce cardiac or overall mortality, and it is likely that it only relieves symptoms.[51,52]

The prognosis of patients with AV block largely depends on the level of the block. Patients with AV nodal block, in general, are less frequently symptomatic, have less often and less severe organic heart disease, have lower risk for developing high-degree and complete AV block, and, as a result of all this, better prognosis than those with His–Purkinje block. Most often the site of block (AV node or His–Purkinje system) can be determined from the surface ECG.[53] EP study may be indicated in symptomatic patients with the second degree AV block in whom His–Purkinje block is suspected, but has not been established, as well as those who continue to be symptomatic after pacemaker implantation, possibly owing to ventricular tachyarrhythmias.[48]

In patients with bifascicular block (e.g. left bundle branch block or right bundle branch block with left anterior or left posterior fascicular block), the HV interval is a measure of the conduction time through the remaining functioning fascicle. Although in patients with bifascicular block generally prolonged HV interval (>55 ms) is associated with increased risk for development of complete AV block,[54,55] the specificity of the test is low (63%) with higher sensitivity (82%).[56] This reflects the fact that, although an HV interval of >55 ms is a frequent finding in those patients, the rate of development of complete AV block in those with prolonged HV (>55 ms) is low, about 2–3% annually.[54,55] However, significantly prolonged HV interval (e.g. >100 ms) carries significantly worse prognosis for development of complete AV block – it developed in 25% of the patients during follow-up of 22 months in one study.[57]

The specificity of the test can be increased by rapid atrial pacing. Development of block within or below the His bundle during atrial pacing with 1:1 AV nodal conduction in these patients is finding with low sensitivity, but with high positive predictive value for development of complete AV block.[58] Intravenous application of ajmaline[34,35] procainamide,[36] or disopyramide[37] may be used to provoke extreme prolongation of the HV interval (>100 or >120 ms) or infra- or intra-His block in patients with bundle branch block, and thus identify patients at risk for complete AV block. In one study in which 73 patients with bifascicular block were followed up for a median period of 23 months,[59] the disopyramide test had a sensitivity of 100% and specificity of 94%, for prediction of high-grade AV block, whilst baseline HV interval >70 ms and/or a His–Purkinje block at atrial pacing had a sensitivity of 30% and specificity of 90%. However, the test carries a risk by itself, since disopyramide can cause severe hypotension as a result of myocardial depression.[60]

In an unknown, but apparently substantial proportion of symptomatic patients with bifascicular blocks, symptoms are due to ventricular tachyarrhythmias rather than high-degree AV block.[61] These patients have an increased risk for sudden tachyarrhythmic, rather than bradyarrhythmic death. Therefore, the electrophysiological evaluation of symptomatic patients with bifascicular block should also include programmed ventricular stimulation.[48]

Risk stratification of patients with tachyarrhythmias

In patients with tachycardias and tachyarrhythmias, the EP study can be used to make a prognosis about the risk of their recurrence, or of the occurrence of other serious tachyarrhythmias. Supraventricular arrhythmias are rarely life-threatening, and therefore the main goal of their treatment is to relieve symptoms and to improve the quality of life. Unlike supraventricular, sustained ventricular arrhythmias, particularly those in patients with heart disease, are usually life-threatening, and therefore the main goal of the treatment is to prevent their occurrence or recurrence.

The EP study is sometimes needed in patients with the Wolff–Parkinson–White (WPW) syndrome who have survived cardiac arrest or have unexplained syncope, presumably owing to very rapid conduction of atrial tachyarrhythmias via the accessory pathway and development of ventricular fibrillation. Atrial fibrillation occurs in 11.5–32% of patients with WPW.[62,63] However, the annual rate of sudden cardiac death in patients with WPW syndrome is 0.15%,[64] i.e. about the same as the sudden cardiac death rate in the general adult population.

The shortest RR during pre-excited atrial fibrillation is strongly related to the risk of development of ventricular fibrillation during atrial fibrillation in patients with WPW syndrome.[65,66] Different cut-off values, such as <250 ms[65] or ≤200 ms[66] have been proposed, but there is an overlap between symptomatic and asymptomatic patients. During the EP study, both the shortest pre-excited RR interval during induced atrial fibrillation, as well the anterograde RP of the accessory pathway must be determined.[67,68] The effect of autonomic tests (i.e. infusion of isoprenaline)

and/or drugs that influence the conduction via the accessory pathway (e.g. ajmaline, procainamide) may also be useful.[67]

Asymptomatic patients with ventricular pre-excitation who are engaged in high-risk occupations or activities (e.g. aircrew, fire-fighters, etc.) can also be studied to determine the electrophysiological properties of the accessory pathway or the propensity for development of supraventricular tachycardia.[48,67]

Risk stratification for sudden cardiac death and sustained ventricular arrhythmias

The main goal of the EP study in patients with sustained ventricular arrhythmias (documented, suspected, or likely to occur) is to assess the risk for their recurrence, and, ultimately, the risk for sudden arrhythmic death. However, clinical experience, as well as the results of clinical trials, such as CASH,[69] the Steinbeck study,[70] and the ESVEM trial[71] has shown that recurrences of ventricular tachycardia do not equate with (and therefore cannot be used as a surrogate for) sudden cardiac death.

The identification of the potential victims of sudden cardiac death continues to be an unresolved issue, despite enormous effort in research and technical advance. The dilemma can be summarised by several well-known figures. Sudden cardiac death claims each year 0.1–0.2% of the general adult population in developed countries. Even if it was possible to recognise all potentials victims (i.e. if risk stratifiers both applicable for general screening and possessing 100% positive predictive value were available), to save them using the best available therapy, the present rate of ICD implantation in the USA, for example, would have to be increased about 10 times. However, the positive predictive value of all available tests including EP study, alone or in combination, is at best 30%.[72]

Besides, most available tools for risk stratification are applicable and can help to identify only a minority of the potential victims within relatively small groups of high-risk patients, most of them with advanced heart disease (e.g. survivors of out-of-hospital cardiac arrest, comprising about 1% of all victims of sudden cardiac death[73]). They are also the patients most likely to benefit from the ICD therapy.[74,75] The vast majority of ("healthier") victims remain dispersed and unidentified within much larger groups of low-risk patients and apparently healthy individuals.[76] In these latter groups, the presently available risk stratifiers, including the EP study, are ineffective, of unknown value, or inapplicable. Even when identified, however, the best therapeutic strategy for the "healthier" potential victims is less clear. Finally, reliable criteria for the efficacy of antiarrhythmic drug therapy are also largely lacking.

The clinical value of the EP study has been studied most extensively and is best established for ventricular arrhythmias in patients with chronic ischaemic heart disease, especially in survivors of myocardial infarction (MI). The application of the EP study in patients with ventricular arrhythmias in the absence of ischaemic heart disease, where the arrhythmia substrate is less known, is still less clear.

Myocardial infarction and in chronic ischaemic heart disease

Patients without major arrhythmic events. Soon after the introduction into clinical practice of the EP study, it was realised that, in patients with heart disease, and especially in those with chronic ischaemic heart disease, spontaneously occurring sustained ventricular arrhythmias can be reproduced repeatedly by programmed stimulation in almost all of the cases. Therefore, it was quite natural to suggest that programmed stimulation could also be used to assess the risk of arrhythmia occurrence in all patients with arrhythmogenic substrate, including those who had not suffered major arrhythmic events.

Many studies in the 1980s and early 1990s addressed the role of the EP study as a risk stratifier in the general population of survivors of myocardial infarction.

Richards *et al.*[77] performed EP study before hospital discharge in 361 patients with acute MI. They were selected out of 612 survivors of the first 5 days after acute MI, with no heart failure, no persistent myocardial ischaemia, and no cardioactive medications other than digoxin. Patients were followed up for as long as 775 days (median 740 days). Patients with inducible ventricular tachycardias were 15.2 times more likely to suffer electrical events, than patients without inducible ventricular tachycardias. At multivariate analysis only delayed ventricular activation, low ejection fraction and inducible ventricular tachycardia had independent predictive value for arrhythmic events, and the value of the latter (sensitivity, specificity, positive and negative predictive value of 58%, 95%, 30% and 98%, respectively) was highest. Of note, only ventricular tachycardia of at least 10 seconds duration and with cycle length ≥ 230 ms, induced with up to three extrastimuli was considered an abnormal finding. Other studies, however, did not confirmed these findings.[78–80]

Despite all uncertainties with its classification, it is clear that the rate of sudden cardiac death in survivors of myocardial infarction has decreased significantly in the thrombolytic era, to about 2% during the first year.[81,82] The same trend is observed in the rate of non-fatal ventricular arrhythmias.[83] Given this low rate of major arrhythmic events, the low positive predictive value of the EP study of ≈30%,[84] the still unresolved issue of the significance of a negative EP study, the invasive character and the possible side effects of the EP study and eventually, of ICD implantation, it is unacceptable to perform programmed stimulation in all survivors of acute myocardial infarction.[85] Obviously, the general post-myocardial infarction patient population must be screened by more applicable and of higher predictive value tools for risk stratification. Until they become available, subgroups of survivors of myocardial infarction known to be at increased risk must be targeted with the available tools for risk stratification, including the EP study.

Patients with left ventricular dysfunction and non-sustained ventricular tachycardia. Left ventricular systolic dysfunction,[77,86] and increased ventricular ectopy (increased number of premature beats[87,88] and/or non-sustained ventricular tachycardia[89]) are considered the two most powerful independent predictors of total mortality and sudden cardiac death in post-myocardial infarction patients. Survivors of the acute phase of myocardial infarction with significant left ventricular dysfunction have a 6-month mortality rate ≥10%,[90] with sudden cardiac death accounting for at least one-third of the deaths. Post-myocardial infarction patients with both risk factors are of particularly increased risk for sudden cardiac death.[86,88,91] The incidence of sudden death in post-myocardial infarction patients with both left ventricular dysfunction and frequent ventricular premature beats (usually dichotomised at 10/hour) can be 11 times higher than that in patients with neither of these findings.[92] The presence of a positive signal averaged ECG (SAECG) further increases the 2-year risk for suffering major arrhythmic events to 40–50%.[93]

Post-myocardial infarction patients with preserved ventricular function without frequent ventricular ectopy are at low risk for arrhythmic death (<2% during the first year after myocardial infarction).[88,94,95] There is generally a consensus that programmed stimulation is not warranted in such patients.[96,97]

The results of two recent trials supported the value of the EP study in patients with left ventricular dysfunction and non-sustained ventricular arrhythmias.

The Mulicenter Automatic Defibrillator Implantation Trial (MADIT)[98] enrolled 196 post-myocardial infarction patients with asymptomatic non-sustained ventricular tachycardia, left ventricular dysfunction (ejection fraction ≤35%) and inducible and non-suppressible at EP study ventricular tachycardias. The patients were randomly assigned to conventional antiarrhythmic therapy (N = 101) or ICD (N = 95). After mean follow-up of 27 months there were 39 deaths in the conventional-therapy group and 15 in the ICD-group (54% reduction in all-cause mortality by ICD, P = 0.009).

A subsequent analysis[99] compared the outcome of patients screened for MADIT who met all eligibility criteria except that they were not inducible (N = 85), with the inducible and non-suppressible patients who were randomised to conventional therapy (N = 101). The adjusted risk of death was 4.24 times greater (8% versus 39%, P <0.001) in the group of patients with inducible and non-suppressible tachycardias.

The long-awaited results of the MUSTT were published recently[100]: 704 patients after myocardial infarction with asymptomatic non-sustained ventricular arrhythmias (VA) and left ventricular dysfunction (LVEF ≤40%) and with inducible sustained ventricular arrhythmias, were randomised to electrophysiologically-guided therapy (antiarrhythmic drugs or implantable defibrillator) or no antiarrhythmic therapy. After median follow-up of 39 months, patients with electrophysiologically-guided therapy had significantly lower 5-year rate of cardiac arrest or death from arrhythmia (25%) compared to those randomised to no therapy (32%) (P = 0.04), representing 27% reduction of the risk of development of arrhythmia.

However, the reduction in arrhythmia occurrence was solely attributable to the ICDs, which were implanted in 58% of the patients randomised to antiarrhythmic therapy. The 5-year rate of cardiac arrest or death from arrhythmia was 9% in those who received defibrillators and 37% in those who did not (P = 0.001). Of note, the 5-year overall mortality rate was also significantly lower in those who received defibrillators than on those who did not (24% versus 55%).

The results of MUSTT suggested that serial testing of antiarrhythmic drugs does not improve survival. The 5-year rate of cardiac arrest or death from arrhythmia was 37% in those patients who received electrophysiologically-guided drug therapy and 32% in those assigned to no antiarrhythmic therapy. The overall mortality rates in the former group also tended to be higher.

Both trials confirmed that EP study could identify a high-risk subset of patients within post-MI patients with left ventricular dysfunction and non-sustained ventricular tachycardia, who would benefit from the implantation of defibrillator.

As the rate of sudden cardiac death and symptomatic ventricular arrhythmias in post-myocardial infarction patients will probably continue to fall with improvement of general treatment strategies (early revascularisation, beta-blockers, ACE-inhibitors, angiotensin-antagonists, etc.), the identification of the potential victims will require more powerful risk stratifiers. The role of EP study for risk stratification is likely to be either restricted to a second-step tool in relatively small high-risk groups of patients preselected by non-invasive tests, or questioned for use at all.

Pedretti *et al.*[101] showed that low ejection fraction, prolonged filtered QRS on the SAECG, reduced HRV, and detection of ≥2 runs of non-sustained ventricular tachycar-

dias were independent predictors of sudden death or sustained ventricular arrhythmias in a cohort of patients with acute myocardial infarction. The combination of ≥2 risk factors out of ejection fraction <40%, filtered QRS ≥106 ms, or ≥2 runs of non-sustained ventricular tachycardia, predicted arrhythmic events with a sensitivity of 87%, specificity of 88%, positive predictive accuracy of 30%, and negative predictive accuracy of 99%. The addition of EP study increased the positive predictive accuracy to 65% (probably one of the highest reported!), whilst sensitivity, specificity, and negative predictive accuracy were 81%, 97%, and 99%, respectively.

More recently, Andresen *et al.*[82] tested a two-step risk-stratification approach on 657 post-MI patients (10–14 days after the event), 61% of them having received thrombolysis. Patients with left ventricular ejection fraction ≤40% or increased ventricular ectopy on Holter monitoring (≥20 ventricular ectopic beats/hour and/or ≥10 ventricular couplets per day, and/or ventricular tachycardia with a cycle length ≤600 ms) underwent programmed stimulation with up to two extrastimuli. Patients were followed up for a minimum of 2 years (mean 37 ± 17 months). Low left ventricular ejection fraction and/or increased ventricular ectopy were significantly related with increased rate of arrhythmic events (3.4% versus 6.6% in those without both markers, P = 0.05). Induction of sustained ventricular tachycardia (sustained monomorphic ventricular tachycardia of at least 10 s duration and a cycle length of ≥230 ms) in the high-risk group was also associated with increased risk of arrhythmic events (18.2% versus 4% in those that were non-inducible). However, the positive predictive value of programmed stimulation in this study was very low (18%), probably owing to the application of less aggressive stimulation protocol (up to two extrastimuli), as well as to quite stringent criteria for inducibility: sustained polymorphic ventricular tachycardia and ventricular fibrillation, plus sustained monomorphic ventricular tachycardia with cycle length <230 ms were not considered an abnormal finding.

Two ongoing trials are expected to have great impact on the primary prevention strategy in post-MI patients. The Sudden Cardiac Death in Heart Failure Trial[102] and the Multicenter Automatic Defibrillator Implantation Trial II (MADIT II)[103] will test the effect of ICD and non-ICD therapy on arrhythmia and total mortality in post-MI patients with ventricular dysfunction (symptomatic heart failure and left ventricular ejection fraction <36% in SCD-Heft, left ventricular ejection fraction <30% in MADIT-II). Most importantly, unlike MADIT and MUSTT, patients will not be preselected with an EP study or non-invasive tests. However, the predictive value of arrhythmia inducibility will also be assessed in MADIT-II, by device-based programmed ventricular stimulation during implantation in patients randomised to ICD.

Patients with major arrhythmic events (arrhythmic death, sustained monomorphic ventricular tachycardia). Spontaneously occurring sustained monomorphic ventricular tachycardias in patients with chronic ischaemic heart disease can be reproduced repeatedly in more than 90%.[96,104] In patients presenting with cardiac arrest, sustained ventricular arrhythmias (sustained monomorphic ventricular tachycardia, sustained polymorphic ventricular tachycardia, or ventricular fibrillation) can also be induced reproducibly with programmed stimulation, although with lesser rate ($\approx$ 50%),[105,106] than in those presenting with sustained monomorphic ventricular tachycardia.

Patients with symptomatic sustained ventricular arrhythmias are at particularly high risk for life-threatening arrhythmias.[107–109] Studies in the 1970s have found a recurrence rate of 30% at 1 year and 45% at 2 years.[110,111] The empiric use of class I antiarrhythmic drugs in survivors of out-of-hospital cardiac arrest was found to be associated with arrhythmia recurrence and mortality rates similar or higher than those in patients who were not treated with antiarrhythmic drugs.[112,113] Therefore the 1980s witnessed the widespread use of non-invasive (Holter monitoring) and invasive (programmed stimulation) techniques to guide antiarrhythmic therapy in those patients.

Multiple studies have shown that inducibility of sustained ventricular tachycardias in this patient population is a powerful predictor of arrhythmia recurrence.[106,114,115] Failure to suppress the inducible arrhythmia by drugs or surgery was proved to be a strong independent predictor of recurrent major cardiac events. For example, in the study of Wilber *et al.*[114] on 166 survivors of out-of-hospital cardiac arrest, those with inducible and non-suppressible arrhythmias had a recurrence rate of 33% during follow-up of 21 months, compared to 12% in those with inducible and suppressible arrhythmias and 17% in those with non-inducible arrhythmias. Persistence of inducible sustained ventricular tachycardia carried 3.97 relative risk (CI 1.8–8.75) for recurrence of cardiac arrest.

Troup[116] summarised the results of 18 studies of EP-guided therapy in 1681 patients altogether, half of them cardiac arrest survivors, who were followed up for a mean of 20 months. The rates of sudden cardiac death and of non-fatal arrhythmia recurrences in patients discharged on antiarrhythmic treatment found to be effective during EP study were 9% and 7%, respectively, whilst in those who were discharged on non-effective treatment the rates were 28% and 34%, respectively.

Antiarrhythmic drug that effectively suppress arrhythmia inducibility can be identified in 26–80%, according to different studies, but the average values are about 30%.[105,106,114,115,117,118] The estimated probability of arrhythmia recurrence also depends on the criteria of non-inducibility.[119] After 30 years of programmed stimulation the latter continue to vary between different laboratories, attesting their arbitrariness.

More importantly, none of the available studies, most of them retrospective, and none randomised, including the placebo-control group, has actually proven the beneficial effect of suppression of arrhythmia inducibility by antiarrhythmic drugs on patients' outcome.

The 1990s witnessed significant decline in the use of programmed stimulation both for risk stratification, as well as for guiding drug therapy in patients with major arrhythmic events. The pharmacological therapy of malignant ventricular arrhythmias has generally been redirected from class I drugs, the backbone of EP-guided therapy during the 1970s and 1980s, to class III drugs. Empiric therapy with amiodarone[120] and EP-guided therapy with sotalol[71] has been shown to be superior to EP-guided therapy with a class I drug. However, adequate comparison of EP-guided versus empiric therapy with class III drugs has not been performed.

Apparently, (more or less) arbitrarily chosen criteria for antiarrhythmic drug efficacy, such as suppression of inducibility at EP study or reduction of premature beats at Holter monitoring, do not (adequately) reflect the effect of the drug on patients' outcome. Not only suppression of arrhythmia inducibility during EP study, but even suppression of arrhythmia recurrence by antiarrhythmic drugs does not necessarily mean improvement of outcome.

For example, Böcker *et al.*[121] compared in a case-controlled study 50 patients with chronic ischaemic heart disease and a history of sustained ventricular tachycardia or ventricular fibrillation, who were rendered non-inducible by sotalol, with 50 patients treated with ICD because of drug-refractory ventricular tachycardia/ventricular fibrillation. Both groups were matched for age, sex, ejection fraction, extent of coronary artery disease, and presenting arrhythmia. Sotalol was superior to ICD in suppressing ventricular arrhythmias: whereas 83% of the patients in the sotalol group were free of sudden death and non-fatal ventricular tachycardias during a period of 3 years, only 33% of those treated with an ICD did not receive appropriate therapy by the device. However, 3-year overall survival rate of patients with ICDs was significantly better than in those treated with sotalol (85% versus 75%, $P = 0.02$).

Antz *et al.*[122] also demonstrated in a prospective randomised study that significant reduction of arrhythmia inducibility by oral sotalol in patients with documented sustained ventricular tachycardias does not correlate with clinical outcome.

The role of the EP study was further undermined by small studies,[123–125] as well as recently published results of randomised trials, such as AVID,[126] CASH,[127] CIDS,[128] and some others,[129] which have shown that the implantable cardioverter–defibrillator is superior to empiric or EP-guided antiarrhythmic drug therapy in reducing total mortality in these patients.

In addition, value of the negative EP study is still an unresolved issue. Earlier studies have found very high negative predictive value of EP study. Kowey et al.[130] performed meta-analysis on the results of 12 studies published between 1986 and 1990 with a total of 926 patients with non-sustained ventricular tachycardia. Patients with inducible sustained ventricular tachycardia had 2.5 times higher risk for sudden cardiac death or major arrhythmic event compared with those who were non-inducible (18% versus 7%, *P* <0.001), despite (or probably also owing to) the fact that 83% of patients in the former group were treated with antiarrhythmic drugs, compared with only 13% in the latter. The sensitivity, specificity, positive and negative predictive value of EP study were 54%, 70%, 18%, and 93%, respectively.

However, data from recent studies do not confirm the high negative predictive value of EP study. Kim et al.[131] performed a retrospective study on a small sample size of 55 men followed up for 15.4 ± 9.8 months. Inclusion criteria were coronary artery disease with left ventricular ejection fraction <40% at the time of EP study, no history of cardiac arrest or syncope, no inducible sustained monomorphic ventricular tachycardia on EP study, and asymptomatic non-sustained ventricular tachycardia. Analysis showed that 22 of 55 of the patients (42%) had sudden cardiac death or sustained ventricular arrhythmia in a mean follow-up of only 15.4 ± 9.8 months. The authors concluded that patients with ischaemic cardiomyopathy who have severely depressed left ventricular ejection fraction, asymptomatic non-sustained ventricular tachycardia, and negative EP study may not be at low risk for future arrhythmic events.

The outcome of patients without inducible ventricular arrhythmias in the MUSTT trial was also not quite favourable – the 2-year and 5-year rate of arrhythmic events was 12% and 24%, respectively.[132] The fate of the non-inducible patients who met the entry criteria for MADIT study was somewhat better – 8% total mortality for 27 months.[99] However, both trials enrolled patients with only asymptomatic non-sustained ventricular arrhythmias. In comparison, the recurrence rate of sudden cardiac death of non-inducible survivors of out-of-hospital cardiac arrest followed up for the same average period of 27 months in the trial of Wilber et al.[114] was twice-higher (17%).

Cardiomyopathies

Potentially lethal ventricular arrhythmias occur frequently in hypertrophic cardiomyopathy (HCM).[133] The risk of sudden cardiac death in HCM ranges between 3 and 5%,[134,135] and is particularly high in young patients, with annual rates as high as 6%.[136] Polymorphic ventricular tachycardia or ventricular fibrillation is much more often the cause of sudden cardiac death in patients with HCM than sustained monomorphic ventricular tachycardia.[96] It seems that ICD implantation is highly effective for sudden cardiac death prevention in selected high-risk patients,[133,137] although its use in HCM is still not generally accepted.[49] The risk stratification of patients with HCM, especially young ones, is still an unresolved issue.[138]

The role of EP study in identifying patients with HCM at risk for sudden cardiac death is much less defined than in IHD, but is generally considered to be lower than in ischaemic heart disease.[139] Polymorphic ventricular tachycardia or ventricular fibrillation are much more frequently induced in patients with HCM than sustained monomorphic ventricular tachycardia. Watson et al.[43] reported that polymorphic ventricular tachycardia that deteriorated to ventricular fibrillation was induced by programmed ventricular stimulation in 8 (44%) of 18 patients with HCM at increased risk of sudden death (with prior cardiac arrest or syncope, non-sustained ventricular tachycardia on Holter, or a family history of sudden death). Notably, no sustained monomorphic ventricular tachycardia was induced.

On the other hand, Fananapazir et al.[140] reported that sustained ventricular arrhythmias were induced significantly more frequently in patients with cardiac arrest than in those with syncope, in patients with syncope than in those with presyncope, and in the latter compared with asymptomatic patients. Induction of ventricular tachycardia in symptomatic HCM patients (syncope or sudden cardiac death) identifies a subgroup of patients at high risk for subsequent cardiac events, with particularly high negative predictive value.[141] However, in more than three-quarters of the cases, the induced sustained ventricular tachycardia is polymorphic ventricular tachycardia or ventricular fibrillation,[140,142] and aggressive stimulation (three extrastimuli) is often required for induction.[141]

On the contrary, Kuck et al.[143] reported that inducibility in patients with HCM does not depend on the presence or absence of symptoms or spontaneous ventricular arrhythmias. Several cases of induction of VF by rapid atrium stimulation in patients with HCM have been described,[143–145] but the significance of this finding is not known.

Most of the available data suggests that the EP study is of limited value for the risk stratification of patients with idiopathic dilated cardiomyopathy.[146–148]

Poll et al.,[149] however, reported that the response to programmed ventricular stimulation in patients with idiopathic dilated cardiomyopathy is related to the clinical arrhythmia. They studied 47 patients with non-ischaemic dilated cardiomyopathy and were able to induce sustained monomorphic ventricular tachycardia in all 13 patients who presented with this arrhythmia, but in only one of 14 survivors of cardiac arrest, and in only two of 20 patients with non-sustained ventricular tachycardia.

In a retrospective analysis of six studies of 288 patients with idiopathic dilated cardiomyopathy altogether, Wilber et al.[150] showed that, although induction of sustained ventricular tachycardia in these patients identifies a high-risk group of sudden death and major arrhythmic events, the predictive value is low and 75% of the victims were not identified.

The role of EP study in arrhythmogenic right ventricular cardiomyopathy[151] is not yet established. Sotalol has been found to be highly effective in both inducible and non-inducible patients.[152] ICD implantation has been recommended in patients in whom antiarrhythmic drugs are ineffective, associated with side effects, or their effect is uncertain due to non-inducibility.[153] However, the development of the disease and the risk of sudden death is largely unpredictable and reliable risk-stratifiers have not been identified.[154,155]

Other cardiac diseases

Ischaemic heart disease and the cardiomyopathies together account for 90–95% of all cases of sudden cardiac death. The other 5–10% are due to valvular heart disease, possibly some forms of mitral valve prolapse, several congenital abnormalities including tetralogy of Fallot, transposition of the great arteries, aortic stenosis and pulmonary vascular obstruction, the congenital long QT syndrome and torsade de pointes induced by drugs or other substances, several types of idiopathic polymorphic ventricular tachycardia, the Brugada syndrome, the so-called "idiopathic ventricular fibrillation", and possibly some other disorders. The role of the EP study for risk stratification in most of them is not well established.

Generally, EP study with programmed ventricular stimulation is indicated in all patients who have survived cardiac arrest without evidence of acute Q wave myocardial infarction,[48] acute reversible cause, or primary repolarisation abnormality, such as congenital long QT syndrome, or drug-induced torsade de pointes. Programmed ventricular stimulation using both standard stimulation protocol, as well as modified protocols including abrupt changes in the cycle length ("short-long-short" sequence protocols[156]) with or without isoproterenol infusion is of limited value in patients with the long QT syndrome and is not generally recommended.[48,96]

In symptomatic patients with Brugada syndrome induction of sustained polymorphic ventricular tachycardia by programmed electrical stimulation is a rule.[157] The annual rate of sudden cardiac death in untreated symptomatic patients is 40%[157] and ICD is the only available treatment

with excellent results. Some experts suggest that asymptomatic patients with family history of sudden cardiac death should also undergo programmed stimulation and, if sustained ventricular tachycardia is induced, an ICD implanted.[157]

Unexplained syncope

In patients without structural heart disease or manifest cardiac arrhythmias the most common cause of unexplained syncope appears to be neurocardiogenic syncope. However, in subjects with cardiac disease the most common cause of unexplained syncope are bradyarrhythmias owing to either sinus node dysfunction or AV block, or more frequently, tachyarrhythmias. Syncope carries significantly worse prognosis in patients compared with those without heart disease – the 1-year mortality in the former group is 19–30%, whilst in the latter it is 1–12%.[50] In patients with unexplained syncope and structural heart disease, in whom general neurological and thorough non-invasive cardiac evaluation has not given results, the EP study may be needed to establish the cause of syncope, and, consequently, to determine the prognosis. It is estimated that, whilst in patients with heart disease the EP study may establish the cause of unexplained syncope in about 70%, in those without heart disease the diagnostic yield is only about 12%.[50] Sinus node dysfunction is a rare finding in patients with unexplained syncope during EP study – it has been found in 6% of patients with unexplained syncope with no evidence of SND during ambulatory monitoring.[158–160] The prognostic significance of abnormal SNRT is not firmly established, but it appears that only significantly prolonged SNRT >2 s, preferably with reproduction of symptoms is likely to identify the cause of syncope, and consequently, to predict alleviation of symptoms after pacemaker implantation.[161]

It is obvious, however, that the reproduction of the symptoms of a clinical arrhythmia in the artificial setting of the electrophysiological laboratory is less reliable than the reproduction of the arrhythmia itself.

As previously mentioned, significantly prolonged HV interval patients with bifascicular block is associated with increased risk for development of complete AV block.[57] In patients with unexplained syncope and no documented intermittent heart block, the isolated finding of prolonged HV >60 ms identifies those with increased risk of developing complete heart block who can benefit from pacemaker implantation.[162]

Ventricular tachycardia is the most common abnormality found during EP study in patients with cardiac disease and unexplained syncope, and it is induced in 36–53% of the patients.[158–160] The prognostic significance of ventricular tachycardia induced during EP study in patients with unexplained syncope is uncertain. Whilst sustained monomorphic ventricular tachycardia is practically always specific, clinically significant finding, non-sustained ventricular tachycardia and sustained polymorphic ventricular tachycardia are likely to be a non-specific finding, and their interpretation as a cause of the syncope is not justified.[159] However, induction of sustained polymorphic ventricular tachycardia or ventricular fibrillation in patients in whom this is likely to be the clinical arrhythmia, especially when achieved with less aggressive stimulation protocol (≤ 2[161] or ≤ 3[96] extrastimuli, with a coupling interval of ≥ 200[161] or > 180 ms[96]), may have clinical significance.

Conclusions: the electrophysiologic study as a risk stratifier today and tomorrow

For three decades the clinical practice of direct recording of cardiac potentials and diagnostic stimulation have changed fundamentally the knowledge of cardiac arrhythmias and the concepts of their management. The very existence of modern non-pharmacological therapy of arrhythmias (multichamber physiological antibradycardia pacing, implantable cardioverter–defibrillators, catheter ablations, and what has survived of arrhythmia surgery) would have been virtually impossible without the knowledge from EP study.

Because of its invasive nature and possible side effects, the role of the EP study as a diagnostic and prognostic tool has been restricted to relatively small groups of patients preselected by clinical variables and non-invasive tests. In recent years its role has been further limited by general development of non-invasive electrocardiology, deeper insight into the surface ECG (accumulated from correlation of surface and intracardiac recordings), and changes in the basic concepts of arrhythmia management. Today patients with bradyarrhythmias are evaluated by clinical and non-invasive tests, and the EP study tends to be preserved only for exceptional cases.

The concept of management of malignant ventricular arrhythmias has changed dramatically in the last decade. Reliable methods to identify the vast majority of potentials victims are still lacking. Even if identified, however, therapy of proven efficacy for this majority is not available, since ICD implantation will continue to be confined to a small subset of high-risk patients. Finally, reliable methods for assessment of the efficacy of the only available therapy for this majority of potential victims, i.e. antiarrhythmic drug therapy, are also lacking.

A decade ago antiarrhythmic drug therapy of malignant ventricular arrhythmias was dominated by class I drugs and arbitrary methods for assessment of their efficacy, such as suppression of spontaneous ventricular ectopy or arrhythmia inducibility. It is clear now that class I drugs do not prevent sudden cardiac death, and suppression of

arrhythmia inducibility does not adequately reflect patients' outcome. It is likely that programmed stimulation will preserve some limited role in the near future for risk stratification of patients likely to benefit from ICD implantation, as suggested by recent primary and secondary prevention trials. The non-ICD and the combined ICD-pharmacological therapy of ventricular arrhythmias, however, will be dominated in the near future by available and newly emerging[163] drugs with class III or similar effect. Apparently, to assess both their efficacy adequately, as well as their potential for arrhythmogenic effect, newer methods are needed that would more deeply or more directly reflect the process of spontaneous arrhythmogenesis.

References

1. Scherlag BJ, Lau SH, Helfant RH, Berkowitz WD, Stein E, Damato AN. Catheter technique for recording His bundle activity in man. *Circulation* 1969;**39**:13–18.
2. Durrer D, Schoo L, Schuilenberg RM *et al.* The role of premature beats in the initiation and termination of supraventricular tachycardia in the Wolff–Parkinon–White syndrome. *Circulation* 1967;**36**:644.
3. Coumel PH, Cabrol C, Fabiato A *et al.* Tachycardia permanente par rhythme réciproque. *Arch Mal Coeur* 1967;**60**:1830.
4. Wellens HJJ, Schuilenburg RM, Durrer D. Electrical stimulation of the heart in patients with ventricular tachycardia. *Circulation* 1972;**46**:216–26.
5. Buxton AE, Lee KL, Fisher JD, Josephson ME, Prystowski EN, Hafley G for the Multicenter Unsustained Tachycardia Trial Investigators. A randomized study of the prevention of sudden death in patients with coronary artery disease. *N Engl J Med* 1999;**341**:1882–90.
6. Cardiac Arrhythmia Suppression Trial (CAST) Investigators. Preliminary report: effect of encainide and flecainide on mortality in a randomized trial of arrhythmia suppression after myocardial infarction. *N Engl J Med* 1989;**321**:406–12.
7. Samojloff A. Weitere Beitrage zur Elektrophysiologie des Herzens. *Pflügers Arch* 1910;**135**:417.
8. Olsson SB, Varnauskas E, Korsgren M. Further improved method for measuring monophasic action potentials of the intact human heart. *J Electrocardiol* 1971;**4**:19–23.
9. Franz MR. Long-term recording of monophasic action potentials from human endocardium. *Am J Cardiol* 1983;**51**:1629–34.
10. Frohlich R, Wetzig T, Bolz A, Schaldach M. Measurement and analysis of monophasic action potentials using fractally coated electrodes: I. *Biomed Technol Berlin* 1995;**40**:154–9.
11. Olsson SB, Yuan S. Technique and use of monophasic action potential recordings. In: Mandel WJ ed. *Cardiac arrhythmias*. Philadelphia: JB Lippincott 1995, pp. 785–810.

12. Ino T, Karagueuzian HS, Hong K, Meesmann M, Mandel WJ, Peter T. Relation of monophasic action potential recorded with contact electrode to underlying transmembrane action potential properties in isolated cardiac tissues: a systematic microelectrode validation study. *Cardiovasc Res* 1988;**22**:255–64.

13. Josephson ME. Electrophysiological investigation: general concepts. In: ME Josephson ed. *Clinical cardiac electrophysiology: techniques and interpretation*. Malvern, Pennsylvania: Lea & Febiger, 1993, pp. 417–615.

14. Gupta PK, Lichstein E, Chadda KD. Chronic His bundle block. Clinical, electrocardiographic, electrophysiological, and follow-up studies on 16 patients. *Br Heart J* 1976;**38**:1343.

15. Amat-Y-Leon F, Dhingra R, Denes P, Wyndham C, Chuquimia R, Rosen KM. The clinical spectrum of chronic His bundle block. *Chest* 1976;**70**:747.

16. Josephson ME. Intraventricular conduction disturbances. In: Josephson ME ed. *Clinical cardiac electrophysiology: techniques and interpretation*. Malvern, Pennsylvania: Lea & Febiger, 1993, pp. 117–49.

17. Saumarez RC, Camm AJ, Panagos A *et al*. Ventricular fibrillation in hypertrophic cardiomyopathy is associated with increased fractionation of paced right ventricular electrograms. *Circulation* 1992;**86**:467–74.

18. Saumarez RC, Slade AK, Grace AA *et al*. The significance of paced electrograms fractionation in hypertrophic cardiomyopathy. A prospective study. *Circulation* 1995;**91**:2762–8.

19. Saumarez RC, Heald S, Gill J *et al*. Primary ventricular fibrillation is associated with increased paced right ventricular electrogram fractionation. *Circulation* 1995;**92**:2565–71.

20. Vassalle M. Electrogenic suppression of automaticity in sheep and dog Purkinje fibers. *Circ Res* 1970;**27**:361.

21. Vassalle M. The relationship among cardiac pacemakers. Overdrive suppression. *Circ Res* 1977;**41**:269.

22. Mandel WJ, Hayakawa H, Allen HN, Danzig R, Marcus HS. Evaluation of sinoatrial node function in man by overdrive suppression. *Circulation* 1971;**44**:59.

23. Mandel WJ, Hayakawa H, Allen HN, Danzig R, Kermaier AI. Assessment of sinus node function in patients with the sick sinus syndrome. *Circulation* 1972;**46**:761.

24. Breithardt G, Seipel L, Loogen F. Sinus node recovery time and calculated sinoatrial conduction time in normal subjects and patients with sinus node dysfunction. *Circulation* 1977;**56**:43.

25. Kulbertus HE, Leval-Rutten F, Mary L, Casters P. Sinus node recovery time in the elderly. *Br Heart J* 1975;**37**:420.

26. Narula OS, Samet P, Javier RP. Significance of the sinus node recovery time. *Circulation* 1972;**45**:140.

27. Josephson ME. Sinus node function. In: Josephson ME ed. *Clinical cardiac electrophysiology: techniques and interpretation*. Malvern, Pennsylvania: Lea & Febiger, 1993, pp. 71–95.

28. Characteristics of extracellular potentials recorded from the sinoatrial pacemaker of the rabbit. *Circ Res* 1977;**41**:292.

29. Strauss HC, Bigger JT, Saroff AL, Giardina EGV. Electrophysiologic evaluation of sinus node function in patients with sinus node dysfunction. *Circulation* 1976;**53**:763.

30. Narula OS, Shanto N, Vasquez M, Towne WD, Linhart JW. A new method for measurement of sinoatrial conduction time. *Circulation* 1978;**58**:706.

31. Strauss HC, Saroff AL, Bigger JT, Giardina EGV. Premature atrial stimulation as a key to the understanding of sinoatrial conduction in man. *Circulation* 1973;**47**:86.

32. Kerr CR, Strauss HC. The measurement of sinus node refractoriness in man. *Circulation* 1983;**68**:1231.

33. Dhingra RC, Wyndham C, Bauernfield R *et al*. Significance of block distal to the His bundle induced by atrial pacing in patients with chronic bifascicular block. *Circulation* 1979;**60**:1455.

34. Kaul U, Dev V, Narula J *et al*. Evaluation of patients with bundle branch block and "unexplained syncope": A study based on comprehensive electrophysiologic testing and ajmaline test. *Pacing Clin Electrophysiol* 1988;**11**:289–96.

35. Wunderlich E, Hetze A. Provocation of higher-degree atrioventricular blocks by ajmaline and rapid ventricular pacing in patients with fascicular block. *Cor Vasa* 1984;**26**:281–8.

36. Tonkin AM, Heddle WF, Tornos P. Intermittent atrioventricular block: Procainamide administration as a provocative test. *Aust N Z J Med* 1978;**8**:594–602.

37. Bergfeldt L, Rosenqvist M, Vallin H *et al*. Disopyramide induced second and third degree atrioventricular block in patients with bifascicular block. An acute stress test to predict atrioventricular block progression. *Br Heart J* 1985;**53**:328–34.

38. Dangman KH, Hoffman BF. Studies on overdrive stimulation of canine cardiac fibres: Maximum diastolic potential as a determinant of the response. *J Am Coll Cardiol* 1983;**2**:1183.

39. Hoffman BF, Dangman KH. Are arrhythmias caused by automatic impulse generation? In: de Carvalho AP, Hoffman BF, Lieberman M (eds): *The symposium on normal and abnormal conduction of the heart beat*. Mount Kisco, NY: Fututra, 1982, pp 429–48.

40. Segers M. Le role des potentiels tardifs du coeur. *Mem Acad R Med Belg (Series II)* 1941;**1**:1–30.

41. Wit AL, Cranfield PF. Triggered activity in cardiac muscle fibers of the simian mitral valve. *Circ Res* 1976;**38**:85–98.

42. Wit AL, Cranfield PF. Triggered and automatic activity in the canine coronary sinus. *Circ Res* 1977;**41**:435–45.

43. Watson RM, Schwartz JL, Maron BJ, Tucker E, Rosing DR, Josephson ME. Inducible polymorphic ventricular tachycardia and ventricular fibrillation in a subgroup of patients with hypertrophic cardiomyopathy at high risk for sudden death. *J Am Coll Cardiol* 1987;**10**:761–74.

44. Yuan S, Blomström-Lundqvist C, Pehrson S, Pripp C-M, Wohlfart B, Olsson SB. Dispersion of repolarisation following double and triple programmed stimulation. A clinical study using the monophasic action potential recording technique. *Eur Heart J* 1996;**17**:1080–91.

45. Andersen HR, Nielsen JC, Thomsen PEB *et al*. Atrioventricular conduction during long-term follow-up of patients with sick sinus syndrome. *Circulation* 1998;**98**:1315–21.

46. Brandt J, Anderson H, Fahraeus T, Schuller H. Natural history of sinus node disease treated with atrial pacing in 213 patients: implications for selection of stimulation mode. *J Am Coll Cardiol* 1992;**20**:633–9.

47. Dhingra RC, Wyndham C, Amat-y-Leon F *et al*. Incidence and site of atrioventricular blcok in patients with chronic bifascicular block. *Circulation* 1979;**59**:238–46.

48. ACC/AHA Task Force Report. Guidelines for clinical intracardiac electrophysiological and catheter ablation procedures. A report of the American College of Cardiology/American Heart Association Task Force on Practice Guidelines (Committee on Clinical Intracardiac Electrophysiologic and Catheter Ablation Procedures), developed in collaboration with the North American Society of Pacing and Electrophysiology. *J Am Coll Cardiol* 1995;**26**:555–73.

49. ACC/AHA Practice Guidelines. ACC/AHA Guidelines for implantation of cardiac pacemakers and antiarrhythmia devices. A report of the American College of Cardiology/American Heart Association Task Force on Practice Guidelines (Committee on Pacemaker Implantation). *J Am Coll Cardiol* 1998;**31**:1175–209.

50. Zipes DP. Genesis of cardiac arrhythmias: electrophysiological considerations. In: Braunwald E ed. *Heart disease. a textbook of cardiovascular medicine*. Philadelphia: W.B. Saunders Co., 1997, pp.548–92.

51. Shaw DB, Holman RR, Gowers JI. Survival in sinoatrial disorder (sick sinus syndrome). *BMJ*1980;**280**:139–41.

52. Rasmussen K. Chronic sinus node disease: natural course and indications for pacing. *Eur Heart J* 1981;**2**:455–9.

53. Zipes DP. Second-degree atrioventricular block. *Circulation* 1979;**60**:465–72.

54. McAnulty JH, Rahimtoola SH, Murphy E *et al*. Natural history of "high risk" bundle branch block. Final report of a prospective study. *N Engl J Med* 1982;**307**:137.

55. Scheinman MM, Peters RW, Modin G, Brennan M, Mies C, O'Young J. Prognostic value of infranodal conduction time in patients with chronic bundle branch block. *Circulation* 1977;**56**:240–4.

56. Dhingra RC, Palileo E, Strasberg B *et al*. Significance of the HV interval in 517 patients with chronic bifascicular block. *Circulation* 1981;**64**:1265.

57. Scheinman MM, Peters RW, Sauve MJ *et al*. Value of the H-Q interval in patients with bundle branch block and the role of prophylactic permanent pacing. *Am J Cardiol* 1982;**50**:1316.

58. Dhingra RC, Wyndham C, Bauernfeind R *et al*. Significance of block distal to the His bundle induced by atrial pacing in patients with chronic bifascicular block. *Circulation* 1979;**60**:1455.

59. Englund A, Bergfeldt L, Rosenqvist M. Disopyramide stress test: A sensitive and specific tool for predicting impending high degree atrioventricular block in patients with bifascicular block. *Br Heart J* 1995;**74**:650–5.

60. Jordaens L. Are there any useful investigations that predict which patients with bifascicular block will develop third degree atrioventricular block? *Heart* 1996;**75**:542–3.

61. Ezri M, Lerman BB, Marchlinski FE, Buxton AE, Josephson ME. Electrophysiologic evaluation of syncope in patients with bifascicular block. *Am Heart J* 1983;**106**:693.

62. Campbell RWF, Smith RA, Gallagher JJ, Pritchett ELC, Wallace AG. Atrial fibrillation in the pre-excitation syndrome. *Am J Cardiol* 1977;**40**:514–20.

63. Robinson K, Rowland E, Krikler DM. Wolff–Parkinson–White syndrome: atrial fibrillation as the presenting arrhythmia. *Br Heart J* 1988;**59**:578–80.

64. Munger TM, Packer DL, Hammill SC *et al*. A population study of the natural history of Wolff–Parkinson–White syndrome in Olmsted county, Minnesota, 1953–1989. *Circulation* 1993;**87**:866–73.

65. Klein GJ, Bashore TM, Sellers TD, Pritchett ELC, Smith WM, Gallagher JJ. Ventricular fibrillation in the Wolff–Parkinson–White syndrome. *N Engl J Med* 1979;**301**:1080–5.

66. Paul T, Guccione P, Garson A. Relation of syncope in young patients with Wolff–Parkinson–White syndrome to rapid ventricular response during atrial fibrillation. *Am J Cardiol* 1990;**65**:318–21.

67. Toff WD, Camm AJ. Ventricular pre-excitation and professional aircrew licensing. *Eur Heart J* 1992;**13**(Suppl. H):**149**:161.

68. Wellens HJJ, Durrer D. Relation between the refractory period of the accessory pathway and ventricular frequency during atrial fibrillation in patients with the Wolff–Parkinson–White syndrome. *Am J Cardiol* 1974;**33**:178.

69. Siebels J, Kuck KH, and the CASH Investigators. Implantable cardioverter defibrillator compared with antiarrhythmic drug treatment in cardiac arrest survivors (the Cardiac Arrest Study Hamburg). *Am Heart J* 1994;**127**:1139–44.

70. Steinbeck G, Greene HL. Management of patients with life-threatening sustained ventricular tachyarrhythmias – the role of guided antiarrhythmic drug therapy. *Prog Cardiovasc Dis* 1996;**38**:419–28.

71. Mason JW, for the ESVEM Investigators. A comparison of electrophysiologic testing with Holter monitoring to predict antiarrhythmic-drug efficacy for ventricular tachyarrhythmias. *N Engl J Med* 1993;**329**:445–51.

72. Zipes DP, Wellens HJJ. Sudden cardiac death. *Circulation* 1998;**98**:2334–51.

73. Myerburg RJ, Interian A Jr, Mitrani RM, Kessler KM, Castellanos A. Frequency of sudden death and profiles of risk. *Am J Cardiol* 1997;**80**(Suppl.):10F–19F.

74. Sheldon R, Connolly S, Krahn A, Roberts R, Gent M, Gardner M, on behalf of the CIDS Investigators. Identification of patients most likely to benefit from implantable cardioverter–defibrillator therapy. The Canadian Implantable Defibrillator Study. *Circulation* 2000;**101**:1660–4.

75. Moss AJ. Implantable cardioverter defibrillator therapy. The sickest patients benefit the most. *Circulation* 2000;**101**:1638–40.

76. Myerburg RJ, Kessler KM, Castellanos A. Sudden cardiac death: Structure, function and time-dependence of risk. *Circulation* 1992;**85**(Suppl. I):1–2.

77. Richards DA, Byth K, Ross DL, Uther JB. What is the best predictor of spontaneous ventricular tachycardia and sudden death after myocardial infarction? *Circulation* 1991;**83**:756–63.

78. Marchlinski F, Buxton A, Waxman H *et al*. Identifying patients at risk of sudden death after myocardial infarction: Value of the response to programmed stimulation, degree

of ventricular ectopic activity and severity of left ventricular dysfunction. *Am J Cardiol* 1983;**52**:1190–6.

79. Doevendans PA, Cheriex EC, van der Zee R *et al*. Risk stratification in the thrombolytic era: Results of a prospective study. *Cardiologie* 1996;**3**:319–23.

80. Roy D, Marchand E, Theroux P *et al*. Programmed ventricular stimulation in survivors of an acute myocardial infarction. *Circulation* 1985;**72**:487–94.

81. Andresen D, Steinbeck G, Brüggemann T *et al*. Risk stratification following myocardial infarction in the thrombolytic era. A two-step strategy using noninvasive and invasive methods. *J Am Coll Cardiol* 1999;**33**:131–8.

82. Andresen D, Brüggemann T, Behrens S, Ehlers C. Risk of ventricular arrhythmias in survivors of myocardial infarction. *Pacing Clin Electrophysiol* 1997;**20**(Pt II):2699–705.

83. McClements BM, Adgey J. Value of signal-averaged electrocardiography, radionuclide ventriculography, Holter monitoring and clinical variables for prediction of arrhythmic events in survivors of acute myocardial infarction in the thrombolytic era. *J Am Coll Cardiol* 1993;**21**:1419–27.

84. Bhandari A, Hong R, Kotlewski A *et al*. Frequency and significance of induced sustained ventricular tachycardia or fibrillation 2 weeks after acute myocardial infarction. *Am J Cardiol* 1985;**5**:737–42.

85. Anderson KP, Shusterman V, Brode S, Gottipaty V, Schwartzman D, Weiss R. Noninvasive testing for selection of patients for electrophysiological study. *Ann Noninvas Electrocardiol* 1999;**4**:434–42.

86. Bigger JT, Fleiss J, Kleiger R, Miller J, and the Multi-Center Post-Infarction Research Group. The relationship between ventricular arrhythmias, left ventricular dysfunction, and mortality on the two years after myocardial infarction. *Circulation* 1984;**69**:250–8.

87. Kostis JB, Byington R, Friedman LM *et al*. Prognostic significance of ventricular ectopic activity in survivors of acute myocardial infarction. *J Am Coll Cardiol* 1987;**10**:231–42.

88. Bigger JT Jr, Weld FM, Rolnitzky LM. Prevalence, characteristics and significance of ventricular tachycardia (three or more complexes) detected by ambulatory electrocardiographic recording in the late hospital phase of acute myocardial infarction. *Am J Cardiol* 1981;**48**:815–23.

89. Tavazzi L, Volpi A for the GISSI Investigators. remarks about postinfarction prognosis in light of the experience with the Gruppo Italiano per lo Studio della Sopravvivenza nell' Infarto Miocardico (GISSI) Trials. *Circulation* 1997;**95**:1341–5.

90. Bigger JT Jr, Fleiss JL, Rolnitzky LM and the Multi-Center Post-Infarction Research Group. Prevalence, characteristics, and significance of ventricular tachycardia detected by 24–hour continuous electrocardiographic recording in the late hospital phase of acute myocardial infarction. *Am J Cardiol* 1986;**58**:1151–60.

91. Mukharji J, Rude RE, Poole WK *et al*. Risk Factors for sudden death after acute myocardial infarction: two-year follow-up. *Am J Cardiol* 1984;**54**:31–6.

92. Gomes JA, Winters SL, Stewart D *et al*. A new noninvasive index to predict sustained ventricular tachycardia and sudden death in the first year after myocardial infarction: based on signal-averaged electrocardiogram, radionuclide

ejection fraction and Holter monitoring. *J Am Coll Cardiol* 1987; 10:349–57.

93. Multicenter Posinfarction Research Group. Risk stratification and survival after after myocardial infarction. *N Engl J Med* 1983;**309**:331–6.

94. Mukharji J, Rude RE, Poole WK *et al*. Risk factors for sudden death after acute myocardial infarction: two year follow-up. *Am J Cardiol* 1984;**54**:31–6.

95. Davis HT, DeCamilla J, Bayer LW, Moss AJ. Survivorship patterns in the posthospital phase of myocardial infarction. *Circulation* 1979;**60**:1252–8.

96. Josephson ME. Recurrent ventricular tachycardia. In: Josephson ME. *Clinical cardiac electrophysiology: techniques and interpretation*. Malvern, Pennsylvania: Lea & Febiger, 1993, pp. 417–615.

97. Middlekauuff HR, Stevenson WG, Tillisch JH. Prevention of sudden death in survivors of myocardial infarction: A decision analysis approach. *Am Heart J* 1992;**123**:475–80.

98. Moss AJ, Hall WJ, Cannom DS *et al*. for the Multicenter Automatic Defibrillator Implantation Trial (MADIT). Improved survival with and implanted defibrillator in patients with coronary disease at high risk for ventricular arrhythmia. *N Engl J Med* 1996;**335**:1933–40.

99. Daubert JP, Higgins SL, Zareba W, Wilbert DJ. Comparative survival of MADIT-eligible but noninducible patients. *J Am Coll Cardiol* 1997;**29**(Suppl.):78A(Abstr.)

100. Buxton AE, Lee KL, Fisher JD, Josephson ME, Prystowski EN, Hafley G for the Multicenter Unsustained Tachycardia Trial Investigators. A randomized study of the prevention of sudden death in patients with coronary artery disease. *N Engl J Med* 1999;**341**:1882–90.

101. Pedretti R, Etro MD, Laporta A *et al*. Prediction of late arrhythmic events after acute myocardial infarction from combined use of noninvasive prognostic variables and inducibility of sustained monomorphic ventricular tachycardia. *Am J Cardiol* 1993;**71**:1131–41.

102. Bardy GH, Lee KL, Mark DB and the SCD-Heft Pilot Investigators. The Sudden Cardiac Death in Heart Failure Trial: pilot study. *Pacing Clin Electrophysiol* 1997;**20**: 1148(Abstr.)

103. Moss AJ, Cannom DS, Daubert JP *et al*. for the MADIT II Investigators. Multicenter Automatic Defibrillator Implantation Trial II (MADIT II): design and clinical protocol. *Ann Noninvas Electrocardiol* 1999;**4**:83–91.

104. Josephson ME, Almendral JM, Marchlinski FE. Mechanisms of ventricular tachycardia. *Circulation* 1987; **75**:41.

105. Roy D, Waxman HL, Kienzle MC, Buxton AE, Marchlinski FE, Josephson ME. Clinical characteristics and long-term follow-up in 119 survivors of out-of-hospital cardiac arrest: relation to inducibility at electrophysiologic testing. *Am J Cardiol* 1983;**52**:969–74.

106. Morady F, Scheinmann MM, Hess DS, Sung RJ, Shen E, Shapiro W. Electrophysiologic testing in the management of survivors of out-of-hospital cardiac arrest. *Am J Cardiol* 1983;**51**:85–9.

107. Baum RS, Alvarez H, Cobb LA. Survival after resuscitation from out-of-hospital ventricular fibrillation. *Circulation* 1974;**50**:1231–5.

108. Schaffer WA, Cobb LA. Recurrent ventricular fibrillation and mode of death in survivors of out of hospital ventricular fibrillation. *N Engl J Med* 1975;**293**:259–62.

109. Myerburg RJ, Kessler KM, Estes D *et al*. Long-term survival after prehospital cardiac arrest: analysis of outcome during an 8 year study. *Circulation* 1984;**70**:538–46.

110. Liberthson RR, Nagel EL, Hirschman JC, Nussenfeld SR. Prehospital ventricular defibrillation: prognosis and follow-up course. *N Engl J Med* 1974;**291**:317–21.

111. Schaffer WA, Cobb LA. Recurrent ventricular fibrillation and modes of death in survivors of out-of-hospital ventricular fibrillation. *N Engl J Med* 1975;**293**:259–62.

112. Weaver WD, Cobb LA, Hallstrom AP. Ambulatory arrhythmias in resuscitated victims of cardiac arrest. *Circulation* 1982;**66**:212–18.

113. Moosvi AR, Goldstein S, Vanderburg-Medentorp S *et al*. Effect of empiric antiarrhythmic therapy in resuscitated out-of-hospital cardiac arrest victims with coronary artery disease. *Am J Cardiol* 1990;**65**:1192–7.

114. Wilber DJ, Garan H, Finkelstein D *et al*. Out-of-hospital cardiac arrest. Use of electrophysiologic testing in the prediction of long-term outcome. *N Engl J Med* 1988;**318**:19–24.

115. Ruskin JN, DiMarco JP, Garan H. Out of hospital cardiac arrest: electrophysiologic observations and selection of long-term antiarrhythmic therapy. *N Engl J Med* 1980;**303**:607–13.

116. Troup PJ. Programmed stimulation-guided therapy compared with implantable cardioverter–defibrillator device therapy in the treatment of ventricular tachyarrhythmias. *Pacing Clin Electrophysiol* 1991;**14**:267–72.

117. Benditt DG, Benson DW Jr, Klein GJ, Pritzker MR, Kriett JM, Anderson RW. Prevention of recurrent sudden cardiac arrest: role of provocative electropharmacologic testing. *J Am Coll Cardiol* 1983;**2**:418–25.

118. Skale BT, Miles WM, Heger JJ, Zipes DP, Prystowsky EN. Survivors of cardiac arrest: prevention of recurrence by drug therapy as predicted by electrophysiologic testing or electrocardiographic monitoring. *Am J Cardiol* 1986;**57**:113–19.

119. Mitchell LB, Sheldon RS, Gillis AM *et al*. Definition of predicted effective antiarrhythmic drug therapy for ventricular tachyarrhythmias by the electrophysiologic study approach: randomized comparison of patient response criteria. *J Am Coll Cardiol* 1997;**30**:1346–53.

120. The CASCADE Investigators. Randomized antiarrhythmic drug therapy in survivors of cardiac arrest (the CASCADE study). *Am J Cardiol* 1993;**72**:280–7.

121. Böcker D, Haverkamp W, Block M, Borggrefe M, Hammel D, Brethardt G. Comparison of d,l-sotalol and implantable defibrillators for treatment of sustained ventricular tachycardia or fibrillation in patients with coronary artery disease. *Circulation* 1996;**94**:151–7.

122. Antz M, Cappato R, Kuck KH. Metoprolol versus sotalol in the treatment of sustained ventricular tachycardia. *J Cardiovasc Pharmacol* 1995;**26**:627–35.

123. Newman D, Sauve MJ, Herre J *et al*. Survival after implantation of the cardioverter defibrillator. *J Am Cardiol* 1992;**69**:899–903.

124. Fogoros RN, Fiedler SB, Elson JJ. The automatic implantable cardioverter–defibrillator in drug-refractory ventricular tachyarrhythmias. *Ann Intern Med* 1987;**107**:635–40.

125. Böcker D, Haverkamp W, Block M, Hammel D, Borggrefe M, Breithardt G. Comparison of d,l-sotalol and implantable defibrillators for treatment of sustained ventricular tachycardia or fibrillation in patients with coronary artery disease. *Circulation* 1996;**94**:151–7.

126. The Antiarrhythmic versus Implantable Defibrillators (AVID) Investigators. A comparison of antiarrhythmic drug therapy with implantable defibrillators in patients resuscitated from near-fatal ventricular arrhythmias. *N Engl J Med* 1997;**337**:1576–83.

127. Kuck KH on behalf of the CASH Investigators. The CASH study: final results. Oral presentation at the *Annual Session of the American College of Cardiology meeting*, Atlanta, March 29–April 1, 1998.

128. Connolly SJ, Gent M, Roberts RS *et al*. for the CIDS Investigators. Canadian Implantable Defibrillator Study (CIDS). A randomized trial of the implantable cardioverter defibrillator against amiodarone. *Circulation* 2000;**101**:1297–302.

129. Wever EFD, Hauer RNW, van Capelle FJI *et al*. Randomized study of implantable defibrillator as first-choice therapy versus conventional strategy in postinfarct sudden death survivors. *Circulation* 1995;**91**:2195–203.

130. Kowey PR, Taylor JE, Marinchak RA, Rials SJ. Does programmed stimulation really help in the evaluation of patients with nonsustained ventricular tachycardia? Results of a meta-analysis. *Am Heart J* 1992;**123**:481–5.

131. Kim MH, Bruckman D, Kirsh MM, Kou WH. Outcome of men with ischemic cardiomyopathy, asymptomatic nonsustained ventricular tachycardia, and negative electrophysiologic study. *Am J Cardiol* 2000;**85**:119–21.

132. Buxton AE for the MUSTT Investigators. Multicentered Unsustained Tachycardia Trial (MUSTT): Utility of electrophysiologic testing to identify patients with coronary artery disease at rusk for sudden death (oral presentation). *North American Society for Pacing and Electrophysiology 20th Scientific Sessions*, May 12–15, 1999, Toronto, Canada.

133. Maron BJ, Shen W-K, Link MS *et al*. Efficacy of implantable cardioverter–defibrillators for the prevention of sudden death in patients with hypertrophic cardiomyopathy. *N Engl J Med* 2000;**342**:365–73.

134. Goodwin JF, Krikler DM. Arrhythmias as a cause of sudden death in hypertrophic cardiomyopathy. *Lancet* 1976;**2**:937–40.

135. Hardarson T, de la Calzada CS, Curiel R *et al*. Prognosis and mortality of hypertrophic obstructive cardiomyopathy. *Lancet* 1973;**2**:1462–7.

136. Clark AL, Coats AJ. Screening for hypertrophic cardiomyopathy. *BMJ* 1993;**306**:409.

137. Elliott PM, Sharma S, Varnava A, Poloniecki J, Rowland E, McKenna WJ. Survival after cardiac arrest or sustained ventricular tachycardia in patients with hypertrophic cardiomyopathy. *J Am Coll Cardiol* 1999;**33**:1596–601.

138. Evaluation of the risk of sudden death in hypertrophic cardiomyopathy. *Arch Mal Coeur Vas* 1999;**1**:65–73 (in French).

139. Wynne J, Braunwald E. The cardiomyopathies and myocarditides. In: Braunwald E ed. *Heart disease. A textbook of cardiovascular medicine*. Philadelphia: WB Saunders, 1997, pp. 1404–63.

140. Fananapazir L, Tracy CM, Leon MB *et al*. Electrophysiologic abnormalities in patients with hypertrophic cardiomyopathy. A consecutive analysis of 155 patients. *Circulation* 1989;**80**:1259–68.

141. Fananapazir L, Chang AC, Epstein SE, McAreavey D. Prognostic determinants in hypertrophic cardiomyopathy. Prospective evaluation of a therapeutic strategy based on clinical, Holter, hemodynamic, and electrophysiologic findings. *Circulation* 1992;**86**:730–40.

142. Fananapazir L, Epstein SE. Hemodynamic and electrophysiologic evaluation of patients with hypertrophic cardiomyopathy surviving cardiac arrest. *Am J Cardiol* 1991;**67**:280–7.

143. Kuck KH, Kunze KP, Schlüter M *et al*. Programmed electrical stimulation in patients with hypertrophic cardiomyopathy. Results in patients with and without cardiac arrest or syncope. *Eur Heart J* 1988;**9**:177–85.

144. Wellens HJJ, Bär FW, Vanagt RJ *et al*. Medical treatment of ventricular tachycardia: Considerations in the selection of patients for surgical treatment. *Am J Cardiol* 1982;**49**:186–93.

145. Stafford WJ, Trohman RG, Bilsker M *et al*. Cardiac arrest in an adolescent with atrial fibrillation and hypertrophic cardiomyopathy. *J Am Coll Cardiol* 1986;**7**:701–4.

146. Milner PG, Dimarco JP, Lerman BB. Electrophysiological evaluation of sustained ventricular tachyarrhythmias in idiopathic dilated cardiomyopathy. *Pacing Clin Electrophysiol* 1988;**11**:562–8.

147. Turrito G, Ahuja RK, Caref EB, El-Sherif N. Risk stratification for arrhythmic events in patients with nonischaemic dilated cardiomyopathy and nonsustained ventricular tachycardia: role of programmed ventricular stimulation and the signal averaged electrocardiogram. *J Am Coll Cardiol* 1994;**24**:1523–8.

148. Meinertz T, Treese N, Kasper W *et al*. Determinants of prognosis in idiopathic dilated cardiomyopathy as determined by programmed electrical stimulation. *Am J Cardiol* 1985;**56**:337–41.

149. Poll DS, Marchlinski FE, Buxton AE, Josephson ME. Usefulness of programmed stimulation in idiopathic dilated cardiomyopathy. *Am J Cardiol* 1986;**58**:992–7.

150. Wilber DM. Evaluation and treatment of nonsustained ventricular tachycardia. *Curr Opin Cardiol* 1996;**11**:23–31.

151. Marcus FI, Fontaine G, Guiraudon G *et al*. Right ventricular dysplasia: a report of 24 adult cases. *Circulation* 1982;**65**:384–98.

152. Wichter T, Borggrefe M, Haverkamp W, Chen X, Breihardt G. Efficacy of antiarrhythmic drugs in patients with arrhythmogenic right ventricular disease. Results in patients with inducible and noninducible tachycardia. *Circulation* 1992;**86**:29–37.

153. Pinamonti B, Sinagra G, Camerini F. Clinical relevance of right ventricular dysplasia/cardiomyopathy. *Heart* 2000;**83**:9–11.

154. Pinamonti B, Di Lenarda A, Sinagra G, Silvestri F, Bussani R, Camerini F and The Heart Muscle Disease Study Group. *Am Heart J* 1995;**129**:412–15.

155. Blomstrom-Lundqvist S, Sabel SG, Olsson SB. A long-term follow-up of 15 patients with arrhythmogenic right ventricular dysplasia. *Br Heart J* 1987;**58**:477–88.

156. Denker S, Lehmann M, Mahmud R, Gilbert C, Akhtar M. Facilitation of ventricular tachycardia induction with abrupt changes in ventricular cycle length. *Am J Cardiol* 1984;**53**:508.

157. Brugada J, Brugada P, Brugada R.. The syndrome of right bundle branch block, ST segment elevation in V1 to V3 and sudden cardiac death – the Brugada syndrome. *Europace* 1999;**1**:156–66.

158. Di Marco JP, Garan H, Harthorne JW, Ruskin JN. Intracardiac electrophysiologic techniques in recurrent syncope of unknown cause. *Ann Intern Med* 1981;**95**:542.

159. Morady F, Shen E, Schwartz A *et al*. Long-term follow-up of patients with recurrent unexplained syncope evaluated by electrophysiologic testing. *J Am Coll Cardiol* 1983;**2**:1053.

160. Akhtar M, Shenasa M, Denker S *et al*. Role of cardiac electrophysiologic studies in patients with unexplained recurrent syncope. *Pacing Clin Electrophysiol* 1983;**6**:192.

161. Morady F. Electrophysiologic testing in the management of patients with unexplained syncope. In: Mandel WJ ed. *Cardiac arrhythmias*, 3rd edn. Philadelphia: JB Lippincott Co., 1995, pp. 863–78.

162. Altschuler H, Fisher JD, Furman S. Significance of isolated H-V interval prolongation in symptomatic patients without documented heart block. *Am Heart J* 1979;**97**:19–26.

163. Camm AJ, Yap YG. What should we expect from the next generation of antiarrhythmic drugs? *J Cardiovasc Electrophysiol* 1999;**10**:307–17.

10 QT dispersion

Velislav Batchvarov and Marek Malik

The attempts to characterise and quantify the abnormalities of ventricular repolarisation from the surface electrocardiogram (ECG) have a long history. Applications of precise mathematical methods, such as principal component analysis, can be traced back to the 1960s.[1] In clinical practice, however, the ECG-based assessment of ventricular repolarisation has been limited to the measurement of the QT interval and its heart rate correction, and to the description of the polarity of the T wave and shape often using vague terms such as "nonspecific ST-T wave changes".

It had been noticed some time ago that the duration of the QT interval varies between individual leads of the standard surface ECG[2] and it has been suggested that these variations may reflect a physiological phenomenon.[3] The old idea was revived in 1990 by the group of the late Professor Campbell and the interlead differences of the QT interval duration (QT interval range), termed "QT dispersion", were proposed as an index of the spatial dispersion of the ventricular recovery times.[4] The cardiological community welcomed the idea. Apparently, the methodological simplicity and the promise of a solution to the old and much debated problem of regional information within the standard surface ECG was appealing to the clinician.

Since that first publication, the cardiological literature has been flooded by articles reporting QT dispersion in practically every cardiac, as well as many non-cardiac, syndrome or disease. However, voices of concern about the validity of the concept and the methodology of the measurement were raised repeatedly. Now, some conclusions may be drawn from the wide spectrum of opinions, ranging from sheer enthusiastic approval to verdicts of "the greatest fallacy in ECG in the 1990s".[5]

The concept

The initial concept of QT dispersion seemed to be based on sound logic. The link between the dispersion of ventricular recovery times and arrhythmias had been repeatedly demonstrated.[6-8] It was generally believed that the standard surface ECG contains regional information. Therefore, when increased QT dispersion in particular groups, in whom the heterogeneity of the ventricular recovery times was previously established, was found, it was assumed that QT dispersion is a reflection of the dispersion of ventricular recovery times. The validity of the concept further seemed to be consolidated by studies correlating intracardiac monophasic action potentials (MAPs) with QT dispersion indices.

Higham et al.[9] found a high positive correlation between ECG dispersion indices and dispersion of recovery times measured directly from epicardial MAPs recorded during sinus rhythm and during ventricular pacing in patients undergoing cardiac surgery.

Zabel et al.,[10] using a custom-built rabbit heart set up with simultaneous recording of MAP and 12-lead ECGs, showed that the dispersion of the QT and JT intervals were significantly correlated with the dispersion of 90% duration of the action potential duration (ADP_{90}) and with the dispersion of recovery times. Later, the same authors confirmed this in patients with 12-lead ECGs recorded within 24 hours of the MAP recordings.[11] These studies were generally accepted as a proof that QT dispersion reflects directly the regional variations of the ventricular recovery times.

However, serious arguments against this concept originated from the ECG lead theory. If the majority of the information about the ventricular electrical activity is contained in the spatial QRS and T loops, the major reason for the differences between separate leads has to be the loss of information resulting from the projection of the loop into the separate leads.[12] Two original studies published in 1998 supported this idea.

Macfarlane et al.[13] and Lee et al.[14] showed independently that QT dispersion can also be found in the so-called "derived" 12-lead ECGs, i.e. ECGs reconstructed from the XYZ leads, which, naturally, contain no regional information. In both studies the QT dispersion in the originally recorded and in the "derived" 12 leads was surprisingly similar (29.1 ± 10.2 versus 27.5 ± 10.8 ms and 41 ± 18 versus 40 ± 20 ms, respectively).

Kors et al.[15] studied the link between the morphology of the T loop and QT dispersion. They found that QT dispersion was significantly different between patients with narrow (54.2 ± 27.1 ms) and wide T loops (69.5 ± 33.5 ms, P <0.001). They also showed that in each of the six limb as well as six precordial leads, the difference between the QT interval in a lead and the maximum QT interval in all six leads was the greatest when the angle between the axis of that lead and the axis of the terminal part of the T loop was the greatest.

Punske *et al.*[16] compared the spatial distribution of the QT intervals from high-resolution maps of human body surface, of the surface of a tank containing an isolated canine heart, and of the surface of exposed canine hearts, with the potential distributions on cardiac and body surfaces, and with recovery times on cardiac surfaces. They showed that on the body and tank surface, as well as on the epicardium, the "zero" potential line, i.e. the line of no potential difference relative to the reference electrode, stabilises for 10–30 ms at the end of repolarisation. This stabilisation of the "zero line" in a given location results in isoelectric terminal portions of the T wave for leads in the vicinity. Regions of shortest QT intervals always coincided with the location of the zero potential line on the cardiac and body surfaces. In addition, there were no consistent regions of earliest recovery times on the cardiac surface that coincided with the location of the zero potential line or shortest QT intervals.

These studies showed rather convincingly that the interlead differences of the QT intervals can be a reflection of (and could be quantified from) the morphology of the T wave loop.

Recently, Malik *et al.*[17] proposed an ECG processing technique to distinguish the T wave signals representing the three-dimensional movement of the ECG dipole from the non-dipolar components likely to be related to regional heterogeneity of myocardial repolarisation. Although the non-dipolar components differed between the different clinical groups, there was very little correlation between the relative amount of the non-dipolar components and QT dispersion measured in the same ECGs (r = −0.086, 0.379, −0.100, and 0.120, in normal subjects, hypertrophic cardiomyopathy patients, dilated cardiomyopathy patients, and survivors of acute myocardial infarction, respectively).

Therefore, it is reasonable to conclude that the dispersion of ventricular recovery times measured with MAPs and QT dispersion are direct and indirect expressions of repolarisation abnormalities, which are likely to correlate even without any mechanistic link. General abnormalities of ventricular repolarisation, not only those leading to regional dispersion of recovery times, modify the spatial T wave loop. Any abnormality may cause the projections of the loop into the individual ECG leads to become less normal and the terminal points of the T wave in the ECG tracings more difficult to be localised. The effect of local

dispersion of repolarisation on the morphology of the T wave loop, explain the (indirect) link between MAP recordings and QT dispersion. Thus, T wave loop dynamics and the variable projections of the loop into individual ECG leads seem to be the true mechanistic background of QT dispersion.

The studies of the link between the T loop morphology and QT dispersion proved an old idea empirically known to ECG readers some time ago: the more abnormal the T wave morphology in separate leads, the more difficult and unreliable the localisation of the T wave offset in each lead and, consequently, the greater the likelihood of increased interlead variation of the QT duration. As Kors *et al.* demonstrated,[15] variations of the T loop morphology lead to variations in the *practically unmeasurable* final part of the T wave, i.e. the proportion of the signal falling within the noise band (Fig 10.1). Thus, variations of the T

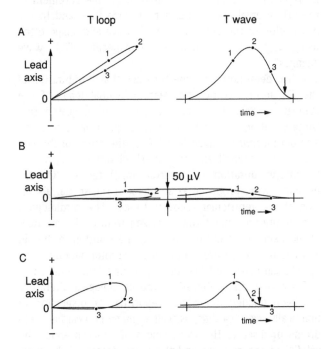

Figure 10.1 Effect of the shape of the T loop on the QT interval measurement in a hypothetical lead. Projections of T loops with different shape and at different angles to the axis of the lead results in T waves with different amplitude and morphology. Only insignificant proportion of the final part of a T wave with high amplitude may be unmeasurable because of falling into the noise band (A). T waves with smaller amplitude as a result of wider T loop (C) or elongated loop at different angle (B), have greater proportion of their final parts falling into the noise band. Thus, the measurable QT interval can almost coincide with the real end of repolarisation (A), or be significantly smaller (B,C). Points 1, 2 and 3 indicate three time instants of the T loop and of the T wave. (Reproduced with permission from Kors JA *et al.*, reference 15.)

loop morphology may lead to both variations in the length of the projections of the T loop into the separate leads, as well as to practically unmeasurable (or measurable with increased error) final proportions of the T wave i.e. *measurement-related* variations in the QT interval (Fig. 10.2).

Thus it seems now to be clear that QT dispersion is a crude and indirect general measure of the repolarisation abnormalities. However, independent of the crudeness of the expression, abnormalities of the T wave loop are of significant importance.[18,19] Even a very indirect measure of T wave loop abnormalities may still have some limited informative value.

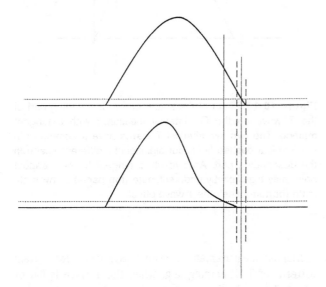

Figure 10.2 QT dispersion as a result of both different real duration and different measurable duration of QT intervals. Two hypothetical T waves of the same amplitude can have different offset (dashed lines) when the heart vector becomes perpendicular to the axis of one of the leads. This results in "real" dispersion of the QT intervals (vertical dashed lines). In addition, a different proportion of the final part of the two T waves is below the threshold level (e.g. with an automatic threshold method). This leads to the measured dispersion of the QT intervals (vertical solid line) which is different from the real dispersion.

Measurement of QT dispersion

General problems

It has been known for decades that the manual determination of the end of the T wave and, consequently, the measurement of the QT interval is very unreliable.[20] Unfortunately, the available automatic methods have far from proven their superiority. The main sources of error, both for human observer and computer are specific mor-

phological patterns, low T wave amplitude,[21,22] and merging of the T wave with U wave or P wave. The morphology of the T wave strongly influences any human measurement of the QT interval, as well as any computer algorithm.

Several basic methods for automatic determination of the T wave end are available (Fig. 10.3). The threshold methods localise the T offset as an interception of the T wave or one of its differentials with a threshold above the isoelectric line, usually expressed as a percentage of the T wave amplitude. Obviously, the amplitude of the T wave influences the measurement results with this method. The other major group of algorithms determines the T offset as an interception between a line, characterising the slope of the descending part of the T wave with the isoelectric line, or a threshold line above it. The slope characterising line can be the steepest tangent, a straight line through the inflex point and the peak of the T wave, a straight line fitted through a region around the inflex point, and possibly others. Obviously, the measured values of the QT interval will depend on the shape of the descending part of the T wave (Fig. 10.4).

The amplitude of the T wave strongly influences the reliability of both automatic[21,23] and manual[22] measurement. Obviously, one and the same tangent method, applied to T waves with different amplitudes (lower T waves are flatter, i.e. have less steep downslope) will produce different measurement error.

The origin of the U wave is still disputed. The popular theory that attributed the U wave to the delayed repolarisation of the His–Purkinje fibres[24] was superseded by the M-cell theory by Antzelevich *et al.*[25] However, later experiments by the same group showed that, what is often interpreted as a "pathologically augmented U wave" or "T-U complex", is in fact a prolonged biphasic T wave with an interrupted ascending or descending limb.[26]

It practice it is often very difficult, if not directly impossible, to separate the end even of a normal T wave from an obvious U wave. Already in 1952, Lepeschkin and Surawicz[27] described and classified the various patterns of T and U wave merging, and suggested methods for determining the end of the T wave when it is "buried" within the U wave. They showed that, depending on the pattern of T-U wave merging, either the point of intersection of the tangent to the downslope steepest point and the isoelectric line, or the nadir between the T and the U wave is closer to the "real" T wave end. Half a century later published reports on manual QT measurements continue to refer to the tangent method without any justification. However, the tangent method was proposed by the authors merely as "... an attempt to determine the true end of the T wave in cases of partial merging of T and U."[27] No elaborate method was actually proposed by them for cases of a simple T wave with no apparent U wave.

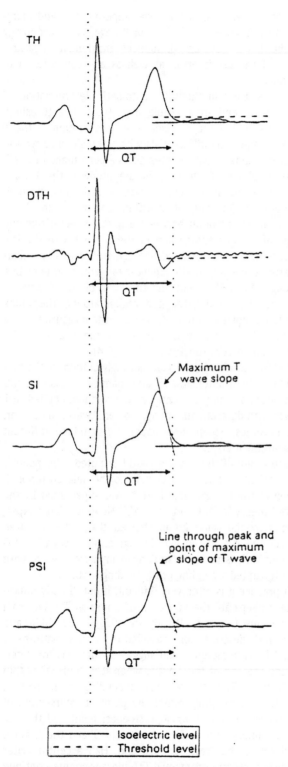

Figure 10.3 Main automatic QT measurement techniques. From top to bottom: threshold method applied to the original T wave (TH), or to its differential (DTH), tangent method with a tangent to the steepest point of the descending limb of the T wave (SI), tangent method with a line through the T wave peak and the maximum slope point (PSI). (Reproduced with permission from McLaughlin NB *et al.*, reference 62).

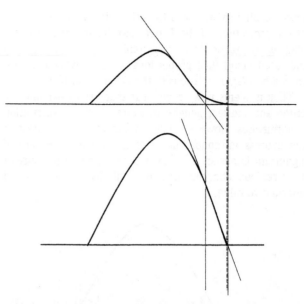

Figure 10.4 Effect of the shape of the descending part of the T wave on the QT interval measured with a tangent method. The two hypothetical T waves have a common offset (vertical dashed line), but significantly different shape in the descending part. As a result, a tangent to the steepest point may significantly underestimate (top panel) or overestimate (bottom panel) the T wave offset.

Manual measurement is even less reliable for certain patterns of T-U merging, e.g. when the T wave is flat or inverted and the U wave augmented. Repolarisation patterns of complex morphology are frequently classified differently by different observers leading to substantial variability of the measurement.[28]

The dispersion of the Q wave, although significantly smaller than the T wave offset dispersion, may still influence QT dispersion.[29,30] Traditional manual measurement, as well as those of some computer algorithms, assess the Q wave onset separately in each lead,[31] while other computer algorithms use a common, lead independent Q onset.[32,33] This may account for part of the variability of the results with different computer algorithms.

Theoretically, an accurate assessment of QT dispersion requires all 12 leads of the ECG to be recorded simultaneously in order to avoid the effect on QT dynamicity of heart rate changes. However, the dynamicity of the QT interval is normally rather slow.[34] Therefore, from a practical point of view, the differences between QT dispersion measurements based on simultaneous recording of three or six leads and on simultaneous recording of all leads during ectopic-free sinus rhythm are probably negligible.

Many studies, including large prospective evaluations,[35,36] used the so-called "corrected QT dispersion", i.e. the dispersion of the QT intervals corrected for heart rate by some correction formula. While the application of linear formulae for heart rate correction of the QT interval, such as those proposed by Hodges *et al.*[37] and in the Framingham Study,[38] renders identical values for QT dispersion and QTc dispersion, this is not true for the non-linear formulae. Although experimental and clinical data show that the heart rate can influence the dispersion of the ventricular recovery times,[39–41] this has never been shown for QT dispersion. Clinical[42,43] and experimental[44] studies have failed to find significant correlation between heart rate and the dispersion of ventricular recovery times measured with MAPs or QT dispersion. However, it has been shown that QT dispersion is increased in premature, compared to normal sinus beats.[45,46]

The exact relation between the heart rate and the dispersion of recovery times is still an unresolved issue. It is certain, however, that QT dispersion measured in the standard 12-lead ECG does not depend on (and therefore should not be corrected for) the heart period in the same way as the QT interval. Even more importantly, it has been demonstrated that the dispersion of the corrected QT intervals may differ between different clinically defined groups of patients, simply as a result of the application of Bazett formula in the presence of difference in the heart rates.[47]

Lead systems for measurement of QT dispersion

In addition to the original expression of QT dispersion as the range of QT interval duration in all measurable leads, many other measurement possibilities have also been proposed. To mitigate the effect of outliers in the QT interval data, standard deviation of the QT interval duration in all leads[48] or coefficient of variation (SD of QT/QT average × 100, the so-called "relative QT dispersion"[49]) have been used. However, the range and standard deviation values correlate very closely.[48,50]

The number of measurable leads in a standard ECG also influences the range of QT interval durations. Some researchers proposed a correction factor dividing QT interval range by the square root of the number of measurable ECG leads, the so-called "adjusted QT dispersion".[51] Hnatkova *et al.*[48] showed that this formula leads to a reasonable correction in normal ECGs. However, they also showed that, whilst the correction leads to maintenance of mean values, the individual errors caused by omitting separate leads are very substantial. Consequently, it is not appropriate to compare results based on QT interval values measured in ECGs of very different number of measurable leads.

Many clinical studies have measured QT dispersion in the six precordial instead of the 12 standard, showing that the clinical value of QT dispersion, whatever this might

be, can be found in the precordial leads. In addition, other lead combinations, such as the orthogonal XYZ or "quasiorthogonal" I,aVF,V_2 leads, have also been studied. It was reported that although, as one would expect, QT dispersion is decreased when a smaller number of leads are used for QT measurement, QT dispersion differences between different patients groups can still be detected in the three leads (AVF, V_1,V_4) among the 12 leads that are most likely to contribute to QT dispersion,[52] in the limb leads,[53] in the orthogonal (X,Y,Z),[54,55] or the "quasi-orthogonal leads" (I,AVF,V_2).[52–54]

Obviously, practically any lead combination may detect general abnormalities of repolarisation (i.e. in the morphology of the T loop) and translate them into increased values of QT dispersion. On the other hand, the more projections of the T loop into different leads with different axes are used, the more likely it is to find an increased QT dispersion. Unfortunately, as already mentioned, this does not directly translate into an increased regional heterogeneity of recovery times. Therefore it seems that there is little point in continuing the quest for the "perfect lead combination" for QT dispersion measurement.

Reliability of measurement of QT dispersion

Many studies have shown high inter- and intra-observer variability of manually measured QT dispersion, with errors reaching the order of the differences between normal subjects and patients with various cardiac diseases. Relative errors of 25–40% of inter-observer and intra-observer variability of manual measurement of QT dispersion have been reported,[28,56] as opposed to relative errors of <6%, for manual measurement of the QT interval.[56] Occasionally, substantially better reproducibility of manual measurement of QT dispersion has also been reported, with interobserver variability of 13–18%[57] and even <5%.[58] Explanations of these discrepancies can only be very speculative.

In addition to differences in the investigated populations, the variations of the results can be attributed to differences in the measurement method (manual measurement with calliper or ruler,[59] application of a digitising board with or without magnification, on-screen measurement with electronic callipers, etc.), the noise level, and the paper speed at which the ECGs were recorded.[22] In a technical study, Malik and Bradford[60] showed that even "gold standard" manual interval measurement using the digitising board, can produce interobserver variations corresponding to purely error-related QT dispersion >40 ms and >60 ms, in 20% and 10% of observers, respectively.

The available automatic methods for QT measurement

have not shown a superior reproducibility. For example, Yi *et al.*[61] reported that the immediate reproducibility (i.e. measurement of sequentially recorded ECGs) of various QT dispersion indices, measured with a downslope tangent method in healthy volunteers, varied between 16% and 44%.

As previously mentioned, most available computer algorithms determine the end of the T wave either as an intersection between a tangent to the descending part of the T wave and the isoelectric line, or as a point at which the T wave (or its differential) falls below a given threshold.[62] Variations include signal processing options, the way in which the tangent is characterised, the definition of an isoelectric line, the threshold level, etc. Some software packages offer a great variety of parameter settings. For instance, one of the versions of the QT Guard software package (Marquette G.E.)[32] offers over 100 programmable options for the T wave end localisation.

Many studies have tried to validate automatic algorithms against manual measurement by experienced ECG readers. The results were disappointing showing very significant difference.[23,63–65] For example, Savelieva *et al.*[64] investigated the agreement between automatic (downslope inflex tangent method, QT Guard) and manual QT measurement in normal subjects and patients with hypertrophic cardiomyopathy (HCM). The agreement between the two methods, expressed as a correlation coefficient, was lower in normal subjects ($r^2 = 0.10$–0.25 in the separate leads) than in HCM patients ($r^2 = 0.46$–0.67). Not surprisingly, even worse was the agreement between automatic and manual measurement of QT dispersion ($r^2 = 0.06$ in HCM patients and $r^2 = 0.00$ in normal subjects) (Fig. 10.5).

Relatively few studies have compared different algorithms for automatic QT measurement. McLaughlin *et al.*[62] compared two threshold- and two slope-based techniques, and a validated manual measurement. The results of the mean measurements with different algorithms varied up to 62 ms, which was greater than the manual interobserver variability. The threshold algorithm demonstrated largest variability and its results depended on filtering and algorithm parameters. In another study[66] the same authors showed that the variability of automatic QT measurement in cardiac patients was twice that in normal subjects, and that it was significantly increased with the decrease of the T wave amplitude.

In a study, only part of which was published Batchvarov *et al.*[67] evaluated the multiple parameter options in the QT Guard package. The differences between the downslope tangent method using different number of samples around the inflex point for computation of the tangent and the modifications of the threshold method were substantial. The results varied significantly less with the different settings of the tangent method than with the

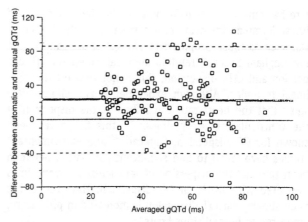

Figure 10.5 Agreement between automatic and manual measurement of QT dispersion in patients with hypertrophic cardiomyopathy. The differences between the measurements are plotted against the mean value from the two measurements (Bland–Altman plot). Most of the differences are within 2 SD from the mean differences (dashed line), which is approximately ±60 ms, obviously an unacceptably high measurement error. There is also no correlation between the two sets of measurements ($r^2 = 0.00$). (Reproduced with permission from Savelieva I *et al.*, reference 64).

threshold methods. The QT measurements changed significantly with the threshold level. Changes in the permissible range of the settings of the package led to differences of up to 60 ms in normal subjects and up to 70 ms in patients with hypertrophic cardiomyopathy. Hence, only comparison of results obtained with the same automatic methods and with the same parameter setting is appropriate.

Clinical studies

A review of the extreme abundance of clinical studies on QT dispersion published over the past decade reveals an amazingly wide range of QT dispersion values in both "positive" and "negative" studies, and a complete lack of any tendency towards establishing of reference values. For example, large studies[68] or literature reviews,[69] suggesting QT dispersion of 65 ms as an upper normal limit in healthy subjects, were published alongside reports claiming QT dispersion ≥40 ms to have 88% sensitivity and 57% specificity for prediction of inducibility of sustained VT during an electrophysiology study.[70] Most of the studies with "positive" results published QT dispersion data well within the demonstrated measurement error of both manual and automatic measurement. As if to further confuse the reader, even large recently published prospective studies[35,36] provide only data for the heart-rate "corrected" QT dispersion (see previous section).

QT dispersion in normal subjects and in the general population

Literature reviews found QT dispersion to vary mostly between 30 and 60 ms in normal subjects,[71,72] although average values of around 70 ms were also reported. In 51 studies, 40 of which were published in the last three years, in which QT dispersion was measured in 56 groups with total of 8455 healthy control subjects of various ages (including three large studies of healthy children[73-75]), we found mean QT dispersion values (QT maximum–QT minimum) to range from 10.5 ± 10.0 ms to 71 ± 7 ms in.[76,77] The weighted mean ±SD from all these studies was 33.4 ± 20.3 ms (Fig. 10.6), while the median was 37 ms. Moreover, most researchers reported a wide overlap of values between normal individuals and different patient groups (Figs 10.6 and 10.7). Therefore all values proposed for upper normal limit in healthy subjects have subsequently turned out to be unreliable.

Published reports show either no statistically significant difference in QT dispersion between the genders,[13,74] or marginally greater values in men.[78,79]

Age-related differences of <10 ms were also reported and appeared to be statistically significant in some studies,[80,81] but not in others.[73,74] For example, in the study of Savelieva et al.[82] on more than 1000 healthy subjects, QT dispersion was 29.1 ± 17.8 ms in the age group of 17–29 years, and 21.7 ± 13.3 ms in the age group of 50–80 years ($P < 0.0001$). On the other hand, in another large study, Macfarlane et al.[13] found no significant age differences (QT dispersion of 23.6 ± 7.7 ms, 24.8 ± 8.2 ms, 24.8 ± 8.5 ms, and 24.5 ± 9.8 ms in the age groups of <30, 30–40, 40–50 and >50 years, respec-

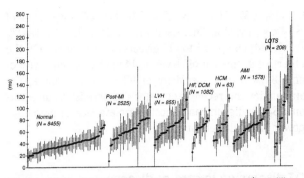

Figure 10.7 Mean ±SD of the QT dispersion (in milliseconds) from the reviewed studies of normal subjects, and patients with chronic myocardial infarction, left ventricular hypertrophy, heart failure and dilated cardiomyopathy, hypertrophic cardiomyopathy, acute myocardial infarction, and long QT syndrome. Abbreviations as in Figure 10.6. See the text for details.

tively). In this study, no age differences of QT dispersion were also found in 1784 neonates, infants and children divided in 16 age groups from <24 h to >15 years of age. QT dispersion was 27.2 ± 10.5 ms in neonates during the first day of life and 28.6 ± 8.5 ms in the group of children above the age of 15 years. The average QT dispersion in the adult group (24.5 ± 8.2 ms) and in the children group as a whole (24.5 ± 8.7 ms) were also surprisingly similar. In both studies the QT parameters were measured automatically.

Several large prospective studies published recently assessed the predictive value of QT dispersion for cardiac and all-cause mortality in the general population. In the Rotterdam study[35] the "corrected" QT dispersion was found to predict cardiac mortality in a general population of 5812 adults of 55 years or older, followed up for 3–6.5 (mean 4) years. In the Strong Heart Study[36] the predictive value of the QTc dispersion was assessed in 1839 American Indians followed up for 3.7 ± 0.9 years. Multivariate analysis showed QTc dispersion of >58 ms (the upper 95th percentile in a separate population of normal subjects) to be associated with a 3.2-fold increased risk of cardiovascular mortality (95% CI 1.8–5.7).

Unfortunately, neither values for the uncorrected QT dispersion, nor for the simple resting heart rate were provided in the report of both studies. The report of the Rotterdam Study, however, briefly mentioned that the results with the uncorrected QT dispersion were similar, but with broader CI.[35]

The West of Scotland Coronary Prevention Study (WOSCOPS)[83] included 6595 middle-aged men with moderately raised cholesterol but no previous myocardial infarction. In a multivariate analysis an increment of 10 ms in QT dispersion increased the risk for death of coronary heart disease or non-fatal myocardial infarction

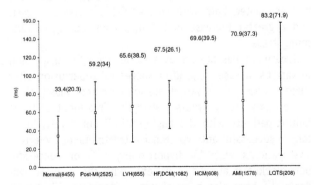

Figure 10.6 Weighted mean ±SD values of QT dispersion (in milliseconds) from reviewed studies in normal subjects, patients with chronic myocardial infarction (chr.MI), left ventricular hypertrophy (LVH) of various aetiology except hypertrophic cardiomyopathy, in heart failure and dilated cardiomyopathy (HF,DCM), in hypertrophic cardiomyopathy (HCM), in acute myocardial infarction (acute MI), and in long QT syndrome (LQTS). See text for details.

by 13% (95% CI 4–22%, P = 0.0041). QT dispersion of >44 ms carried an increased risk of 36% (95% CI 2–81%, P = 0.034) compared to QT dispersion of <44 ms. On the other hand, this cut-off level of 44 ms had a sensitivity of only 8.8% with a specificity of 93.8%. Furthermore, the area under the receiver operator characteristic curve was only 54% indicating an almost complete lack of predictive power of QT dispersion.

QT dispersion in cardiac disease

The majority of studies have shown increased QT dispersion in various cardiac diseases. We have pooled data from 18 studies with a total of 2525 post-myocardial infarction (MI) patients, 16 studies with 855 patients with left ventricular hypertrophy (LVH) of various origin, excluding hypertrophic cardiomyopathy (HCM), eight studies with 1082 patients with heart failure, including idiopathic dilated cardiomyopathy (DCM), 11 studies with 635 patients with HCM, 16 studies with a total of 1578 patients with acute MI, and 10 studies with 208 patients with long QT syndrome of various genotype (Fig. 10.6).

There is a clear tendency towards increase of QT dispersion in various cardiac diseases, with highest mean values reported in the long QT syndrome "the pure global repolarisation disease" (Figs 10.6 and 10.7). On the other hand, the overlap of values between patients with different cardiac diseases, between patients and normal subjects, as well as the wide variation of values within each cardiac disease renders any attempt at establishing of reference values fruitless. However, it should be also acknowledged that patients with various clinical symptoms, with and without arrhythmias, on and off various medications, have been included in these pooled studies, which probably accounts for a part of the variation.

Generally, QT dispersion is increased in acute MI, although mean values from 40 ± 18 to 162.3 ± 64.8 ms have been reported. [76,84] Although QT dispersion is increased in the chronic phase of MI and in other chronic forms of ischaemic artery disease, there seems to be a trend towards lower values of QT dispersion compared to the acute phase of MI, possibly due to the spontaneous dynamicity or to revascularisation procedures. Some authors did not find significant differences in QT dispersion between patients with chronic MI or other forms of chronic CAD and normal subjects. [85,86]

Compared to healthy controls, an increased QT dispersion has been reported in heart failure and left ventricular dysfunction of various aetiology, [87–90] including highly trained athletes, [91–93] in left ventricular hypertrophy of various origin, [94–98] and even in patients with arterial hypertension irrespective of the presence or absence of hypertrophy, [99] in patients with hypertrophic cardiomyopathy compared to healthy controls, [100–103] in the long QT syndrome, [104–107] and in many other cardiac and even non-cardiac diseases. However, some studies have found QT dispersion values not significantly different between healthy subjects and patients with heart failure [108] or LV hypertrophy as a result of physical training, [109–111] or between patients with and without LV hypertrophy. [112]

Many studies tried to correlate QT dispersion with the extent or the localisation of the pathological process of various diseases. Some studies have shown greater QT dispersion in anterior compared to inferior MI, [113–115] correlation between QT dispersion in MI and indirect measures of infarct size, such as ejection fraction [116,117] or the amount of viable myocardium in the infarct region. [118] Similarly, significant correlation between QT dispersion and left ventricular mass index in hypertensive patients with LV hypertrophy was found in some studies, [119,120] but not in others. [121]

Changes of QT dispersion have been shown to follow the spontaneous or induced dynamicity of the pathological process in some cardiac diseases. For instance, QT dispersion seems to undergo dynamic changes during the first day, [122] as well as during the following days [123,124] of acute MI. It increases significantly during ischaemia induced by balloon inflation during angioplasty, [125–127] by exercise stress testing [128] or atrial pacing, [129] during reperfusion following angioplasty, [130] or by myocardial microcirculatory disturbances induced by coronary rotational atherectomy. [131] It has also been shown to correlate with the improvement of left ventricular contractility on the echocardiogram after the infarction, [132] and with the degree of improvement of left ventricular function after revascularisation. [133,134] A recent study [135] reported that the presence of viable myocardium in post-MI patients, assessed by low-dose dobutamine stress echocardiography, was associated both with smaller QT dispersion at rest, and a greater increase in QT dispersion during dobutamine stress.

Treatment has been shown to decrease QT dispersion in various diseases, e.g. after successful reperfusion after thrombolysis, [136,137] revascularisation with angioplasty, [138–140] or coronary artery bypass grafting. [134] Treatment of heart failure patients with the angiotensin-II antagonist, losartan, [141] successful antihypertensive treatment of hypertensive patients with LV hypertrophy, [142–145] or successful beta-blocker treatment of patients with the long-QT syndrome, [146] have also been shown to decrease QT dispersion.

In general, the impression from all these studies fits with the concept of QT dispersion expressing general repolarisation abnormality. However, the variety of "positive" and "negative" studies, practically balanced in many diseases, probably reflects more variations in the measurement mode, the degree of influence upon the operator of the T wave morphology, and other technical factors, rather than real physiological differences in the studied patient groups.

Prognostic value of QT dispersion

Many studies addressed the value of QT dispersion for the prediction of ventricular arrhythmias or other adverse events in various cardiac diseases. The results are again controversial.

We have pooled data from 23 studies on patients with and without serious ventricular arrhythmias in various cardiac diseases, most of them with ischaemic heart disease. Altogether, 490 patients with and 1341 patients without serious ventricular arrhythmias were included. Although most studies show significantly greater QT dispersion in patients with ventricular arrhythmias, the values are largely overlapping (Fig. 10.8).

Many studies, most of them retrospective, have found that patients with acute[147–149] or chronic MI[150–153] with ventricular arrhythmias have significantly higher QT dispersion than patients without arrhythmias. However, the first prospectively analysed study in post-MI patients reported by Zabel et al.[154] showed that none of the 26 ventricular dispersion indices that were tested had any predictive value for an adverse outcome in 280 consecutive MI survivors followed up for 32 ± 10 months. Newer studies[155] support these findings.

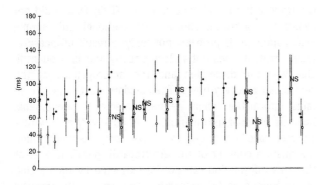

Figure 10.8 Mean and standard deviations of QT dispersion in patients with (closed circles) and without (opened circles) serious ventricular arrhythmias. In one study patients with ventricular fibrillation (closed square) and sustained monomorphic ventricular tachycardias (closed circle) were compared separately with patients without sustained ventricular arrhythmias. * $P < 0.05$ between groups with and without serious ventricular arrhythmias; NS = statistically non-significant difference between groups with and without serious ventricular arrhythmias.

However, one most recently published prospective study deserves attention. Dabrowski et al.[45] measured QT dispersion (manual measurement on four-fold enlarged ECGs) in ventricular premature beats, and in the last preceding sinus beat in 148 patients with remote myocardial infarction. QT-dispersion was significantly greater in ventricular premature beats, compared to the preceding sinus beats (83 ± 33 versus 74 ± 34 ms, $P = 0.001$). Both QT dispersion in sinus, as well as in premature beats, were significantly increased in patients with, compared with those without major arrhythmic events (sustained ventricular tachycardia, ventricular fibrillation, or sudden death) during follow-up of 35 ± 17 months. However, only QT dispersion of ≥ 100 measured in ventricular premature bpm, was an independent predictor of arrhythmic events in univariate and multivariate analysis, with sensitivity, specificity, positive and negative predictive values of 67%, 75%, 41% and 90%, respectively.

Some studies showed that QT dispersion can predict inducibility of ventricular arrhythmias during electrophysiology (EP) study[157–159] while others failed to observe this.[160–162]

Several studies[163–165] showed significant correlation between QT dispersion and outcome in patients with heart failure. Analysis[166] from the ELITE heart failure study, in which heart failure patients treated with the angiotensin-II antagonist losartan, had reduction of sudden cardiac death compared with those treated with captopril,[167] showed that captopril but not losartan increased QT dispersion. A recent prospective study[168] suggested that increase in QTc dispersion by exercise might have predictive power for sudden cardiac death in patients with heart failure. On the other hand, substudies of the DAMOND-CHF Study,[169] the UK-HEART study,[170] as well as other large prospective study,[171] failed to show any power of QT dispersion for predicting outcome in heart failure patients. Available studies also failed to show independent predictive value of QT dispersion for sudden cardiac death and cardiac mortality in patients with LV hypertrophy.[172]

Several authors reported significantly higher QT dispersion in hypertrophic cardiomyopathy patients with ventricular arrhythmias compared with those without arrhythmias.[173–175] Larger studies, however, did not confirm these initial findings.[176,177]

In the long QT syndrome, the diagnostic value of increased QT dispersion seems undisputed. On the other hand, although Priori et al.[178] reported that patients not responding to beta-blockers had a significantly higher QT dispersion than responders (137 ± 52 versus 75 ± 38 ms, $P < 0.05$), no other presently available data suggest that QT dispersion has any prognostic value in long QT syndrome patients.

Generally, the positive results of small retrospective studies conducted in the years of initial enthusiasm were later confirmed only in some very large prospective studies. However, even in the latter, patients groups with adverse outcomes often had QT dispersion values well within both the measurement error and the range of values in healthy subjects reported in other studies. Thus, if we are allowed to paraphrase Surawicz,[179] the positive results can be interpreted as indicating an "indifferent" QT dispersion, which does not signify lack of clinical importance. It points to the fact that increased QT dispersion in these patient groups merely signifies general repolarisation abnormality, in the majority (if not all) of the cases already visible from abnormal T wave morphology and/or increased QT interval, does not necessitate a specific therapeutic action, and in practice does not help in the risk stratification of the patients.

Effect of drugs on QT dispersion and the risk of torsade de pointes tachycardia

The limitations of both the presence and the degree of QT interval prolongation for prediction of torsade de pointes are well known.[180] Consequently, the potential role of QT dispersion for the prediction of drug-induced torsade de pointes has been addressed in several studies.

Quinidine increases QT dispersion[181-183] and, unlike the corrected QTc interval, increased QT dispersion seems to have some predictive value for development of torsade de pointes during quinidine therapy.[182,183] A recent study examined the effect of quinidine on QT dispersion in patients with inducible ventricular tachycardia during baseline EP study.[184] QT dispersion was significantly increased in patients in whom the drug failed to suppress inducibility (from 78 ± 28 ms at baseline to 113 ± 40 ms after treatment, P <0.05), but not in those who responded to treatment (81 ± 26 versus 83 ± 42 ms).

Sotalol has been shown to decrease[185] or not to change[186] QT dispersion in patients with ischaemic heart disease. However, Hohnloser et al.[187] reported that QT dispersion was significantly increased in 11 patients who developed torsade de pointes from a group of 50 patients treated for ventricular tachycardia/fibrillation with sotalol.

In clinical studies, amiodarone has been reported to decrease[181,186,188] or not to change[182,189,190] QT dispersion. It is known that amiodarone can be administered relatively safely in patients who had experienced torsade de pointes during antiarrhythmic therapy with other drugs,[191] and this effect is paralleled by a decrease in QT dispersion.[182] However, cases of an excessive increase of QT dispersion and induction of torsade de pointes by amiodarone have also been reported.[192] On the other hand, it has been demonstrated that increase in QTc and QT dispersion during chronic amiodarone treatment does not affect survival and is independent of the decrease in arrhythmia risk.[193]

Propafenone,[194] disopyramide,[195] and almokalant (blocker of the rapid component of the delayed rectifier, I_{Kr})[196] have been shown to increase QT dispersion, whilst in one study dofetilide infusion did not produce increase of the dispersion of repolarisation between two right ventricular endocardial sites.[197] A significant decrease of QT and QTc dispersion after treatment with azimilide[198] and magnesium[199] have also been reported.

In addition to the long QT syndrome,[146] beta-blockers have been shown to decrease QT dispersion in patients with syndrome X,[200] heart failure,[201] but not in hypertrophic cardiomyopathy.[176]

It seems that ECG monitoring of the effect of drugs that prolong ventricular repolarisation is the only area in which QT dispersion preserved (some) immediate clinical significance. Again, if we can paraphrase Surawicz,[179] grossly abnormal values (e.g. ≥100 ms,[202] quite unlikely to be due to measurement error) during treatment with drugs effecting repolarisation signify "bad QT dispersion", which probably should prompt urgent assessment of the drug effect with superior diagnostic methods and, eventually, considering treatment. On the other hand, lack of abnormal QT dispersion value is by no means a reassuring sign of therapeutic safety. Generally, the ECG detection of increased risk of torsade de pointes during treatment with repolarisation active drugs is still an unresolved issue, and most probably even here QT dispersion will have only some supportive value.

Conclusions

Contrary to the initial expectations, QT dispersion did not evolve into a useful clinical tool. Although this simple ECG parameter is probably not (only) a result of measurement error, it does not reflect directly and in a quantifiable way the dispersion and the heterogeneity of the ventricular recovery times. The standard 12-lead ECG contains information about regional electrical phenomena, but this regional information, as Abildskov et al.[203] wrote 13 years ago, continues to be part of "the unidentified information content of the electrocardiogram". It is clear that this information can not be extracted by such a simple technique as QT dispersion assessment. Its practical value, if any, will probably remain as a marker of global, rather than localised repolarisation abnormality.

However, even general repolarisation abnormalities are reflected indirectly and approximately in QT dispersion. Therefore, in clinical practice, probably only grossly abnormal values of QT dispersion, clearly outside the possible measurement error, e.g. ≥100 ms, may have significance merely by signalling that the repolarisation is abnormal. It seems therefore that the clinical significance will be limited to diseases and syndromes in which such values are likely to be encountered, e.g. drug-induced torsade de pointes. Of course, one can wonder what is the likelihood of finding such extreme values in ECGs with normal T wave morphology, i.e. how likely is QT dispersion to offer any additional information to the traditional diagnosis of the T wave abnormality. Even in the long QT syndrome, i.e. in the case of the "pure global repolarisation disease", QT dispersion failed to add substantial additional information to that provided by the general observation of abnormal TU complexes.

In addition, not only the magnitude of dispersion of recovery times, but the distance over which they are dispersed is important for arrhythmogenesis. In a similar way as we distinguish, though arbitrarily, "micro re-entry" from "macro re-entry", it seems logical to distinguish dispersion of recovery times of adjacent areas (local dispersion) from dispersion over large areas (global dispersion), and, possibly, from dispersion between both ventricles (interventricular dispersion). Clearly, such a scale of distinction is beyond the resolution power of the standard surface ECG. Local dispersion of recovery times created by MI is no more visible on the standard surface ECG than the delayed conduction created by the same infarct.

The very idea of detecting and quantifying only the dispersion of the end of repolarisation, i.e. the dispersion of the complete recovery times, seems also questionable. Action potentials of different duration usually have very different shape, particularly during phase 3. Such a "phase 3 dispersion", i.e. the dispersion of the partial recovery times, has direct relation to arrhythmogenesis. Whilst it is reflected in the shape of the T wave, it does not contribute to the dispersion of the ends of the MAPs, let alone the dispersion of the QT intervals.

Older concepts of quantification of the repolarisation abnormalities, as well as newer ideas, deserve more attention than parameters based on duration of repolarisation intervals.

Principal component analysis (PCA) has been used for decades in the analysis of ECG signals from body surface potential mapping for reduction of the redundancy of the data.[1] Recently it has also been implemented to assess the complexity of the T wave from standard 12-lead ECG and from 12-lead digital Holter recordings. The method has been shown to differentiate between normal subjects and patients with the long QT syndrome from 12-lead Holter ECGs,[204] in patients with hypertrophic cardiomyopathy,[205] and arrhythmogenic right ventricular dysplasia.[206] In general, the method defines the principal, non-redundant spatial components (or "factors"), into which the T wave could be decomposed and which contribute (in descending order of significance) to the morphology of the T wave. The significance of each component is measured by its eigenvalue. When the repolarisation is uniform, i.e. the T wave is smooth, without notches, most of the informa-

tion about its morphology is contained in the first, main principal component. When the T wave becomes more complex, the relative value of the next, smaller components of T wave increases (i.e. their eigenvalues increase). Details about PCA of the ECG waveforms can be found elsewhere.[1,204] Although PCA is already included in some commercially available programs for automatic repolarisation analysis, such as the QT Guard (Marquette, GE), its clinical role is still not well defined.

Recently, frontal and horizontal T wave axis has also been demonstrated to be predictive of cardiac mortality.[207] Most probably, other wavefront direction parameters, based on measurement of vector time integrals (i.e. QRST areas) will also be studied in the near future.

Recently, a concept of measuring the T wave "morphology dispersion" in surface electrocardiograms has been proposed by Acar *et al.*[208] Based on single value decomposition of simultaneously recorded 12-lead ECGs and on the computation of the eigenvalues of the signal, they proposed several indices characterising the sequence of repolarisation changes through the ventricular myocardium, including parameters describing the dissimilarities of the shape of the T wave in individual ECG leads. Comparison of normal and abnormal ECGs of hypertrophic cardiomyopathy patients showed that indices of T wave morphology separated these two groups more powerfully than both QT dispersion and rate-corrected QT interval duration. The concept was subsequently applied to the ECGs database of the first prospective study on QT dispersion in survivors of myocardial infarction by Zabel *et al.*[154] They showed that, unlike QT dispersion,[19] selected indices of T wave morphology characteristics obtained from single beat resting 12-lead ECGs are powerful and independent predictors of adverse events during follow-up.

In summary, further elaboration on the concept or measurement technology of QT dispersion (or dispersion of other repolarisation intervals), as well as large prospective evaluations, are likely to be unproductive. Future efforts should concentrate on more focused and more detailed technologies for repolarisation assessment. The available technologies (e.g. principal component analysis, T wave loop descriptors, T wave morphology "dispersion") should be subjected to evaluation in existing ECG databases and in ECG collections of new studies. At the same time, efforts should be put into the development of new ECG processing concepts addressing detailed aspects of repolarisation characteristics and repolarisation changes.

References

1. Horan LG, Flowers NC, Brody DA. Principal factor waveforms of the thoracic QRS complex. *Circ Res* 1964;**15**:131–45.

2. Wilson FN, Macleod AG, Barker PS, Johnston FD. Determination of the significance of the areas of the ventricular deflections of the electrocardiogram. *Am Heart J* 1934;**10**:46–61.

3. Cowan C, Yusoff K, Moore M *et al*. Variability in QT interval measurement. In: GS Butrous, PJ Schwartz eds. *Clinical aspects of ventricular repolarization*. London: Farrand Press, 1989, pp. 49–55.

4. Day CP, McComb LM, Campbell RWF. QT dispersion: an indication of arrhythmia risk in patients with long QT intervals. *Br Heart J* 1990;**63**:342–4.

5. Rautaharju PM. QT and dispersion of ventricular repolarization: the greatest fallacy in electrocardiography in the 1990s. *Circulation* 1999;**18**:2477–8.

6. Han J, Moe GK. Nonuniform recovery of excitability in ventricular muscle. *Circ Res* 1964;**14**:44.

7. Allessie MA, Bonke FIM, Schopman FJG. Circus movement in rabbit atrial muscle as a mechanism of tachycardia. II: The role of nonuniform recovery of excitability in the occurrence of unidirectional block, as studied with multiple microelectrodes. *Circ Res* 1976;**39**:168–77.

8. Kuo C-S, Munakata K, Reddy P, Surawicz B. Characteristics and possible mechanism of ventricular arrhythmia dependent on the dispersion of action potential durations. *Circulation* 1983;**67**:1356–67.

9. Higham PD, Hilton CJ, Aitcheson JD, Furniss SS, Bourke JP, Campbell RWF. Does QT dispersion reflect dispersion of ventricular recovery? *Circulation* 1992;**86**(Suppl. I): 392(Abstr.).

10. Zabel M, Portnoy S, Franz MR. Electrocardiographic indexes of dispersion of ventricular repolarization: an isolated heart validation study. *J Am Coll Cardiol* 1995;**25**:746–52.

11. Zabel M, Lichtlen PR, Haverich A, Franz MR. Comparison of ECG variables of dispersion of ventricular repolarization with direct myocardial repolarization measurements in the human heart. *J Cardiovasc Electrophysiol* 1998;**9**:1279–84.

12. Coumel P, Maison-Blanche P, Badilini F. Dispersion of ventricular repolarization. Reality? Illusion? Significance? *Circulation* 1998;**97**:2491–3.

13. Macfarlane PW, McLaughlin SC, Rodger C. Influence of lead selection and population on automated measurement of QT dispersion. *Circulation* 1998;**98**:2160–7.

14. Lee KW, Kligfield P, Okin PM, Dower GE. Determinants of precordial QT dispersion in normal subjects. *J Electrocardiol* 1998;**31**(Suppl.):128–33.

15. Kors JA, van Herpen G, van Bemmel JH. QT dispersion as an attribute of T-loop morphology. *Circulation* 1999;**99**:1458–63.

16. Punske BB, Lux RL, MacLeod RS *et al*. Mechanisms of the spatial distribution of QT intervals on the epicardial and body surfaces. *J Cardiovasc Electrophysiol* 1999;**10**:1605–18.

17. Malik M, Acar B, Yap Y-G, Yi G. QT dispersion does not express spatial heterogeneity of ventricular refractoriness in 12 lead ECGs. *Circulation* 1999;**100**(Suppl. I):245 (Abstr.).

18. Kors JA, de Bruyne MC, Hoes AW *et al*. T axis as an indicator of risk of cardiac events in elderly people. *Lancet* 1998;**352**:601–4.

19. Zabel M, Acar B, Waktare JEP *et al*. Twelve-lead T wave morphology analysis for risk stratification in post myocardial infarction patients. *Circulation* 1999;**100**(Suppl. I):509(Abstr.).

20. Taran L, Szilagyi N. The measurement of the QT interval in acute heart disease. *Bull St Francis Sanatorium* 1951;**8**:13.

21. McLaughlin NB, Campbell RWF, Murray A. Influence of T wave amplitude on automatic QT measurement. In: *Computers in cardiology 1995*, Vienna: IEEE Computer Society Press, 1995, pp. 777–80.

22. Murray A, McLaughlin NB, Bourke JP, Doig JC, Furniss SS, Campbell RWF. Errors in manual measurement of QT intervals. *Br Heart J* 1994;**71**:386–90.

23. Kors JA, van Herpen G. Measurement error as a source of QT dispersion: a computerised analysis. *Heart* 1998;**80**:453–8.

24. Watanabe Y. Purkinje repolarization as a possible cause of the U wave in the electrocardiogram. *Circulation* 1975;**51**: 1030–7.

25. Anzelevich C, Nesterenko VV, Yan GX. The role of M cells in acquired long QT syndrome, U waves and torsade de pointes. *J Electrocardiol* 1996;**28**(Suppl.):131–8.

26. Yan G-Y, Antzelevich C. Cellular basis for the normal T wave and the electrocardiographic manifestations of the long-QT syndrome. *Circulation* 1998;**98**:1928–36.

27. Lepeschkin E, Surawicz B. The measurement of the QT interval of the electrocardiogram. *Circulation* 1952;**6**:378–88.

28. Kautzner J, Yi G, Kishore R *et al*. Interobserver reproducibility of QT interval measurement and QT dispersion in patients after acute myocardial infarction. *Ann Noninvas Electrocardiol* 1996;**1**:363–74.

29. Cowan JC, Yusoff K, Moore M, Amos PA, Gold AE, Bourke JPl. Importance of lead selection in QT interval measurement. *Am J Cardiol* 1988;**61**:83–7.

30. Mirvis DM. Spatial variation of QT intervals on normal persons and patients with acute myocardial infarction. *J Am Coll Cardiol* 1985;**5**:625–31.

31. Macfarlane PW, Devine B, Latif S, McLaughlin S, Shoat DB, Watts MP. Methodology of QRS interpretation in the Glasgow program. *Methods Inf Med* 1990;**29**:354–61.

32. Xue Q, Reddy S. New algorithms for QT dispersion analysis. *Proceedings of the Marquette 14th ECG Analysis Seminar* 1996, pp. 20–3.

33. Van Bemmel JH, Kors JA, Van Herpen G. Methodology of the modular ECG analysis system MEANS. *Methods Inf Med* 1990;**29**:346–53.

34. Lau CP, Freedman AR, Fleming S, Malik M, Camm AJ, Ward DE. Hysteresis of the ventricular paced QT interval in response to abrupt changes in pacing rate. *Cardiovasc Res* 1987;**22**:67–72.

35. De Bruyne MC, Hoes AW, Kors JA, Hofman A, van Bemmel JH, Grobbee DE. QTc dispersion predicts cardiac mortality in the elderly. The Rotterdam Study. *Circulation* 1998;**97**:467–72.

36. Okin PM, Devereux RB, Howard BV, Fabsitz RR, Lee ET, Welty TK. Assessment of QT interval and QT dispersion for prediction of all-cause and cardiovascular mortality in American Indians. The Strong Heart Study. *Circulation* 2000;**101**:61–6.

37. Hodges M, Salerno D, Erlinen D. Bazett's QT correction reviewed: evidence that a linear QT correction for heart rate is better. *J Am Coll Cardiol* 1983;**1**:694(Abstr.).

38. Sagie A, Larson MG, Goldberg RJ, Bengtson JR, Levy D. An improved method for adjusting the QT interval for heart rate (The Framingham Heart Study). *Am J Cardiol* 1992;**70**:797–801.

39. Han J, Millet D, Chizzonitti B, Moe GK. Temporal dispersion of recovery of excitability in atrium and ventricle as a function of heart rate. *Am Heart J* 1966;**71**:481–7.

40. Mitchell LB, Wyse DG, Duff HJ. Programmed electrical stimulation for ventricular tachycardia induction in humans. I.The role of ventricular functional refractoriness in tachycardia induction. *J Am Coll Cardiol* 1986;**8**:567–75.

41. Morgan JM, Cunningham D, Rowland E. Dispersion of monophasic action potential duration: demonstrable in humans after premature ventricular extrastimulation but not in steady state. *J Am Coll Cardiol* 1992;**19**:1244–53.

42. Maarouf N, Aytemir K, Gallagher M, Yap YG, Camm AJ, Malik M. Is QT dispersion heart rate dependent? What are the values of correction formulas for QT interval? *J Am Coll Cardiol* 1999;**33**(Suppl. A):113A-114A(Abstr.).

43. Savelieva I, Reddy SB, Camm AJ, Malik M. Does dispersion of repolarization depend on cardiac cycle length and should it be rate-corrected? Observations in 1096 healthy subjects. *J Am Coll Cardiol* 2000;**35**(Suppl.A):143A(Abstr.)

44. Zabel M, Woosley RL, Franz MR. Is dispersion of ventricular repolarization rate dependent? *PACE* 1997;**20**:2405–11.

45. Dabrowski A, Kramarz E, Piotrowicz, Kubik L. Predictive power of increased QT dispersion in ventricular extrasystoles and in sinus beats for risk stratification after myocardial infarction. *Circulation* 2000;**101**:1693–7.

46. Day CHP, McComb JM, Campbell RWF. QT dispersion in sinus beats and ventricular extrasystoles in normal hearts. *Br Heart J* 1992;**67**:39–42.

47. Malik M, Camm AJ. Mystery of QTc interval dispersion. *Am J Cardiol* 1997;**79**:785–7.

48. Hnatkova K, Malik M, Yi G, Camm AJ. Adjustment of QT dispersion assessed from 12 lead electrocardiograms for different number of analysed electrocardiographic leads: comparison of stability of different methods. *Br Heart J* 1994;**72**:390–6.

49. Hailer B, Van Leeuwen P, Lange S, Pilath M, Wehr M. Coronary artery disease may alter the spatial dispersion of the QT interval at rest. *Ann Noninvas Electrocardiol* 1999;**4**:267–73.

50. Yi G, Guo X-H, Crook R, Hnatkova K, Camm AJ, Malik M. Computerised measurements of QT dispersion in healthy subjects. *Heart* 1998;**80**:459–66.

51. Day CP, McComb JM, Mathews J, Campbell RW. Reduction of QT dispersion by sotalol following myocardial infarction. *Eur Heart J* 1991;**12**:423–7.

52. Glancy JM, Garratt CJ, Woods KL, De Bono DP. Three-lead measurement of QTc dispersion. *J Cardiovasc Electrophysiol* 1995;**6**:987–92.

53. Zareba W, Moss A. Dispersion of repolarization evaluated in three orthogonal-type electrocardiographic leads: L1, aVF, V2. *PACE* 1995;**18**:895(Abstr.).

54. Saint Beuve C, Badilini F, Maison-Blanche P, Kedra A, Coumel P. QT dispersion: comparison of orthogonal, quasi-orthogonal, and 12-lead configurations. *Ann Noninvas Electrocardiol* 1999;**4**:167–75.

55. Macfarlane PW, McLaughlin SC, Rodger C. Influence of lead selection and population on automated measurement of QT dispersion. *Circulation* 1998;**98**:2160–7.

56. Kautzner J, Yi G, Camm AJ, Malik M. Short- and long-term reproducibility of QT, QTc, and QT dispersion measurement in healthy subjects. *PACE* 1994;**17**:928–37.

57. Perkiömäkki JS, Kiostinen MJ, Yli-Mäyry S, Huikuri HV. Dispersion of the QT interval in patients with and without susceptibility to ventricular tachyarrhythmias after previous myocardial infarction. *J Am Coll Cardiol* 1995;**26**:174–9.

58. Halle M, Huonker M, Hohnloser SH, Alivertis M, Berg A, Keul J. QT dispersion in exercise-induced myocardial hypertrophy. *Am Heart J* 1999;**138**:309–12.

59. Tran HT, Fan C, Tu WQ, Kertland H, Li L, Kluger J, Chow MSS. QT measurement: a comparison of three simple methods. *Ann Noninvas Electrocardiol* 1998;**3**:228–31.

60. Malik M. Bradford A. Human precision of operating a digitizing board: implications for electrocardiogram measurement. *PACE* 1998;**21**:1656–62.

61. Yi G, Guo X-H, Crook R, Hnatkova K, Camm AJ, Malik M. Computerised measurements of QT dispersion in healthy subjects. *Heart* 1998;**80**:459–66.

62. McLaughlin NB, Campbell RWF, Murray A. Comparison of automatic QT measurement techniques in the normal 12 lead electrocardiogram. *Br Heart J* 1995;**74**:84–9.

63. Murray A, McLaughlin NB, Campbell RWF. Measuring QT dispersion: man versus machine. *Heart* 1997;**77**:539–42.

64. Savelieva I, Yi G, Guo X-H, Hnatkova K, Malik M. Agreement and reproducibility of automatic versus manual measurement of QT interval and QT dispersion. *Am J Cardiol* 1998;**81**:471–7.

65. Vloka ME, Babaev A, Ehlert FA, Narula DD, Steinberg JS. Poor correlation of automated and manual QT dispersion measurements in patients and normal subjects. *J Am Coll Cardiol* 1999;**33**(Suppl. A):350A(Abstr.).

66. McLaughlin NB, Campbell RWF, Murray A. Accuracy of four automatic QT measurement techniques in cardiac patients and healthy subjects. *Heart* 1996;**76**:422–6.

67. Batchvarov V, Yi G, Guo X-H, Savelieva I, Camm AJ, Malik M. QT interval and QT dispersion measured with the threshold method depend on threshold level. *PACE* 1998;**21**:2372–5.

68. Zaidi M, Robert A, Fesler R, Derwael C, Brohet C. Dispersion of ventricular repolarisation: a marker of ventricular arrhythmias in patients with previous myocardial infarction. *Heart* 1997;**78**:371–5.

69. Surawicz B. Will QT dispersion play a role in clinical decision-making? *J Cardiovasc Electrophysiol* 1996;**7**:777–84.

70. Goldner B, Brandspiegel HZ, Horwitz L, Jadonath R, Cohen T. Utility of QT dispersion combined with the signal-averaged electrocardiogram in detecting patients susceptible to ventricular tachyarrhythmia. *Am J Cardiol* 1995;**76**:1192–4.

71. Kautzner J, Malik M. QT dispersion and its clinical utility. *PACE* 1997;**20**:2625–40.

72. Statters DJ, Malik M, Ward DE, Camm AJ. QT dispersion: problems of methodology and clinical significance. *J Cardiovasc Electrophysiol* 1994;**5**:672–85.

73. Berul CI, Sweeten TL, Hill SL, Vetter VL. Provocative tests in children with suspect congenital long QT syndrome. *Ann Noninvas Electrocardiol* 1998;**3**:3–11.

74. Tutar H, Öcal B, Imamoglu A, Atalay S. Dispersion of QT and QTc interval in healthy children, and effects of sinus arrhythmia on QT dispersion. *Heart* 1998;**80**:77–9.

75. Macfarlane PW, McLaughlin SC, Devine B, Yang TF. Effects of age, sex, and race on ECG interval measurements. *J Electrocardiol* 1994;**27**:14–19.

76. Shah CP, Thakur RK, Reisdorff EJ, Lane E, Aufderheide TP, Hayes OW. QT dispersion may be a useful adjunct for detection of myocardial infarction in the chest pain center. *Am Heart J* 1998;**136**:496–8.

77. Davey PP, Bateman J, Mulligan IP, Forfar C, Barlow C, Hart G. QT interval dispersion in chronic heart failure and left ventricular hypertrophy: relation to autonomic nervous system and Holter tape abnormalities. *Br Heart J* 1994;**71**:268–73.

78. Challapalli S, Lingamneni R, Horvath G, Parker M, Goldberger JJ, Kadish A. Twelve-lead QT dispersion is smaller in women than in men. *Ann Noninvas Electrocardiol* 1998;**3**:25–31.

79. Savelieva I, Camm AJ, Malik M. Gender-specific differences on QT dispersion measured in 1100 healthy subjects. *PACE* 1999;**22**:885(Abstr.).

80. Savelieva I, Camm AJ, Malik M. Do we need age-adjustment of QT dispersion? Observations from 1096 normal subjects. *Heart* 1999;**81**(Suppl. 1):P47(Abstr.).

81. Zhang N, Ho TF, Yip WCL. QT dispersion in healthy Chinese children and adolescents. *Ann Noninvas Electrocardiol* 1999;**4**:281–5.

82. Savelieva I, Camm AJ, Malik M. Do we need age-adjustment of QT dispersion? Observations from 1096 normal subjects. *Heart* 1999;**81**(Suppl. 1):P47(Abstr.).

83. Macfarlane PW on behalf of the WOSCOPS. QT dispersion – lack of discriminating power. *Circulation* 1998;**98**(Suppl.): I-81(Abstr.).

84. Glancy JM, Garrat CJ, de Bono DP. Dynamics of QT dispersion during myocardial infarction and ischemia. *Int J Cardiol* 1996;**57**:55–60.

85. Ashikaga T, Nishizaki M, Arita M et al. Effect of dipyridamole on QT dispersion in vasospastic angina pectoris. *Am J Cardiol* 1999;**84**:807–10.

86. Sporton SC, Taggart P, Sutton PM, Walker JM, Hardman SM. Acute ischemia: a dynamic influence on QT dispersion. *Lancet* 1997;**349**:306–9.

87. Fei L, Goldman JH, Prasad K et al. QT dispersion and RR variations on 12-lead ECGs in patients with congestive heart failure secondary to idiopathic dilated cardiomyopathy. *Eur Heart J* 1996;**17**:258–63.

88. Pye M, Quinn AC, Cobbe SM. QT interval dispersion: a non-invasive marker of susceptibility to arrhythmia in patients with sustained ventricular arrhythmias? *Br Heart J* 1994;**71**:511–14.

89. Zaidi M, Robert A, Fesler R, Derwael C, Brohet C. Dispersion of ventricular repolarization in dilated cardiomyopathy. *Eur Heart J* 1997;**18**:1129–34.

90. Bonnar CE, Davie AP, Caruana L et al. QT Dispersion in patients with chronic heart failure: beta-blockers are associated with a reduction in QT dispersion. *Heart* 1999;**81**:297–302.

91. Muir DF, Love MWA, MacGregor GD, McCann GP, Hillis WS. Athletic left ventricular hypertrophy is associated with increased QT dispersion: an observational study. *J Am Coll Cardiol* 1999;**33**(Suppl. A):510A(Abstr.).

92. Mandecki T, Szulc A, Kastelik J, Mizia-Stec K, Szymanski L. The observation of the QT dispersion in left ventricular hypertrophy in weight lifters. *Ann Noninvas Electrocardiol* 1998;**3**:S18(Abstr.).

93. Simoncelli U, Rusconi C, Nicosia F, Drago F, Marchetti A. QT dispersion in endurance athletes. *Int J Sports Cardiol* 1998;**7**:63–7.

94. Davey PP, Bateman J, Mulligan IP, Forfar C, Barlow C, Hart G. QT interval dispersion in chronic heart failure and left ventricular hypertrophy: relation to autonomic nervous system and Holter tape abnormalities. *Br Heart J* 1994;**71**:268–73.

95. Ichkhan K, Molnar J, Somberg J. Relation of left ventricular mass and QT dispersion in patients with systemic hypertension. *Am J Cardiol* 1997;**79**:508–11.

96. Perkiömäki JS, Ikäheimo MJ, Pikkujämsä SM et al. Dispersion of the QT interval and autonomic modulation of heart rate in hypertensive men with and without left ventricular hypertrophy. *Hypertension* 1996;**28**:16–21.

97. Maheshwari VD, Girish MP. QT dispersion as a marker of left ventricular mass in essential hypertension. *Ind Heart J* 1998;**50**:414–17.

98. Tomiyama H, Doba N, Fu Y et al. Left ventricular geometric patterns and QT dispersion in borderline and mild hypertension: their evolution and regression. *Am J Hypertens* 1998;**11**:286–92.

99. Özerkan F, Zoghi M, Gürgün C, Yavuzgil O, Kaylikçioglu, Önder R. QT dispersion in hypertensive patients who had normal coronary angiogram with or without left ventricular hypertrophy. *Eur Heart J* 1999;**20**(Suppl.):85(Abstr.).

100. Yi G, Elliott P, McKenna WJ et al. QT dispersion and risk factors for sudden cardiac death in patients with hypertrophic cardiomyopathy. *Am J Cardiol* 1998;**82**:1514–19.

101. Calo L, Sciarra L, Sabina F et al. QT dispersion and late potentials in hypertrophic cardiomyopathy. *J Am Coll Cardiol* 1996;**27**(Suppl. A):59A(Abstr.).

102. Dritsas A, Sbarouni E, Gilligan D, Nihoyannopoulos P, Oakley CM. QT-interval abnormalities in hypertrophic cardiomyopathy. *Clin Cardiol* 1992;**15**:739–42.

103. Zaidi M, Robert A, Fesler R, Derwael C, Brohet C. Dispersion of ventricular repolarization in hypertrophic cardiomyopathy. *J Electrocardiol* 1996;**29**(Suppl.):89–94.

104. Zareba W, Moss AJ, Locati EH et al. ECG predictors of follow-up cardiac events in long QT syndrome probands. *Circulation* 1997;**96**(Suppl.):I-325(Abstr.).

105. Priori SG, Napolitano C, Diehl L, Schwartz PJ. Dispersion of the QT interval. A marker of therapeutic efficacy in the idiopathic long QT syndrome. *Circulation* 1994;**89**:1681–9.

106. Gavrilescu S, Luca C. Right ventricular monophasic action

potentials in patients with long QT syndrome. *Br Heart J* 1978;**40**:1014–18.

107. Bonatti V, Rolli A, Botti G. Recording of monophasic action potentials of the right ventricle in long QT syndromes complicated by severe ventricular arrhythmias. *Eur Heart J* 1983;**4**:168–79.

108. Yap YG, Yi G, Aytemir K, Goa X-H, Camm AJ, Malik M. Comprehensive assessment of QT dispersion in various at risk groups including acute myocardial infarction, unstable angina, hypertrophic cardiomyopathy, idiopathic dilated cardiomyopathy, and healthy controls. *PACE* 1999;**22**:A38(Abstr.).

109. Zoghi M, Gürgün C, Ercan E *et al*. QT dispersion in patients with different aetiology of left ventricular hypertrophy. *Eur Heart J* 1999;**20**(Suppl.):335(Abstr.).

110. Halle M, Huonker M, Hohnloser SH, Alivertis M, Berg A, Keul J. QT dispersion in exercise-induced myocardial hypertrophy. *Am Heart J* 1999;**138**:309–12.

111. Mayet J, Kanagaratnam P, Shahi M *et al*. QT dispersion in athletic left ventricular hypertrophy. *Am Heart J* 1999;**137**:678–81.

112. Bugra Z, Koylan N, Vural A *et al*. Left ventricular geometric patterns and QT dispersion in untreated essential hypertension. *Am J Hypertens* 1998;**11**:1164–70.

113. Yap YG, Yi G, Guo X-H, Aytemir K, Camm AJ, Malik M. Dynamic changes of QT dispersion and its relationship with clinical variables and arrhythmic events after myocardial infarction. *J Am Coll Cardiol* 1999;**33**(Suppl. A):107A(Abstr.).

114. Bennemeier H, Hartmann F, Giannitsis E *et al*. Effects of primary angioplasty on the course of QT dispersion after myocardial infarction and its association with infarct size. *PACE* 1999;**22**:A19(Abstr.).

115. Paventi S, Bevilacqua U, Parafati MA, Di Luzio E, Rossi F, Pelliccioni PR. QT dispersion and early arrhythmic risk during acute myocardial infarction. *Angiology* 1999;**50**:209–15.

116. Puljevic D, Smalcelj A, Durakovic Z, Goldner V. Effects of postmyocardial infarction scar size, cardiac function, and severity of coronary artery disease on QT interval dispersion as a risk factor for complex ventricular arrhythmia. *PACE* 1998;**21**:1508–16.

117. Kluger J, Hathaway L, Giedrimiene D. Does left ventricular function influence QT dispersion in patients with previous myocardial infarction and ventricular tachyarrhythmias? *J Am Coll Cardiol* 1997;**29**(Suppl. A):510A(Abstr.).

118. Schneider CA, Voth E, Baer FM, Horst M, Wagner R, Sechtem U. QT dispersion is determined by the extent of viable myocardium in patients with chronic Q-wave myocardial infarction. *Circulation* 1997;**96**:3913–20.

119. Clarkson PBM, Naas AAO, McMahon A, MacLeod C, Struthers AD, MacDonald TM. QT dispersion in essential hypertension. *Qu J Med* 1995;**88**:327–32.

120. Kohno I, Takusagawa M, Yin D *et al*. QT dispersion in dipper- and nondipper-type hypertension. *Am J Hypertens* 1998;**11**:280–5.

121. Bugra Z, Koylan N, Vural A *et al*. Left ventricular geometric patterns and QT dispersion in untreated essential hypertension. *Am J Hypertens* 1998;**11**:1164–70.

122. Higham PD, Furniss SS, Campbell RWF. QT dispersion and components of the QT interval in ischemia and infarction. *Br Heart J* 1995;**73**:32–6.

123. Yap YG, Yi G, Guo X-H, Aytemir K, Camm AJ, Malik M. Dynamic changes of QT dispersion and its relationship with clinical variables and arrhythmic events after myocardial infarction. *J Am Coll Cardiol* 1999;**33**(Suppl. A):107A(Abstr.).

124. Glancy JM, Garrat CJ, de Bono DP. Dynamics of QT dispersion during myocardial infarction and ischemia. *Int J Cardiol* 1996;**57**:55–60.

125. Aytemir K, Bavafa V, Ozer N, Aksoyek S, Oto A, Ozmen F. Effect of balloon inflation-induced acute ischemia on QT dispersion during percutaneous transluminal coronary angioplasty. *Clin Cardiol* 1999;**22**:21–4.

126. Okishige K, Yamashita K, Yoshinaga H, Azemagi K, Satoh T, Goseki Y, Fujii S, Ohira H, Satake S. Electrophysiological effects of ischemic preconditioning on QT dispersion during coronary angioplasty. *J Am Coll Cardiol* 1996;**28**:70–3.

127. Tarabey R, Sukenik D, Milnar J, Somberg JC. Effect of intracoronary balloon inflation at percutaneous transluminal coronary angioplasty on QT dispersion. *Am Heart J* 1998;**135**:519–22.

128. Yi G, Crook R, Guo H, Staunton A, Camm AJ, Malik M. Exercise-induced changes in the QT interval duration and dispersion in patients with sudden cardiac death after myocardial infarction. *Int J Cardiol* 1998;**63**:271–9.

129. Sporton SC, Taggart P, Sutton PM, Walker JM, Hardman SM. Acute ischemia: a dynamic influence on QT dispersion. *Lancet* 1997;**349**:306–9.

130. Michelucci A, Padeletti L, Frati M *et al*. Effects of ischemia and reperfusion on QT dispersion during coronary angioplasty. *PACE* 1996;**19**:1905–8.

131. Tomoda H, Aoki N. Prolonged QT interval and QT dispersion induced by coronary rotational atherectomy. *J Am Coll Cardiol* 2000;**35**(Suppl.A):88A(Abstr.).

132. Gabrielli F, Balzotti L, Bandiera A. QT dispersion variability and myocardial viability in acute myocardial infarction. *Intern J Cardiol* 1997;**61**:61–7.

133. Nakajima T, Fujimoto S, Uemura S *et al*. Does increased QT dispersion in the acute phase of anterior myocardial infarction predict recovery of left ventricular wall motion? *J Electrocardiol* 1998;**31**:1–8.

134. Schneider CA, Voth E, Baer FM, Horst M, Wagner R, Sechtem U. QT dispersion is determined by the extent of viable myocardium in patients with chronic Q-wave myocardial infarction. *Circulation* 1997;**96**:3913–20.

135. Ikonomidis I, Athanassopoulos G, Karatasakis G *et al*. Dispersion of ventricular repolarization is determined by the presence of myocardial viability in patients with old myocardial infarction. A dobutamine stress echocardiography study. *Eur Heart J* 2000;**21**:446–56.

136. Moreno FL, Villanueva T, Karagounis LA, Anderson JL. Reduction of QT interval dispersion by successful thrombolytic therapy in acute myocardial infarction. TEAM-2 Study Investigators. *Circulation* 1994;**90**:94–100.

137. Karagounis LA, Anderson JL, Moreno FL, Sorensen SG for the TEAM-3 Investigators. Multivariate associates of QT dispersion in patients with acute myocardial infarction: pri-

macy of patency status of the infarct-related artery. *Am Heart J* 1998;**135**:1027–35.

138. Kelly RF, Parillo JE, Hollenberg SM. Effect of coronary angioplasty on QT dispersion. *Am Heart J* 1997;**134**:399–405.

139. Szydlo K, Trusz-Gluza M, Drzewiecki J, Wozniak-Skowerska I, Szczogiel J. Correlation of heart rate variability parameters and QT interval in patients after PTCA of infarct related coronary artery as an indicator of improved autonomic regulation. *PACE* 1998;**21**:2407–10.

140. Choi K-J, Lee C-W, Kang D-H *et al*. Change of QT dispersion after PTCA in angina patients. *Ann Noninvas Electrocardiol* 1999;**4**:195–9.

141. Brooksby P, Robinson PJ, Segal R, Klinger G, Pitt B, Cowley AJC on behalf of the ELITE study group. Effects of losartan and captopril on QT dispersion in elderly patients with heart failure. *Lancet* 1999;**534**:395–6.

142. Mayet J, Shahi M, McGrath K *et al*. Left ventricular hypertrophy and QT dispersion in hypertension. *Hypertension* 1996;**28**:791–6.

143. Lim PO, Nys M, Naas AAO, Struthers AD, Osbakken M, MacDonald T. Irbesartan reduces QT dispersion in hypertensive individuals. *Hypertension* 1999;**33**:713–18.

144. Karpanou EA, Vyssoulis GP, Psichogios A *et al*. Regression of left ventricular hypertrophy results in improvement of QT dispersion in patients with hypertension. *Am Heart J* 1998;**136**:765–8.

145. Gonzalez-Juanatey JR, Garcia-Acuna JM, Pose A *et al*. Reduction of QT and QTc dispersion during long-term treatment of systemic hypertension with enalapril. *Am J Cardiol* 1998;**81**:170–4.

146. Priori SG, Napolitano C, Diehl L, Schwartz PJ. Dispersion of the QT interval. A marker of therapeutic efficacy in the idiopathic long QT syndrome. *Circulation* 1994;**89**:1681–9.

147. Barbato G, Franco N, di Niro M, Pavesi PC, Bracchetti D. Correlation between dispersion of ventricular repolarization and malignant arrhythmias during acute myocardial infarction. *Eur Heart J* 1995;**16**(Suppl.):446(Abstr.).

148. Zaputovic L, Mavric Z, Zaninovic-Jurjevic T, Matana A, Bradic N. Relationship between QT dispersion and the incidence of early ventricular arrhythmias in patients with acute myocardial infarction. *Int J Cardiol* 1997;**62**:211–16.

149. Papandonakis E, Tsoukas A, Christakos S. QT dispersion as a noninvasive arrhythmogenic marker in acute myocardial infarction. *Ann Noninvas Electrocardiol* 1999;**4**:35–8.

150. Zareba W, Moss AJ, le Cessie S. Dispersion of ventricular repolarization and arrhythmic cardiac death in coronary artery disease. *Am J Cardiol* 1994;**74**:550–3.

151. Pye M, Quinn AC, Cobbe SM. QT interval dispersion: a noninvasive marker of susceptibility to arrhythmia in patients with sustained ventricular arrhythmias? *Br Heart J* 1994;**71**:511–14.

152. Shulan Z, Yin'an S, Huixian H. Prediction value of ventricular arrhythmia of patients with acute myocardial infarction by QT dispersion. *J Xi'An Med Univ* 1998;**19**:616–17.

153. Zhao L-x, Ozawa Y, Watanabe I, Saito S, Kanmatsuse. Prognostic significance of QTc dispersion in patients after myocardial infarction with and without late potentials, ven-

tricular tachycardia and sudden cardiac death. *J Am Coll Cardiol* 2000;**35**(Suppl. A):121A(Abstr.).

154. Zabel M, Klingenheben T, Franz MR, Hohnloser SH. Assessment of QT dispersion for prediction of mortality or arrhythmic events after myocardial infarction. *Circulation* 1998;**97**:2543–50.

155. Tavernier R, Jordaens L. Repolarisation characteristics and sudden death after myocardial infarction: a case control study. *J Am Coll Cardiol* 1999;**33**(Suppl. A):146A (Abstr.).

156. Moenning G, Haverkamp W, Schulte H *et al*. Prognostic value of QT-interval and dispersion in apparently healthy individuals. results from the Münster Heart Study (PROCAM). *J Am Coll Cardiol* 1999;**33**(Suppl. A):333A (Abstr.).

157. Lee KW, Okin PM, Kligfield P, Stein KM, Lerman BB. Precordial QT dispersion and inducible ventricular tachycardia. *Am Heart J* 1997;**134**:1005–13.

158. Gillis AM, Trabousli M, Hii JTY *et al*. Antiarrhythmic drug effects on QT interval dispersion in patients undergoing electropharmacologic testing for ventricular tachycardia and fibrillation. *Am J Cardiol* 1998;**81**:588–93.

159. Berul CI, Michaud GF, Lee VC, Hill SL, Mark Estes III, Wang PJ. A comparison of T-wave alternans and QT dispersion as noninvasive predictors of ventricular arrhythmias. *Ann Noninvas Electrocardiol* 1999;**4**:274–80.

160. Zabel M, Klingenheben T, Sticherling C, Franz MR, Hohnloser SH. QT-dispersion does not predict inducibility or adequate device treatment in patients with malignant ventricular tachyarrhythmias. *Eur Heart J* 1998;**19**(Suppl.):600(Abstr.).

161. Armoundas AA, Osaka M, Mela T *et al*. T-wave alternans and dispersion of the QT interval as risk stratification markers in patients susceptible to sustained ventricular arrhythmias. *Am J Cardiol* 1998;**82**:1127–9.

162. De Sutter J, Tavernier R, van de Wiele C *et al*. QT dispersion is not related to infarct size or inducibility in patients with coronary artery disease and life threatening ventricular arrhythmias. *Heart* 1999;**81**:533–8.

163. Fu G-S, Meissner A, Simon R. Repolarization dispersion and sudden cardiac death in patients with impaired left ventricular function. *Eur Heart J* 1997;**18**:281–9.

164. Galinier M, Vialette J-C, Fourcade J *et al*. QT interval dispersion as a predictor of arrhythmic events in congestive heart failure. Importance of aetiology. *Eur Heart J* 1998;**19**:1054–62.

165. Anastasiou-Nana MI, Nanas JN, Karagounis LA *et al*. Dispersion of QRS and QT in patients with advanced congestive heart failure: relation to cardiac and sudden cardiac death mortality. *Eur Heart J* 1999;**20**(Suppl.):117(Abstr.).

166. Brooksby P, Robinson PJ, Segal R, Klinger G, Pitt B, Cowley AJC on behalf of the ELITE study group. Effects of losartan and captopril on QT dispersion in elderly patients with heart failure. *Lancet* 1999;**534**:395–6.

167. Pitt B, Segal R, Martinez FA *et al*. Randomised trial of losartan versus captopril in patients over 65 with heart failure. *Lancet* 1997;**349**:747–52.

168. Ogita H, Fukunami M, Shimonagata T *et al*. An increase in corrected QT dispersion on exercise predicts sudden death in patients with chronic heart failure – a prospective study. *J Am Coll Cardiol* 2000;**35**(Suppl. A):187A(Abstr.).

169. Brendorp B, Elming H, Køber L, Malik M, Jun L, Torp-Pedersen C for the Diamond Study Group. Prognostic implications of QT interval and dispersion in patients with congestive heart failure. *PACE* 1999;**22**:259(Abstr.).

170. Brooksby P, Batin PD, Nolan J *et al.* The relationship between QT intervals and mortality in ambulant patients with chronic heart failure. The United Kingdom Heart Failure Evaluation and Assessment of Risk Trial (UK-HEART). *Eur Heart J* 1999;**20**:1335–41.

171. Radmanabhan S, Amin J, Silvet H, Pai RG. QT dispersion has no impact on mortality in patients with moderate and severe left ventricular dysfunction: results from a cohort of 2263 patients. *J Am Coll Cardiol* 1999;33(Suppl. A):107A(Abstr.).

172. Galinier M, Balanescu S, Fourcade J *et al.* Prognostic value of arrhythmogenic markers in systemic hypertension. *Eur Heart J* 1997;**18**:1484–91.

173. Buja G, Miorelli M, Turrini P, Melacini P, Nava A. Comparison of QT dispersion in hypertrophic cardiomyopathy between patients with and without ventricular arrhythmias and sudden death. *Am J Cardiol* 1993;**72**:973–6.

174. Miorelli M, Buja G, Melacini P, Fasoli G, Nava A. QT-interval variability in hypertrophic cardiomyopathy patients with cardiac arrest. *Int J Cardiol* 1994;**45**:121–7.

175. Baranowski R, Malecka L, Poplawska W *et al.* Analysis of QT dispersion in patients with hypertrophic cardiomyopathy – correlation with clinical data and survival. *Eur Heart J* 1998;**19**(Suppl.):428(Abstr.).

176. Yi G, Elliott P, McKenna WJ *et al.* QT dispersion and risk factors for sudden cardiac death in patients with hypertrophic cardiomyopathy. *Am J Cardiol* 1998;**82**:1514–19.

177. Maron BJ, Leyhe MJ, Gohman TE, Casey SA, Crow RS, Hodges M. QT dispersion is not a predictor of sudden cardiac death in hypertrophic cardiomyopathy as assessed in an unselected patient population. *J Am Coll Cardiol* 1999;**33**(Suppl. A):128A(Abstr.).

178. Priori SG, Napolitano C, Diehl L, Schwartz PJ. Dispersion of the QT interval. A marker of therapeutic efficacy in the idiopathic long QT syndrome. *Circulation* 1994;**89**:1681–9.

179. Surawicz B. Long QT: good, bad, indifferent and fascinating. *ACC Current J Rev* 1999;19–21.

180. Moss AJ. Drugs that prolong the QT interval: regulatory and QT measurement issues from the United States and European perspectives. *Ann Noninvas Electrocardiol* 1999;**4**:255–6.

181. Cui G, Sager P, Singh BN, Sen L. Effects of amiodarone and quinidine on depolarisation, JT interval and dispersion in patients with intraventricular conduction delay. *J Am Coll Cardiol* 1994;179A(Abstr.).

182. Hii JTY, Wyse DG, Gillis AM, Duff HJ, Solylo MA, Mitchell LB. Precordial QT interval dispersion as a marker of torsade de pointes. Disparate effects of class Ia antiarrhythmic drugs and amiodarone. *Circulation* 1992;**86**:1376–82.

183. Hohnloser SH, van de Loo A, Baedeker F. Efficacy and proarrhythmic hazards of pharmacologic cardioversion of atrial fibrillation: prospective comparison of sotalol versus quinidine. *J Am Coll Cardiol* 1995;**26**:852–8.

184. Kertland H, White CM, Chow MSS, Kluger J. QT disper-sion as a marker for response to quinidine in patients with ventricular tachyarrhythmias. *ANE* 2000;**5**:39–44.

185. Day CP, McComb JM, Mathews J, Campbell RWF. Reduction in QT dispersion by sotalol following myocardial infarction. *Eur Heart J* 1991;**12**:423–7.

186. Cui G, Sen L, Sager P, Uppal P, Singh BN. Effects of amio-darone, sematilide, and sotalol on QT dispersion. *Am J Cardiol* 1994;**74**:896–900.

187. Hohnloser SH, van de Loo, Kalusche D, Arendts W, Quart B. Does sotalol-induced alteration of QT-dispersion predict drug effectiveness or proarrhythmic hazards? *Circulation* 1993;**88**(Suppl. I):397(Abstr.).

188. Dritsas A, Gilligan D, Nihoyannopoulos P, Oakley CM. Amiodarone reduces QT dispersion in patients with hyper-trophic cardiomyopathy. *Int J Cardiol* 1992;**36**:345–9.

189. Meierhenrich R, Helguera ME, Kidwell GA, Tebbe U. Influence of amiodarone on QT dispersion in patients with life-threatening ventricular arrhythmias and clinical out-come. *Int J Cardiol* 1997;**60**:289–94.

190. Grimm W, Steder U, Menz V, Hoffmann J, Maisch B. Effect of amiodarone on QT dispersion in the 12-lead stan-dard electrocardiogram and its significance for subsequent arrhythmic events. *Clin Cardiol* 1997;**20**:107–10.

191. Van de Loo A, Klingenheben T, Hohnloser SH. Amiodarone therapy after sotalol-induced torsade de pointes: prolonged QT interval and QT dispersion in differentiation of pro-arrhythmic effects. *Z Kardiolog* 1994;**83**:887–90.

192. Tran HT, Chow MS, Kluger J. Amiodarone induced tor-sades de pointes with excessive QT dispersion following quinidine induced polymorphic ventricular tachycardia. *PACE* 1997;**20**:2275–8.

193. Yadav A, Paquette M, Newman D, Connolly SJ, Dorian P. Amiodarone is associated with increased QT dispersion but low mortality in a CIDS cohort. *PACE* 1999;**22**:896(Abstr.).

194. Faber TS, Zehender M, Krahnfeld O, Daisenberger K, Meinetz T, Just H. Propafenone during acute myocardial ischemia in patients: a double-blind, randomized, placebo-controlled study. *J Am Coll Cardiol* 1997;**29**:561–7.

195. Trusz-Gluza M, Świderska E, Śmieja-Jaroczynska B, Wozniak-Skowerska I, Filipecki A. Factors influencing dis-persion of repolarisation under antiarrhythmic treatment. *Ann Noninvas Electrocardiol* 1998;**3**:S18(Abstr.).

196. Houltz B, Darpö B, Edvardsson N *et al.* Electrocardiographic and clinical predictors of torsades de pointes induced by almokalant infusion in patients with chronic atrial fibrilla-tion of flutter: a prospective study. *PACE* 1998;**21**:1044–57.

197. Sedwick ML, Rasmussen HS, Cobbe SM. Effects of the class III antiarrhythmic drug dofetilide on ventricular monophasic action potential duration and the QT interval dispersion in stable angina pectoris. *Am J Cardiol* 1992;**70**:1432–7.

198. Brum J, Alkhalidi H, Karam R, Marcello S. Effects of azim-ilide, an IKs/IKr blocking anti arrhythmic on QT and QTc dispersion, in patients with ventricular tachycardia (VT). *PACE* 1999;**22**:A13(Abstr.).

199. Parikka H, Toivonen L, Naukkarinen V *et al.* Decreases by magnesium of QT dispersion and ventricular arrhythmias in

patients with acute myocardial infarction. *Eur Heart J* 1999;**20**:111–20.

200. Leonardo F, Fragasso G, Rosano GMC, Pagnotta P, Chierchia SL. Effect of atenolol on QT interval and dispersion in patients with syndrome X. *Am J Cardiol* 1997;**80**:789–90.

201. Bonnar CE, Davie AP, Caruana L *et al*. QT dispersion in patients with chronic heart failure: beta-blockers are associated with a reduction in QT dispersion. *Heart* 1999;**81**:297–302.

202. Committee for Proprietary Medicinal Products. *Points to consider: the assessment of the potential for QT interval prolongation by non-cardiovascular medicinal products*. The European Agency for the Evaluation of Medicinal Products. December, 1997.

203. Abildskov JA, Burgess MJ, Urie PM, Lux RL, Wyatt RF. The unidentified information content of the electrocardiogram. *Circ Res* 1977;**40**:3–7.

204. Priori SG, Mortara DW, Napolitano C *et al*. Evaluation of the spatial aspects of T-wave complexity in the long-QT syndrome. *Circulation* 1997;**96**:3006–12.

205. Yi G, Prasad K, Elliott P *et al*. T wave complexity in patients with hypertrophic cardiomyopathy. *PACE* 1998;**21**:2382–6.

206. De Ambroggi LD, Aime E, Ceriotti C, Rovida M, Negroni S. Mapping of ventricular repolarization potentials in patients with arrhythmogenic right ventricular dysplasia. Principal component analysis of the ST-T waves. *Circulation* 1997;**96**:4314–18.

207. Kors JA, de Bruyne MC, Hoes AW *et al*. T axis as an indicator of risk of cardiac events in elderly people. *Lancet* 1998;**352**:601–4.

208. Acar B, Yi G, Hnatkova K, Malik M. Spatial, temporal and wavefront direction characteristics of 12-lead T wave morphology. *Med Biol Eng Comput* 1999;**37**:574–84.

11 Electrocardiographic assessment of myocardial ischaemia (with a note on the ischaemia–arrhythmia connection)

Shlomo Stern

The downward shift of the ST segment on the electrocardiogram (ECG) after exercise had already noted by Einthoven himself, but a search into history to find out who described first the significance of ST depression as a sign of myocardial ischaemia is not in the scope of this chapter. It could be stated, however, that the first link between this ECG phenomenon and ischaemia of the myocardium was established in the classic study of Pardee in 1920,[1] and Feil and Siegel in 1929 assumed that these changes were induced by a reduction in coronary blood flow.[2]

ST depression in the resting 12-lead ECG

A permanent ST segment depression is not specific for myocardial ischaemia, as many pharmacological, extracardiac or even cardiac abnormalities other than ischaemia, are possible causes.[3] The division of the ST segment abnormalities into secondary and primary ones, was advocated by Grant in the early 1950s[4] and was recently concisely and precisely reviewed by Hurst.[5,6] We can safely state that, if the so called "secondary" causes are ruled out, ST depression in the resting 12-lead ECG points to an ischaemic mechanism and, if this change appears in subjects with coronary risk factors, typical clinical picture of angina, etc., the diagnosis of angina pectoris seems to be clinched. It has been stated that although this ECG abnormality is only occasionally detected during a routine 12–lead ECG recording, its frequency was estimated to be 50% during an anginal episode in patients who have a normal resting ECG.[7]

If the resting ECG, even when used as a screening method, shows ST depression, this will carry prognostic value.[8-11] Interestingly, the resting ECG may more frequently disclose signs of ischaemia in totally asymptomatic subjects, who are siblings of a parent who died prematurely from coronary disease.[12] ST-T segment abnormalities recorded in the resting 12-lead ECG in the chronic stage of myocardial infarction (1–6 months after the event), was the only non-invasive test variable that identified a significantly increased risk for recurrent cardiac event, whilst exercise testing, ambulatory ECG monitoring, and thallium stress testing, all failed to do so.[13]

ST depression during spontaneous chest pain

We are on more firm ground with a transient ST depression, when it appears under the watchful eyes of the doctor. Such transient ST depression can be observed when the patient, while being examined, suffers from precordial pain, when exercised for diagnostic purposes, or when the stress is induced pharmacologically; each of these situations deserve to be addressed separately. ST depression if observed in unstable angina patients hospitalised in an ICCU bed or in an ambulatory patient detected in retrospect on a Holter ECG, with the clinical picture of chest pain, the concomitant ST depression confirms the ischaemic nature of the pain.

Somewhat different is the interpretation if the ST depression episode under ambulatory conditions appears without accompanying chest pain. This "silent" ST depression episodes, if recorded in patients with risk for ischaemic heart disease and recorded under perfect technical conditions, are confirmed by many studies not only as being an expression of ischaemia, but also as a representation of a poor prognosis, as discussed below.

ST depression provoked by physical exercise

An extensive amount of investigations were devoted to this topic since its description by Arthur Master in the late 1920s. A meta-analysis was really needed to compile these data, which was done excellently by Gianrossi and co-workers.[14] It seems to be somewhat disappointing that exercise-induced ST depression's mean sensitivity was found to be only 68% (23–100%), its specificity somewhat higher (77%; 17–100%), using coronary arteriography as the gold standard. If women and men are matched for the presence and severity of coronary artery disease, the ECG stress test will perform similarly, independent of the gender of the examinee.[15]

Interestingly, not only the development of ≥1 mm flat or downsloping ST depression during the treadmill test had prognostic significance in the study of Rywik and co-workers,[16] but also ST depression developing during recovery in apparently healthy individuals, had adverse effect on the prognosis of future coronary events, presaging a ~2.5-fold independent risk. On the other hand, neither the ECG changes nor exercise-induced angina were associated with prognosis in a population-based cohort, which included many symptomatic individuals, some with history of previous MIs and various other definite risk factors.[17] The Bayesian theory explains this wide variations in the specificity and sensitivity of exercise testing and the different conclusions reached concerning its predictive value. Differences in the clinical status of the patients referred for the test influence the reliability of the test: the older the patient, the more risk factors are carried, the more the sensitivity will increase; the specificity will be lower in patients with other forms of heart disease, left ventricular hypertrophy from different causes, digitalis therapy, etc. All these obviously influence the use of exercise testing as a prognostic tool. Interestingly, the presence or absence of chest pain in patients with an ischaemic ST response to exercise testing did not alter the risk during a 2-year follow-up period, as shown by Callaham *et al.*[18]

Thus, although exercise ECG's role seemed to be "changing," as Chaitman stated in his excellent review in 1986,[19] one can safely say that, during the last decade, ECG recording during stress, physical or mental, proved further its unique and essential role in the assessment of myocardial ischaemia. Resting versus dynamic recordings, in- and out-of-hospital monitorings, exercising already in the Emergency Department,[20] computer-assisted, multilead recordings, use of artificial neural networks,[21] taking into consideration postexercise HRV changes,[21] and many other innovations will give more and more significance to this venerable tool of diagnostic cardiology.

Quantitative value of ST depression in measuring ischaemia

Whilst ST depression, both in stable and in unstable coronary artery disease, represents a bad prognostic omen, as compared to the same clinical picture but without this ECG alteration, its use for quantitation still seems to be a "high hurdle". The situation is more complicated, as not only the depth of the ST depression (and also of a T wave inversion) but also its duration, the number of leads in which it appears, are all important factors as well.

Experimental observations confirm the progressive nature of the ST-T abnormalities, which start (following ligation of a coronary artery) with inversion of the T wave; successively, ST depression develops and progresses. However, in the clinical setting, a direct relationship between the intensity of the ischaemia and the degree of ST depression can rarely be documented, not even if we study a dynamic continuous Holter or overhead monitor leads, let alone a 12-lead ECG routine recording.

Somewhat better is the situation when the ECG under scrutiny is recorded during a stress testing. Although the identification of the site of the ischaemia and/or identification of the diseased coronary artery were proven to be goals inaccessible by the localisation and measuring the degree of ST depression, newer and more complicated methods introduced and advocated by several investigators improve our knowledge. Although R and Q wave amplitude criteria and/or maximal ST/heart rate slope increase the sensitivity (and decrease the specificity), a quantitative risk stratification based on the ECG only, rather than on the exercise work load or length of exercise performance, is still disappointing. Bogaty and co-workers[23] studied ECG indexes during exercise testing in patients with proven coronary artery disease. Maximal ST depression could not quantify the number of diseased vessels, was not related to vessel disease score, to maximal thallium deficit, nor to redistribution gradient; it was, however, related to the extent of a perfusion abnormality. Interestingly, in this study an upsloping ST segment depression had similar significance as a horizontal or a downsloping one. The quantitative significance of the ST depression was better in the study of Kaul and co-workers,[24] who found that a ≥2 mm ST depression was a marker of high risk in acute coronary syndromes.

It is possible that, by the use of more sophisticated ECG parameters, such as linear regression analysis of the heart rate-related change in ST depression, as proposed by Okin and co-workers,[25] or a score integrating ST segment altitude and slope changes as done by Hollenberg *et al.*,[26] better quantitative value will be obtained in the future. In the meantime, one can agree with Lindahl[27] that, as far as ST depression is concerned, "more is worse."

Spontaneous ST depression episodes during daily activity

Although ambulatory ECG monitoring "provides accurate and clinically meaningful information about myocardial ischaemia in patients with coronary disease," as stated by the ACC/AHA Guidelines,[28] it has not reduced the need for exercise testing as a first-line screening method. It is rare to detect ischaemic episodes in persons with a negative exercise test, but even in such cases it may reveal important information if variant angina is suspected, in patients with chest pain who cannot exercise, in patients with coronary artery disease and atypical chest pain, or in patients with episodic chest pain "not otherwise explained," as stated in the Guidelines.

Daily life ischaemia, as assessed by ambulatory Holter monitoring at the entry of patients to the ACIP investigation, provided independent prognostic information.[29] This seems to be now the latest data on that subject, confirming many previous investigations,[30–37] but in contrast with a few others.[38–40]

During mental stress test, more than half of the patients with documented coronary disease in the PIMI study[41] developed either reversible left ventricular dysfunction or ST depression. The ST depression to mental stress was more predictive of ischaemic episodes during routine daily activities than other laboratory-based ischaemic markers. The intriguing subject of mental stress-induced ischaemia, its characteristics, the haemodynamic and neurohormonal responses and its prognostic value, were recently reviewed by Gottdiener *et al.*[42]

ECG's contribution in acute coronary syndromes

In patients with unstable angina, several studies demonstrated that ST depression episodes, a majority of which are silent, relate to the clinical outcome of the patients. In such patients, 12-lead ECG monitoring, with computer-assisted continuous ST segment recordings, in the CAPTURE-study demonstrated a reduction in ischaemic burden by abciximab.[43] The ischaemic burden was calculated either as the total duration of ST depression episodes per patient, the area under the curve of the ST vector magnitude during episodes, or the sum of the areas under the curves of 12-leads during the episodes. This method of continuous 12-lead ST segment analysis was used in the TAMI 7 and other studies for diagnosis and quantification of myocardial ischaemia and detection of myocardial infarction.[44–47] Computerised ST depression analysis was shown to improve risk stratification for cardiovascular and total mortality,[48] compared with standard visual Minnesota Coding.

In unstable coronary syndromes, ST depression on admission is known to be an important indicator of poor outcome.[49] Cannon and co-workers[50] demonstrated in the TIMI III Registry that, even ≥0.5 mm ST segment deviation on admission identifies high-risk patients, and is an independent predictor of 1-year outcome. In a recent study of Holmvang and co-workers,[51] investigating not only baseline ST-T changes but also troponin T and I, myoglobin and creatine kinase MB, on multivariate analysis only the admission ECG carried independent prognostic value.

The value of continuous 12-lead monitoring of the ST segment was documented by Jernberg and co-workers,[52] who demonstrated that ST deviation in patients with non-diagnostic ECG but symptoms suggestive of acute coronary syndrome provides important prognostic information and improves early risk stratification. These studies reinforce the previous observations, obtained by the use of the two- or three-lead Holter-technique, that, in unstable coronary syndromes, the presence of ischaemic ST depression episodes, frequently silent, are related to worse outcome.[53–56] However, owing to the relatively low sensitivity of the continuous ST-segment monitoring in most studies, regardless of the method used,[57] clinical data and the use the older or the newer biochemical markers are essential additions, and this combination promises "powerful and accurate"[58] risk stratification in unstable coronary disease.

Not only the appearance but also the resolution of the deviation of the ST segment is turning into a prognostic sign in acute infarction: Shah and co-workers[59] have shown that a continuous analysis of the resolution provides prognostic information about in-hospital mortality.

Exercise-induced ST segment elevation

Although a 1 mm ST elevation 60–80 ms after J-point in three consecutive leads is considered an abnormal response, both in Q and non-Q leads,[60–62] the true meaning and mechanism of this ECG abnormality has so far not been fully elucidated. The classic conclusion of Chahine and co-workers,[63] that this commonly reflects severe coronary disease with associated left ventricular aneurysm, and is relating more to abnormal wall motion than to the ischaemia *per se*, is certainly valid. This notion was supported by these authors' observation, that chest pain occurrence is less frequent in these patients than in those who exhibit the more common exercise-induced ST depression. In a recent study in patients with Q wave infarction and single-vessel disease, Margonatoel *et al.*[64] demonstrated a high specificity and acceptable sensitivity of exercise-induced ST elevation in infarct-related leads for the detection of residual viability, and the use of ECG for this purpose has been called "simple, inexpensive, and widely available."

The possible concomitant reciprocal ST-segment depression has also been addressed in the literature, and a similar value for detecting residual myocardial viability has been reported[65] in patients with previous ST depression. The sensitivity, specificity, and accuracy were 84%, 100%, and 90%, respectively. In patients with inferior Q wave infarction, ST depression during dobutamine stress testing in the high lateral leads is seen as a reciprocal change to ST elevation in the inferior leads by Elhandy and co-workers,[66] but, in the anterior leads, the ST depression seemed to be a sign of myocardial ischaemia. The extension of the area of data collection to the posterior (V_{7-9}) chest leads, proved itself also useful, as ST elevation in these leads revealed acute posterior infaction in the investigation of Matetzky and co-workers.[67] The addition of such leads to the routine ECG evaluation of patients with acute infarction has already been advocated years ago,[68,69] but even the conventional leads still provide localising information about the occlusion site in the left anterior descending artery in an acute anterior infarction, as shown recently by Engelen and co-workers.[70]

Myocardial ischaemia and its relation to arrhythmias

Disturbances in the heart rhythm as a reaction to ischaemia were known since Mac William called attention to the fact that asphyxia makes the myocardium unduly "excitable", and ventricular fibrillation is easily induced even if gentle digital pressure is applied to it.[71] The cellular electrophysiological effects of ischaemia have been intensely studied during the last few decades, from the early works of Harris[72] through several excellent experimental studies of recent years,[73] and our understanding of the complex and multiple factors governing this phenomenon is ever growing. In the clinical setting as well, it has been known for many years that ischaemia is a significant harbinger of ventricular arrhythmias. This clinical information is becoming more and more supported by well-based and controlled observations, accumulated during recent years.

Ventricular arrhythmias in the acute and chronic phase of myocardial infarction (AMI)

A wide variety of ectopic activities have been described to originate when a coronary artery occludes and infarction of the myocardium starts. Premature ventricular complexes are observed in the majority of patients with AMI.[74] Non-sustained ventricular tachycardia (NSVT) has been reported to occur in about 1% to 7% of the patients,[75,76] and usually no adverse effect was attributed neither on in-hospital nor on 1-year survival. This prevailing opinion was confirmed by Cheema and co-workers[77] only if the NSVT occurred within the first several hours of presentation; if, however, it was diagnosed beyond the first several hours after the acute event, it was associated with substantial increases in relative risk. Its occurrence became significant after 13 hours, plateauing at ~24 hours. It is probable that NSVTs occurring during the first few hours (the first 13 hours, according to the last quoted

study) may have a mechanism which were identified in animal models as "phase 2" arrhythmias, while during the ensuing hours they are due to other mechanisms that are associated with a poor prognosis. These other mechanisms may be an ongoing ischaemia, left ventricular dysfunction, or some other cause for electrical instability.

Thus, the achievement of electrical stability as early as possible, the "open artery hypothesis",[78] is certainly desirable. The theory that reperfusion increases the electrical stability of the heart, independently of myocyte salvage, could be confirmed in animal studies.[79] In this study, a "dramatic" reduction in the incidence and duration of VT and VF was observed after either early or late reperfusion. Thus, the reopening of an occluded coronary artery may probably reduce the risk of future arrhythmic events in the clinical setting as well, as a consequence of the increased electrical stability, which is strongly affected by the sympathetic/parasympathetic balance of the autonomic nervous system. The reperfusion itself, however, carries a certain arrhythmic risk, as reported by Alexopoulos et al.[80] after comparing arrhythmic events in streptokinase-treated and placebo-treated patients; the former group had, on Holter, during the first 24 hours, more ventricular pairs, runs, and repetitive arrhythmias than the latter group; the more frequent myocardial perfusion achieved by streptokinase seems to be a plausible hypothesis for this phenomenon.

In the late hospital phase of AMI, a careful detection of ventricular and supraventricular arrhythmias was advocated by Berisso et al.,[81] since their occurrence may suggest underlying cardiac dysfunction. These arrhythmias, however, were not independently related to subsequent cardiac death. As to the chronic phase of MI, experimental studies support the assumption that re-entry is the mechanism of VT in these patients.[82] For the first 1 to 2 years, this situation prevails and the patients continue to be at risk for malignant ventricular arrhythmias.[83,84]

Ventricular arrhythmias in chronic ischaemic heart disease

In chronic ischaemic heart disease, 35% of ischaemic episodes were associated ventricular arrhythmias, as described by Carboni and co-workers[85] who even found Lown grade 3–5 arrhythmias during ischaemic episodes. We found only low-level ventricular ectopic activity during ischaemia in about 75% of our prospectively studied examinees, who were carefully selected as ones who had no previously known ventricular arrhythmias.[86] The Holter-disclosed ventricular ectopy increased during the ischaemia in 6% of the episodes. In our study, as well as in the investigation of Carboni et al., the increased ventricular ectopic activity appeared mostly during the last phase of the ischaemic episode, when the ST segment started to return towards the isoelectric line. It is an open question whether this observation points to a mechanism of "reperfusion" following the subendocardial ischaemia similar to the well-documented reperfusion arrhythmias after transmural ischaemia. The duration of the ischaemic episode had no influence on the increase of the ventricular ectopic activity in neither of these studies. On the other hand, Bayes de Luna and co-workers found[87] in patients with Prinzmetal's angina that, during long attacks of >4 mm ST elevation or more, ventricular arrhythmias occurred rather than when the ST elevation was <4 mm or the attacks were brief.

Circadian variations in ischaemia and in arrhythmias

Holter ambulatory monitoring provided the opportunity to detect circadian variations both in ischaemic events and in arrhythmic episodes. A double-peaked curve was described for ischaemia, with predominance in the early morning hours and a smaller peak in the afternoon by Mulcahy and co-workers[88] and was later confirmed by several investigators.[89–92] Englund and co-workers in their recent study,[93] using recording by an implanted defibrillatior, confirmed the double-peaked pattern, both in ischaemic and non-ischaemic heart disease patients, suggesting that the trigger mechanisms of the initiation of ventricular tachyarrhythmias may be similar, irrespective of the underlying heart disease; this points probably to the possibility that mechanisms other than ischaemia play the dominant role in these circadian variations.

Ischaemia in the genesis of arrhythmic death

The underlying mechanisms of spontaneous VT and VF has been studied extensively.[94–96] A recent experimental investigation confirmed, on an isolated Langendorff model, that acute global ischaemia significantly increased the width of the vulnerable window of the myocardium, confirming again that acute ischaemia facilitates the initiation of ventricular fibrillation.[97] Still it is obviously difficult to obtain reliable information concerning the presence of acute or enhanced chronic ischaemia in patients who were resuscitated from sudden VF-induced death. Gomes *et al.*[98] found more connection with an arrhythmic substrate (presence of late potentials or a positive EP study) than with silent ischaemia, as this last phenomenon preceded the VT in only 14% of patients wearing a Holter during the sudden death episode. On the other hand, both Goldstein *et al.*[99] and Pepine *et al.*[100] found, in about

one-third of their patients, ischaemia preceding the sudden death. The largest review so far on this subject is from Bayes de Luna and co-workers[101] whose results were similar to those of Gomes *et al.*

Thus, in spite of the experimental evidence proving the ischaemia–arrhythmia connection, in the clinical setting there is no firm evidence for a considerable part, let alone for an exclusive role of preceding ischaemia in inducing sudden death, and the link between these two phenomena is still "elusive".[102] If, in the future, the monitoring capabilities of the implantable defibrillators could be expanded also for reliable ST segment monitoring (and first steps towards this goal have already been made[103]), such new modalities could provide an answer for this controversy.

Summary

The use of ECG for evaluation of myocardial ischaemia was gaining gradually in importance throughout the 20th century, and in the meantime there is no other non-invasive, easily applied, and inexpensive method in view that could take its place. If today more than 50 million ECG tests are daily performed all over the world, this number can safely be expected to grow. The limitations of using ST segment depression for assessing, diagnosing, or quantifying ischaemia are well-known, but its strengths and advantages are more and more apparent and it seems that it will remain a first-line diagnostic method also through the 21st century.

References

1. Pardee HEB. An electrocardiographic sign of coronary artery obstruction. *Arch Int Med* 1920;**26**:244.
2. Feil H, Siegel M. Electrocardiographic changes during attacks of angina pectoris. *Am J Med Sci* 1929;**177**:223–42.
3. Frisch C. Electrocardiography. In: Braunwald E ed. *Heart disease*. Philadelphia: WB Saunders, 1997; pp. 108–52.
4. Grant RP. *Clinical electrocardiography*. New York: McGraw-Hill, 1957, pp. 101–7.
5. Hurst JW. Abnormalities of the ST segment – part I. *Clin Cardiol* 1997;**20**:511–20.
6. Hurst JW. Abnormalities of the ST segment – part II. *Clin Cardiol* 1997;**20**:595–600.
7. Gibbons RT, Chair. ACC/AHA/ACP/ASIM Guidelines for the management of patients with chronic stable angina. *J Am Coll Cardiol* 1999;**33**:2092–197.
8. Kannel W, Anderson K, McGee D *et al.* Non-specific electrocardiographic abnormality as a predictor of coronary heart disease: The Framingham Heart Study. *Am Heart J* 1987;**113**:370–6.
9. Liao Y, Liu K, Dyer A *et al.* Major and minor electrocardio-

graphic abnormalities and risk of death from coronary heart disease, cardiovascular diseases, and all causes in men and women. *J Am Coll Cardiol* 1988;**12**:1494–500.

10. Sigurdsson E, Sigfusson N, Sigvaldason H, Thorgeirsson G. Silent ST-T changes in an epidemiologic cohort study – a marker of hypertension or coronary heart disease: or both: the Reykjavik study. *J Am Coll Cardiol* 1996;**27**:1140–7.

11. De Bacquer D, De Backer G, Kornitzer M *et al.* Prognostic value of ischemic electrocardiographic findings for cardiovascular mortality in men and women. *J Am Coll Cardiol* 1998;**32**:680–5.

12. De Bacquer D, De Backer G, Kornitzer M, Blackburn H. Parental history of premature coronary heart disease mortality and signs of ischaemia on the resting electrocardiogram. *J Am Coll Cardiol* 1999;**33**:1491–8.

13. Moss AJ, Goldstein RE, Hall WJ *et al.* Detection and significance of myocardial ischaemia in stable patients after recovery from an acute coronary event. *JAMA* 1993;**18**:2418–19.

14. Gianrossi R, Detrano R, Mulvihill D. Exercise-induced ST depression in the diagnosis of coronary artery disease. *Circulation* 1989;**80**:87–98.

15. Weiner DA, Ryan TJ, McCabe CH. Exercise stress testing: Correlations among history of angina, ST-segment response and prevalence of coronary artery disease in the Coronary Artery Surgery Study. *New Engl J Med* 1989;321:320–4.

16. Rywik TM, Zink RC, Gittings NS *et al.* Independent prognostic significance of ischaemic ST-segment response limited recovery from treadmill exercise in asymptomatic subjects. *Circulation* 1998;**97**:2117–22.

17. Roger VL, Jacobsen SJ, Pellikka PA *et al.* Prognostic value of exercise testing: A population based study in Olmsted County, Minnesota. *Circulation* 1998;**98**:2836–41.

18. Callaham PR, Froelicher VF, Klein J, Risch M, Dubach P, Friis R. Exercise-induced silent ischaemia: age, diabetes mellitus, previous myocardial infarction and prognosis. *J Am Coll Cardiol* 1989;**14**:1175–80.

19. Chaitman BR. The changing role of the electrocardiogram as a diagnostic and prognostic test for chronic ischaemic heart disease. *J Am Coll Cardiol* 1986;8:1195–210.

20. Lewis WR, Amsterdam E, Turnipseed S, Kirk JD. Immediate exercise testing of low risk patients with known coronary disease presenting to the emergency department with chest pain. *J Am Coll Cardiol* 1999;**33**:1843–7.

21. Heden B, Ohlsson M, Rittner R *et al.* Agreement between artificial neural networks and experienced electrocardiographer on electrocardiographic diagnosis of healed myocardial infarction. *J Am Coll Cardiol* 1996;**28**:1012–16.

22. Cole CR, Dresing TJ, Robbins MA, Snader C, Marwick TH, Lauer MS. Heart rate variability immediately following exercise testing predicts mortality independent of thallium perfusion defects. *J Am Coll Cardiol* 1999;**33**:561–2.

23. Bogaty P, Guimond J, Bobitaille NM *et al.* A reappraisal of exercise electrocardiographic indexes of the severity of ischaemic heart disease: angiographic and scintigraphic correlates. *J Am Coll Cardiol* 1997;**29**:1497–504.

24. Kaul P, Fu Y, Ching Chang W *et al.* The ST depression ≥2 mm sign: An ominous prognosis in acute coronary syndromes. *Circulation* 1999;**100**:432.

25. Okin PM, Kligfield P, Ameisen O, Goldberg HL, Borer JS. Improved accuracy of the exercise electrocardiogram: identification of three-vessel coronary disease in stable angina pectoris by analysis of peak rate-related changes in ST segments. *Am J Cardiol* 1985;**55**:271–6.

26. Hollenberg M, Budge WR, Wisneski JA, Gertz EW. Treadmill score quantifies electrocardiographic response to exercise and improves test accuracy and reproducibility. *Circulation* 1980;**61**:276–85.

27. Lindahl B. More is worse – ST segment deviation in unstable coronary artery disease. *Eur Heart J* 1999;**20**:1611–12.

28. Crawford MH, Chair. ACC/AHA Guidelines for ambulatory electrocardiography. *J Am Coll Cardiol* 1999;**34**:912–48.

29. Pepine CJ, Sharaf B, Andrews TC *et al.* Relation between clinical, angiographic and ischaemic findings at baseline and ischaemia-related adverse outcomes one year in the asymptomatic cardiac ischaemia pilot study. *J Am Coll Cardiol* 1997;**29**:1483–9.

30. Stern S, Tzivoni S. Early detection of silent ischaemic heart disease by 24-hour electrocardiographic monitoring of active subjects. *Br Heart J* 1974;**36**:481–6.

31. Rocco MB, Nabel EG, Campbell S *et al.* Prognostic importance of myocardial ischaemia detected by ambulatory monitoring in patients with stable coronary artery disease. *Circulation* 1988;**78**:877–84.

32. Tzivoni D, Weisz G, Gavish A, Zin D, Keren A, Stern S. Comparison of mortality and myocardial infarction rates in stable angina pectoris with and without ischaemic episodes during daily activities. *Am J Cardiol* 1989;**63**:273–6.

33. Deedwania PC, Carbajal EV. Silent ischaemia during daily life is an independent predictor of mortality in stable angina. *Circulation* 1990;**81**:748–56.

34. Yeung AC, Barry J, Orav J, Bonassin E, Raby KE, Selwyn AP. Effects of asymptomatic ischaemia on long-term prognosis in chronic stable coronary disease. *Circulation* 1991;**83**:1598–604.

35. de Marchena E, Asch J, Martinez J *et al.* Usefulness of persistent silent myocardial ischaemia in predicting high cardiac event rate in men with medically controlled stable angina pectoris. *Am J Cardiol* 1994;**73**:390–2.

36. Von Arnim T for the TIBBS Investigators. Prognostic significance of transient ischaemic episodes: response to treatment shows improved prognosis. Results of the Total Ischaemic Burden Bisoprolol Study (TIBBS) follow-up. *J Am Coll Cardiol* 1996;**28**:20–4.

37. Pepine CJ, Cohn PF, Deedwania PC *et al.* For the ASIST Study Group. Effects of treatment on outcome in asymptomatic and mildly symptomatic patients with ischaemia during daily life: the Atenolol Silent Ischaemia Study (ASIST). *Circulation* 1994;**90**:762–8.

38. Quyyumi AA, Panza JA, Diodati JG, Callahan TS, Bonow RLO, Epstein SE. Prognostic implications of myocardial ischaemia during daily life in low risk patients with coronary artery disease. *J Am Coll Cardiol* 1993;**21**:700–8.

39. Dargie HJ, Ford I, Fox KM on behalf of TIBET study group. Effects of ischaemia and treatment with atenolol, nifedipine SR and their combination on outcome in patients with chronic stable angina. *Eur Heart J* 1996;**17**:104–12.

40. Mulcahy D, Husain S, Zalos G *et al.* Ischaemia during

ambulatory monitoring as a prognostic indicator in patients with stable coronary artery disease. *JAMA* 1997;**277**:318–24.

41. Stone PH, Krantz DS, McMahon RP *et al.* Relationship among mental stress-induced ischemia and ischemia during daily life and during exercise: the psychophysiologic investigations of myocardial ischemia (PIMI) study. *J Am Coll Cardiol* 1999;**33**:1476–84.

42. Gottdiener JS, Kop WJ, Krantz DS. Mental stress and silent myocardial ischemia: evidence, mechanisms, and clinical implications. In: Stern S ed. *Silent myocardial ischaemia.* London: Martin Dunitz, 1998, pp. 175–99.

43. Klootwijk P, Meij S, Melkert R, Lenderink T, Simoons ML. Reduction of recurrent ischaemia with abciximab during continuous ECG – ischaemia monitoring in patients with unstable angina refractory to standard treatment (CAPTURE). *Circulation* 1998;**98**:1358–64.

44. Krucoff MW, Croll MA, Pope JE *et al.* Continuous 12-lead ST segment recovery analysis in the TAMI 7 study: performance of a noninvasive method for real-time detection of failed myocardial reperfusion. *Circulation* 1993;**88**:437–46.

45. Dellborg M, Steg PG, Simoons M *et al.* Vectorcardiographic monitoring to assess early vessel patency after reperfusion therapy for acute myocardial infarction. *Eur Heart J* 1995;**16**:21–9.

46. Klootwijk P, Langer A, Meij S *et al.* Non-invasive prediction of reperfusion and coronary artery patency by continuous ST segment monitoring in the GUSTO-1 trial. *Eur Heart J* 1996;**17**:689–98.

47. Klootwijk P, Meij S, von Es GA *et al.* Comparison of usefulness of computer assisted continuous 48 hours 3-lead with 12-lead ECG ischaemia monitoring for detection and quantitation of ischaemia in patients with unstable angina. *Eur Heart J* 1997;**18**:931–40.

48. Okin PM, Howard BV, Kors JA, Herpen G, Crow RS, Fabsitz RR. Computerized ST depression analysis improves prediction of cardiovascular morbidity and mortality in American Indians: the Strong Heart Study. *Circulation* 1999;**100**:104.

49. Nyman I, Areskog M, Areskog NH, Swahn E, Wallentin L. Very early risk stratification by electrocardiagram at rest in men with suspected unstable coronary heart disease. *J Intern Med* 1993;**234**:293–301.

50. Cannon CP, McCabe CH, Stone PH *et al.* The electrocardiogram predicts one-year outcome of patients with unstable angina and non-Q wave myocardial infraction: results of the TIMI III Registry ECG Ancillary Study. *J Am Coll Cardiol* 1997;**30**:133–40.

51. Holmvang L, Luscher MS, Clemmensen P, Thygesen K, Grande P. Very early risk stratification using combined ECG and biochemical assessment in patients with unstable coronary artery disease (a thrombin inhibition in myocardial ischaemia [TRIM] substudy). *Circulation* 1998;**98**:2004–9.

52. Jernberg T, Lindahl B, Wallentin L. ST-segment monitoring in continuous 12-lead ECG improves early risk stratification in patients with chest pain and ECG nondiagnostic of acute myocardial infarction. *J Am Coll Cardiol* 1999;**34**:1413–19.

53. Johnson SM, Mauritson DR, Winniford MD *et al.* Acute myocardial

54. Gottlieb SO, Weisfeldt ML, Ouyang P, Mellits ED, Gerstenblith G. Silent ischaemia as a marker for early unfavorable outcomes in patients with unstable angina. *New Engl J Med* 1986;**314**:1214–19.

55. Gill JB, Cairns JA, Roberts RS *et al.* Prognostic importance of myocardial ischaemia detected by ambulatory monitoring early after acute myocardial infarction. *N Engl J Med* 1996;**334**:65–70.

56. Patel DJ, Knight CJ, Holdright DR *et al.* Long-term prognosis in unstable angina. The importance of early risk stratification using continuous ST-segment monitoring. *Eur Heart J* 1998;**19**:240–9.

57. Krucoff MW, Wagner NB, Pope JE *et al.* The portable programmable microprocessor-driven real-time 12-lead electrocardiographic monitor: a preliminary report of a new device for the noninvasive detection of successful reperfusion of silent coronary reocclusion. *Am J Cardiol* 1990;**52**:936–42.

58. Norgaard BL, Anderson K, Dellborg M, Abrahamsson P, Ravkilde J, Thygesen K. Admission risk assessment by cardiac troponin T in unstable coronary artery disease: additional prognostic information from continuous ST segment monitoring. *J Am Coll Cardiol* 1999;**33**:1519–27.

59. Shah A, Wagner GS, Califf RM *et al.* Comparative prognostic significance of simultaneous versus independent resolution of ST segment depression relative to ST segment elevation during acute myocardial infarction. *J Am Coll Cardiol* 1997;**30**:1478–83.

60. Fortuin NJ, Friesinger GC. Exercise-induced ST segment elevation: clinical, electrocardiographic and arteriographic studies in twelve patients. *Am J Med* 1970;**49**:459–64.

61. Feyter PJD, Majid PA, Eenige MJV, Wardeh R, Wempe FN, Roos JP. Clinical significance of exercise-induced ST segment elevation: correlative angiographic study in patients with ischaemic heart disease. *Br Heart J* 1981;**46**:84–92.

62. Fox KM, Jonathan A, Selwyn A. Significance of exercise induced ST segment elevation in patients with previous myocardial infarction. *Br Heart J* 1983;**49**:15–19.

63. Chahine RA, Raizner AE, Ishimori T. The clinical significance of exercise-induced ST-segment elevation. *Circulation* 1976;**54**:209–13.

64. Margonato A, Chierchia SL, Xuereb RG *et al.* Specificity and sensitivity of exercise-induced ST segment elevation for detection of residual viability: comparison with fluorodeoxyglucose and positron emission tomography. *J Am Coll Cardiol* 1995;**25**:1032–8.

65. Nakano A, Lee JD, Shimizu H *et al.* Reciprocal ST-segment depression associated with exercise-induced ST-segment elevation indicates residual viability after myocardial infarction. *J Am Coll Cardiol* 1999;**33**:620–6.

66. Elhendy A, van Domburg RT, Bax JJ, Roelandt JRTC. The significance of stress-induced ST segment depression in patients with inferior Q wave myocardial infarction. *J Am Coll Cardiol* 1999;**33**:1909–15.

67. Matezky S, Freimark D, Feinberg M *et al.* Acute myocardial

infarction with isolated ST-segment elevation in posterior chest leads V_{7-9}: hidden ST- segment elevations revealing acute posterior infarction. *J Am Coll Cardiol* 1999;**34**:748–53.

68. Zalenski RJ, Cooke D, Rydman R *et al.* Assessing the diagnostic value of an ECG containing leads V_{4R}, V_8, and V_9: the 15-lead ECG. *Ann Emerg Med* 1993;**22**:786–93.

69. Zalenski RJ, Rydman RJ, Sloan EP *et al.* Value to posterior and right ventricular leads in comparison to the standard 12-lead electrocardiogram in evaluation of ST-segment elevation in suspected acute myocardial infarction. *Am J Cardiol* 1997;**79**:1579–85.

70. Engelen DJ, Gorgels AP, Cheriex EC *et al.* Value of the electrocardiogram in localizing the occlusion site in the left anterior descending coronary artery in acute anterior myocardial infarction. *J Am Coll Cardiol* 1999;**34**:389–95.

71. Mac William JA. Fibrillar contraction of the heart. *J Physiol* 1887;**8**:296.

72. Harris AS. Delayed development of ventricular ectopic rhythms following experimental coronary occlusion. *Circulation* 1950;**1**:1318.

73. Wit AL, Janse JJ. Experimental models of ventricular tachycardia and ventricular fibrillation caused by ischaemia and infarction. *Circulation* 1992;**85**:32–4.

74. Bigger J, Dresdale R, Heissenbuttel R, Weld F, Witt A. Ventricular arrhythmias in ischaemic heart disease: mechanism, prevalence, significance, and management. *Prog Cardiovasc Dis* 1977;**19**:255–300.

75. Campbell R, Murray A, Julian D. Ventricular arrhythmias in the first 12 hours of acute myocardial infarction. *Br Heart J* 1981;**46**:351–7.

76. de Soyza N, Bissett J, Kane J, Murphy M, Doherty J. Ectopic ventricular prematurity and its relationship to ventricular tachycardia in acute myocardial infarction in men. *Circulation* 1974;**50**:529–33.

77. Cheema AN, Sheu K, Parker M, Kadish A, Goldberger JJ. Nonsustained ventricular tachycardia in the setting of acute myocardial infarction: tachycardia characteristics and their prognostic implications. *Circulation* 1998;2030–6.

78. Braunwald E. Myocardial reperfusion, limitation of infarct size, reduction of left ventricular dysfunction, and improved survival: should the paradigm be expanded? *Circulation* 1989;**79**:441–4.

79. Opitz CF, Finn PV, Pfeffer MA, Mitchell GF, Pfeffer JM. Effects of reperfusion on arrhythmias and death after coronary artery occlusion in the rat: increased electrical stability independent of myocardial salvage. *J Am Coll Cardiol* 1998;**32**:261–7.

80. Alexopoulos D, Collins R, Adamopoulos S, Peto R, Sleight P. Holter monitoring of ventricular arrhythmias in a randomised, controlled study of intravenous streptokinase in acute myocardial infarction. *Br Heart J* 1991;**65**:9–13.

81. Berisso MZ, Carratino L, Ferroni A, Mela GS, Mazzotta G, Vecchio C. Frequency, characteristics and significance of supraventricular tachyarrhythmias detected by 24-hour electrocardiographic recording in the late hospital phase of acute myocardial infarction. *Am J Cardiol* 1990;**65**:1064–70.

82. De Bakker JMT, Van Capelle FJL, Janse MJ *et al.* Reentry as a cause of ventricular tachycardia in patients with chronic ischaemic heart disease: electrophysiologic and anatomic correlation. *Circulation* 1988;**77**:589–606.

83. Bigger JT, Fleiss JL, Kleiger R *et al.* The relationships between ventricular arrhythmias, left ventricular dysfunction, and mortality in the two years after myocardial infarction. *Circulation* 1984;**69**:250.

84. Kostis JB, Byington R, Friedman LM *et al.* Prognostic significance of ventricular ectopic activity in survivors of acute myocardial infarction. *J Am Coll Cardiol* 1987;**10**:231.

85. Carboni GP, Lahiri A, Cashman PMM, Raftery EB. Mechanism of arrhythmias accompanying ST-segment depression on ambulatory monitoring in stable angina pectoris. *Am J Cardiol* 1987;**60**:1246–53.

86. Stern S, Banai S, Keren A, Tzivoni D. Ventricular ectopic activity during myocardial ischaemic episodes in ambulatory patients. *Am J Cardiol* 1989;**65**:412–16.

87. Bayes de Luna A, Carreras F, Clandellas M, Oca F, Sages F, Garcia Moll M. Holter ECG study of the electrocardiographic phenomena in Prinzmetal angina attacks with emphasis on the study of ventricular arrhythmias. *J Electrocardiol* 1985;**18**:267–76.

88. Mulcahy D, Keean J, Cunningham D *et al.* Circadian variation of total ischaemic burden and its alteration with antianginal agents. *Lancet* 1988;**2**:755–9.

89. Pepine CJ. Circadian variations in myocardial ischaemia. Implications for management. *JAMA* 1991;**265**:386–90.

90. Benhorin J, Banai S, Moriel M, Stern S. Circadian variations in ischaemic threshold and their relation to the occurrence of ischaemic episodes. *Circulation* 1993;**87**:808–14.

91. Hausmann D, Lichtlen PR, Nikutta P, Wenzlaff P, Daniel WG. Circadian variation of myocardial ischaemia in patients with stable coronary artery disease. *Chronobiol Int* 1991;**8**:385–98.

92. Hausmann D, Nikutta P, Trappe HJ, Daniel WG, Wenzlaff P, Lichtlen PR. Circadian distribution of the characteristics of ischaemic episodes in patients with stable coronary artery disease. *Am J Cardiol* 1990;**66**:668–72.

93. Englund A, Behrens S, Wegscheider K, Rowland E. Circadian variation of malignant ventricular arrhythmias in patients with ischaemic and nonischaemic heart disease after cardioverter defibrillator implantation. *J Am Coll Cardiol* 1999;**34**:1560–8.

94. Pogwizd SM, Corr PB. Mechanisms underlying the development of ventricular fibrillation during early myocardial ischaemia. *Circ Res* 1990;**66**:672–95.

95. Gettes LS, Cascio WE, Sanders WE. Mechanism of sudden cardiac death. In: Zipes DP, Jalife J eds. *Cardiac electrophysiology: from cell to bedside.* Philadelphia: WB Saunders, 1995, pp. 527–38.

96. Janse MJ, Opthof T. Mechanisms of ischaemia-induced arrhythmias. In: Zipes DP, Jalife J eds. *Cardiac electrophysiology: from cell to bedside.* Philadelphia: WB Saunders, 1995, pp. 489–96.

97. Behrens S, Li C, Franz M. Effects of myocardial ischaemia on ventricular fibrillation inducibility and defibrillation efficacy. *J Am Coll Cardiol* 1997;**29**:817–24.

98. Gomes JA, Alexopoulos D, Winters SL, Deshmukh P, Fuster

V, Suh K. The role of silent ischaemia, the arrhythmia substrate and the short-long sequence in the genesis of sudden cardiac death. *J Am Coll Cardiol* 1989;**14**:1618–25.

99. Goldstein S, Medendorp SV, Landis JR *et al*. Analysis of cardiac symptoms preceding cardiac arrest. *Am J Cardiol* 1996;**58**:1195–8.

100. Pepine CJ, Gottlieb SO, Morganroth J. Ambulatory ischaemia and sudden death: an analysis of 35 cases of death during ambulatory ECG monitoring. *J Am Coll Cardiol* 1991;**17**:63A.

101. Bayes de Luna A, Coumel P, Leclercq JF *et al*. Ambulatory sudden cardiac death: Mechanisms of production of fatal arrhythmia on the basis of data from 157 cases. *Am Heart J* 1989;117:151–9.

102. Podrid P. Silent ischaemia, ventricular arrhythmia and sudden cardiac death. *J Am Coll Cardiol* 1990;**16**:55–6.

103. Grom A, Faber TS, Macharzina R. Detection of localized myocardial ischaemia by ECG leads available in the implantable cardioverter–defibrillator. *Circulation* 1999; **100**(Suppl. I):786(Abstr.).

12 Exercise electrocardiography for the assessment of arrhythmias

Michael Cusack and Simon Redwood

Since the advent of the electrocardiogram (ECG) in 1903,[1] it has become the most widely used non-invasive cardiovascular investigation. Subsequent developments in recording of the ECG have made it relatively easy and inexpensive to perform. The information provided by the ECG is extremely reproducible. In the diagnosis of arrhythmias, the sensitivity of the ECG is high, though specificity may vary as a result of underlying pathophysiological factors.[2]

Although it is more commonly seen as a tool in the assessment of ischaemia in patients with coronary artery disease, exercise testing is being increasingly used to extend the role of ECG in the diagnosis and management of arrhythmias. The physiological effects of exercise may assist in diagnosis by arrhythmia provocation and may allow the effectiveness of treatment to be determined.

A number of physiological changes occur in response to exercise. In response to both the anticipation of physical exertion and onset of the exercise itself, there is an increase in efferent sympathetic traffic and in the level of circulating catecholamines. There is a rise in heart rate, systolic blood pressure, and force of contractility, which results in an increase in myocardial oxygen demand, and, among patients with an impaired coronary blood supply, this results in myocardial ischaemia. Within the heart there is increased catecholamine stimulation of the beta$_1$-adrenoceptor. Ischaemia causes local acidosis and alterations in ion fluxes, resulting in extracellular hyperkalaemia. These changes within the milieu of the cardiocyte alter electrophysiological properties; with loss of the resting membrane potential, a reduction in the refractory period and an increase in automaticity.

Mechanical stresses within the heart during exercise may not be uniform, giving rise to local alterations in refractoriness and increased automaticity.[3] In addition, differences in regional myocardial blood flow result in heterogeneity in local conditions.[4] The resultant loss of electrophysiological uniformity provides an important mechanism for re-entry. Thus exercise enhances arrhythmogenesis by several well-described mechanisms[5] (Box 12.1).[6] These effects are particularly seen within diseased myocardium where the effects of ischaemia and altered mechanical forces are likely to coincide.

Box 12.1 Potential mechanisms of enhanced arrhythmogenesis during exercise

- Loss of resting membrane potential
- Reduction in refractory period
- Heterogeneity in refractoriness
- Enhanced automaticity

Exercise test protocols

The exercise test itself may be conducted on a treadmill or bicycle ergometer, or by step testing. A progressive treadmill exercise test creates a greater physiological stress, and maximal oxygen uptake is higher than with other forms of exercise testing. There are a number of exercise test protocols available (Table 12.1). However, as the higher stages of the Bruce protocol are more physically demanding than those of the other protocols, it tends to be the most frequently used. Bicycle ergometry, although less stressful, often has less electrical interference during the test than other modes of testing, and tends to be used when low voltage electrical parameters are to be recorded. The 6-minute walk test is the least stressful of all protocols as the patient merely walks at their own pace for 6 minutes. This, however, may be useful when detailed ECG recording is not required, and is often employed to determine rate response to exercise.

Atrial arrhythmias

Atrial extrasystoles

Supraventricular arrhythmias are relatively common during exercise. The most frequently encountered are premature beats which have been reported to occur in 5–27%[7,8] of all exercise tests. They have a positive relationship with age, occurring more frequently with advancing age. In addition, they are seen more frequently among patients with underlying heart disease. In a review of 650 patients undergoing exercise testing, 5% of normal individuals had

Table 12.1   Commonly used exercise test protocols

	Test							
	Naughton		Sheffield		Ellesta		Bruce	
Stage	(%)	(mph)	(%)	(mph)	(%)	(mph)	(%)	(mph)
1	0.0	1.0	0.0	1.7	10.0	1.7	10.0	1.7
2	0.0	2.0	5.0	1.7	10.0	3.0	12.0	2.5
3	0.0	2.0	10.0	1.7	10.0	4.0	14.0	3.4
4	3.5	2.0	12.0	2.5	10.0	5.0	16.0	4.2
5	7.0	2.0	14.0	3.4	15.0	5.0	18.0	5.0
6	10.5	2.0	16.0	4.2	15.0	6.0	20.0	5.5
7	14.0	2.0	18.0	5.0	–	–	22.0	6.0

supraventricular ectopic beats compared to 40% of those with documented heart disease.[9] Although common among patients with heart disease, because of the frequency with which this arrhythmia occurs in normal individuals their presence cannot be used as a predictor for heart disease. As these ectopic beats are usually asymptomatic, they rarely require treatment.

Tachycardias

The frequency of supraventricular tachycardias during exercise testing is somewhat less than that of ectopic beats and has been estimated to be between 0.1% and 2.8%.[10,11] Atrial fibrillation has been reported to occur in 0.3–1.1%[7,11,12] of tests. The capacity of the exercise test to reproduce atrial arrhythmias reliably is relatively poor, although there are few data to precisely define this. However, it is no surprise that patients with a previous history of supraventricular tachyarrhythmias are more

likely to encounter these during the exercise test than those who do not. Among those patients with exercise-induced supraventricular arrhythmias, exercise testing whilst the patients are on antiarrhythmic drug therapy may allow the efficacy of treatment to be assessed, although poor reproducibility means this is not a precise tool with which to guide drug therapy.

Exercise testing in the presence of an accessory pathway

Patients with Wolff–Parkinson–White syndrome (WPW) may be assessed with exercise testing. Such patients may be at risk if they develop atrial fibrillation, which can cause rapid ventricular stimulation via the accessory pathway, potentially resulting in ventricular fibrillation. Among patients who have pre-excitation on their resting ECG, exercise testing may be used to determine to some degree the refractory period of the accessory pathway[13] (Fig.12.1).

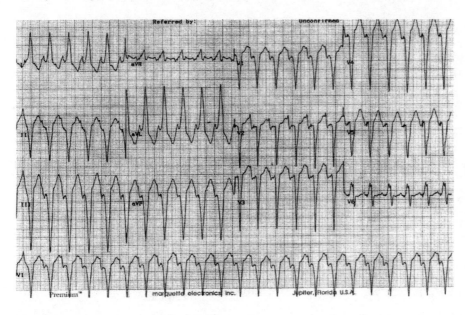

Figure 12.1   Persistent pre-excitation in the inferolateral ECG leads in a Wolff–Parkinson–White patient with an exercise-induced heart rate of 140 bpm.

During exercise testing, as the refractory periods of the AV node and accessory pathway alter, several changes in the surface ECG may be seen[14] (Box 12.2)

Box 12.2 Surface ECG changes during exercise in the presence of an accessory pathway

- Persistence of the delta-wave throughout associated with a greater reduction in the accessory pathway effective refractory period (AERP) compared with that of the AV node.
- Diminution of the delta-wave without complete disappearance implying comparable reductions in the AERP and AV nodal conduction time.
- Disappearance of the delta-wave which may be abrupt or more gradual

---

These modifications in delta-wave morphology during exercise result from relative differences in the effects of sympathetic stimulation on the refractory periods of the AV node and the accessory pathway. As a result, exercise testing alone has not been considered sufficiently reliable to define the risk of sudden death among these patients.[14,15] The predictive accuracy of exercise testing in this regard has been compared with that of invasive electrophysiological (EP) testing. Among 67 patients, including nine with previous ventricular fibrillation (VF), EP testing was used to define a high-risk group. Here, those with a coupling interval of less than 250 ms between two consecutive pre-excited beats during induced atrial fibrillation were taken to be at risk of VF.[16] The sensitivity of EP testing for identifying the group who had previous VF was found to be 87.5%, with a specificity of only 48.3%. In the same study, continuous pre-excitation, which persisted following administration of i.v. disopyramide (2 mg/kg), had a sensitivity of 71.4% but a

low specificity of 26.1% in identifying these patients. When the data from disopyramide infusion was combined with the presence of continuous pre-excitation on exercise testing, the sensitivity and specificity were both 66.7% among these patients. In a similar study among WPW syndrome patients, EP testing was used to determine those at high risk. Persistence of pre-excitation on an exercise test showed a sensitivity of 96% and again a low specificity of 17% in identifying this group.[17] Thus both invasive and non-invasive testing appear to have a good sensitivity but a low specificity in identifying patients with WPW syndrome at risk of sudden death.

Atrial fibrillation

Among patients with permanent atrial fibrillation the ventricular response is governed by the effective refractory period of the AV node. Satisfactory control of the ventricular rate at rest does not necessarily equate to adequate control during exercise; thus the exercise test, along with Holter recording, is frequently employed to assess the control of the ventricular response during physical activity. The aim of therapy here is to ensure an appropriate ventricular rate during exercise, which is important in achieving optimal ventricular function among these patients.[18] In addition, chronic poor control of ventricular rate in permanent atrial fibrillation may result in a progressive decline in systolic ventricular function.[19] On exercise, patients with atrial fibrillation tend to display an initial delayed acceleration in heart rate followed by an exaggerated heart rate response (Fig. 12.2). Following the cessation of exercise a prolonged tachycardia often persists. Treatment with AV nodal blocking drugs, either alone or in combination, may be titrated to the ventricular

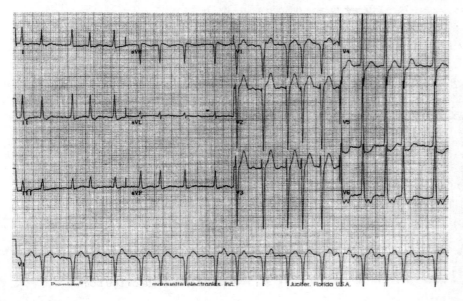

Figure 12.2 This 62-year-old man with good left ventricular function underwent a Bruce protocol exercise test while under investigation for breathlessness and poor exercise tolerance. He was known to have permanent atrial fibrillation controlled with digoxin and beta-blockade. After 90 seconds of the test he had developed a ventricular rate of 113 bpm, which represented an inappropriate acceleration of his heart rate.

response seen on exercise testing, thus allowing therapy to be optimised for each individual. However, despite treatment, the majority of patients still demonstrate an abnormal chronic chronotropic response to exercise.[20]

Bradycardias

These are generally due to dysfunction of the sinoatrial node, which represents a spectrum of disease (Box 12.3).

Box 12.3 Spectrum of sino-atrial node disease

- Inappropriate bradycardia
- Inappropriate decelerations in heart rate
- Chronotropic incompetence on exercise
- Sinus pauses and sinus arrest

The presence of a sinus bradycardia at rest may be indistinguishable from that seen in those with a high vagal tone. Although it is commonly seen with increasing age it is not unusual among younger individuals.

Patients with sinus node dysfunction on exercise are found to have a heart rate that is low for all levels of exercise.[21,22] There is a smaller increase in heart rate than would be expected and a reduced exercise tolerance compared with normal controls (Fig. 12.3).[23] In a significant number of patients with sinus node dysfunction, the reduction in heart rate following cessation of exercise occurs more rapidly than in normal subjects. Combining the peak heart rate attained during exercise with the decrease in rate following exercise increases the sensitivity of the exercise test in identifying sinus node dysfunction, and may allow its use as a screening test.[24]

Chronotropic incompetence may be used as a marker of

sinus node disease but is not diagnostic. It is commonly defined as a failure to achieve 85% of the age-predicted heart rate on exercise in the absence of rate limiting drugs.[25] Others have used a definition of a heart rate response of less than 100 bpm on maximal exercise which has greater specificity but is less sensitive.[26]

It is well documented that sick sinus syndrome often occurs in association with tachyarrhythmias. These are usually supraventricular in nature, reflecting a disease process more widespread within the atrium than merely in the region of the sinoatrial node. Ventricular arrhythmias are occasionally associated with sick sinus syndrome. It has been noted that patients with sick sinus syndrome often do not show normal shortening of the QT interval corrected for heart rate according to Bazett's formula (QTc). In a study of 40 patients with sick sinus syndrome, 24 (60%) showed an increase of their QTc during exercise. One patient showed no variation in the QTc and the remainder had the usual shortening in QTc. As the QTc was corrected for heart rate, this effect was unlikely to be due to these patients exhibiting a blunted chronotropic response. The abnormality in ventricular repolarisation observed among some of these patients has not been explained, and may have a role in arrhythmogenesis among some of these patients.

Where significant symptoms attributable to sinus node disease are present, permanent physiological pacing is indicated (AAIR or DDDR mode).

Pacemaker assessment

Exercise testing may be used, particularly among patients with sinus node dysfunction, to identify patients who are likely to benefit from permanent cardiac pacing. Physiological pacing, preserving AV synchrony where pos-

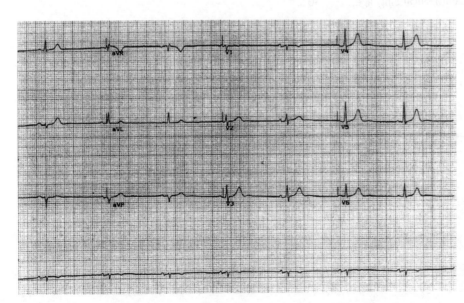

Figure 12.3 Persistent sinus bradycardia recorded in a 77-year-old man after 4 minutes of a Bruce protocol exercise test, who had complained of fatigue and poor exercise tolerance.

sible, is increasingly seen as the goal of treatment. This has been shown to increase effort tolerance significantly when compared to ventricular pacing.[27] In addition, atrial synchronous pacing reduces patient morbidity, principally by reducing the incidence of atrial fibrillation, and mortality compared to ventricular pacing.[28]

Increasingly, pacemaker rate adaptation appears to be of importance particularly among patients with chronotropic incompetance. The increase in cardiac output, which occurs on exercise, is due to both an increase in stroke volume but principally is the result of the rise in heart rate:

$$\text{cardiac output} = \text{stroke volume} \times \text{heart rate}$$

Among patients with both sick sinus syndrome and AV block, programming of the pacemaker to a VVI mode results in a significant reduction in exercise tolerance as determined by exercise testing.[29] Exercise testing among patients with dual-chamber pacemakers showed those with DDDR systems to have a higher maximal heart rate and greater exercise capacity than those with DDD systems irrespective of the indication for pacing.[30] An exercise test may be used to determine the appropriate degree of pacemaker rate response that should be programmed for patients to optimise their exercise capacity, although a formal test is often not required as sufficient data can be obtained from a 6-minute walk.[31]

Ventricular arrhythmias

Ventricular arrhythmias are commonly seen on exercise. The incidence of simple ventricular premature beats (VPBs) during exercise testing has been reported to be between 5% and 35% depending on the patient population studied.[8,9] This frequency increases with advancing age,

with VPBs occurring in approximately 50% of those over 50 years of age.[32,33] These arrhythmias are more common in men than in women,[32] and the age-related increase in frequency is more often seen among men.[33] Exercise-induced ventricular arrhythmias are most commonly seen in patients who have underlying coronary artery disease, with simple VPBs occurring on exercise in up to 50% of those with coronary disease.[8,9] Among these patients, the degree of ventricular ectopy on exercise is often related to ischaemic ST-segment shifts during exercise and the degree of underlying coronary disease that is present.[34,35] In addition, a relationship has also been seen between the presence of VPBs during exercise and left ventricular dysfunction[36] or more extensive wall motion abnormalities.[35]

Complex or repetitive ventricular premature beats during exercise are less common than simple VPBs. Among normal subjects they have been reported to occur in 0–2.4% of exercise tests.[8,35] In patients with underlying coronary disease, their incidence is considerably greater, being seen in up to 31% of tests (Fig.12.4).[37]

The reproducibility of these ventricular arrhythmias during exercise is relatively low, but greatest among those with underlying coronary disease,[38] particularly in those with higher grade arrhythmias.[39]

Tachyarrhythmias

Ventricular tachycardia has been defined as three or more consecutive ventricular complexes occurring at a rate of greater than 100 bpm. Episodes of ventricular tachycardia on exercise testing have been reported to occur with an incidence of 0.8–1.7%.[40,41] It has been subdivided into non-sustained ventricular tachycardia, lasting for less than 30 s, and sustained tachycardia lasting for more than 30 s.[42]

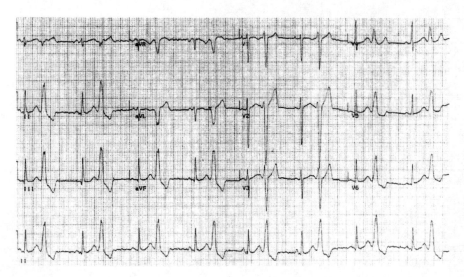

Figure 12.4 Bigemini occurring in the exercise test recovery period in a patient with known triple vessel coronary artery disease.

Sustained ventricular arrhythmias that develop during exercise are uncommon, even among those with underlying coronary disease (Table 12.2).

Table 12.2 Incidence of sustained ventricular arrhythmia on exercise

Study	No. of patients studied	No. with arrhythmia
Codine *et al.*[40]	5730	47 (0.8%)
Gooch and McConnell[41]	713	12 (1.7%)
Yang *et al.*[33]	3351	5 (0.15%)
Detry *et al.*[66]	7500	19 (0.25%)

Tachycardias in patients with right ventricular outflow tract (RVOT) ventricular tachycardia and idiopathic non-ischaemic ventricular tachycardia are often exercise induced. In a series of 23 patients with RVOT ventricular tachycardia, reported by Buxton *et al.*,[43] 14 patients had a tachycardia inducible on exercise. Similar observations have been made among patients with idiopathic non-ischaemic ventricular tachycardia.[44] Unlike patients with underlying coronary disease, exercise-induced ventricular tachycardia in these groups is as high as 62%.[44]

Mechanisms

The mechanisms of re-entry, enhanced automaticity and triggered automaticity underlie most exercise induced ventricular arrhythmia (Box 12.4).[5,6,45]

Box 12.4 Mechanisms of ventricular arrhythmia

- ***Re-entry*** requires a delay in impulse conduction in one area and unidirectional conduction block in another. This may occur in the setting of regional myocardial ischaemia induced by exercise or previous ventricular scar.
- ***Enhanced automaticity*** on exercise may occur from myocardial ischaemia or as a result of a direct effect of enhanced catecholamine stimulation of the myocardium, producing late potentials[6] and after-depolarisations[67].
- ***Triggered activity*** is due to fluctuations in the membrane potential during repolarisation. These fluctuations are the result of previous depolarisations and tend to occur at particular heart rates. During exercise they may be induced by direct sympathetic stimulation of the heart, and do not necessarily require an ischaemic substrate.

In addition, changes in blood potassium levels during and following exercise may contribute to these mechanisms of arrhythmia. During exercise, arterial potassium levels rise. Following exercise, arterial potassium levels decrease rapidly. Hypokalaemia is known to decrease the threshold for ventricular fibrillation in the myocardium during ischaemia.[46] This may account for the finding that, among patients with coronary artery disease, ventricular arrhythmias occur most commonly early in the recovery period following exercise (Fig. 12.5).[12,47,48]

Although underlying ischaemic heart disease is the most frequent cause of ventricular arrhythmias on exercise, there are a number of other conditions associated with this (Box 12.5).

Box 12.5 Conditions associated with ventricular arrhythmias on exercise

- Ischaemic heart disease
- Idiopathic
- Aortic stenosis
- Cardiomyopathy
  - hypertrophic
  - dilated
- Myocardial infiltrations
  - sarcoid
  - amyloid
  - haemachromatosis
- Digitalis toxicity
- Hypokalaemia
- Prolonged Q-T interval
  - idiopathic
    - Romano–Ward syndrome
    - Jervil and Lange-Nielson syndrome
  - drug-related
    - class 1 antiarrhythmic agents
    - phenothiazines
    - antihistamines
    - antibiotics
- Congenital abnormalities
  - right ventricular dysplasia
  - corrected tetralogy of Fallot

Prognosis

The underlying cardiac disease often determines the prognosis among patients with ventricular arrhythmias. Much of the data available for prognosis following the occurrence of exercise-induced ventricular arrhythmias has been derived from patients with coronary artery disease. In patients undergoing predischarge exercise testing following myocardial infarction, those with exercise-induced ventricular arrhythmias had a mortality at 1 year of 15%, compared to 7% in those without ventricular arrhythmias during exercise.[49] In this study, those with exercise-induced arrhythmias tended to have had more extensive infarctions with worse ventricular function. Among these patients, the most accurate predictor of subsequent mor-

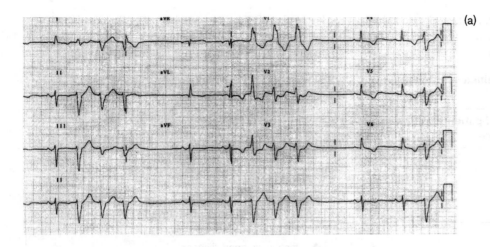

(a)

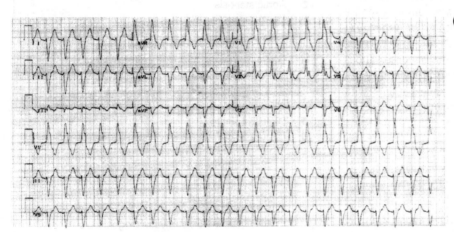

(b)

Figure 12.5 Tracings (a) and (b) were recorded from a 71-year-old woman with a history of palpitations and unexplained syncope. An ECG recorded 2 minutes following the start of a Bruce protocol exercise test (a) showed repetitive ventricular ectopic activity. The patient managed to exercise for 6 minutes and 30 seconds without further arrhythmia or symptoms. Following 45 seconds of recovery she developed sustained ventricular tachycardia (b), which responded to an i.v. bolus of 100 mg lignocaine.

tality was left ventricular function. In a similar study, the mortality 1 year after a myocardial infarction rose from 4% for those without VPBs on exercise to 12% in those patients who had exercise-induced VPBs.[50]

Following myocardial infarction exercise-induced changes in the QT interval may provide prognostic information. Prolongation of the QT interval corrected for heart rate (Bazett and Fridericia's correction) have been shown to differentiate patients at high risk of sudden cardiac death from those at low risk.[51] Exercise-induced changes in QT dispersion, which reflect inhomogeneities in ventricular repolarisation, have been found in some studies to be predictive of future arrhythmic events.[52] However, the study by Yi *et al*.[52] failed to identify such an association. It has been suggested that these inconsistencies may reflect differing methodologies in recording this parameter.[53]

Among patients with documented coronary disease but without recent myocardial infarction a similar relationship between exercise-induced arrhythmia and mortality has been described. Over a 3-year follow-up period there was

a 10% mortality among patients with coronary disease who did not develop VPBs on exercise testing.[34] In the same study, those who had simple VPBs induced by exercise had a 17% mortality and those with complex VPBs had a 25% mortality during the three years. Among patients with coronary disease who develop ischaemic ST-segment changes during exercise testing, the presence of exercise-induced ventricular arrhythmia allows further risk stratification during 1-year follow-up (Table 12.3).[54]

Table 12.3   One-year mortality rates determined by exercise testing in patients with coronary artery disease[55]

	Induced arrhythmia		
ST changes	No VPBs (%)	Simple VPBs (%)	Complex VPBs (%)
Present	10	33	42
Absent	2	15	29

Although the association between exercise-induced ventricular arrhythmias and subsequent mortality among patients with coronary disease appears to be significant, it is not a consistent finding in all studies.[36]

In those without underlying heart disease who have exercise-induced ventricular tachycardia, the prognosis is somewhat better. In several small studies, no sudden deaths were reported among such patients on long-term follow-up.[44,55,56]

Although the exercise test can provide useful prognostic information, a significant number of individuals at risk of serious arrhythmia are not identified by this or other non-invasive investigations. Recently, it has become possible to record T wave alternans during exercise with the use of sensitive spectral processing techniques.[57] This parameter recorded during pacing has been reported to be an accurate predictor of subsequent ventricular arrhythmic events. However, the variation in the T wave may be only of the order of a few microvolts and is difficult to detect. In a group of 27 patients, who also underwent electrophysiological evaluation for sustained ventricular arrhythmia, T wave alternans on bicycle exercise had an overall predictive accuracy of 80% for arrhythmic vulnerability.[58]

Management

Exercise testing is widely used for the assessment of the patient with suspected coronary artery disease. When ventricular arrhythmias occur on exercise in association with myocardial ischaemia, treatment should be directed to preventing the ischaemia either medically or with revascularisation. However, exercise-induced ventricular arrhythmias may become more frequent or appear for the first time following coronary artery bypass surgery owing to perioperative myocardial injury.[59] Patients with preoperative ventricular wall motion abnormalities as a result of previous myocardial infarction are the most likely to have persistence of exercise-induced arrhythmias following bypass grafting.[35] The same study demonstrated that persistent ischaemia on exercise testing after revascularisation was also associated with recurrence of exercise-induced ventricular arrhythmias. These findings are likely to be due to persistence of the arrhythmic substrate.

Where no evidence of myocardial ischaemia is found to account for exercise-induced arrhythmia, further assessment with electrophysiological study is often useful. This has greater reproducibility than exercise testing and may provide information as to the substrate underlying the arrhythmia. It may be also used to guide drug or defibrillator therapy among these patients. Despite limited reproducibility, exercise testing may be used to assess the efficacy of long-term treatment among patients with serious ventricular arrhythmia. It is particularly useful in patients with catecholamine-dependent ventricular arrhythmias where ambulatory monitoring or electrophysiological study may not generate the circumstances necessary for induction of the arrhythmia. Among patients with ventricular arrhythmias, who were considered controlled on ambulatory monitoring, 15% still had significant arrhythmias inducible on exercise testing.[60]

Pro-arrhythmia due to treatment with antiarrhythmic agents is well described.[61] Exercise testing may have a role in determining the safety of antiarrhythmic drug therapy. Patients with subclinical abnormalities of ventricular repolarisation may be at increased risk of arrhythmia when using Class IA agents. These patients may exhibit failure of shortening of the QT interval on exercise, which may be used to identify this subgroup. A paradoxical increase in the QT interval on exercise has also been reported among those in whom ventricular arrhythmias are aggravated by the use of Class IA drugs.[62]

Safety

Exercise testing among individuals with possible underlying cardiac disease for investigation and management of arrhythmias raises issues over the safety of the test. The incidence of serious ventricular arrhythmia on exercise testing has been reported to be 4.7 per 10 000 tests with 0.5 deaths occurring per 10 000 tests.[63] A review of 71 914 individuals undergoing maximal exercise testing demonstrated a complication rate as low as 0.8 per 10 000 tests.[64] In a study of 263 patients with a previous history of malignant ventricular arrhythmias undergoing exercise testing, a serious arrhythmia requiring immediate treatment occurred in 24 patients (9.1%).[65] All of these patients were successfully resuscitated and no deaths or long-term sequelae occurred among these patients as a result of the exercise test.

Therefore the risk of an adverse event as a result of exercise testing in the general population is extremely low. Among patients deemed to be at high risk based on their previous history, the risk of arrhythmia is somewhat higher. An exercise test may still however, be safely conducted in this group, provided that the facilities and expertise for resuscitation are immediately available.

Summary

Exercise testing remains an important tool for the non-invasive evaluation of patients with suspected arrhythmia. It is an investigation that is readily available in most hospitals and has a good safety record. Although it has limited reproducibility, it may be effectively combined with other investigations such as Holter recording and electrophysiological study in both the diagnosis and management of these patients. It is likely in the future that additional information derived from the test, such as the behaviour of the QTc, dispersion of the QT interval, and T wave alternans on exercise will be more commonly available. In generating such information, the exercise test will probably be able to provide increasingly powerful prognostic information among patients with heart disease.

Acknowledgements

Dr Cusack and Dr Redwood are supported by a British Heart Foundation Project Grant.

References

1. Einthoven W. Die galvanometrische Registerung des menschlichen Elektrocardiogramms; Zugleich eine Beurteilung der Anwendung des Capillar-Elektrometers in der Physiologie. *Pflügers Arch ges Physiol* 1903;**99**:72–80.
2. Fisch C. Evolution of the clinical electrocardiogram. *J Am Coll Cardiol* 1989;**14**:1127–38.
3. Dean JW, Lab MJ. Arrhythmia in heart failure: role of mechanically induced changes in electrophysiology. *Lancet* 1989;**10**:1309–12.
4. Watanabe I, Johnson TA, Buchanan J, Angle CL, Gettes L. Effect of graded coronary flow reduction on ionic, electrical and mechanical indices of ischaemia in the pig. *Circulation* 1987;**76**:1127–34.
5. Wit A, Rosen MR. Pathophysiological mechanisms of cardiac arrhythmias. *Am Heart J* 1983;**106**:798–811.
6. Hoffman BF, Rosen MR. Cellular mechanisms for cardiac arrhythmias. *Circ Res.* 1981;**49**:1–15.
7. Master AM. Cardiac arrhythmias elicited by the two-step exercise test. *Am J Cardiol* 1973;**32**:766–71.
8. Whinnery JE. Dysrrhythmia comparison in apparently healthy males during and after treadmill and accelerated stress test. *Am J Cardiol* 1983;**105**:732–7.
9. McHenry PL, Fisch C, Jordan JW, Corya, BR. Cardiac arrhythmias observed during maximal treadmill exercise testing in clinically normal men. *Am J Cardiol* 1972;**29**:331–6.
10. Beard EF, Owen CA. Cardiac arrhythmias during exercise stress testing in healthy men. *Aerosp Med* 1973;**44**:286–9.
11. Gooch AS, McConnell D. Analysis of transient arrhythmia and conduction disturbances during submaximal treadmill exercise testing. *Prog Cardiovasc Dis* 1970;**13**:293–307.
12. Jelinek MV, Lown B. Exercise stress testing for the exposure of cardiac arrhythmia. *Prog Cardiovasc Dis* 1974;**16**:497–522.
13. Melon P, Lancellotti P, Kulbertus H. How I study the assessment of the risk of sudden death in Wolff–Parkinson–White syndrome. *Rev Med Liege* 1998;**53**:218–19.
14. Daubert C, Ollitrault J, Descaves C, Mabo P, Ritter P, Gouffault J. Failure of the exercise test to predict the anterograde refractory period of the accessory pathway in Wolff–Parkinson–White syndrome. *Pacing Clin Electrophysiol* 1988;**11**:1130–8.
15. German LD, Gallagher JJ, Broughton A, Guarnieri T, Trantham JL. Effects of exercise and isoproterenol during atrial fibrillation in patients with Wolff–Parkinson–White syndrome. *Am J Cardiol* 1983;**51**:1203–6.
16. Sharma AD, Yee R, Guiraudon G, Klein GJ. Sensitivity and specificity of invasive and non-invasive testing for risk of sudden death in Wolff–Parkinson–White syndrome. *J Am Coll Cardiol* 1987;**10**:373–81.
17. Gaita F, Giustetto C, Riccardi R, Mangiardi L, Brusca A. Stress and pharmacologic tests as methods to identify patients with Wolff–Parkinson–White syndrome at risk of sudden death. *Am J Cardiol* 1989;**64**:487–90.
18. Lang R, Klein HO, Di SE et al. Verapamil improves exercise capacity in chronic atrial fibrillation: double-blind crossover study. *Am Heart J* 1983;**105**:820–5.
19. Peters KG, Kienzle MG. Severe cardiomyopathy due to chronic rapidly conducted atrial fibrillation: complete recovery after restoration of sinus rhythm. *Am J Med* 1988;**85**:242–4.
20. Corbelli R, Masterson M, Wilkoff BL. Chronotropic response to exercise in patients with atrial fibrillation. *Pacing Clin Electrophysiol* 1990;**13**:179–87.
21. Crook B, Nijhof P, van dK, Jennison C. The chronotropic response of the sinus node to exercise: a new method of analysis and a study of pacemaker patients. *Eur Heart J* 1995;**16**:993–8.
22. Shimizu A, Fukatani M, Kitano K et al. The total heart beats per 24 hours by ambulatory ECG and the changes of heart rate by treadmill exercise test in sick sinus syndrome. *Jap Circ J* 1988;**52**:139–48.
23. Johnston FA, Robinson JF, Fyfe T. Exercise testing in the diagnosis of sick sinus syndrome in the elderly: implications for treatment. *Pacing Clin Electrophysiol* 1987:**10**(4 Pt. 1):831–8.
24. Shul'man VA, Kusaev VV, Matiushin GV, Kostiuk FF. Use of a physical exertion test for the diagnosis of the sick sinus syndrome. *Terapevtich Arkh* 1985;**57**:116–19.
25. Ellestad MH, Wan MK. Predictive implications of stress testing. Follow-up of 2700 subjects after maximum treadmill stress testing. *Circulation* 1975;**51**:363–9.
26. Dreifus LS, Fisch C, Griffin JC, Gillette PC, Mason JW, Parsonnet V. Guidelines for implantation of cardiac pacemakers and antiarrhythmia devices. A report of the American College of Cardiology/American *Heart* Association Task Force on Assessment of Diagnostic and Therapeutic Cardiovascular Procedures. (Committee on Pacemaker Implantation.) *Circulation* 1991;**84**:455–67.
27. Sutton R, Perrins EJ, Morley C, Chan SL. Sustained improvement in exercise tolerance following physiological cardiac pacing. *Eur Heart J* 1983;**4**:781–5.
28. McComb JM, Gribbin GM. Effect of pacing mode on morbidity and mortality: update of clinical pacing trials. *Am J Cardiol* 1999:**83**(5B):211D–3D.
29. Heinz M, Worl HH, Alt E, Theres H, Blomer H. Which

patient is most likely to benefit from a rate responsive pacemaker?. *Pacing Clin Electrophysiol* 1988:**11**:1834–9.

30. Capucci A, Boriani G, Specchia S, Marinelli M, Santarelli A, Magnani B. Evaluation by cardiopulmonary exercise test of DDDR versus DDD pacing. *Pacing Clin Electrophysiol* 1992:**15**:1908–13.

31. Provenier F, Jordaens L. Evaluation of six minute walking test in patients with single chamber rate responsive pacemakers. *Br Heart J* 1994;**72**:192–6.

32. Ekblom B, Hartley LH, Day WC. Occurrence and reproducibility of exercise-induced ventricular ectopy in normal subjects. *Am J Cardiol* 1979;**43**:35–40.

33. Yang JC, Wesley RCJ, Froelicher VF. Ventricular tachycardia during routine treadmill testing. Risk and prognosis. *Arch Intern Med* 1991:**151**:349–53.

34. Califf RM, McKinnis RA, McNeer JF et al. Prognostic value of ventricular arrhythmias associated with treadmill exercise testing in patients studied with cardiac catheterization for suspected ischemic heart disease. *J Am Coll Cardiol* 1983:**2**:1060–7.

35. Weiner DA, Levine SR, Klein MD, Ryan TJ. Ventricular arrhythmias during exercise testing: mechanism, response to coronary bypass surgery and prognostic significance. *Am J Cardiol* 1984:**53**:1553–7.

36. Sami M, Chaitman B, Fisher L, Holmes D, Fray D, Alderman E. Significance of exercise-induced ventricular arrhythmia in stable coronary artery disease: a coronary artery surgery study project. *Am J Cardiol* 1984:**54**:1182–8.

37. Poblete PF, Kennedy HL, Caralis DG. Detection of ventricular ectopy in patients with coronary heart disease and normal subjects by exercise testing and ambulatory electrocardiography. *Chest* 1978:**74**:402–7.

38. Faris JV, McHenry PL, Jordan JW, Morris SN. Prevalence and reproducibility of exercise-induced ventricular arrhythmias during maximal exercise testing in normal men. *Am J Cardiol* 1976;**37**:617–22.

39. Saini V, Graboys TB, Towne V, Lown B. Reproducibility of exercise-induced ventricular arrhythmia in patients undergoing evaluation for malignant ventricular arrhythmia. *Am J Cardiol* 1989:**63**:697–701.

40. Codini MA, Sommerfeldt L, Eybel CE, Messer JV. Clinical significance and characteristics of exercise-induced ventricular tachycardia. *Catheter Cardiovasc Diag* 1981:**7**:227–34.

41. Gooch AS, McConnell D. Analysis of transient arrhythmias and conduction disturbances occurring during submaximal treadmill exercise testing. *Prog Cardiovasc Dis* 1970;**13**:293–307.

42. O'Hara GE, Brugada P, Rodriguez LM et al. Incidence, pathophysiology and prognosis of exercise-induced sustained ventricular tachycardia associated with healed myocardial infarction. *Am J Cardiol* 1992;**70**:875–8.

43. Buxton AE, Waxman HL, Marchlinski FE, Simson MB, Cassidy D, Josephson ME. Right ventricular tachycardia: clinical and electrophysiologic characteristics. *Circulation* 1983:**68**:917–27.

44. Mont L, Seixas T, Brugada P et al. Clinical and electrophysiologic characteristics of exercise-related idiopathic ventricular tachycardia. *Am J Cardiol* 1991;**68**:897–900.

45. Spear JF, Moore EN. Mechanisms of cardiac arrhythmias. *Ann Rev Physiol* 1982;**44**:485–97.

46. Hohnloser SH, Verrier RL, Lown B, Raeder EA. Effect of hypokalemia on susceptibility to ventricular fibrillation in the normal and ischemic canine heart. *Am Heart J* 1986:**112**:32–5.

47. Goldschlager N, Cake D, Cohn K. Exercise-induced ventricular arrhythmias in patients with coronary artery disease. Their relation to angiographic findings. *Am J Cardiol* 1973;**31**:434–40.

48. Thomson A, Kelly DT. Exercise stress-induced changes in systemic arterial potassium in angina pectoris. *Am J Cardiol* 1989:**63**:1435–40.

49. Fioretti P, Deckers J, Baardman T, Beelen A, ten KH, Brower RW, Simoons ML. Incidence and prognostic implications of repetitive ventricular complexes during predischarge bicycle ergometry after myocardial infarction. *Eur Heart J* 1987:8(Suppl. D):51–4.

50. Weld FM, Chu KL, Bigger JTJ, Rolnitzky LM. Risk stratification with low-level exercise testing 2 weeks after acute myocardial infarction. *Circulation* 1981;**64**:306–14.

51. Yi G, Crook R, Guo XH, Staunton A, Camm AJ, Malik M. Exercise-induced changes in the QT interval duration and dispersion in patients with sudden cardiac death after myocardial infarction. *Int J Cardiol* 1998;**63**:271–9.

52. Yu GL, Cheng IR, Zhao SP, Zhuang HP, Cai XY. Clinical significance of QT dispersion after exercise in patients with previous myocardial infarction. *Int J Cardiol* 1998;**65**:255–60.

53. Kautzner J, Malik M. QT interval dispersion and its clinical utility. *Pacing Clin Electrophysiol* 1997:**20**:2625–40.

54. Udall JA, Ellestad MH. Predictive implications of ventricular premature contractions associated with treadmill stress testing. *Circulation* 1977;**56**:985–9.

55. Fleg JL, Lakatta EG. Prevalence and prognosis of exercise-induced non-sustained ventricular tachycardia in apparently healthy volunteers. *Am J Cardiol* 1984;**54**:762–4.

56. Lemery R, Brugada P, Bella PD, Dugernier T, van dD, Wellens HJ. non-ischemic ventricular tachycardia. Clinical course and long-term follow-up in patients without clinically overt heart disease. *Circulation* 1989;**79**:990–9.

57. Albrecht P, Arnold J, Krishnamachari S, Cohen RJ. Exercise recordings for the detection of T wave alternans. Promises and pitfalls. *J Electrocardiol* 1996:29 Suppl:46–51.

58. Estes NA, Michaud G, Zipes DP et al. Electrical alternans during rest and exercise as predictors of vulnerability to ventricular arrhythmias. *Am J Cardiol* 1997:**80**:1314–18.

59. Mathes P. The effect of coronary revascularization on exercise-induced ventricular arrhythmias. *Eur Heart J* 1987:8(Suppl. D):79–81.

60. Lown B, Podrid PJ, De SR, Graboys TB. Sudden cardiac death-management of the patient at risk. *Curr Probl Cardiol* 1980:**4**(12):1–62.

61. Falk RH. Flecainide-induced ventricular tachycardia and fibrillation in patients treated for atrial fibrillation. *Ann Intern Med* 1989:**111**:107–11.

62. Kadish AH, Weisman HF, Veltri EP, Epstein AE, Slepian, MJ, Levine JH. Paradoxical effects of exercise on the QT interval in patients with polymorphic ventricular tachycar-

dia receiving type Ia antiarrhythmic agents. *Circulation* 1990;**81**:14–19.

63. Stuart RJJ, Ellestad MH. National survey of exercise stress testing facilities. *Chest* 1980;**77**:94–7.

64. Gibbons L, Blair SN, Kohl HW, Cooper K. The safety of maximal exercise testing. *Circulation* 1989;**80**:846–52.

65. Young DZ, Lampert S, Graboys TB, Lown B. Safety of maxi-

mal exercise testing in patients at high risk for ventricular arrhythmia. *Circulation* 1984;**70**:184–91.

66. Detry JM, Abouantoun S, Wyns W. Incidence and prognostic implications of severe ventricular arrhythmias during maximal exercise testing. *Cardiology* 1981;**68**(Suppl. 2):35–43.

67. Cranefield PF, Wit AL. Cardiac arrhythmias. *Ann Rev Physiol* 1979;**41**:459–72.

13 Analysis of monophasic action potentials

Peter Taggart and Peter Sutton

If two extracellular electrodes are placed lightly on the heart close together, a bipolar electrogram may be recorded. If gentle pressure is then exerted on one of the electrodes the electrogram waveform changes into a signal, which is similar in shape to the intracellular action potential. This signal known as the monophasic action potential (MAP) has been validated as providing a reliable measure of the time course of repolarisation of the intracellular action potential. The method of acquiring the signal enables recordings to be made *in vivo* in a vigorously beating heart. The technique is readily applicable to humans, and the MAPs may be conveniently incorporated into routine clinical procedures such as cardiac catheterisation or cardiac surgery. The direct determination of repolarisation in patients has a wide range of applications, including:

- assessment of antiarrhythmic drugs;
- arrhythmia mechanisms;
- cycle length dependent effects on repolarisation;
- local ischaemia;
- dispersion of repolarisation;
- mechanical/electrical interactions, etc.

In recent years, there has been a growing interest in MAP recordings, and recordings in humans in particular, perhaps owing to an awareness of the need for acquiring basic electrophysiological information directly from individual patients.

Historical note

In 1882, Burden-Sanderson and Page published the first description of a cardiac monophasic action potential obtained from a frog ventricle.[1] Although the electrocardiogram was developed around the turn of the century, it was not until the 1930s that experiments were performed using the MAP signal.[2] Up to this time, severe tissue injury at one electrode site was thought to be a prerequisite for obtaining MAP recordings. Soon after this, the first recordings were made without creating severe injury to the myocardium either by the use of suction[3] or by

pressure.[4] Some while after this the technique for direct recording of transmembrane action potentials was developed[5–7] which represented a milestone in our understanding of basic cellular electrophysiology. In 1959 Hoffman and Cranefield compared the MAP to the now "gold standard" of the intracellular action potential, showing that the repolarisation time course of the MAP paralleled that of the intracellular action potential.[8] In 1966 the first recording was made in humans, from the right atrial endocardium, using a specially designed cardiac catheter.[9] Subsequently, the technique for recording in patients was developed and largely pioneered by Olsson.[10–13] However, the technique incorporated suction through the lumen of the catheter in order to create local injury on the myocardial surface. This posed some limitations on the length of time for which the catheter tip could safely be left in position in humans with the suction applied, estimated at about 2 minutes. Olsson had observed that good quality signals could be obtained using the suction electrode catheter without applying suction but by gently increasing the contact pressure between the tip electrode and the myocardium.

With this approach, MAPs were recorded from the human right ventricle (Fig.13.1).[14] In the example shown, two MAPs were recorded simultaneously from the right

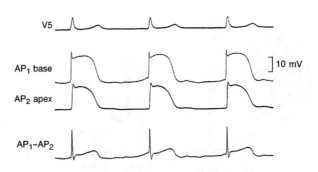

Figure 13.1 Monophasic action potentials from the base (AP$_1$) and apex (AP$_2$) of the right ventricular septum from a patient aged 32 with a normal heart. The algebraic sum of the signals (AP$_1$–AP$_2$) results in the ECG like waveform. V5 = V5 precordial ECG.

ventricular endocardium. The algebraic subtractions of the MAP waveforms for base and apex resulted in an ECG-like waveform. In view of the potential problems with suction, i.e. time limitation and complexity of apparatus requiring the catheter to be fluid-filled to avoid the introduction of air (Fig. 13.2), the pressure contact electrode was developed. Several different types and designs have evolved.

Recordings during cardiac catheterisation

MAPs may be recorded from the endocardium of the right atrium, right ventricle or left ventricle by a catheter electrode introduced percutaneously via the femoral vein or femoral artery as appropriate. A contact electrode catheter designed for the purpose is shown in Fig. 13.3. The electrodes are made from non-polarisable silver/silver chloride pellets. The tip electrode makes direct contact with the endocardium and the reference (indifferent) electrode situated about 5 mm proximal on the shaft completes the circuit via the intracavity blood. Detailed tests in animals have shown that silver/silver chloride electrodes are free from toxic effects and the technique was passed for use in human hearts in the USA by the federal Food and Drug Administration (FDA) in 1985. The catheter is introduced into the heart under fluoroscopy and positioned with the tip in as near perpendicular apposition to the endocardium as possible. A gentle curved lie of the catheter within the heart together with the flexible nature of the catheter itself helps to stabilise the tip during the volume and shape changes of the chambers during the cardiac cycle. One catheter manufactured by EP technologies, Boston Scientific Ltd, incorporates a steering device enabling the tip to be bent through an arc of 180°. An additional feature of this catheter is the ability to pace from two pacing electrodes situated between the tip recording electrode and the reference electrode. The con-

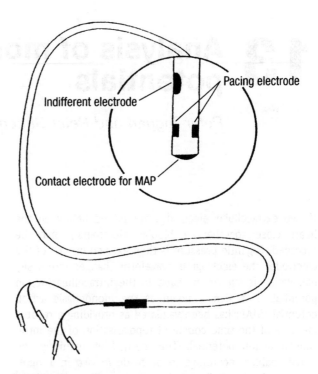

Figure 13.3 Franz contact electrode catheter for recording MAP signals.

tact pressure is important. Sufficient pressure is necessary to create the local depolarisation under the electrode necessary to generate the MAP signal. On the other hand too strong a pressure may cause damage to the myocardium. Monitoring of the ST segment in a unipolar electrogram obtained from the indifferent electrode on the MAP catheter has been advocated. In this way ST segment elevation (in the absence of ischaemia) may provide an indication of excessive local contact pressure. Given the appropriate amount of curve in the catheter and positioning of the tip, good quality MAP signals of between 10–40 mV are usually obtained and stable signals for up to several hours have been reported.

Recordings during cardiac surgery

MAPs may be recorded from the epicardium during cardiac surgery with pressure contact electrodes applied directly to the heart by a hand-held probe. Several designs have been used, usually consisting of a short spatula-like handle with an electrode mounted on the end (Fig. 13.4). A different design used by the authors is shown in Fig. 13.5. The electrodes are mounted in an acrylic holder. The part of the holder surrounding the electrodes forms a cup. The rim of the cup ensures perpendicular apposition of the electrode to the epicardium and a stable pressure.

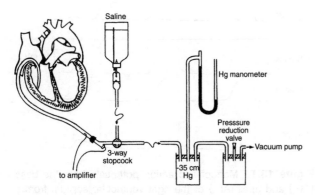

Figure 13.2 Diagram of the apparatus used to generate suction through the fluid filled MAP catheter as developed by Olsson *et al.* (reference 11).

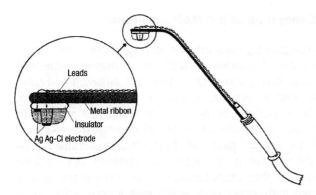

Figure 13.4 Hand-held probe for recording MAP signals from the epicardium in patients as used by Franz *et al.* (reference 71).

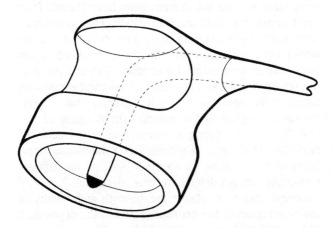

Figure 13.5 Hand-held probe for recording MAP signals from the epicardium in patients as used by the authors (reference 15).

The reference electrode makes contact with the epicardium through a saline-soaked sponge. The sides of the holder are grooved to allow it to be gripped between the surgeon's index and middle fingers. This enables the surgeon to position the electrode by sliding the hand between the heart and surrounding structures and placed on lateral, inferior, and posterior aspects without direct vision.

Research laboratory studies

The contact electrode designs for use on the endocardium during cardiac catheterisation and on epicardium during cardiac surgery are also suitable for hearts of large animal species. An example of recording obtained from epicardium in canine and humans is shown in Fig. 13.6. A spring cantilever design for epicardial recordings, which may be table-mounted, is commercially available (EP

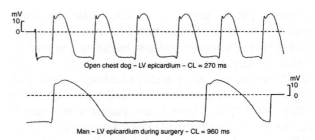

Figure 13.6 Example of monophasic action potential recordings: Top: recording from the left ventricular (LV) epicardium of a dog at cycle length (CL) of 270 ms. Bottom: recording from LV epicardium of a patient during open heart surgery (reference 15). CL = 960 ms; zero and 10 mV calibration signals.

Technologies). Small suction electrodes are also used for epicardial MAP studies. Either suction or pressure contact recordings may be made in small hearts and in Langendorff preparations. An apparatus for combining up to 10 MAPs from endocardium and epicardium together with three ECG electrodes in the Wilson or Einthoven configuration is shown in Fig. 13.7.

The MAP waveform

The MAP waveform is of lower amplitude than the intracellular action potential, i.e. 10–40 mV and approximately 120 mV respectively. In DC recordings, zero potential is

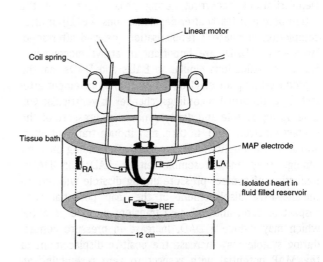

Figure 13.7 Diagram of apparatus for recording MAPs from multiple right and left ventricular epicardial and endocardial sites simultaneously in Langendorff perfused small animal hearts. Only two MAP electrodes are included in the figure for clarity. ECG electrodes, RA, LA, LF, REF record in the Wilson and Einthoven configuration (reference 16).

closer to plateau potentials in intracellular recordings compared to the MAP. The reason for both these amplitude-related differences probably relates to the way in which the MAP waveform is generated (see below). The MAP therefore does not provide a quantitative measure of amplitude or resting membrane potential, although under stable recording conditions useful qualitative information may be obtained for both of these parameters (see below).

Several studies have validated the MAP as providing an accurate measure of the repolarisation time course of the intracellular action potential and therefore an accurate measure of action potential duration.[8,17-19] The end of the repolarisation phase is difficult to define. Consequently, total APD is more commonly reported at 90% repolarisation (measured from the peak of the plateau to the baseline) rather than to the junction of the end of the MAP with the baseline. APD is conventionally measured with reference to dV/dt max of the MAP upstroke or the notch on the upstroke if present.

The MAP upstroke velocity is also less than the intracellular action potential (about 7 V/s and 200 V/s respectively). The difference is probably due to the large number of cells from which the MAP signal is derived and the normal variation in activation time of the cells within the field of recording. The upstroke velocity is therefore somewhat dependent on conduction sequence. With these reservations in mind, a decrease in Vmax of the MAP upstroke has been shown to provide a marker of myocardial ischaemia.[20] In addition, changes in Vmax in the MAP have been used to classify use dependent properties of Class I antiarrhythmic drugs.

MAP recordings will detect after-depolarisations. Depolarisations occurring during phase 2 or 3 of the action potential (early after-depolarisations – EAD) or after completion of phase 3 repolarisation (delayed after-depolarisations – DAD) are important in arrhythmogenesis.[21] However, deflections similar to EADs and DADs may be reproduced by poor electrode contact and movement artefact. In endocardial recordings, changes in ventricular volume during systole and diastole may alter pressure of the contact electrode and, in turn, may induce transient alterations in the amplitude of the signal. Depending on their timing, they may resemble either EADs or DADs. Reduction of contact pressure during diastole will reduce the negative displacement of the map potential with respect to zero, and induce a transient positive potential which may induce a DAD. Increase in pressure contact during systole may increase the positive displacement of the MAP potential with respect to zero resembling an EAD. Consequently, despite the use of special measurement criteria to help differentiate true after-depolarisations from artefact by some authors,[22] a general consensus is that the interpretation of "humps" resembling after-depolarisations needs care.

Generation of the MAP waveform

With growing popularity and increasing use of the MAP, a number of theories to explain the derivation of the MAP signal have evolved. One hypothesis proposed by Franz[23] to explain pressure contact recordings is as follows. Gentle pressure of the electrode against the myocardium results in depolarisation of cells under the electrode. These cells are electrically frozen at zero potential and are unresponsive to the activation wavefront. An electrical gradient then exists between these cells and the immediately surrounding cells, which have normal action potentials and depolarise and repolarise normally. During diastole the normal cells have a resting potential of about −90 mV. The depolarised cells at 0 mV are therefore relatively more positive and current flows intracellularly from the depolarised cells to the normal cells. The current then returns extracellularly from the normal cells to the depolarised cells creating a sink in the depolarised region under the pressure contact electrode. With the arrival of the activation wave and the onset of electrical systole, the normal cells depolarise to about +30 mV. This reverses the electrical gradient and reverses the direction of current flow, now creating a source over the depolarised cells. The MAP signal is recorded as a differential signal between the pressure tip electrode and the immediately surrounding myocardium (reference electrode). The MAP waveform therefore reflects the strength and polarity of the currents across the boundary between the depolarised and normal regions. A point of discussion is commonly whether the MAP signal is generated in the central depolarised zone or in the surrounding normal myocardium. According to this hypothesis, both would appear to be the case, i.e. the MAP signal would be expected to register changes in the normal cells surrounding the electrode but both the depolarised and surrounding normal cells participate in the currents which form the MAP potential.

Antiarrhythmic drugs evaluation

MAP recordings enable the action of antiarrhythmic drugs to be evaluated in vivo.[24] This is particularly useful for drugs with class I or class III action. Several factors which coexist *in vivo* influence class III action. Class III drug action involves the prolongation of APD as a result of block of K channels and hence prolongation of the refractory period. The effect is more pronounced at slow heart rates and reduced at fast heart rates, a phenomenon known as "reverse use dependence". There is, however, some variability among class III agents in this regard,[25,26] Amiodarone, for example, showing little, if any, rate dependence.[26] Another *in vivo* influence is the autonomic nervous system. The effect of class III agents has been shown to be reduced with enhanced sympathetic tone,[27-29] possibly as a result of upregulation of iK_s which is unopposed by selective iK_r blockers such as *d*-sotalol. Drug action *in vivo* is dependent on myocardial uptake. As a result, myocardial uptake, particularly after intravenous administration, may be inhomogeneous and is known to correlate poorly with blood levels.[30] The MAP therefore provides a means of directly assessing drug action on a regional basis.

A disadvantage of class III agents is the development of early after-depolarisations (EADs) and torsade de pointes arrhythmias. Several studies using MAP recordings *in vivo* and in isolated animal heart models have demonstrated the development of torsade de pointes following the appearance of drug-induced deflections in the MAP resembling EADs.[31-33] After critical evaluation, these deflections have been accepted as representing true EADs. These studies therefore are an example of the usefulness of the MAP to demonstrate after-depolarisations.

Class I antiarrhythmic agents depress sodium channels and slow conduction, and are thereby thought to exert an antiarrhythmic action by converting unidirectional block to bidirectional block. In addition, sodium channel block also depresses excitability as a result of which refractoriness may no longer correspond to action potential repolarisation but be delayed, known as "post-repolarisation refractoriness".[34] Post-repolarisation refractoriness also occurs with class III agents, which prolong refractory period more than the prolongation of APD. The Franz MAP catheter described earlier has the dual facility for pacing and the recording of the MAP signals. The positioning of the pacing electrodes (see Fig. 13.3) enables very low current strengths to be used with consequently only a very small stimulus artefact and so minimal interference with the MAP upstroke. The proximity of the pacing and MAP recording electrodes ensures that the pacing stimulus is delivered as close to the MAP recording site as possible. This allows the simultaneous determination of APD and refractory period at the same site and hence an evaluation of the relationship between repolarisation and refractoriness.[35,36]

Mechano-electric feedback

Altering the mechanical load on myocardial fibres may alter the electrophysiology of the cells known as "mechano-electric feedback" (MEF).[37-40] Several clinical conditions associated with sudden cardiac death owing to arrhythmia are frequently accompanied by abnormalities of ventricular wall loading and stretch.[40] The MAP is particularly suited to the study of mechanical/electrical interactions in whole heart models and much of our knowledge of MEF has been acquired using MAP record-

ings. Mechanical interventions have been shown to result in depolarisation of the resting potential and either a shortening or lengthening of APD and ERP depending on the nature of the intervention. As indicated earlier, whereas the MAP does not provide quantitative information on resting potential, useful qualitative information may be obtained. An example is shown in Fig. 13.8 from an isolated rabbit heart model with heart block. Transient stretch pulses were introduced by inflating a balloon in the left ventricle. Pulses of low volume (lower trace) resulted in barely detectable depolarisations of the diastolic baseline of the MAP recording (upper trace). As the pulse volume was increased, the depolarisation amplitude increased until threshold was reached and a regular sequence of MAPs ensued.[41] Computer simulations have been able to reproduce this sequence as a result of stretch activation of stretch-activated channels.[42] These depolarisations should not be confused with after-depolarisations, which by definition occur "after" an action potential and probably occur by a different mechanism.

MEF however may also induce after-depolarisations. In Fig. 13.9, MAP signals were recorded from the right ventricular endocardium in patients undergoing pulmonary artery valvuloplasty.[43] The procedure involves the positioning of an inflatable balloon within the narrowed pulmonary valve orifice. As the balloon is inflated for several seconds to stretch open the valve, right ventricular pressure and volume increase. During this time, deflections resembling EADs were seen in the MAP recordings (arrowed in Fig. 13.9) often followed by a premature beat. It is likely that these deflections represent EADs. This study also noted a shortening of APD during the increase in pressure/volume in the right ventricle.

A similar shortening of APD was observed on the epicardium in patients undergoing coronary artery surgery during the pressure/volume changes accompanying weaning off cardiopulmonary bypass (Fig. 13.10). During this period, of about 30 s, as volume and pressure within the ventricles increase (lower trace), APD in the left ventricular epicardial MAP shortens progressively (upper trace).[44]

The MAP has been used in a variety of models to examine mechanical/electrical relations including animal models of acute and chronic overload as well as human hearts.

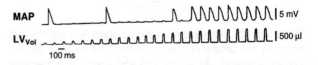

Figure 13.8 Incremental volume pulses (lower trace) in the left ventricle of an isolated rabbit heart with heart block, which reach threshold and trigger action potentials after the 3rd idioventricular beat (upper trace) (reference 41).

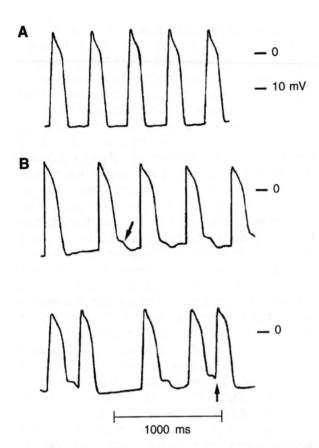

Figure 13.9 Monophasic action potentials from the right ventricular endocardium in a patient undergoing pulmonary valvuloplasty for pulmonary stenosis (see text). During obstruction of the right ventricular outflow tract, deflections resembling after-depolarisations are seen (arrows) from which premature action potentials arise (lower trace) (reference 43).

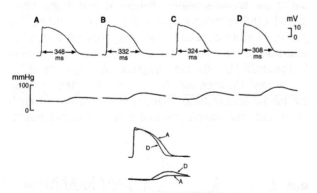

Figure 13.10 Monophasic action potentials from the left ventricular epicardium in a patient during discontinuing cardiopulmonary bypass. As the volume and pressure in the ventricle increase, radial artery pressure rises (middle panel) and MAP duration shortens (top panel). Superimposition of the first and last MAPs and pressure traces in the sequence are shown below (reference 44).

Experimental work [37] and computer modelling[42,45] indicate that the timing of stretch in relation to the phase of the action potential at which the stretch occurs may influence the effect on repolarisation, inducing either a shortening or lengthening of APD (see figure 5, reference 40). This may partly relate to the timing in relation to the reversal potential for stretch-activated channels, which occurs in the region of −30 to −50 mV. The MAP is established as providing a reliable measure of APD at all levels of repolarisation. Therefore, provided repolarisation shape changes from movement artefact are excluded, the MAP may be a sensitive means of discriminating between changes affecting early and late repolarisation.

Ischaemia

The effects of ischaemia on the action potential are well-known[21] and include loss of resting membrane potential, loss of amplitude, slowing of upstroke velocity, and shortening of action potential duration. The MAP reflects all these changes in a qualitative manner and provides a quantitative measure of changes in repolarisation. In animal models, the MAP enables comparisons to be made between repolarisation changes in an ischaemic areas and other physiological parameters, such as extracellular potassium[46] and catecholamines.[47] Coronary artery angioplasty of the left anterior descending coronary artery provides the opportunity to obtain MAP recordings from an area of regional ischaemia in patients. During the procedure when the balloon is inflated within the narrowed segment of the coronary artery in order to dilate the stenosis, the myocardium served by the vessel is rendered ischaemic. During this time, usually 1–3 minutes, the MAP recordings may be obtained from the ischaemic area by a catheter positioned on the right ventricular septum.[48] An example is shown in Fig. 13.11. The top trace shows the MAP recorded from the right ventricular septum; the middle trace is an epicardial electrogram recorded from the angioplasty catheter guide wire in the coronary artery; and the lower trace is ECG lead V5. During occlusion of the artery the MAP shows the effects of ischaemia on the action potential described above. After 2¾ minutes alternans develops followed by a tachyarrhythmia. Following release of the occlusion the deformed action potentials regain normal contour and the tachyarrhythmia self-terminates (within one beat). The APD remains short and, after a period of stable rhythm for about 30 seconds, two non-sustained salvos of ventricular premature beats occur, followed by ventricular fibrillation requiring defibrillation. Ventricular fibrillation is uncommon during angioplasty, which usually provides a relatively stable opportunity to study short periods of ischaemia. One study used this "model" to investigate the effects of ischaemia on the

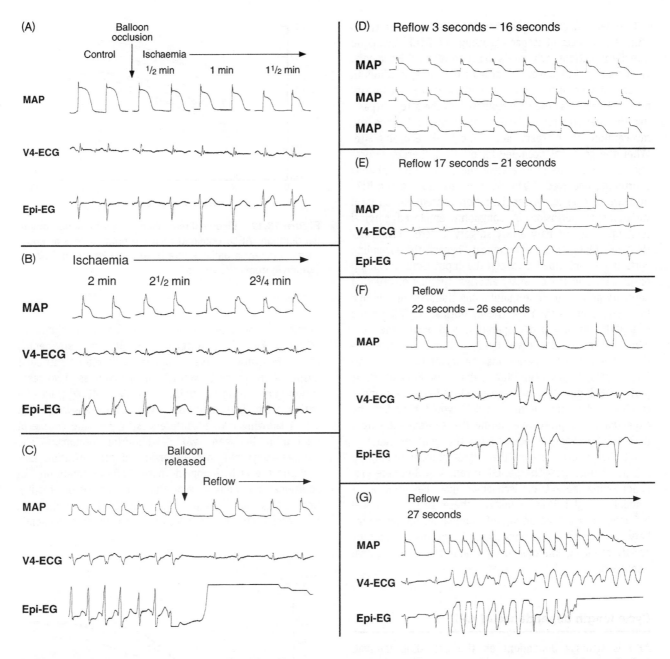

Figure 13.11 Monophasic action potential (MAP) from the right ventricular septum and electrogram from the angioplasty catheter guide wire in the left anterior descending coronary artery (Epi-EG) during an angioplasty procedure (see text). Inflation of the balloon within the artery occludes the lumen (balloon occlusion) (A) and induces ischaemia with loss of MAP amplitude and shortening of MAP duration and ST elevation on the Epi-EG. By 2.75 minutes alternans is present (B), followed by a tachy-arrhythmia and a disorganised MAP configuration (C). Within one beat of deflation of the balloon (balloon released) (C), the arrhythmia self-terminates and MAP configuration normalises. The MAP remains stable for 16 s (D). Two short runs of non-sustained VT then occur (E, F) followed by ventricular fibrillation (G), which was cardioverted to sinus rhythm (not shown).

cycle length dependence of action potential duration (electrical restitution).[49] Although repeated occlusions of the artery are normally undertaken as part of the routine procedure, comparisons made between successive periods of ischaemia involve uncertainties with regard to collateral blood flow and make interpretation more complex. MAPs may be combined with other methods of creating regional ischaemia. Atrial pacing to the angina threshold may be used with nuclear imaging to define regions of ischaemia.[50-52]

Coronary artery surgery affords the opportunity to study the effects of ischaemia using the MAP technique directly in patients who are subject to regional ischaemia. In one study, MAPs were recorded from the epicardium in an area downstream from a stenosis in a major coronary artery. A graft was then anastomosed to the artery bypassing the stenotic region and thereby revascularising the myocardium downstream, i.e. at the MAP recording site. When the graft was occluded for 60–90 s, thereby returning perfusion to its preoperative anatomy, significant APD shortening occurred.[53] The MAP is therefore a sensitive measure of changes in repolarisation consequent on local variations in perfusion. A commonly employed surgical technique for coronary artery surgery is "cross-clamp fibrillation". Once on cardiopulmonary bypass, the ascending aorta is cross-clamped between the input from the pump oxygenator and the coronary arteries, thereby obstructing coronary perfusion while maintaining the systemic circulation. The heart is then electrically fibrillated. This results in a still heart and a dry operating field during the time while the anastomoses are being fashioned by the surgeon. The ischaemic period may be maintained for up to 15 minutes. It has been shown that a preliminary short period of 3 minutes, ischaemia induced in this manner results in preconditioning,[54] which would therefore be expected to be protective during the subsequent longer periods of ischaemia required for the graft procedures. Since the cellular changes that effect preconditioning do not occur until *after* the period of reflow, a 3-minute preconditioning period of ischaemia may be used as a "model" of global ischaemia in these patients. Global ischaemia has the advantage of eliminating border zones between ischaemic and non-ischaemic regions and thereby greatly reducing inhomogeneity characteristic of regional ischaemia.[55]

Cycle length dependence of APD

APD is strongly dependent on the preceding interval. Following an abrupt alteration in cycle length, such as a premature beat, a short coupling interval is followed by an action potential with a short APD. With longer coupling intervals the subsequent APD is correspondingly longer. The relationship between APD and the preceding interval is known as the "electrical restitution curve".[56] Examples of restitution curves obtained from right ventricular endocardium in humans using the Franz catheter electrode are shown in Fig. 13.12.[57] The slope of the restitution curve is thought to be important in the development of ventricular fibrillation.[58–61] A steep slope is thought to facilitate the break up of spiral waves after the first few rotations of a re-entrant circuit, and result in the formation of ventricular fibrillation. Recordings made using MAP electrodes in

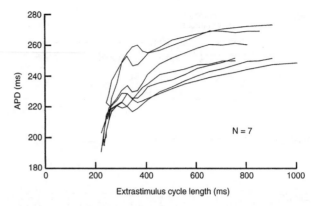

Figure 13.12 Electrical restitution curves for action potential duration (APD) obtained from the right ventricular endocardium in seven patients at a base cycle length of 600 ms. (Redrawn from reference 57.)

porcine epicardium during infusion of adrenaline are shown in Fig. 13.13. Adrenaline resulted in a steepening of the restitution curve.[62] Patients with right ventricular dysplasia are prone to ventricular arrhythmias. Two restitution curves from the right ventricular outflow tract in a patient with right ventricular dysplasia are shown in Fig. 13.14 showing marked differences in the time course of restitution between two neighbouring regions.[63] The authors suggested that dispersion of repolarisation may underlie the arrhythmogenic nature of the condition. An additional possibility may be the steepness of the restitution curves may be important. Using MAP recordings on the porcine epicardium, it has been shown that ischaemia

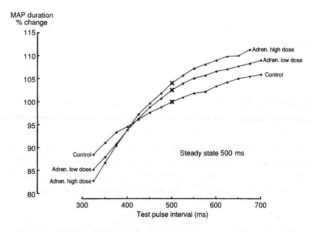

Figure 13.13 Electrical restitution curves for action potential duration obtained from MAP recordings on porcine epicardium at a basic stimulation cycle length of 500 ms. Intravenous adrenaline (Adren) infusion resulted in a steepening of the restitution curve which was dose related (reference 62).

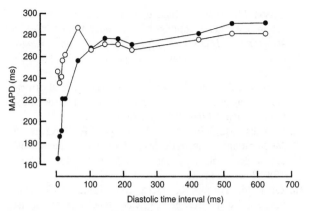

Figure 13.14 Two electrical restitution curves from nearby sites in the right ventricular outflow tract of a patient with right ventricular disease and complicating ventricular tachycardia. A marked dispersion of action potential duration is seen at short interbeat intervals (reference 63).

flattens the electrical restitution curve.[64] This has been confirmed in humans by MAP recording during angioplasty.[49] As steepening of the restitution curve is thought to underlie degeneration of an arrhythmia into ventricular fibrillation, flattening of the curve might be construed as protective. However, it is also in keeping with the concept that spiral wave break-up does not occur in the ischaemic zone, but in the normal myocardium surrounding the ischaemic region. It is evident from these studies that the MAP technique is eminently suited to this promising line of investigation.

Dispersion of repolarisation and the T wave

It is well-established that enhanced dispersion of repolarisation facilitates re-entrant arrhythmias.[21,65,66] A key study employed multiple MAP recordings on the epicardium in canine hearts. As APD is sensitive to temperature, prolonging with cooling and shortening with warming, dispersion of APD was created by perfusing part of the heart at different temperatures.[66,67] When APD dispersion, i.e. the difference between the longest and shortest MAP durations, reached 120 ms, re-entrant arrhythmias could be induced. Several workers have recorded MAPs from two or three endocardial sites simultaneously in patients, such as from the right ventricular outflow tract in patients with right ventricular dysplasia[63] or from ischaemic and non-ischaemic region.[50–52] Dispersion of repolarisation is a function not only of APD at different sites but also the time required for the activation wavefront to reach those sites. As the upstroke of the MAP is a reliable measure of the time of activation, MAP measurements at several sites provide information on activation time, APD and repolari-

sation.[68] With these three parameters, it has been shown that not only that dispersion of repolarisation is increased in patients with ventricular tachycardia/fibrillation, but also that this was due to an increase in both activation time and MAP duration in patients with polymorphic ventricular tachycardia and/or fibrillation, but mainly due to increased activation time in patients with monomorphic ventricular tachycardia.[69,70]

A problem with dispersion of repolarisation is that there is an intrinsic variation of APD from site to site in the left ventricle ranging over about 40 ms in the human left ventricle.[71,72] Any assessment of dispersion should therefore ideally incorporate measurements at multiple sites. This is not possible on human endocardium and difficult on epicardium. QT dispersion in the ECG is now widely used as a surrogate marker for dispersion of repolarisation with the tacit assumption that QT intervals represent underlying APDs. However, the relationship between APD and the T wave has fascinated physiologists for decades and the derivation of the T wave remains an unresolved issue.[73,74] A relationship has been demonstrated between activation time and MAP duration such that areas of the left ventricle activated earliest have the longest APDs and areas activated latest have the shortest APDs.[71,72] On the basis of theoretical concepts,[75,76] this relationship has been suggested to underly the polarity of the T wave, a connotation supported by the loss of the relationship in patients with T wave inversion due to left ventricular hypertrophy.[72] On the other hand, rather than lateral gradients, i.e. base/apex differences, transmural repolarisation gradients, have been proposed as the main source of the T wave. Evidence for this is derived from *in vitro* differences in APD within the ventricular wall and MAP recordings within the wall in arterially perfused canine wedge preparations. However, whether sufficient repolarisation gradients could exist *in vivo* when cells are electrically and mechanically well coupled is a matter of continuing debate.[77,78] In addition the method for recording MAPs from within the ventricular wall is different to the conventional technique and may be prone to artefact (see earlier). Thus while the origin of the T wave remains an enigma, evidence based on MAP recordings continue to play a leading role in this arena of discussion.

Atrial MAPs

The majority of the foregoing has focused on ventricular MAPs. Historically, the MAP technique was first used to record atrial MAPs. There are many applications for MAP recordings in atrium including:

● looking at the mechanisms of drug actions, particularly in atrial fibrillation;

- defining the relationship between APD and refractory period;
- studying the effects of drugs on the refractory period/APD ratio;
- as an aid to distinguishing between atrial fibrillation and other arrhythmias;
- studying atrial remodelling in chronic atrial fibrillation.[79]

Miscellaneous

Other applications of the MAP recording technique include study of:

- ventricular fibrillation;
- long QT syndrome, and
- monitoring of radiofrequency ablation.

References

1. Burdon-Sanderson J, Page FJM. On the time-relations of the excitatory process in the ventricle of the heart of the frog. *J Physiol (Lond)* 1882;**2**:385–412.
2. Schütz E. Einphasische Aktionsströme vom in situ durchbluteten Säugetierherzen. *Zeitschr Biol* 1932;**92**:441–52.
3. Schütz E. Elektrophysiologie des Herzens bei einphasischer Ableitung. *Ergebn Physiol Exper Pharmakol* 1936;**38**:493–620.
4. Jochim K, Katz LN, Mayne W. The monophasic electrogram obtained from the mammalian heart. *Am J Physiol* 1935;**111**:177–86.
5. Ling G, Gerard RW. The normal membrane potential of frog sartorius fibers. *J Cell Comp Physiol* 1949;**34**:383–96.
6. Woodbury LA, Woodbury JW, Hecht HH. Membrane resting and action potentials from single cardiac muscle fibers. *Circulation* 1950:1:264–6.
7. Draper MH, Weidmann S. Cardiac resting and action potentials recorded with an intracellular electrode. *J Physiol (Lond)* 1951;**115**:74–94.
8. Hoffman BF, Cranefield PF, Lepeschkin E, Surawicz B, Herrlich H. Comparison of cardiac monophasic action potentials recorded by intracellular and suction electrodes. *Am J Physiol* 1959;**196**:1296–301.
9. Korsgren M, Leskinen E, Sjostrand U, Varnauskas E. Intracardiac recording of monophasic action potentials in the human heart. *Scand J Clin Lab Invest* 1966;**18**; 561–4.
10. Olsson SB, Varnauskas E. Monophasic action potentials from intact human heart. Effect of different heart rates. *Circulation* 1969;39–**40**:111–57(Abstr.).
11. Olsson SB, Varnauskas E, Korsgren M. Further improved method for measuring monophasic action potentials of the intact human heart. *J Electrocardiol* 1971;**4**:19–23.
12. Olsson SB. Estimation of ventricular repolarization in man by monophasic action potential recording technique. *Eur Heart J* 1985;**6**(Suppl. D):71–9.
13. Olsson SB, Yuan S. Technique and use of monophasic action potential recordings. In: Mandel WJ ed. *Cardiac arrhythmias. Their mechanisms, diagnosis, and management*. 3rd edn. Philadelphia: Lippincott, 1995, pp. 785–810.
14. Emanuel RW, Noble D, Taggart P. Simulation of electrocardiogram by algebraic sum of monophasic action potentials in man. *J Physiol (Lond)* 1980;**312**:36–37P.
15. Runnalls ME, Sutton PMI, Taggart P, Treasure T. Modifications of electrode design for recording monophasic action potentials in animals and humans. *Am J Physiol* 1987;**253**:H1315–20.
16. Zabel M, Portnoy S, Franz MR. Electrocardiographic indices of dispersion of ventricular repolarization: an isolated heart validation study. *J Am Coll Cardiol* 1995;**25**:746–52.
17. Franz MR, Burkhoff D, Spurgeon H, Weisfeldt ML, Lakatta EG. In vitro validation of a new cardiac catheter technique for recording monophasic action potentials. *Eur Heart J* 1986;**7**:34–41.
18. Ino T, Karagueuzian HS, Hong K, Meesmann M, Mandel WJ, Peter T. Relation of monophasic action potential recorded with contact electrode to underlying transmembrane action potential properties in isolated cardiac tissues: a systematic microelectrode validation study. *Cardiovasc Res* 1988;**22**:255–64.
19. Franz MR, Burkhoff D, Lakatta EG, Weisfeldt ML, Monophasic action potential recording by contact electrode technique: in vitro validation and clinical applications. In: Butrous GS, Schwartz PJ, eds. *Clinical aspects of ventricular repolarization*. London: Farrand Press, 1989, pp. 81–92.
20. Franz MR, Flaherty JT, Platia EV, Bulkley BH, Weisfeldt ML. Localization of regional myocardial ischemia by recording of monophasic action potentials. *Circulation* 1984;**69**:593–604.
21. Janse MJ, Wit AL. Electrophysiological mechanisms of ventricular arrhythmias resulting from myocardial ischemia and infarction. *Physiol Rev* 1989;**69**:1049–69.
22. de Groot SH, Vos MA, Gorgels AP, Leunissen JD, van der Steld BJ, Wellens HJ. Combining monophasic action potential recordings with pacing to demonstrate delayed afterdepolarizations and triggered arrhythmias in the intact heart. Value of diastolic slope. *Circulation* 1995;**92**:2697–704.
23. Franz MR. Current status of monophasic action potential recordings: theories measurements and interpretations. *Cardiovasc Res* 1999;**41**:25–40.
24. O'Donoghue S, Platia EV. Monophasic action potential recordings: evaluation of antiarrhythmic drugs. *Cardiovasc Dis* 1991;**34**:1–14.
25. Schmitt C, Brachmann J, Karch M *et al.* Reverse use dependence of sotalol demonstrated by recording monophasic action potentials of the right ventricle. *Am J Cardiol* 1991;**68**:1183–7.
26. Huikuri HV, Yli-Mayryr S. Frequency dependent effects of d-sotalol and amiodarone on the action potential duration of the human right ventricle. *PACE* 1992;**15**:2103–6.
27. Shenasa H, Shenasa M. Reversibility of antiarrhythmic effects of sotalol by isoproterenol in patients with ventricular tachycardia. In: Vereecke PP, van Bogaert PP, Verdouck

F eds. *Potassium channels in normal and pathological conditions*. Leuven: Leuven University Press, 1995, pp. 400–6.

28. Sager PT, Follmer C, Uppal P, Pruitt C, Godfrey R. The effects of beta-adrenergic stimulation on the frequency-dependent electrophysiologic actions of amiodarone and sematilide in humans. *Circulation* 1994;**90**:1811–19.

29. Vanoli E, Priori SG, Nakagawa H *et al*. Sympathetic activation, ventricular repolarization and IKr blockade: implications for antifibrillation efficacy of potassium channel blocking agents. *J Am Coll Cardiol* 1995;**24**:1609–14.

30. Franz MR, Behrens S, Li C. Myocardial tissue concentrations of amiodarone and desethyl amiodarone after chronic treatment: correlation with local action potential duration (abstract). *J Am Coll Cardiol* 1997:**27**(Suppl.):344A.

31. El-Sherif N, Zeilor RH, Craelius W, Gough WB, Henkin R. QTU prolongation and polymorphic ventricular arrhythmias due to bradycardia dependent early after depolarizations. *Circ Res* 1988;**63**:286–305.

32. Vos MA, Verduyn SC, Gorgels A, Lipesei GC, Wellens H. Reproducible induction of early afterdepolarizations and torsade de pointes arrhythmias by d-sotalol and pacing in dogs with chronic atrioventricular block. *Circulation* 1995;**91**:864–72.

33. Zabel M, Hohnloser SH, Behrens S, Li YG, Woosley RL, Franz MR. Electrophysiologic features of torsade de pointes: insights from a new isolated rabbit heart model. *J Cardiovasc Electrophysiol* 1997;**8**:1148–58.

34. Natel S, Zeng FD. Frequency dependent effects of antiarrhythmic drugs on action potential duration and refractoriness of canine cardiac Purkinje fibers. *J Pharmacol Exp Ther* 1984;**229**:283–91.

35. Franz MR, Costard A. Frequency dependent effects of quinidine on the relationship between action potential duration and refractoriness. *Circulation* 1988;**77**:1177–84.

36. Lee RJ, Liem LB, Cohen TJ, Franz MR. Relation between repolarization and refractoriness in the human ventricle: cycle length dependence and effect of procainamide. *J Am Coll Cardiol* 1992;**19**:614–18.

37. Lab MJ. Contraction excitation feedback in myocardium. Physiological basis and clinical relevance. *Circ Res* 1982;**50**:757–66.

38. Lab MJ. Mechanoelectric feedback (transduction) in heart: concepts and implications. *Cardiovasc Res* 1996;**32**:3–14.

39. Franz MR. Mechano-electrical feedback in ventricular myocardium. *Cardiovasc Res* 1996;**32**:15–24.

40. Taggart P, Sutton PMI. Cardiac mechano-electric feedback in man: clinical relevance. *Prog Biophys Mol Biol* 1999;**71**: 139–54.

41. Franz MR, Cima R, Wang D, Profitt D, Kurz R. Electrophysiological effects of myocardial stretch and mechanical determinants of stretch-activated arrhythmias. *Circulation* 1992;**86**:968–78 (published erratum appears in *Circulation* 1992;**86**:1663).

42. Kohl P, Day K, Noble D. Cellular mechanisms of cardiac mechano-electric feedback in a mathematical model. *Can J Cardiol* 1998;**14**:111–19.

43. Levine JH, Guarnieri T, Kadish AH, White RI, Calkins H, Khan JS. Changes in myocardial repolarization in patients undergoing balloon valvuloplasty for congenital pulmonary stenosis: evidence for contraction-excitation feedback in humans. *Circulation* 1988;**77**:70–7.

44. Taggart P, Sutton PMI, Treasure T *et al*. Monophasic action potentials at discontinuation of cardiopulmonary bypass: evidence for contraction-excitation feedback in man. *Circulation* 1988;**77**:1266–75.

45. Zabel M, Koller BS, Sachs F, Franz MR. Stretch-induced voltage changes in the isolated beating heart: importance of the timing of stretch and implications for stretch-activated ion channels. *Cardiovasc Res* 1996;**32**:120–30.

46. Donaldson RM, Nashat FS, Noble D, Taggart P. Differential effects of ischaemia and hyperkalaemia on myocardial repolarisation and conduction times in the dog. *J Physiol (Lond)* 1984;**353**:393–403.

47. Taggart P, Sutton P, Spear DW, Drake HF, Swanton RH, Emanuel RW. Simultaneous endocardial and epicardial monophasic action potential recordings during brief periods of coronary ligations: influence of adrenaline, beta-blockade and alpha-blockade. *Cardiovasc Res* 1988;**22**:900–9.

48. Taggart P, Sutton PMI, John R, Hayward R, Swanton RH. The epicardial electrogram: a quantitative assessment during balloon angioplasty incorporating monophasic action potential recordings. *Br Heart J* 1989;**62**:342–52.

49. Taggart P, Sutton PMI, Boyett MR, Lab M, Swanton H. Human ventricular action potential duration during short and long cycles. Rapid modulation by ischemia. *Circulation* 1996;**94**:2526–34.

50. John RM, Taggart PI, Sutton PM, Ell PJ, Swanton H. Direct effect of dobutamine on action potential duration in ischemic compared with normal areas in the human ventricle. *J Am Coll Cardiol* 1992;**20**:896–903.

51. John RM, Taggart PI, Sutton PM, Costa DC, Ell PJ, Swanton H. Vasodilator myocardial perfusion imaging: demonstration of local electrophysiological changes of ischaemia. *Br Heart J* 1992;**68**:21–30.

52. John RM, Taggart PI, Sutton PM, Costa DC, Ell PJ, Swanton H. Endocardial monophasic action potential recordings for the detection of myocardial ischemia in man: a study using atrial pacing stress and myocardial perfusion scintigraphy. *Am Heart J* 1991;**122**:1599–609.

53. Taggart P, Sutton P, Runnalls M *et al*. Use of monophasic action potential recordings during routine coronary artery bypass surgery as an index of localised myocardial ischaemia. *Lancet* 1996;**1**:1462–5.

54. Yellon DM, Alkhulaifi AM, Pugsley WB. Preconditioning in human myocardium. *Lancet* 1993;**342**:276–7.

55. Coronel R, Wilms-Schopman FJG, Opthof T, Van Capelle FJL, Janse MJ. Injury current and gradients of diastolic stimulation threshold. TQ potential and extracellular potassium concentration during acute regional ischemia in the isolated perfused pig heart. *Circ Res* 1991;**68**:1241–9.

56. Boyett MR, Jewell BR, Analysis of the effects of changes in rate and rhythm upon the electrical activity in the heart. *Prog Biophys Mol Biol* 1980;**36**:1–52.

57. Franz MR, Swerdlow CD, Liem LB, Schaefer J. Cycle length dependence of human action potential duration in vivo: effects of single extrastimuli, sudden sustained rate acceleration and deceleration, and different steady-state frequencies. *J Clin Invest* 1988;**82**:972–9.

58. Gilmour RF, Chialvo DR. Electrical restitution, critical mass and the riddle of fibrillation. *Cardiovasc Electrophysiol* 1999;**10**:1087–9.

59. Qu Z, Weiss JN, Garfinkel A. Cardiac electrical restitution properties and stability of reentrant spiral waves: a simulation study. *Am J Physiol* 1999;**45**:H269–83.

60. Pastore JM, Girouard SD, Laurita KR, Akar FG, Rosenbaum DS. Mechanism linking T wave alternans to the genesis of cardiac fibrillation. *Circulation* 1999;**99**:1385–94.

61. Koller ML, Riccio ML, Gilmour RF. Dynamic restitution of action potential duration during electrical alternans and ventricular fibrillation. *Am J Physiol* 1998;**275**:H1635–42.

62. Taggart P, Sutton P, Lab M, Dean J, Harrison F. Interplay between adrenaline and interbeat interval on ventricular repolarisation in intact heart in vivo. *Cardiovasc Res* 1990;**24**:884–95.

63. Morgan JM, Cunningham D, Rowland E. Dispersion of monophasic action potential duration: demonstrable in humans after premature ventricular extrastimulation but not in steady state. *J Am Coll Cardiol* 1992;**19**:1244–53.

64. Dilly SG, Lab MJ. Electrophysiological alternans and restitution during acute regional ischaemia in myocardium of anaesthetized pig. *J Physiol (Lond)* 1988;**402**:315–33.

65. Han J, Moe GK. non-uniform recovery of excitability in ventricular muscle. *Circ Res* 1964;**14**:44–54.

66. Kuo CS, Munakata K, Reddy CP, Surawicz B. Characteristics and possible mechanism of ventricular arrhythmia dependent on the dispersion of action potential duration. *Circulation* 1983;**67**:1356–67.

67. Kuo CS, Atarashi H, Reddy CP, Surawicz B. Dispersion of ventricular repolarization and arrhythmia: study of two consecutive ventricular premature complexes. *Circulation* 1985;72:370–6.

68. Kuo CS, Amlie JP, Munakata K, Reddy CP, Surawicz B. Dispersion of monophasic action potential durations and activation times during atrial pacing, ventricular pacing and ventricular premature stimulation in canine ventricles. *Cardiovasc Res* 1983;**17**:152–61.

69. Yuan S, Blomström-Lundquist C, Pripp CM, Pehrson S, Wohlfart B, Olsson SB. Signed value of monophasic action potential duration difference. A useful measure in evaluation of dispersion of repolarization in patients with ventricular arrhythmias. *Eur Heart J* 1996:**17**(Suppl. 8):275.

70. Yuan S, Blomström-Lundquist C, Pehrson S, Pripp CM, Wohlfart B, Olsson SB. Dispersion of repolarization following double and triple programmed stimulation – a clinical study using the monophasic action potential recording technique. *Eur Heart J* 1996;**17**:1080–91.

71. Franz MR, Bargheer K, Rafflenbeul W, Haverick A, Lichtlen PR. Monophasic action potential mapping in human subjects with normal electrocardiograms: direct evidence for the genesis of the T wave. *Circulation* 1987;**75**:379–86.

72. Cowan JC, Hilton CJ, Griffiths CJ et al. Sequence of epicardial repolarisation and configuration of the T wave. *Br Heart J* 1988;**60**:424–33.

73. Li D, Li CY, Yong AC, Kilpatrick D. The source of electrocardiographic ST changes in subendocardial ischemia. *Circ Res* 1998;**82**:957–70.

74. Kors JA, van Herpen G, van Bemmel JH. QT dispersion as an attribute of T-loop morphology. *Circulation* 1999;**99**:1458–63.

75. Cohen I, Giles W, Noble D. Cellular basis for the T wave of the electrocardiogram. *Nature* 1976;**262**:657.

76. Holland RP, Arnsdorf MF. Solid angle theory and the electrocardiogram: physiologic and quantitative interpretations. *Prog Cardiovasc Dis* 1977;**19**:431–56.

77. Anyukhousky EP, Susunov EA, Gainullin RZ, Rosen MR. The controversial M cell. *J Cardiovasc Electrophysiol* 1999;**10**:244–60.

78. Antzelevitch C, Shimizu W, Yan G-X et al. The M cell: Its contribution to the ECG and to normal and abnormal function of the heart. *J Cardiovasc Electrophysiol* 1999;**10**:1124–52.

79. Franz MR, Karasik PL, Li C, Moubarak J, Chavez M. Electrical remodelling of the human atrium: similar effects in patients with chronic atrial fibrillation and atrial flutter. *J Am Coll Cardiol* 1997;**30**:1785–92.

14 Ventricular signal averaged electrocardiography

Piotr Kulakowski

Re-entry plays a major role in the genesis of most life-threatening ventricular arrhythmias.[1] The prerequisites for re-entry are slow conduction, unidirectional block and recovery of the myocardial cells ahead of the wavefront of excitation.[1] Tissue showing such electrophysiological properties is usually located at the border zone of a remote myocardial infarction.[1] In 1973 Boineau and Cox[2] recorded potentials from ischaemic regions of the canine heart that were delayed far beyond the end of the QRS complex. Subsequent studies in humans demonstrated that these fragmented, low-amplitude signals represent areas of slow conduction in myocardium.[3,4] Because these signals often extend well into the ST segment, they were named ventricular late potentials.[3,4] However, the amplitude of late potentials is too low to be detected on the standard surface ECG. In 1978 Berbari *et al.*[5] first demonstrated that using high-gain amplification, filtering and signal averaging late potentials could be recorded from the body surface (Fig. 14.1). Simson[6] and Breithardt *et al.*[7] were the first investigators to show the clinical value of ventricular signal averaged electrocardiography (ECG) for identification of patients with sustained ventricular tachycardia.

Technical considerations

Recording and analysis of late potentials should be performed according to the "Standards for analysis of ventricular late potentials using high resolution or signal-averaged ECG", published in 1991.[8] The summary of these recommendations is presented below.

Acquisition

Commercially available devices with a low-noise amplifiers are usually used for late potential recording. Late potentials can be also recorded by means of Holter ECG, particularly when solid-state digital recording is used.[9] The most often used technique for recording of late potentials is high-gain amplification (usually × 10 000), complex filter-

ing, and averaging of many identical beats to eliminate the remaining random noise and to improve the signal-to-noise ratio. An orthogonal, bipolar XYZ lead set is most commonly used. Silver–silver chloride electrodes are mandatory to obtain high-quality recordings. The skin is cleansed with alcohol or other solvent and abraded to minimise impedance.

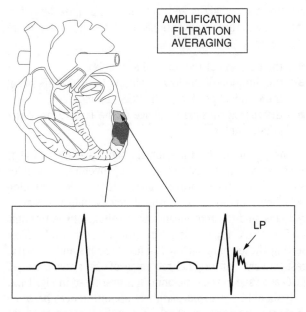

Figure 14.1 Schematic representation of the recording of late potentials. At the top a fragment of the ventricle muscle is depicted. The black area represents a postinfarction scar, surrounded by areas of slow conduction (shaded area) where re-entrant ventricular arrhythmias can arise. The ECG signals are recorded from the body surface and subsequently averaged, amplified, and filtered. The result is the signal-averaged ECG, in which microvolt oscillations at the end and after the high-gain QRS complex can be detected (right, lower part of the diagram). These are ventricular late potentials and they result from the slow conduction in areas of diseased myocardium. The signals recorded from a normal myocardium are not fragmented or delayed and no late potentials are present at the end of the QRS complex (left, lower part of the diagram).

Consecutive cardiac beats are compared with the template QRS complex and accepted or rejected based on a predetermined value for the correlation coefficient (usually r >0.95). The averaging process is ended when the lowest possible noise level is achieved, preferably below 0.3 µV.[10] Usually, 100–300 cardiac cycles are necessary to achieve such a noise level. A computer algorithm is used to identify the onset of the QRS complex and the end of late potentials.

Analysis

Late potentials are most often analysed in the time domain. The signal-averaged ECG recording is filtered between 25 and 250 Hz or between 40 and 250 Hz. Subsequently, the filtered XYZ leads are combined into a vector magnitude:

$$\sqrt{(x^2 + y^2 + z^2)}$$

The advantage of this procedure is to obtain a single waveform for analysis and to reduce the noise level further. Then, three conventional time-domain indexes are calculated:

- the duration of the total QRS complex;
- the duration of the low amplitude ($<40\,\mu V$) signals at the terminal portion of the QRS complex;
- the root-mean-square voltage of the last 40 ms of the QRS complex.

The result of the time-domain signal-averaged ECG is abnormal when at least two of three conventional variables are beyond the normal range: total QRS duration >120 ms; duration of terminal low amplitude signals >40 ms, and the root mean-square voltage of the terminal QRS <25 µV at a 25-Hz filter setting.[11] For a 40-Hz filter setting these values are >114 ms, >38 ms and <20 µV, respectively.[8] An original recording of the signal-averaged ECG analysed in the time-domain is presented in Fig. 14.2.

It should be stressed that there are differences between authors regarding normal values, and these standards were designed in postinfarction patients to identify individuals prone to sustained ventricular tachycardia. Therefore, they may not be applicable in other cardiac disorders. Each laboratory needs to define its own normal values. Moreover, the use of other filter settings or different electrode localisation also influences the results. Patients with bundle branch block are usually excluded from the time-domain analysis; however, some investigators use modified criteria to detect late potentials in such patients.[12,13]

The data so far presented were related to the most widely used technique to detect late potentials, signal averaging in the time domain. There are also different approaches to record and analyse late potentials. One is spatial averaging on a beat-to-beat basis, which allows the detection of transient late potentials.[14] The other approach is to analyse signal averaged ECG in the frequency domain, usually using fast Fourier transform analysis. With this technique, recordings from patients with bundle branch block can be included and the ECG signal is not distorted by high-gain amplification and filtering. Some authors have also demonstrated that late potentials hidden within the QRS complex can be detected using frequency-domain analysis.[15] Various methods of frequency-domain analysis, such as spectral temporal mapping,[16] spectral turbulence analysis,[17] wavelet decomposition,[18] combined spatial and spectral analyses of the entire cardiac cycle,[19] and many others have been introduced. Although initial results were promising,[16,17] other studies failed to show superiority of these techniques over standard time-domain analysis,[20,21] and frequency-domain analysis has not become a standard technique for late potential analysis. There are many reasons for this, including the poor reproducibility of frequency-domain analysis,[22,23] the limitations of the fast Fourier transform when applied to a biological signal[24] and the high complexity of some frequency-domain approaches. Nevertheless, in some clinical situations frequency-domain analysis may add important information to that obtained by the time-domain analysis of the signal-averaged ECG.[25,26]

Clinical value for arrhythmia risk prediction

Evaluation of patients with complex ventricular tachyarrhythmias

Sustained, monomorphic ventricular tachycardia is the most typical ventricular tachyarrhythmia in patients with abnormal signal-averaged ECG, particularly in postinfarction patients with a left ventricular aneurysm.[6,7] Therefore, the signal-averaged ECG may serve as a screening test for inducibility of sustained ventricular tachycardia during electrophysiological studies in high-risk patients.[27] Moreover, this technique is a valuable tool in a common clinical situation; postinfarction patients with complex ventricular arrhythmias detected on ambulatory ECG monitoring and no history of sustained ventricular tachyarrhythmias. In such patients an abnormal signal-averaged ECG identifies those who will have inducible sustained ventricular tachycardia during programmed ventricular stimulation with a sensitivity of 64–100% and a specificity ranging from 46% to 89%.[8–30] Therefore, signal-averaged ECG may be useful in detecting low-risk patients with complex ventricular arrhythmias who may not require invasive electrophysiological testing.

Signal-averaged ECG may also be used for differential

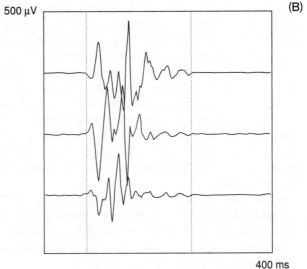

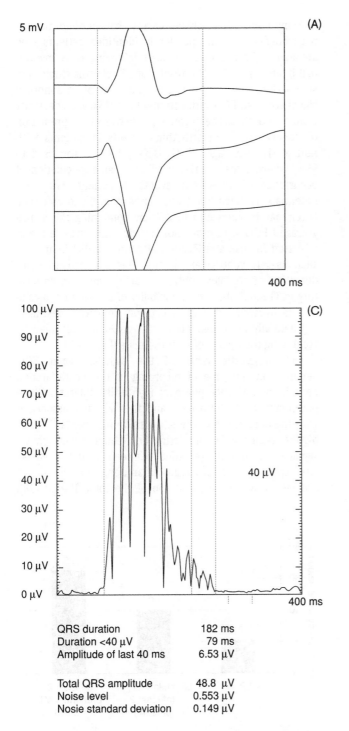

QRS duration	182 ms
Duration <40 μV	79 ms
Amplitude of last 40 ms	6.53 μV
Total QRS amplitude	48.8 μV
Noise level	0.553 μV
Nosie standard deviation	0.149 μV

Figure 14.2 An original signal-averaged ECG recording (obtained using a solid-state ambulatory ECG recorder FD-3 and analysed using the computer software Excel-2, Oxford, UK) from a patient with a history of sustained ventricular tachycardia. Panel A: XYZ leads after averaging.

Panel B: XYZ leads after averaging and high-pass filtering between 25 Hz and 250 Hz. The low-frequency signals of the ST segment and T wave are now reduced and high-frequency components at the end of the QRS complex, representing late potentials, are clearly visible.

Panel C: filtered XYZ leads are now combined into a vector magnitude $\sqrt{(x^2 + y^2 + z^2)}$ to obtain a single waveform for analysis and to reduce the noise level further. Prominent late potentials are present at the end of the QRS complex and all signal-averaged ECG variables are abnormal: (i) duration of the filtered QRS complex is 182 ms; (ii) duration of low-amplitude (less than 40 μV) signals is 79 ms; and (iii) root mean square amplitude (voltage) of the last 40 ms is 6.53 μV. The noise level is 0.553 μV, and the noise standard deviation is 0.149 μV.

diagnosis of broad complex tachycardia.[31] Although the sensitivity of this technique for the diagnosis of ventricular tachycardia is low (ranging from 28% to 45%), specificity is high (96%). Signal averaging in the remote diagnosis of broad complex tachycardia is therefore only useful if late potentials are detected.

In patients with a history of polymorphic ventricular tachycardia or ventricular fibrillation late potentials are

less frequent which reflects the differences in underlying arrhythmogenic substrate between these arrhythmias and monomorphic ventricular tachycardia.[32,33] It has been shown that in patients with a history of out-of-hospital ventricular fibrillation signal-averaged ECG failed to predict inducibility of sustained ventricular arrhythmia,[34,35] which may represent a significant limitation of this technique in identifying patients at risk for sudden death.

Implantation of a cardioverter–defibrillator is currently thought to be the most appropriate mode of treatment in patients with ventricular tachycardia or fibrillation. There is no doubt that any non-invasive method that is to play an important role in arrhythmia risk stratification should be able to identify patients who will benefit from this type of therapy. However, three studies addressing this issue have failed to demonstrate a clinical value of ventricular signal averaging for identification of patients with a cardioverter–defibrillator who will benefit from device implantation or who will have recurrences of arrhythmia after implantation.[36–38]

In summary, although ventricular signal-averaged ECG is helpful for evaluation of patients with ventricular tachyarrhythmias, the value of this technique for establishing the optimal therapeutic strategies in such patients may be limited and has not yet been fully established.

Ventricular signal averaging in risk stratification after myocardial infarction

This is undoubtedly the most important and widely used clinical application of ventricular signal-averaged ECG. Late potentials are present in 12%–50% of patients with acute myocardial infarction.[11,39–55] The prevalence of late potentials is greater in patients with inferior wall infarction than in those with anterior wall infarction, which is probably due to the different activation times of various left ventricular sites.[55] The inferoposterobasal area of the left ventricle (the usual site of inferior infarction) is activated late, and late potentials, even of short duration, may easily extend beyond the QRS complex.

There is also clear evidence that intravenous thrombolysis changes the prevalence of late potentials in patients who survived the acute phase of myocardial infarction.[56–61] The decrease in the incidence of abnormal signal-averaged ECG may be marked, from 43% in patients treated conservatively to 16% in patients who received thrombolytic agents.[57] These[56–61] and other studies[62–68] have also demonstrated that the absence of late potentials seems to be a good non-invasive predictor of the patency of the infarct-related artery: in one study a sensitivity of 81% and a specificity of 90% was reported.[57]

These encouraging results prompted interest in the use of ventricular signal-averaged ECG for the bedside detection of reperfusion during the first 3 hours of acute myocardial infarction. Four studies have recently shown that an abnormal signal-averaged ECG identifies patients without reperfusion, whereas normalisation of signal-averaged ECG following thrombolysis indicates the patency of an infarct-related artery.[69–72] Therefore worsening or non-improvement of ventricular signal-averaged ECG may help in identification of patients who may need invasive treatment.

Many studies have shown clearly that an abnormal signal-averaged ECG independently identifies patients who are at risk of sudden cardiac death following acute myocardial infarction.[11,39–55] The results of 17 relevant studies are summarised in Table 14.1. The sensitivity of an abnormal signal-averaged ECG varies from 44% to 93% and specificity from 61% to 83%. The negative predictive value (prediction of no occurrence of arrhythmic events in patients with normal signal-averaged ECG) is very high – from 89% to 99%, whereas the positive predictive value (prediction of occurrence of arrhythmic events in patients with late potentials) is much lower and varies from 6% to 29%. The latter may be increased to 65% by combining the signal-averaged ECG with other non-invasive and invasive methods used for risk stratification after myocardial infarction, such as left ventricular ejection fraction measurement, detection of complex ventricular arrhythmias on ambulatory ECG monitoring, or inducibility of sustained ventricular tachycardia during electrophysiological testing.[46] Substantially more patients at risk could be identified by combining the results of all these tests (Fig. 14.3).

The prognostic value of the signal-averaged ECG depends on the time of recording in the postinfarction period. In the acute phase of myocardial infarction, late potentials can be transient, and they are not associated with the occurrence of the late arrhythmic events.[43,47] The highest accuracy for predicting arrhythmic events shows signal-averaged ECG recorded between 1 and 4 weeks after the onset of myocardial infarction.[43] Of the signal-averaged ECG indices, duration of the total filtered QRS

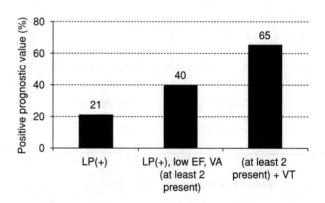

Figure 14.3 Positive predictive value of signal-averaged ECG alone and in combination with other parameters in predicting arrhythmic events following myocardial infarction (combined data from the references 11, 40, 41, 44, 46). By combining the results of all tests, the positive predictive value increases from 21% (signal-averaged ECG analysis alone) to 65% (all tests). Abbreviations: LP(+) = late potentials present; EF = ejection fraction; VA = ventricular arrhythmia on Holter monitoring; VT = ventricular tachycardia inducible at electrophysiological study.

complex is the best parameter for identification of patients at risk of sudden death.[44,45]

Many of the risk-stratification studies were conducted before the widespread use of thrombolysis.[11,39–45,51] Since this therapy decreases the prevalence of late potentials, decreases mortality after myocardial infarction, and also changes arrhythmogenic substrate, the accuracy of signal-averaged ECG in identification of patients at risk may be altered.[73] For example, in the studies performed before the thrombolytic era, the mean value of sensitivity of the signal-averaged ECG was 79%, whereas in the more recent studies it decreased to 62% (Table 14.1). Moreover, sustained monomorphic ventricular tachycardia, the most characteristic arrhythmia for the presence of late potentials, has become rare in the thrombolytic era. The changes in the incidence of arrhythmic events (defined as sudden cardiac death, non-fatal ventricular fibrillation or tachycardia) and episodes of sustained ventricular tachycardia in a postinfarction population are well depicted in Table 14.1. Before the widespread use of thrombolysis,[11,39–45,51] 7% of patients experienced arrhythmic events in comparison with 4% of patients in the thrombolytic era.[46–50,52–54] The same holds true for sustained ventricular tachycardia, 3.4% versus 1.3%, respectively. Moreover, some recent preliminary reports have suggested that the presence of late potentials no longer identifies patients' prone to arrhythmic events after myocardial infarction,[74,75] particularly when a postinfarction population with reduced left ventricular ejection fraction is studied.[52] Therefore, the role of ventricular signal-averaged ECG in risk stratification after myocardial infarction in the 1990s may be less important than previously thought.

For a diagnostic method to find a wide clinical application in risk stratification it is necessary that it has some impact on further therapeutic strategies. However, to date, no convincing data exist suggesting that ventricular signal-averaging has any therapeutic implication. It may be speculated that coexistence of several non-invasive risk markers (including abnormal signal-averaged ECG) following myocardial infarction may better identify a subgroup of patients who should undergo invasive electrophysiological testing, and, if sustained ventricular tachycardia is inducible, prophylactic antiarrhythmic therapy (preferably implantation of a cardioverter–defibrillator) should be instituted. However, the role of signal-averaged ECG in such an approach has not yet been established.

Ventricular signal averaging in risk stratification in other heart diseases

Arrhythmogenic right ventricular disease

Of all cardiomyopathies, late potentials are most common (up to 73% of patients) in patients with arrhythmogenic right ventricular dysplasia (Table 14.2). A fatty fibrous substitution of myocardium forms the substrate for delayed myocardial activation, which may be a source of late potentials. Fontaine *et al.*[76] were the first investigators to demonstrate the presence of late potentials on the surface ECG in this condition. Subsequent studies have shown close correlation between the extent of abnormality of the signal-averaged ECG and the severity of the disease.[77–82] The relationship between abnormal signal-averaged ECG and dangerous ventricular arrhythmias has not been well established: some authors[77,78,80] have found such a relationship whereas others[79,81] did not. Even less information is available on the prognostic value of signal-averaged ECG in this condition,[79] and large studies with a long-term follow-up are needed to clarify this issue. Thus, signal-averaged ECG in arrhythmogenic right ventricular cardiomyopathy may serve as a non-invasive tool for detection of the disease and for assessment of the extent of myocardial abnormality. Some authors have also suggested that progression of the disease may be associated with worsening of the signal-averaged ECG parameters.[77,79] The role of this technique for arrhythmia risk stratification remains to be defined.

Non-ischaemic dilated cardiomyopathy

Late potentials are present in 23% of patients with this condition and are associated with the presence of ventricular tachyarrhythmias[83–88] (Table 14.2). The predictive accuracy of signal-averaged ECG for identification of patients with spontaneous or inducible sustained ventricular tachycardia differs markedly between studies: sensitivity values range from 22% to 83%,[83–85] specificity from 66% to 97%,[83–85] and overall predictive accuracy from 50% to 88%.[85,87] It has been shown that the performance of the time-domain signal-averaged ECG may be improved by using two-dimensional frequency-domain techniques, such as spectral turbulence analysis[85] However, as in patients with arrhythmogenic right ventricular disease, the prognostic value of signal-averaged ECG in non-ischaemic dilated cardiomyopathy remains uncertain. Some authors were able to demonstrate that an abnormal signal-averaged ECG is a marker for future arrhythmic events,[86] others have failed to show the usefulness of signal-averaged ECG for risk stratification in this condition,[87,88] or the number of events during follow-up was too small to draw any meaningful conclusions.[85]

Also, the severity of the disease may be assessed using signal-averaged ECG. Yamada *et al.*[89] have shown a close correlation between the abnormal signal-averaged ECG and the extent of myocardial fibrosis, measured in endomyocardial biopsy samples.

Interesting data have been published on the usefulness of ventricular signal-averaged ECG in the screening of

Table 14.1 Value of ventricular signal-averaged ECG in predicting events after acute myocardial infarction

Author	No. of pts	% of pts with thrombolysis	Follow-up (months)[a]	No. (%) of pts with AE	No. (%) of pts with sVT	Sensitivity (%)	Specificity (%)	PPV (%)	NPV (%)
Breithartdt et al.[39] (1986)	511	NR	18 ± 3	30 (5)	14 (2)	79	63	6	97
Gomes et al.[40] (1987)	102	NR	12 ± 6	15 (15)	10 (9)	87	63	29	96
Kuchar et al.[41] (1987)	210	9	14 (6–24)	15 (7)	7 (3)	93	65	17	99
Cripps et al.[11] (1988)	159	NR	12 ± 6	11 (7)	6 (4)	91	81	26	99
Verzoni et al.[42] (1989)	220	NR	8 ± 4	6 (3)	3 (1)	83	73	8	99
El Sherif et al.[43] (1989)	156	NR	12	12 (7)	8 (5)	75	79	23	97
Steinbert et al.[44] (1992)	182	8	14 ± 7	16 (9)	4 (2)	69	62	15	95
Malik et al.[45] (1992)	332	NR	6	26 (7)	14 (4)	63	78	NR	NR
Pedretti et al.[46] (1993)	305	54	15 ± 7	19 (6)	10 (3)	79	75	17	98
McClements et al.[47] (1993)	301	68	12 (11–18)	13 (4)	2 (0.6)	64	81	11	98
Strasbert et al.[48] (1993)	100	38	24	12 (12)	1 (1)	50	61	15	90
Denes et al.[49] (1994)	787	46	10 ± 3	33 (4)	2 (0.2)	60	98	20	89
Makijarvi et al.[50] (1995)	778	29	6	33 (4)	13 (1)	76	63	8	98
Bloomfield et al.[51] (1996)[b]	177	NR	14 ± 7	16 (9)	4 (2)	69	62	15	95
Fetsch et al.[52] (1997)	856	NR	24	13 (1.5)	NR	NR	NR	NR	NR
Zimmerman et al.[53] (1997)	458	23	70 (15–115)	32 (6)	11 (2)	44	83	20	94
El-Harari et al.[54] (1998)	204	66	12	6 (3)	0	NR	NR	NR	NR

[a]Duration of follow-up calculated as a mean ±SD, or as a median (range), or a number of months when the duration of follow-up was fixed; [b]Data published in 1996 but study population treated between 1986 and 1988.

Abbreviations: AE = arrhythmic events (defined as sudden cardiac death, non-fatal ventricular fibrillation or tachycardia) during follow-up; No. = number; NPV = negative predictive value; NR = not reported; PPV = positive predictive value; pts = patients; sVT = episode of sustained ventricular tachycardia during follow-up.

Table 14.2   The role of ventricular late potentials in patients with cardiomyopathies (combined data from references 77–79, 83–88, 92)

Condition	Prevalence of LP (%)	Identification of pts with VT[a]			Prediction of AE		
		Sens (%)	Spec (%)	Overall PA (%)	Sens (%)	Spec (%)	Overall PA (%)
Arrhythmogenic right ventricular disease	73	70	76	74	Not established		
Non-ischaemic dilated cardiomyopathy	23	44	80	68	32	90	80
Hypertrophic cardiomyopathy	7	11	97	78	No LP in pts with AE		

[a]Sustained VT in patients with arrhythmogenic right ventricular cardiomyopathy and non-ischaemic dilated cardiomyopathy; non-sustained VT in patients with hypertrophic cardiomyopathy.
Abbreviations: LP = ventricular late potentials; PA = predictive accuracy; Sens = sensitivity; Spec = specificity; other abbreviations as in Table 14.1.

familial forms of dilated cardiomyopathy. In the study by Gang Yi et al.,[90] the sensitivity, specificity, and positive predictive accuracy of signal-averaged ECG in the identification of relatives with left ventricular enlargement were 20%, 95%, and 54%, respectively. However, although the specificity was high, the sensitivity and positive predictive accuracy were still too low to recommend the use of this technique as a non-invasive screening test for the early detection of the familial form of dilated cardiomyopathy.

Hypertrophic cardiomyopathy

The usefulness of signal-averaged ECG in this group of patients has not been established. Although initial results were optimistic,[91] a larger study did not confirm these findings.[92] The incidence of late potentials is low, ranging from 6% to 8%[92] (Table 14.2). Since sustained monomorphic ventricular tachycardia is uncommon in hypertrophic cardiomyopathy and the arrhythmogenic substrate for ventricular arrhythmias, myocardial disarray, is usually more widely dispersed than in postinfarction patients, the low incidence of late potentials and lack of their predictive value for arrhythmic events in patients with hypertrophic cardiomyopathy is not surprising.

Patients with ventricular tachycardia and no apparent heart disease

This heterogeneous group of patients includes both subjects with structurally unchanged heart as well as patients with early stages of cardiomyopathies, undetectable using conventional diagnostic techniques. There is strong evidence that signal-averaged ECG is useful in detecting cardiac abnormality in patients with no apparent heart disease and episodes of spontaneous or inducible sustained ventricular tachycardia.[93–95] Although sensitivity of signal-averaged ECG for identification of patients with cardiac involvement, confirmed by abnor-

mal endomyocardial biopsy, or patients with inducible ventricular tachycardia is low, 63% and 37% respectively, specificity for these variables is high, 84% and 100% respectively.[93] According to Leclercq et al.,[96] the predictive value of late potentials for detecting underlying heart disease is even higher: sensitivity – 81%; specificity – 96%; negative predictive value – 97%; and positive predictive value – 76%. Therefore, signal-averaged ECG may serve as a non-invasive screening test for identification of patients with early stages of cardiomyopathy, most often with arrhythmogenic right ventricular disease. However, as in overt forms of cardiomyopathies, the predictive value of signal-averaged ECG for future arrhythmic events is currently unknown.

Tetralogy of Fallot

Ventricular tachyarrhythmias are common following surgical repair of tetralogy of Fallot. Abnormal signal-averaged ECG identifies patients prone to non-sustained ventricular tachycardia with a sensitivity of 100%, and specificity ranging from 75% to 88%.[97,98] Long-term prognostic value of signal-averaged ECG has to be determined.

Cardiac involvement in systemic or muscular diseases

The presence of late potentials has been demonstrated in patients with systemic sclerosis,[99] myotonic dystrophy,[100] and Duchenne muscular dystrophy,[101] particularly in those with depressed left ventricular function or complex ventricular arrhythmias. Also, primary amyloidosis patients with cardiac involvement have abnormal signal-averaged ECG more frequently than patients with normal echocardiography.[102] In this study, the presence of late potentials has been shown to be an independent predictor of adverse prognosis.

Ventricular signal averaging in risk stratification in other clinical situations

Patients presenting with syncope

Syncope of unknown origin is a frequent clinical problem. It has been shown that the signal-averaged ECG might be useful (sensitivity 70–82%, specificity 55–91%) in identifying those patients with recurrent syncope in whom ventricular tachycardia may be the underlying mechanism.[103–106] Therefore, the signal-averaged ECG can serve as a non-invasive test for selecting patients with syncope who should undergo programmed ventricular stimulation.

Patients awaiting heart transplantation

These patients are particularly vulnerable to life-threatening ventricular tachyarrhythmias and the yearly incidence of sudden cardiac death may approach 21%.[107] It has been demonstrated that signal-averaged ECG improves risk

Table 14.3   Clinical use of signal-averaged ECG

Application	Comment
Risk stratification after myocardial infarction	Prognostic value well established but may be limited in the thrombolytic era Widely used in clinical practice So far, no impact on therapeutic strategies
Evaluation of mechanism of cardiac arrest in patients with aborted sudden death	Helps to differentiate between sustained VT and VF as clinical arrhythmia May have prognostic significance May influence further treatment
Evaluation of patients with non-sustained VT	Identification of patients prone to sustained VT Prognostic value established
Evaluation of patients with wide complex tachycardias	Helps to differentiate between supraventricular and ventricular origin of tachycardia
Evaluation of patients with syncope	Identifies patients in whom sustained VT is the most likely underlying mechanism of syncope Prognostic value probable but not examined
Non-invasive assessment of reperfusion in patients with myocardial infarction	Helps to assess efficacy of reperfusion therapies in acute and subacute phase of infarction Clinical value needs to be established
Detection of early stages of cardiomyopathy	Well-established clinical value Prognostic value not yet established
Diagnosis of cardiac involvement in patients with systemic diseases	Well-established clinical value Prognostic value confirmed in amyloidosis
Early detection of rejection episodes in patients after heart transplantation	More research needed to establish clinical value
Evaluation of patients awaiting heart transplantation	Identifies those who are at higher risk of sudden death while awaiting heart transplantation Prognostic value probable Impact on antiarrhythmic strategy probable
Evaluation of candidates for ICD	So far, no data supporting the use of signal-averaged ECG for selecting patients for ICD
Evaluation of patients with ICD	So far, no data showing that signal-averaged ECG identifies patients who will have recurrences of arrhythmia after device implantation

Abbreviations: ICD = implantable cardioverter–defibrillator; VF = ventricular fibrillation; VT = ventricular tachycardia.

stratification in this group of patients, identifying subjects prone to sudden death with low positive predictive accuracy (27%), but high negative predictive accuracy (87%).[107] These results suggest that signal-averaged ECG may be helpful in selecting patients awaiting heart transplantation who will not benefit from prophylactic antiarrhythmic therapy, although this hypothesis needs to be prospectively tested.

Patients after heart transplantation

Detection of heart transplant acute rejection is of vital importance. Endomyocardial biopsy has been routinely used for this purpose but this technique is invasive, cannot be performed on a daily basis, and, therefore, there is a need for other non-invasive methods. Initial results using signal-averaged ECG are promising.[108–110] Sensitivity of this method ranges from 50% to 92%, and specificity from 44% to 87%.[108–110] More research should be done to establish the role of signal-averaged ECG in this setting and to introduce it into clinical practice.

Summary and future perspectives

The clinical utility of signal-averaged ECG is summarised in Table 14.3. Progress in the development of new clinical applications of signal averaging has been a little disappointing and no new technique has gained widespread acceptance in the past few years. Routine time-domain analysis remains the gold standard. However, analysis limited to the terminal portion of the QRS complex may exclude detection of >95% of the signals generated by myocardium responsible for ventricular tachycardia.[111] We are still waiting for new methods enabling the detection of "late potentials" located within the QRS complex. Promising results were recently obtained with body surface potential maps.[112] The question is whether these new and relatively complex techniques will increase significantly the positive predictive accuracy of the test and whether they will gain wider acceptance among clinical cardiologists.

What is then the current role of ventricular signal-averaged ECG? It is used for risk stratification after myocardial infarction, in evaluation of patients with syncope or non-sustained ventricular tachycardia, and for the detection of early stages of cardiomyopathy. However, in the absence of studies demonstrating important clinical applications of this technique, particularly in patients who may benefit from or who already have a cardioverter–defibrillator, and in the screening of patients with systemic diseases or cardiomyopathies, ventricular signal-averaged ECG will remain just one of many non-invasive techniques of little clinical importance.

References

1. El-Sherif N, Scherlag BJ, Lazzara R, Hope RR. Reentrant ventricular arrhythmias in the late myocardial infarction period. I. Conduction characteristics in the infarction zone. *Circulation* 1977;**55**:686–702.
2. Boineau JP, Cox JL. Slow ventricular activation in acute myocardial infarction. A source of reentrant premature ventricular contractions. *Circulation* 1973;**48**:702–13.
3. Josephson ME, Horowitz LN, Farshidi A. Continuous local electrical activity: A mechanism of recurrent ventricular tachycardia. *Circulation* 1978;**57**:658–65.
4. Fontaine G, Giraudon G, Frank R, Vedel J, Grosgogeat Y, Cabrol C. Modern concepts of ventricular tachycardia. *Eur J Cardiol* 1978;**8**:565–80.
5. Berbari EJ, Scherlag BJ, Hope RR, Lazzara R. Recording from the body surface of arrhythmogenic ventricular activity during the S-T segment. *Am J Cardiol* 1978;**41**:697–702.
6. Simson MB. Use of signals in the terminal QRS complex to identify patients with ventricular tachycardia after myocardial infarction. *Circulation* 1981;**64**:235–42.
7. Breithardt G, Becker R, Seipel L, Abendroth RR, Ostermeyer J. Non-invasive detection of late potentials in man – a new marker for ventricular tachycardia. *Eur Heart J* 1981;**2**:1–11.
8. Breithardt G (Chairman), Cain ME, El-Sherif N *et al*. Standards for analysis of ventricular late potentials using high resolution or signal-averaged electrocardiography. A statement by a Task Force Committee between the European Society of Cardiology, the American Heart Association and the American College of Cardiology. *Eur Heart J* 1991;**12**:473–80
9. Kulakowski P, Biedrzycka A, Ceremuzynski L. Late potentials detected by digital Holter ECG: Reproducibility, lead systems, and effects of physical activity. *Ann Noninvas Electrocardiol* 1996;**1**:70–8.
10. Steinberg JS, Bigger JT Jr. Importance of the endpoint of noise reduction in analysis of the signal-averaged electrocardiogram. *Am J Cardiol* 1989;**63**:556–60.
11. Cripps T, Bennett ED, Camm AJ, Ward DE. High gain signal-averaged electrocardiogram combined with 24 hour monitoring in patients early after myocardial infarction for bedside prediction of arrhythmic events. *Br Heart J* 1988;**60**:181–7.
12. Buckingham TA, Thessen CC, Stevens LL, Reed RM, Kennedy HL. Effect of conduction defects on the signal-averaged electrocardiographic determination of late potentials. *Am J Cardiol* 1988;**61**:1265–71.
13. Fontaine JM, Rao R, Henkin R, Suneja R, Ursell SN, El-Sherif N. Study of the influence of left bundle branch block on the signal-averaged electrocardiogram: a qualitative and quantitative analysis. *Am Heart J* 1991;**121**:494–508.
14. Hombach V, Kebbel U, Hopp HW, Winter U, Hirche H. Non-invasive beat by beat registration of ventricular late potentials using high resolution electrocardiography. *Int J Cardiol* 1984;**6**:167–83.
15. Lindsay BD, Markham J, Schechtman KB, Ambos HD, Cain

ME. Identification of patients with sustained ventricular tachycardia by frequency analysis of signal-averaged electrocardiograms despite the presence of bundle branch block. *Circulation* 1988;**77**:122–30.

16. Haberl R, Jilge G, Putler R, Steinbeck G. Spectral mapping of the electrocardiogram with Fourier transform for identification of patients with sustained ventricular tachycardia and coronary artery disease. *Eur Heart J* 1989;**10**:316–22.

17. Kelen GJ, Henkin R, Starr AM, Caref EB, Bloomfield D, El-Sherif N. Spectral turbulence analysis of the signal-averaged electrocardiogram and its predictive accuracy for inducible sustained monomorphic ventricular tachycardia. *Am J Cardiol* 1991;**67**:965–75.

18. Morlet D, Peyrin F, Desseigne P, Touboul P, Rubel P. Wavelet analysis of high resolution signal-averaged ECG in postinfarction patients. *J Electrocardiol* 1993;**26**:311–20.

19. Kavesh NG, Cain ME, Ambos HD, Arthur RM. Enhanced detection of distinguishing features in signal-averaged electrocardiograms from patients with ventricular tachycardia by combined spatial and spectral analyses of entire cardiac cycle. *Circulation* 1994;**90**:254–63

20. Kulakowski P, Malik M, Poloniecki J *et al*. Frequency versus time domain analysis of signal-averaged electrocardiograms. II. Identification of patients with ventricular tachycardia after myocardial infarction. *J Am Coll Cardiol* 1992;**20**:135–43.

21. Odemuyiwa O, Malik M, Poloniecki J *et al*. Frequency versus time domain analysis of signal-averaged electrocardiograms. III. Stratification of postinfarction patients for arrhythmic events. *J Am Coll Cardiol* 1992;**20**:144–50.

22. Emmot W, Vacek JL. Lack of reproducibility of frequency versus time domain signal-averaged electrocardiographic analyses and effects of lead polarity in coronary artery disease. *Am J Cardiol* 1991;**68**:913–17.

23. Malik M, Kulakowski P, Poloniecki J *et al*. Frequency versus time domain analysis of the signal-averaged electrocardiogram. I. Reproducibility of the results. *J Am Coll Cardiol* 1992;**20**:127–34.

24. Parker B. Fourier analysis of electrograms. *PACE* 1979;**2**:246–8.

25. Pierce DL, Easley AR, Windle JR, Engel TR. Fast Fourier transformation of the entire low amplitude late QRS potential to predict ventricular tachycardia. *J Am Coll Cardiol* 1989;**14**:1731–40.

26. Buckingham TA, Greenwalt T, Lingle A *et al*. In anterior myocardial infarction, frequency domain is better than time domain analysis of the signal-averaged ECG for identifying patients at risk for sustained ventricular tachycardia. *PACE* 1992;**15**(Part I):1681–7.

27. Nalos PC, Gang ES, Mandel WJ, Ladenheim ML, Lass Y, Peter T. The signal-averaged electrocardiogram as a screening test for inducibility of sustained ventricular tachycardia in high risk patients: a prospective study. *J Am Coll Cardiol* 1987:**9**:539–48.

28. Buxton AE, Simson MB, Falcone RA, Marchlinski FE, Doherty JU, Josephson ME. Results of signal-averaged electrocardiography and electrophysiologic study in patients with non-sustained ventricular tachycardia after healing of acute myocardial infarction. *Am J Cardiol* 1987;**60**:80–5.

29. Turitto G, Fontaine JM, Ursell SN, Caref EB, Henkin R, El-Sherif N. Value of the signal-averaged electrocardiogram as a predictor of the results of programmed stimulation in non-sustained ventricular tachycardia. *Am J Cardiol* 1988;**61**:1272–8.

30. Winters SL, Steward D, Targonski A, Gomes JA. Role of signal averaging of the surface QRS complex in selecting patients with non-sustained ventricular tachycardia and high grade ventricular arrhythmias for programmed ventricular stimulation. *J Am Coll Cardiol* 1988;**12**:1481–7.

31. Griffith MJ, de Belder MA, Mehta D, Ward DE, Camm AJ. Signal averaging of the electrocardiogram in the remote differential diagnosis of broad complex tachycardias. *Eur Heart J* 1991;**12**:777–83.

32. Freedman RA, Gillis AM, Keren A, Soderholm-Difatte V, Mason JW. Signal-averaged electrocardiographic late potentials in patients with ventricular fibrillation or ventricular tachycardia: correlation with clinical arrhythmia and electrophysiologic study. *Am J Cardiol* 1985;**55**:1350–3.

33. Denniss AR, Ross DL, Richards DA *et al*. Differences between patients with ventricular tachycardia and ventricular fibrillation as assessed by signal-averaged electrocardiogram, radionuclide ventriculography and cardiac mapping. *J Am Coll Cardiol* 1988;**11**:276–83.

34. Dolack GL, Callahan DB, Burdy GH, Greene HL. Signal-averaged electrocardiographic late potentials in resuscitated survivors of out-of-hospital ventricular fibrillation. *Am J Cardiol* 1990;**65**:1102–4.

35. Vaitkus PT, Kindwall E, Marchlinski FE, Miller JM, Buxton AE, Josephson ME. Differences in electrophysiological substrate in patients with coronary artery disease and cardiac arrest or ventricular tachycardia. *Circulation* 1991;**84**:672–8.

36. Epstein AE, Dailey SM, Shepard RB, Kirk KA, Kay GN, Plumb VJ. Inability of the signal-averaged electrocardiogram to determine risk of arrhythmia recurrence in patients with implantable cardioverter defibrillators. *PACE* 1991;**14**:1169–78.

37. Zareba W, Steinberg JS, Moss AJ, Heo M, F. I. Marcus for the MADIT Investigators. Signal-averaged ECG in the Multicenter Automatic Defibrillator Implantation Trial (MADIT). *J Am Coll Cardiol* 1997;**29**:31A(Abstr. 912–16).

38. Cook JR, Flack JE, Gregory CA, Deaton DW, Rousou JA, Engelman RM for The CABG Patch Trial. Influence of the preoperative signal-averaged electrocardiogram on left ventricular function after coronary artery bypass graft surgery in patients with left ventricular dysfunction. *Am J Cardiol* 1998;**82**:285–9.

39. Breithardt G, Borggrefe M. Pathophysiological mechanisms and clinical significance of ventricular late potentials. *Eur Heart J* 1986:7:364–85.

40. Gomes JA, Winters SL, Steward D, Horowitz S, Milner M, Barreca P. A new non-invasive index to predict sustained ventricular tachycardia and sudden death in the first year after myocardial infarction: based on signal-averaged electrocardiogram, radionuclide ejection fraction and Holter monitoring. *J Am Coll Cardiol* 1987;**10**:349–57.

41. Kuchar DL, Thorburn CW, Sammel NL. Prediction of serious arrhythmic events after myocardial infarction; signal-

averaged electrocardiogram, Holter monitoring and radionuclide ventriculography. *J Am Coll Cardiol* 1987:9:531–8.

42. Verzoni A, Romano S, Pozzoni L, Tarricone D, Sangiorgio S, Croce L. Prognostic significance and evolution of late ventricular potentials in the first year after myocardial infarction: a prospective study. *PACE* 1989;**12**:41–51.

43. El-Sherif N, Ursell SN, Bekheit S *et al*. Prognostic significance of the signal-averaged ECG depends on the time of recording in the postinfarction period. *Am Heart J* 1989;**118**:256–64

44. Steinberg JS, Regan A, Sciacca RR, Bigger JT, Fleiss JL. Predicting arrhythmic events after acute myocardial infarction using the signal-averaged electrocardiogram. *Am J Cardiol* 1992;**69**:13–21.

45. Malik M, Odemuyiwa O, Poloniecki J *et al*. Late potentials after acute myocardial infarction. Performance of different criteria for the prediction of arrhythmic complications. *Eur Heart J* 1992;**13**:599–607.

46. Pedretti R, Etro MD, Laporta A, Braga SS, Caru B. Prediction of late arrhythmic events after acute myocardial infarction from combined use of non-invasive prognostic variables and inducibility of sustained monomorphic ventricular tachycardia. *Am J Cardiol* 1993;**71**:1131–41.

47. McClements BM, Adgey AAJ. Value of signal-averaged electrocardiography, radionuclide ventriculography, Holter monitoring and clinical variables for prediction of arrhythmic events in survivors of acute myocardial infarction in the thrombolytic era. *J Am Coll Cardiol* 1993;**21**:1419–27.

48. Strasberg B, Abboud S, Kusniec J *et al*. Prediction of arrhythmic events after acute myocardial infarction using two methods for late potentials recording. *PACE* 1993;**16**:2118–26.

49. Denes P, El-Sherif N, Katz R *et al*. for the Cardiac Arrhythmia Suppression Trial (CAST) SAECG Substudy Investigators. Prognostic significance of signal-averaged electrocardiogram after thrombolytic therapy and/or angioplasty during acute myocardial infarction (CAST Substudy). *Am J Cardiol* 1994;**74**:216–20.

50. Makijarvi M, Fetsch T, Reinhardt L *et al*. for the Postinfarction Late Potential (PILP) study. Comparison and combination of late potentials and spectral turbulence analysis to predict arrhythmic events after myocardial infarction in the Postinfarction Late Potential (PILP) study. *Eur Heart J* 1995;**16**:651–9.

51. Bloomfield DM, Snyder JE, Steinberg JS. A critical appraisal of quantitative spectro-temporal analysis of the signal-averaged ECG: Predicting arrhythmic events after myocardial infarction. *PACE* 1996;**19**:768–77.

52. Fetsch T, Reinhardt L, Borggrefe M *et al*. The role of ventricular late potentials for risk stratification in a postinfarction population with reduced left ventricular function: results from EMIAT. *Circulation* 1997;**96**:I-459(Abstr. 2564).

53. Zimmerman M, Sentici A, Adamec R, Metzger J, Mermillod B, Rutishauser W. Long-term prognostic significance of ventricular late potentials after a first acute myocardial infarction. *Am Heart J* 1997;**134**:1019–28.

54. El-Harari MB, Adams PC, Albers C, Bourke JP. Should routine evaluation of ventricular tachyarrhythmic risk be aban-

doned in postinfarction patients in the late 1990s? *Eur Heart J* 1998;**19**:79(Abstr. P596).

55. Breithardt G, Schwartzmaier J, Borggrefe M, Haerten K, Seipel L. Prognostic significance of late ventricular potentials after acute myocardial infarction. *Eur Heart J* 1983;4:487–95.

56. Gang ES, Lew AS, Hong M *et al*. Decreased incidence of ventricular late potentials after successful thrombolytic therapy for acute myocardial infarction. *New Engl J Med* 1989;**321**:712–16.

57. Chew EW, Morton P, Murtgath JG, Scott ME, OKeeffe B. Intravenous streptokinase for acute myocardial infarction reduces the occurrence of ventricular late potentials. *Br Heart J* 1990;**64**:5–8.

58. Eldar M, Leor J, Hod H *et al*. Effects of thrombolysis on the evolution of late potentials within 10 days of infarction. *Br Heart J* 1990;**63**:273–6.

59. Leor J, Hod H, Rotstein Z *et al*. Effects of thrombolysis on the 12-lead signal-averaged ECG in the early postinfarction period. *Am Heart J* 1990;**120**:495–502.

60. Zimmermann M, Adamec R, Ciaroni S. Reduction in the frequency of ventricular late potentials after acute myocardial infarction by early thrombolytic therapy. *Am J Cardiol* 1991;**67**:697–703.

61. Pedretti R, Laporta A, Etro MD *et al*. Influence of thrombolysis on signal-averaged electrocardiogram and late arrhythmic events after acute myocardial infarction. *Am J Cardiol* 1992;**69**:866–72.

62. Lange RA, Cigarroa RC, Wells PJ, Kremers MS, Hillis LD. Influence of anterograde flow in the infarct artery on the incidence of late potentials after acute myocardial infarction. *Am J Cardiol* 1990;**65**:554–8.

63. Tranchesi B, Verstraete M, Van de Werf F *et al*. Usefulness of high-frequency analysis of signal-averaged surface electrocardiograms in acute myocardial infarction before and after coronary thrombolysis for assessing coronary reperfusion. *Am J Cardiol* 1990;**66**:1196–8.

64. Aguirre FV, Kern MJ, Hsia J *et al*. Importance of myocardial infarct artery patency on the prevalence of ventricular arrhythmia and late potentials after thrombolysis in acute myocardial infarction. *Am J Cardiol* 1991;**68**:1410–16.

65. Vatterott PJ, Hammill SC, Bailey KR, Wiltgen CM, Gersh BJ. Late potentials on signal-averaged electrocardiograms and patency of the infarct-related artery in survivors of acute myocardial infarction. *J Am Coll Cardiol* 1991;**17**:330–7.

66. Moreno FLL, Karagounis L, Marshall H, Menlove RL, Ipsen S, Anderson JL. Thrombolysis-related early patency reduces ECG late potentials after acute myocardial infarction. *Am Heart J* 1992;**124**:557–64.

67. Chillou de C, Rodriguez LM, Doevendans P *et al*. Effects on the signal-averaged electrocardiogram of opening the coronary artery by thrombolytic therapy or percutaneous transluminal coronary angioplasty during acute myocardial infarction. *Am J Cardiol* 1993;**71**:805–9.

68. Steinberg JS, Hochman JS, Morgan CD *et al*. Effects of thrombolytic therapy administered 6 to 24 hours after myocardial infarction on the signal-averaged ECG. *Circulation* 1994;**90**:746–52.

69. Beauregard LM, Waxman HL, Volosin R *et al*. Signal-averaged ECG prior to and serially after thrombolytic therapy for acute myocardial infarction. *PACE* 1996;**19**:883–9.

70. Peters W, Kowallik P, Wilhelm K *et al*. Evolution of late potentials during the first 8 hours of myocardial infarction treated with thrombolysis. *PACE* 1996;**19**(Pt II):1918–22.

71. Kontoyannis DA, Nanas JN, Kontoyannis S.A. *et al*. Evolution of late potential parameters in thrombolyzed acute myocardial infarction might predict patency of the infarct-related artery. *Am J Cardiol* 1997;**79**:570–4.

72. Kulakowski P, Karpinski G, Szymot J, Ceremuzynski L. Signal-averaged ECG in non-invasive assessment of reperfusion in the acute phase of myocardial infarction. *Ann Non-invas Electrocardiol* 1999;**4**:301–8.

73. Malik M, Kulakowski P, Odemuyiwa O *et al*. Effect of thrombolytic therapy on the predictive value of signal-averaged electrocardiography after acute myocardial infarction. *Am J Cardiol* 1992;**70**:21–5.

74. Klingenheben T, Credner S.C., Mauss O, Gronefeld GC, Hohnloser SH. Comparison of measures of autonomic tone and the signal-averaged ECG for risk stratification after myocardial infarction: results of a prospective long-term follow-up trial in 411 consecutive patients. *Eur Heart J* 1999;**20**:342(Abstr. 1799).

75. Kazianis G, Feggos S, Cokkinos DV, Economou A. Is abnormal signal-averaged electrocardiogram in time or frequency domain analysis an independent predictor of mortality post acute myocardial infarction and what is the optimal time of recording? *Eur Heart J* 1999;**20**:342(Abstr. 1800).

76. Fontaine G, Frank R, Gallais-Hamonno F, Allali I, Phan-Thuc H, Grosgogeat Y. Electrocardiographie des potentiels tardifs du syndrome de post-excitation. *Arch Mal Coeur* 1978;**71**:854–64.

77. Blomstrom-Lundqvist C, Olsson SB, Edvardsson N. Follow-up by repeated signal-averaged surface QRS in patients with the syndrome of arrhythmogenic right ventricular dysplasia. *Eur Heart J* 1989;**10**(Suppl. D):54–60.

78. Canciani B, Nava A, Martini B, Buja GF, Thiene G. Signal-averaged electrocardiography in arrhythmogenic right ventricular cardiomyopathy (arrhythmogenic right ventricular dysplasia). *Proceedings of the 10th International Congress "The New Frontiers of Arrhythmias"*, Marilleva, Italy, 1992, pp, 513–17.

79. Leclercq JF, Coumel P. Late potentials in arrhythmogenic right ventricular dysplasia. Prevalence, diagnostic and prognostic values. *Eur Heart J* 1993;**14**(Suppl. E):80–3.

80. Wichter T, Hindricks G, Lerch H *et al*. Regional myocardial sympathetic dysinnervation in arrhythmogenic right ventricular cardiomyopathy. An analysis using ^{123}I-meta-iodobenzylguanidine scintigraphy. *Circulation* 1994;**89**:667–83.

81. Oselladore L, Nava A, Buja G *et al*. Signal-averaged electrocardiography in familial form of arrhythmogenic right ventricular cardiomyopathy. *Am J Cardiol* 1995;**75**:1038–41.

82. Mehta D, Goldman M, David O, Gomes JA. Value of quantitative measurement of signal-averaged electrocardiographic variables in arrhythmogenic right ventricular dysplasia: Correlation with echocardiographic right ventricular cavity dimensions. *J Am Coll Cardiol* 1996;**28**:713–19.

83. Poll D, Marchlinski FE, Falcone RA, Josephson ME, Simson MB. Abnormal signal-averaged electrocardiograms in patients with non-ischemic congestive cardiomyopathy: relationship to sustained ventricular tachycardia. *Circulation* 1985:**6**:1308–13.

84. Denereaz D, Zimmerman M, Adamec R. Significance of ventricular late potentials in non-ischaemic dilated cardiomyopathy. *Eur Heart J* 1992;**13**:895–901.

85. Keeling PJ, Kulakowski P, Gang Z, Slade AKB, Bent S, McKenna WJ. Usefulness of signal-averaged electrocardiogram in idiopathic dilated cardiomyopathy for identifying patients with ventricular arrhythmias. *Am J Cardiol* 1993;**72**:78–84.

86. Mancini DM, Wong KL, Simson MB. Prognostic value of an abnormal signal-averaged electrocardiogram in patients with non-ischemic congestive cardiomyopathy. *Circulation* 1993;**87**:1083–92.

87. Turitto G, Ahuja RK, Caref EB, El-Sherif N. Risk stratification for arrhythmic events in patients with non-ischemic dilated cardiomyopathy and non-sustained ventricular tachycardia: role of programmed ventricular stimulation and the signal-averaged electrocardiogram. *J Am Coll Cardiol* 1994;**24**:1523–8.

88. Grimm W, Hoffman J, Knop U, Winzenburg J, Menz V, Maisch B. Value of time- and frequency-domain analysis of signal-averaged electrocardiography for arrhythmia risk prediction in idiopathic dilated cardiomyopathy. *PACE* 1996;**19**(Pt II):1923–7.

89. Yamada T, Fukunami M, Ohmori M. New approach to the estimation of the extent of myocardial fibrosis in patients with dilated cardiomyopathy: use of signal-averaged electrocardiography. *Am Heart J* 1993;**126**:626–31.

90. Gang Yi, Keeling PJ, Hnatkova K, Goldman JH, Malik M, McKenna WJ. Usefulness of signal-averaged electrocardiography in evaluation of idiopathic-dilated cardiomyopathy in families. *Am J Cardiol* 1997;**79**:1203–7.

91. Cripps TR, Counihan PJ, Frenneaux MP, Ward DE, Camm AJ, McKenna WJ. Signal-averaged electrocardiography in hypertrophic cardiomyopathy. *J Am Coll Cardiol* 1990;**15**:956–61.

92. Kulakowski P, Counihan PJ, Camm AJ, McKenna WJ. The value of time and frequency domain, and spectral temporal mapping analysis of the signal-averaged electrocardiogram in identification of patients with hypertrophic cardiomyopathy at increased risk of sudden death. *Eur Heart J* 1993;**14**:941–50.

93. Mehta D, McKenna WJ, Ward DE, Davies MJ, Camm AJ. Significance of signal-averaged electrocardiography in relation to endomyocardial biopsy and ventricular stimulation studies in patients with ventricular tachycardia without clinically apparent heart disease. *J Am Coll Cardiol* 1989;**14**:372–9.

94. Kulakowski P, Gill J, Camm AJ. Signal-averaged electrocardiography in patients with ventricular tachycardia and no structural heart disease. In: Gomes AJ ed. *Signal-averaged electrocardiography. Concepts, methods and applications. Part IV. The signal-averaged ECG in patients with sustained ventricular tachycardia and no evidence of heart disease.* Dordrecht, Boston, London: Kluwer Academic Publishers, 1993, pp. 345–64.

95. La Vecchia L, Ometto R, Bedogni F *et al*. Ventricular late potentials, interstitial fibrosis, and right ventricular function in patients with ventricular tachycardia and normal left ventricular function. *Am J Cardiol* 1998;**81**:790–2

96. Leclercq JF, Denjoy I, Coumel P, Slama R. Signification of late potentials in patients with ventricular arrhythmias and apparently normal heart. *Proceedings of the 10th International Congress "The New Frontiers of Arrhyhmias"*, Marilleva, Italy, 1992, pp. 735–9.

97. Zimmermann M, Friedli B, Adamec R, Oberhansli I. Ventricular late potentials and induced ventricular arrhythmias after surgical repair of tetralogy of Fallot. *Am J Cardiol* 1991;**67**:873–8.

98. Vaksmann G, El Kohen M, Lacroix D *et al*. Influence of clinical and hemodynamic characteristics on signal-averaged electrocardiogram in postoperative tetralogy of Fallot. *Am J Cardiol* 1993;**71**:317–21.

99. Moser D, Stevenson WG, Woo MA *et al*. Frequency of late potentials in systemic sclerosis. *Am J Cardiol* 1991;**67**:541–3.

100. Baciarello G, Villani M, Di Maio F, Sciacca A. Late surface potentials in myotonic dystrophy with ventricular tachycardia. *Am Heart J* 1986;**111**:413–14.

101. Kubo M, Matsuoka S, Hayabuchi Y, Akita H, Matsuka Y, Kuroda Y. Abnormal signal-averaged electrocardiogram in patients with Duchenne muscular dystrophy: comparison of time and frequency domain analyses from the signal-averaged electrocardiogram. *Clin Cardiol* 1993;**16**:723–8.

102. Dubrey SW, Bilazarian S, LaValley M, Reisinger J, Skinner M, Falk RH. Signal-averaged electrocardiography in patients with AL (primary) amyloidosis. *Am Heart J* 1997;**134**:994–1001.

103. Kuchar DL, Thorburn CW, Sammel NL. Signal averaged electrocardiogram for evaluation of recurrent syncope. *Am J Cardiol* 1986;**58**:949–53.

104. Gang ES, Peter T, Rosenthal ME, Mandel WJ, Lass Z. Detection of late potentials on the surface electrocardiogram in unexplained syncope. *Am J Cardiol* 1986;**58**:1014–20.

105. Winters SL, Steward D, Gomes JA. Signal averaging of the surface QRS complex predicts inducibility of ventricular tachycardia in patients with syncope of unknown origin: a prospective study. *J Am Coll Cardiol* 1987;**10**:775–81.

106. Steinberg JS, Prystowsky E, Freedman RA *et al*. Use of the signal-averaged electrocardiogram for predicting inducible ventricular tachycardia in patients with unexplained syncope: relation to clinical variables in a multivariate analysis. *J Am Coll Cardiol* 1994;**23**:99–106.

107. Lindsay BD, Osborn JL, Schechtman KB, Kenzora JL, Ambos HD, Cain ME. Prospective detection of vulnerability to sustained ventricular tachycardia in patients awaiting cardiac transplantation. *Am J Cardiol* 1992;**69**:619–24.

108. Keren A, Gillis AM, Friedmann RA *et al*. Heart transplant rejection monitored by signal-averaged electrocardiography in patients receiving cyclosporine. *Circulation* 1984:**70**(Suppl. I):124–9.

109. Haberl R, Weber M, Reichenspurner H *et al*. Frequency analysis of the surface electrocardiogram for recognition of acute rejection after orthopic cardiac transplantation in man. *Circulation* 1987;**76**:101–8.

110. Lacroix D, Kacet S, Savard P *et al*. Signal-averaged electrocardiography and detection of heart transplant rejection: comparison of time and frequency domain analyses. *J Am Coll Cardiol* 1992;**19**:553–8.

111. Hood MA, Pogwizd SW, Peirick J, Cain ME. Contribution of myocardium responsible for ventricular tachycardia to abnormalities detected by analysis of signal-averaged electrocardiograms. *Circulation* 1992;**86**:1888–901.

112. Meeder RJJ, Stroink G, Ritcey SP, Gardner MJ, Horacek BM. Low-frequency component of body surface potential maps identifies patients at risk for ventricular tachycardia. *Eur Heart J* 1999;**20**:1126–34.

15 Signal averaged P wave

Antonio Michelucci, Luigi Padeletti, Andrea Colella, Maria Cristina Porciani, Paolo Pieragnoli, Alessandro Costoli and Gian Franco Gensini

The only means at our disposal for interpreting nature are daring ideas, unjustifiable anticipations, and unfounded speculations: they are the only tool, the only instruments that are available to us. And in order to earn our prize we must dare to use them.

Karl R. Popper

P wave signal-averaging represents an important contribution to the field of non-invasive electrocardiology. The improvements in the methodology concerning the recording and the analysis of the atrial depolarisation,[1-3] have led to the widespread use of this test in clinical settings, especially to study patients with atrial fibrillation. This would be desirable considering that this arrhythmia still today represents a great challenge for physicians.[4-7] Yet, despite a considerable body of research, the signal-averaged P wave has not been so far accepted into clinical practice. However, new attempts to refine this technique and other studies concerning its clinical applications have been performed. Namely, adoption of new parameters[8,9] and a more sophisticated usation of the older measurements[10,11] have led to a more comprehensive knowledge of the potential utilisations of this technique. Recent data suggest that the signal-averaged P wave might ultimately find a clinical role, not only as a diagnostic test for atrial fibrillation, but also as an adjunct to its management and an investigational tool that helps to advance our understanding of the arrhythmia in humans. Obviously it is necessary to know what information can be provided by this test in order to define its role in diagnostic and therapeutic procedures. The aim of this paper is to highlight technical and clinical aspects of P wave signal averaging.

Technical aspects

The P wave has an amplitude smaller than that of the QRS complex because the atria have a mass smaller than that of the ventricles. Thus, devices used for P wave must be able to amplify signal more than those for QRS complex. Therefore resolution should be at least 1 µV. Signal averaging technique is based on the exclusion of all that is not repeatable ("noise")[12] (Fig. 15.1). To reach this goal, first, the skin at the site of lead attachment must be abraded to decrease impedance, which generates noise. Second, silver/silver-chloride electrodes should be used because the low half-cell potential also reduces noise. Finally, the signal-averaging process allows a further reduction of noise, which, however, is not complete.[13] An acceptable final noise level should be less than 0.5 µ V.[1,2,14]

Three bipolar orthogonal leads have been generally used for P wave signal averaging[1,2,14-18] (Fig. 15.2). Some innovations have been introduced for P wave signal averaging (Fig. 15.3). Currently it is possible to trigger on the P wave.[1,2,18] Previously, only QRS complex could be used as a trigger and, because of the variability of the PR interval, it was impossible to obtain an optimal alignment of P waves.[1,3] A correct alignment is very important in order to avoid an erroneous evaluation of the P wave duration[1] and presumably a distortion of frequency spectrum. During P wave triggering it is necessary to sample only the desired electrocardiographic signal. For example, in order to record only sinus P waves, it is necessary to exclude atrial ectopic beats, P wave with excessive noise, and T waves.[1,2,18] This is possible by using the "template comparing method" (Fig. 15.4). The latter allows the establishment at the beginning of averaging which wave form must be sampled. So any other wave with characteristics different from those initially defined is excluded. Softwares that contain both P wave triggering and template comparing method are now commercially available[1,2,18] and thus available in clinical settings.

- Pre-existing noise
- Abrasion of skin
- Silver/silver-chloride electrodes
- Number of averaged beats

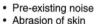

Final noise level

Figure 15.1 Factors involved in the determination of the final noise level during P wave signal-averaging process

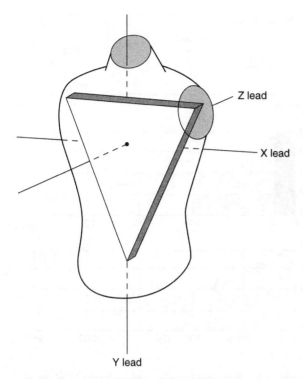

Figure 15.2 Axes of the three orthogonal leads generally used for P wave signal-averaging. X, Y, and Z leads cover horizontal, frontal, and sagittal planes respectively.

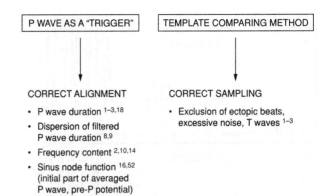

Figure 15.3 Techniques adopted for P wave signal-averaging: P wave triggering and template comparing method. Advantages of these techniques are reported

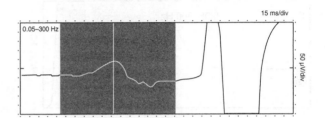

Figure 15.4 Example of a sinus wave used as a trigger during P wave signal-averaging. The black area contains the signal used as a template to obtain better signal alignment and to exclude ectopic atrial beats or T waves.

Averaged P wave can be analysed in the time and frequency domains. By time-domain analysis it is possible to analyse a single lead or, as it was done for QRS complex,[19] vectorial sum of signals recorded by the three ortogonal leads[1,2,17,18] (Fig. 15.5). It is possible to measure amplitude (μV) and duration (ms) of the averaged signal. Evaluation is performed after having filtered the ECG signal.[1,2] The high pass filter should not be less than 40 Hz in order to obtain a clear separation between P and QRS (Figure 15.5). One study[20] evaluated whether the use of different filterings is diagnostically equivalent. P wave duration proved to be longer in patients with paroxysmal atrial fibrillation for all filters and cut-off frequencies studied. The authors, however, underscored that the normality limits derived from one filter cannot be applied directly to recordings obtained from the other filters.

Frequency-domain analysis has been used as an alternative to time-domain analysis[2,14,21] (Fig. 15.6). Devices must sample a signal with a frequency content (0.05–300 Hz) larger than that included in conventional ECG. Frequency analysis generally uses the Fast Fourier Transform method.[2,14,21] The magnitude versus frequency plot curves can be obtained. The magnitude can be given in db or in μV (Fig. 15.6). Some authors[14] performed frequency analysis using only one of the three bipolar orthogonal leads (i.e. that on the sagittal plane), and a 100 ms segment from 75 ms before to 25 ms after the end of the P wave. Using only one lead does not seem justified considering that differences between patients with paroxysmal atrial fibrillation and age-matched normal subjects were observed in more than one orthogonal lead.[2] Thus it seems justified to analyse all orthogonal leads to improve the diagnostic power of this method.[2] Evaluation of a 100 ms segment from 75 ms before to 25 ms after the end of P wave could also be incorrect because, in this way, the frequency components of His bundle are included in the analysed signal. Moreover, the use of only the last 75 ms is known to lead to the exclusion of right atrial components.[22] So, structural changes frequently observed in patients with paroxysmal atrial fibrillation are localised also in the right atrial myocardium[23] as suggested indirectly also by endocavitary studies[24] So on the basis of accumulated experience,[2,11,21] analysis on the entire P wave should be preferred. It does appear useful to evaluate also the diagnostic power of total frequency content of P wave (sum of the three orthogonal leads). This parameter, in fact, has been used with encouraging results for identification of patients at risk of relapse after electrical cardioversion.[10]

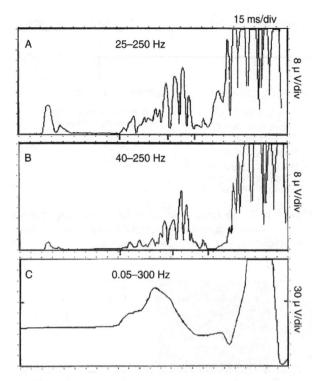

Figure 15.5 Examples (panel A and B) of the averaged P wave analysed in the form of a composite vector, calculated from the three bipolar orthogonal leads combined by the formula $(x^2 + y^2 + z^2)^{\frac{1}{2}}$. The range of frequencies in panel A is between 25 and 250 Hz, and in panel B between 40 and 250 Hz. It is evident in panel B how the use of 40 Hz as a high-pass filter allows a clear separation between the atrial and ventricular waves. In this way a correct analysis of the final part of P wave is possible. Morphology of unfiltered (0.05–300 Hz) averaged P wave recorded on sagittal plane is reported in panel C.

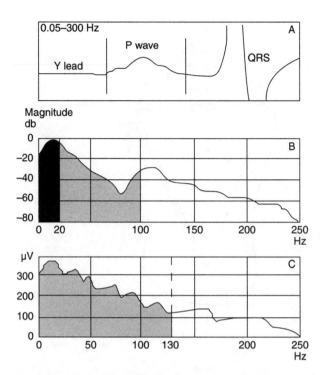

Figure 15.6 Representative recording (panel A) of the signal-averaged non-filtered (0.05–300 Hz) P wave, of one of the three orthogonal leads (Y lead), obtained from a normal volunteer. The two vertical lines (panel A) delimit the entire P wave which should be used for frequency analysis. Then the magnitude versus frequency plot curves can be obtained. The magnitude can be given in db (panel B) or in μV (panel C). The black and grey areas under the curves have been used to evaluate P wave frequency content in each lead. All the components of the signal with a frequency higher than 130–150 Hz have not been used, because a high incidence of noise can be present.

Reproducibility of signal-averaged P wave measurements

The parameter that showed the best reproducibility was the signal-averaged P wave duration.[25–28] Other parameters have been rejected because of poor reproducibility. It should be underscored that frequency analysis might suffer from reproducibility. It has been suggested that this could be due more to spontaneous variation in P wave morphology than to inconsistencies in the P wave averaging system.[29] Thus a correct application of the recording method can contribute significantly to minimising the extent of variation between recording pairs. On the other hand, it is possible that total P wave frequency content (sum of all leads) does not vary, even when P wave morphology changes, allowing a good reproducibility.

Correlation with endocavitary recordings

Some studies[30,31] confirmed the relationship between signal-averaged P wave and atrial conduction delay. Moreover, a link between inducibility of atrial fibrillation and P wave duration has been observed.[32] This is noteworthy considering that only endocavitary electrophysiological studies have been used to show atrial vulnerability.[33]

Clinical results

A number of studies used P wave signal-averaging suggesting the possible present and future indications for this technique (Box 15.1). A significantly longer duration of averaged P wave was observed in patients with paroxysmal

Box 15.1 Possible present and future indications for P wave signal-averaged ECG

- Identification of atrial fibrillation risk
  - coronary bypass surgery[18,37–41]
  - hypertrophic cardiomyopathy[44]
  - congestive heart failure[46]
  - mitral valve prolapse[45]
  - hyperthyroidism[43]
  - arterial hypertension*
  - valvular heart disease*
  - stroke of unknown aetiology*
- Management of patients with already documented atrial fibrillation
  - prediction of relapse after electrical cardioversion[10,11,53,55]
  - evaluation of antiarrhythmic drug efficacy[8,9]
  - identification of a coexistent sinus node dysfunction[16,52]
  - prediction of transition to chronic atrial fibrillation[50]

*Still not evaluated

atrial fibrillation.[1,2,18] Thus this parameter has been advocated in order to prospectively identify patients at risk of this arrhythmia. The 40 Hz high-pass filter showed the best predictive accuracy.[1] Even the root mean square voltage of the terminal segment of averaged P wave has been evaluated. However, conflicting data exist regarding the value of this parameter. In fact, Fukunami et al.[1] have noted that patients with paroxysmal atrial fibrillation had significantly lower voltage in the terminal 10- and 20-ms segments of the vector P wave signal. On the contrary another study[2] has shown that the voltage of terminal 10, 20, 30, and 40 ms of the composite vector P wave did not differ between patients with and without paroxysmal atrial fibrillation. A different age of patients and non-comparable orthogonal leads are likely to explain the different results. Other authors[17,34] have defined additional parameters reporting inconsistent results. In conclusion, it is apparent that the total P wave duration provides the most consistent data. Frequency-domain analysis proved to be useful in identifying patients with high frequency of atrial fibrillation attacks.[2] The frequency content of patients with high frequency of attacks proved to be significantly greater than that of patients with low frequency of attacks. This result is remarkable considering that a possible link between high frequency of atrial fibrillation attacks and higher embolic risk has been suggested.[35,36]

Up to now the most extensive clinical evaluation has been performed in patients undergoing coronary bypass surgery in whom the incidence of atrial fibrillation during the post-surgical period is particularly high (30–50% of cases).[18,29,37–41] The signal-averaged P wave duration emerged as the most potent independent predictor of postoperative atrial fibrillation. The clinical value of the P wave signal-averaging needs to be confirmed in other populations. Suitable candidates include patients with valvular heart disease, arterial hypertension, hyperthyroidism, coronary artery disease, hypertrophic cardiomyopathy, and mitral valve prolapse, especially when heart failure is present.[42–46] Even patients with sinus node dysfunction are at high risk owing to the increased incidence of thromboembolic complications secondary to atrial tachyarrhythmias.[35,47] Finally, even patients with stroke of unknown aetiology (cryptogenic stroke) should be analysed considering that atrial fibrillation is the principal cause of cerebral emboli of cardiac origin.[33] It would be very useful to plan prospective studies in these populations also, because an extensive evaluation of the influence of age,[2] autonomic manipulations,[27] and atrial volume[2,48] on the length and the frequency content of signal-averaged P wave have not been performed. Interestingly, there are studies that examined the influence of coexistent organic heart disease.[18,49,50] Frequency analysis appeared able to differentiate patients with paroxysmal atrial fibrillation from those without arrhythmia, irrespective of the presence of organic heart disease. Instead, time domain analysis appeared able to differentiate only when patients and control group were matched for the prevalence of organic heart disease.

One study[51] analysed the influence of gender. P wave duration was prolonged in patients with paroxysmal atrial fibrillation, but less in women than in men. Thus it was observed that, even with the use of gender-specific values, signal-averaged P wave has a lower sensitivity in women. Two original recent studies[8,9] have suggested that the peculiar atrial electrophysiologic substrate of patients with paroxysmal atrial fibrillation might be reflected on the spatial dispersion of signal-averaged P wave duration on the precordial body surface. They compared results obtained by averaging unipolar P waves recorded from 16 precordial positions with those obtained by P wave duration recorded using the standard vector technique. Results showed that spatial dispersion of signal-averaged P wave would improve the detectability of paroxysmal atrial fibrillation patients.

Usefulness in patients with recent atrial fibrillation

Abe et al.[50] indicated that P wave signal-averaging could be useful to identify patients at risk for the transition from the paroxysmal to the chronic form of atrial fibrillation. Yamada et al.[52] reported that the presence of sinus node dysfunction in patients with paroxysmal atrial fibrillation was detectable. The study was accomplished measuring the root mean square voltage for the initial 30 ms and the duration of initial low amplitude signals of filtered P wave in the vector magnitude. In this regard it should be stressed that a different range of frequencies (0.05–25 Hz) has been used for evaluating sinus node function.[16] This should allow a non-invasive recording of sinus node activity and possibly an evaluation of sinoatrial conduction.

However the main clinical applications of P wave signal-averaging for atrial fibrillation management have been done in two important clinical settings: prediction of relapse after electrical cardioversion and evaluation of antiarrhytmic drug efficacy. Results concerning these two topics are reported in the following paragraphs.

Prediction of relapse after electrical cardioversion

P wave duration proved to be significantly longer in patients with relapse than in patients who maintained sinus rhythm.[53,54] Previous studies evaluated prediction of relapse independently of the time of occurrence. More recently two studies[10,11] have analysed the role of time and frequency domain parameters in predicting early relapse (defined as the reappearance of atrial fibrillation in the first days after cardioversion). The possibility of predicting early relapse is important given that, if properly identified, these are the patients who need prevention immediately after cardioversion. Averaged P wave duration was not different in patients with or without early relapse. Instead, frequency analysis was able to identify patients with early appearance of the arrhythmia. Some aspects of these studies should be emphasised. In one study,[10] total frequency content of P wave, as the sum of the three orthogonal leads, proved to be significantly higher in patients with early relapse. In the other study,[11] P wave frequency content of patients, who remained in sinus rhythm for at least 1 week, showed a fall within the first 24 hours. These results justify further studies in order to assess the real clinical value of the adopted parameters.

Evaluation of antiarrhythmic drugs effects

It has been suggested that P wave signal-averaging is useful for studying drug-induced changes in atrial electrophysiology.[15,55] Recently a new signal-averaging P wave mapping system, which uses 16 unipolar anterior chest leads, has been developed.[8,9] Averaged signals were used to measure P wave dispersion as the difference between the maximal and minimal P wave duration. Dispersion decreased significantly after a single administration of an antiarrhytmic agent in all patients without atrial fibrillation recurrence, in comparison to those with recurrence. Thus it has been suggested that drug efficacy can be predicted by the change in dispersion with a single oral dose. It should be emphasised that in these studies changes in P

wave duration were not different between patients with and without recurrence. These initial data are encouraging and suggest that signal-averaged P wave might ultimately find a clinical role for management of patients with paroxysmal atrial fibrillation.

References

1. Fukunami M, Yamada T, Ohmori M *et al*. Detection of patients at risk of paroxysmal atrial fibrillation during sinus rhythm by P wave-triggered signal-averaged electrocardiogram. *Circulation* 1991;**83**:162–9.
2. Michelucci A, Padeletti L, Chelucci A *et al*. Influence of age, lead axis, frequency of arrhythmic episodes, and atrial dimensions on P wave triggered SAECG in patients with lone paroxysmal atrial fibrillation. *Pacing Clin Electrophysiol* 1996;**19**:758–67.
3. Barbaro V, Bartolini P, Fierli M. New algorithm for the detection of the ECG fiducial point in the averaging technique. *Med Biol Eng Comput* 1991;**29**:129–35.
4. Bialy D, Lehmann MH, Schumaker DN, Steinman RT, Meissmer MD. Hospitalization for arrhythmias in the United States: importance of atrial fibrillation. *J Am Coll Cardiol* 1992;**19**:A41.
5. Lip GYH, Beevers G. ABC of atrial fibrillation: history, epidemiology and importance of atrial fibrillation. *BMJ* 1995;**311**:1361–3.
6. EAFT Study Group. Silent brain infarction in non-rheumathic atrial fibrillation. *Neurology* 1996;**46**:159–65.
7. Lip GYH, Beevers DG, Singh SP, Watson RDS. ABC of atrial fibrillation. Aetiology, pathophysiology, and clinical features. *BMJ* 1995;**311**:1425–8.
8. Kubara I, Ikeda H, Hiraki T, Yoshida T, Ohga M, Imaizumi T. Dispersion of filtered P wave duration by P wave signal-averaged ECG mapping system. *J Cardiovasc Electrophysiol* 1999;**10**:670–9.
9. Yamada T, Fukunami M, Shimonagata T *et al*. Dispersion of signal-averaged P wave duration on precordial body surface in patients with paroxysmal atrial fibrillation. *Eur Heart J* 1999:**20**:211–20.
10. Michelucci A, Padeletti L, Porciani MC *et al*. Prediction of early atrial fibrillation relapse after endocavitary electrical cardioversion by frequency analysis of signal averaged P wave. *G Ital Cardiol* 1998,**28**:440–2.
11. Stafford PJ, Kamalvand K, Tan K, Vincent R, Sulke N. Prediction of maintenance of sinus rhythm after cardioversion of atrial fibrillation by analysis of serial signal-averaged P waves. *Pacing Clin Electrophysiol* 1998:**21**:1387–95.
12. Michelucci A, Padeletti L, Chelucci A *et al*. P wave signal-averaging: technical aspects and clinical usefulness. In: Santini M ed. *Progress in clinical pacing*. Armonk, NY: Futura Media Services, 1995, pp. 29–58.
13. Berbari EJ, Lander P. Principles of noise reduction. In: El-Sherif N, Turitto G eds. *High resolution electrocardiography*. Mount Kisco, NY: Futura Publishing Co., 1992, pp. 51–66.
14. Yamada T, Fukunami M, Ohmori M *et al*. Characteristics of frequency content of atrial signal-averaged electrocardio-

grams during sinus rhythm in patients with paroxysmal atrial fibrillation. *J Am Coll Cardiol* 1992;**19**:559–63.

15. Michelucci A, Padeletti L, Porciani M C, Gensini G F. P wave signal-averaging. *Card Electrophysiol Rev* 1997;**3**:325–28.

16. Michelucci A, Toso A, Mezzani A *et al*. Non-invasive recording of sinus node activity by P wave-triggered signal-averaged electrocardiogram: validation using direct intra-atrial recording of sinus node electrogram. *Am J Non-Inv Cardiol* 1993;**7**:132–7.

17. Stafford PJ, Turner I, Vincent R. Quantitative analysis of signal-averaged P waves in idiopathic paroxysmal atrial fibrillation. *Am J Cardiol* 1991;**68**:751–5.

18. Klein M, Evans SJL, Blumberg S, Cataldo L, Bodenheimer MM. Use of P wave-triggered, P wave signal-averaged electrocardiogram to predict atrial fibrillation after coronary artery bypass surgery. *Am Heart J* 1995;**129**:895–901.

19. Simson MB. Use of signals in the terminal QRS complex to identify patients with ventricular tachycardia after myocardial infarction. *Circulation* 1981;**64**:235–42.

20. Valverde ER, Quinteiro RA, Bertrand GC, Arini PD, Glenny P, Biagetti MO. Influence of filtering techniques on the time-domain analysis of signal-averaged P wave electrocardiogram. *J Cardiovasc Electrophysiol* 1998;**9**:253–60.

21. Stafford P, Denbigh P, Vincent R. Frequency analysis of the P wave: comparative techniques. *Pacing Clin Electrophysiol* 1995;**18**:261–70.

22. Puech P. P wave morphology. *Ann NY Acad Sci* 1990;**601**:1–23.

23. Bharati S, Lev M. Histology of the normal and diseased atrium. In: Falk RH, Podrid PJ eds. *Atrial fibrillation: mechanisms and management*. New York: Raven Press Ltd., 1992, pp. 15–39.

24. Michelucci A, Padeletti L, Porciani MC *et al*. Dispersion of refractoriness and atrial fibrillation. In: Olsson SB, Allessie MA, Campbell RWF eds. *Atrial fibrillation: mechanisms and therapeutic strategies*. Armonk, NY: Futura Publishing, 1994, pp. 81–107.

25. Stafford PJ, Cooper J, Clifford J, Garrat DM. Reproducibility of the signal averaged P wave. *Pacing Clin Electrophysiol* 1996;**19**:586.

26. Steinberg JS, Ehlert FA, Menchavez-Tan E. Immediate and short term reproducibility of the P wave signal-averaged electrocardiogram. *J Am Coll Cardiol* 1994;Feb:252A.

27. Cheema AN, Ahgmed MW, Kadish AH, Goldberger JJ. Effects of autonomic stimulation and blockade on signal-averaged P wave duration. *J Am Coll Cardiol* 1995;**26**:497–502.

28. Villani CQ, Rosi A, Aschieri D, Passerini F, Capucci A. Reproducibility of the P wave averaged ECG parameters in patients with paroxysmal atrial fibrillation. *New Trends Arrhyth* 1996;**XI**:310–11.

29. Stafford PJ, Cooper J, Fothergill J, Schlindwein F, deBono DP, Garrant CJ. Reproducibility of the signal-averaged P wave: time and frequency domain analysis. *Heart* 1997;**77**:412–16.

30. Michelucci A, Padeletti L, Chelucci A *et al*. Relationship between P wave signal-averaging and atrial conduction delay or dispersion of atrial refractoriness. *Pacing Clin Electrophysiol* 1995;**18**:1109.

31. Pellerin D, Attuel P, Davy JM, Slama M, Mottè G. Evaluation of signal-averaged P wave in patients with and without history of atrial arrhythmias. Comparison with ECG and electrophysiological study. *Eur Heart J* 1991;**12**:278.

32. Gencel L, Poquet F, Gosse P, Haissaguerre M, Marcus FI, Clementy J. Correlation of signal-averaged P wave with electrophysiological testing for atrial vulnerability in strokes of unexplained etiology. *Pacing Clin Electrophysiol* 1994;**17**:2118–24.

33. Attuel P, Rancurel G, Delgatte B *et al*. Importance of atrial electrophysiology in the work-up of cerebral ischemic attacks. *Pacing Clin Electrophysiol* 1986;**9**:1121–6.

34. Paylos JM, Cardero B, Lopez de Sa' E *et al*. Spectral temporal mapping of the P wave in subjects with and without paroxysmal atrial fibrillation. *J Am Coll Cardiol* 1993;**21**:181A.

35. Fairfax A, Lambert C, Leatham A. Systemic embolism in chronic sinoatrial disorder. *New Engl J Med* 1976;**295**:190–2.

36. Barold S, Santini M. Natural history of sick sinus syndrome after pacemaker implantation. In: Barold S, Mugica J eds. *New perspectives in cardiac pacing. III.* Mount Kisco, NY: Futura Publishing Co., 1993, pp. 169–81.

37. Stafford PJ, Kolvekar S, Cooper J, Spyt TJ, Garrat CJ. The preoperative signal-averaged P wave compared to clinical, standard electrocardiographic or echocardiographic variables for prediction of atrial fibrillation after coronary bypass grafting. *Eur Heart J* 1996;**17**:124.

38. Steinberg JS, Zelenkofske S, Wong S-C, Gelernt M, Sciacca R, Menchavez E. Value of the P wave signal-averaged ECG for prediction of atrial fibrillation after cardiac surgery. *Circulation* 1993;**88**:2618–22.

39. Chelucci A, Michelucci A, Padeletti L *et al*. Multiparametric evaluation of risk of atrial fibrillation following coronary artery bypass surgery. *New Trends Arrhyth* 1995;**XI**:239–40.

40. Dimmer C, Jordaens L, Gorgov N *et al*. Analysis of the P wave with signal averaging to assess the risk of atrial fibrillation after coronary artery bypass surgery. *Cardiology* 1998;**89**:19–24.

41. Zaman AG, Alamgir F, Richens T, Williams R, Rothman MT, Mills PG. The role of signal averaged P wave duration and serum magnesium as a combined predictor of atrial fibrillation after elective coronary artery bypass surgery. *Heart* 1997;**77**:527–31.

42. Krahn AD, Manfreda J, Tate RB, Mathewson FAL, Cuddy TE. The natural history of atrial fibrillation: incidence, risk factors, and prognosis in the Manitoba follow-up study. *Am J Med* 1995;**98**:476–84.

43. Montereggi A, Marconi P, Olivotto I *et al*. Signal-averaged P wave duration and risk of paroxysmal atrial fibrillation in hyperthyroidism. *Am J Cardiol* 1996;**77**:266–9.

44. Cecchi F, Montereggi A, Olivotto I, Marconi P, Dolara A, Maron B J. Risk of atrial fibrillation in patients with hypertrophic cardiomyopathy assessed by signal averaged P wave duration. *Heart* 1997;**78**:44–9.

45. Pierog M, Banasiak W, Telichowski A *et al*. Significance of atrial signal-averaged electrocardiogram in diagnosis of

paroxysmal atrial fibrillation in patients with mitral valve prolapse syndrome. *Pol Arch Med Wewn* 1997;**97**:232–8.

46. Yamada T, Fukunami M, Shimonagata T *et al*. Prediction of paroxysmal atrial fibrillation in patients with congestive heart failure by P wave signal-averaged ECG: a prospective study. *Circulation* 1998;**98**:I-441.

47. Lip GYH, Lowe GDO. ABC of atrial fibrillation: Antithrombotic treatment for atrial fibrillation. *BMJ* 1996;**312**:45–9.

48. Vainer J, Cheriex EC, Van Der Steld B, Dassen WRM, Smeets JLRM, Wellens HJJ. Effects of acute volume changes on P wave characteristics: correlation with echocardiographic findings in healthy men. *J Cardiovasc Electrophysiol* 1994;**5**:999–1005.

49. Abe Y, Fukunami M, Ohmori M *et al*. Prognostic significance of P wave triggered signal-averaged electrocardiograms in predicting paroxysmal atrial fibrillation: a prospective study. *Circulation* 1993;**88**:I-312.

50. Abe Y, Fukunami M, Yamada T *et al*. Prediction of transition to chronic atrial fibrillation in patients with paroxysmal atrial fibrillation by signal-averaged electrocardiography. A prospective study. *Circulation* 1997;**96**:2612–16.

51. Dhala A, Underwood D, Madu E, Angel J and the Multicenter P HiRes Study. Sex-specific differences in the P wave signal-averaged ECG. Multicenter P HiRes Study. *J Electrocardiol* 1998;**30**:34–5.

52. Yamada T, Fukunami M, Shimonagata T *et al*. Identification of the involvement of sinus node dysfunction in patients with paroxysmal atrial fibrillation by atrial early potentials. *J Am Coll Cardiol* 1999;**33**:143A.

53. Opolski G, Scislo P, Stanislawska J, Gorecki A, Steckiewicz R, Torbicki A. Detection of patients at risk for recurrence of atrial fibrillation after successful electrical cardioversion by signal-averaged P wave ECG. *Int J Cardiol* 1997;**60**:181–5.

54. Ansalone G, Magris B, Auriti G *et al*. Signal-averaged P wave after cardioversion for atrial fibrillation and probability of relapses. *Eur Heart J* 1996;**17**:393.

55. Banasiak W, Telichowski A, Anker S D *et al*. Effects of amiodarone on the P wave triggered signal-averaged electrocardiogram in patients with paroxysmal atrial fibrillation and coronary artery disease. *Am J Cardiol* 1999;**83**:112–14.

16 Non-invasive investigation of Wedensky modulation

Katerina Hnatkova and Marek Malik

Various mechanisms may temporarily improve the depressed state of cardiac conductivity. These include the supernormal phase, Wedensky facilitation, Wedensky effect, and Wedensky inhibition. The Wedensky phenomena were originally described in nervous fibres. However, the evidence is accumulating for their existence in the cardiac tissue. The phenomena appear to play a role, the magnitude of which remains to be defined, in the genesis of some of the clinical arrhythmias. The role of Wedensky phenomena supports the concept that some ectopic rhythms can appear due to a local change in excitability rather than conductivity (re-entry). This not only determines a dependency of some ectopic centres on a dominant impulse but also defines one possible mechanism of such dependency.

Having this in mind, we have compiled this text to describe the essence of Wedensky phenomena and to introduce a possibility of investigating them non-invasively in the human heart.

Supernormal phase

The supernormal phase of conductivity is a very short period of paradoxically improved conduction that may occur during the absolute, or more rarely, relative refractory period. The situation is paradoxical because conduction only occurs during a short critical period, while both earlier and later impulses are either blocked or have a much greater conduction delay. The term is somewhat misleading as the conduction is not supernormal but merely a temporarily improved from a depressed state. The supernormal phase does not occur in the normal heart but only when conductivity is depressed.[1] It lasts only a few tens of milliseconds.[1] The position in the cardiac cycle usually coincides with the U wave or the distal limb of the T wave.

Thus, the supernormal phase of excitability is a brief interval, usually near the end of the T wave, during which a stimulus that is otherwise too weak to evoke a response may do so.

Wedensky effect

In 1886, Wedensky[2] described a relatively long enhancing effect that followed the application of maximal shock or stimulus to a neuromuscular preparation. A sub-threshold stimulus, too small to evoke a response, could do so if preceded by a suprathreshold shock. The phenomenon is graphically illustrated in Fig. 16.1. Wedensky attributed this phenomenon to a relatively prolonged lowered threshold of excitability following the maximum shock. This observation, found in neuromuscular preparation of frogs, was confirmed by other investigators and is termed the "Wedensky effect". In 1930, Samojloff[3] made the observation that the activating effect of a single induction shock lasts a considerable time, with low rates of sub-threshold stimulation for up to 0.5 s, which considerably exceed the duration of supernormal phase.

Goldenberg and Rothberger[4] confirmed the Wedensky effect in excised dog Purkinje fibres. If sub-threshold discharges were used, a single induction shock so lowered the threshold that long groups of 1:1 responses followed. Spontaneous automatic beats had the same activating effect. Applying these findings to clinical ectopic arrhythmias, Goldenberg and Rothberger interpreted them as

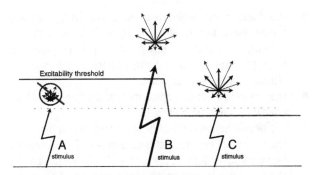

Figure 16.1 Wedensky effect. Stimulus A is the intensity sub-threshold and does not evoke any response. A strong stimulus B is applied thereafter which elicits a response and lowers the intensity threshold. The next stimulus C of the same intensity as stimulus A is applied shortly after B and elicits the response.

indicating the activity of an ectopic centre, located in a branch of the conduction system, the impulses of which become effective only during a certain phase of increased excitability after the preceding beat.

Scherf and Schott[5] first introduced the concept of the Wedensky effect into clinical ECGs. They reported that under certain conditions, one impulse could trigger another impulse without invoking vulnerability or supernormality. They considered that such a mechanism and not a re-entry, could adequately explain the origin of extrasystoles occurring late in the cardiac cycle. In particular, they concluded that extrasystoles were primarily due to a disturbance of cardiac excitability, not of conduction.

In 1966, Castellanos *et al.*[6] first reported a clear evidence for the presence of the Wedensky effect in the human heart. They studied the population of seven patients with atherosclerotic heart disease and complete heart block with slow idioventricular rhythms. Two intracardiac electrical pacemakers were used, one for sub-threshold stimulation and the other for applying one synchronised or unsynchronised strong stimulus with an intensity of about 15 to 20 times the threshold. Supernormal periods ranging from 160 to 195 ms were observed. A true Wedensky effect was found twice: in one patient the previously sub-threshold impulses yielded a response 160–260 ms after the end of the T wave of an electrically-induced beat; in another patient, sub-threshold impulses, also occurring well after the end of supernormality, i.e. 260 ms after the end of the T wave and 740 ms after the strong stimulus, elicited a response when the intensity of the driving stimulus was increased from 2 to 15 times above threshold. These findings supported the hypothesis that a disturbance or excitability rather than abnormality of conductivity can best explain the origin of ventricular extrasystoles occurring late in diastole.

Pertinent to the genesis of cardiac arrhythmias were additional observations which demonstrated that:

- the duration of Wedensky effect is relatively long persisting for a period of as much as 200 ms after the "strong" stimulus in nerve tissue and 160–260 ms after the end of the T wave following the "strong" stimulus in the human heart;
- the magnitude of the phenomenon may be altered by changing the ionic milieu;
- the phenomenon can be elicited by interventions other than "strong" electrical stimulation (e.g. in the case of nerve tissue by local application of NaCl crystals and in the dog heart by systematic administration of digitalis).

Wedensky facilitation

In 1903, Wedensky described another phenomenon explaining another mechanism underlying the origin of some extrasystoles. Wedensky facilitation[7] refers to a phenomenon wherein an impulse arriving proximal to a region of block enhances the region beyond the block by lowering its threshold. Thus the excitability beyond a block may be increased by a proximal stimulus (Fig. 16.2). It was subsequently demonstrated that this increase in excitability beyond the block is due to an extrinsic potential produced by an electrotonic current. Such block can be induced for example by cold, pressure, or using various drugs.

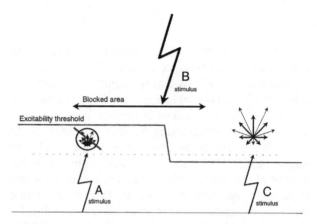

Figure 16.2 Wedensky facilitation. Impulse A is a sub-threshold and does not evoke a response. Impulse B is a stimulus that arrives at a blocked area and lowers the excitability threshold beyond the block. A subsequent stimulus C that is of the same intensity as stimulus A, now becomes threshold and is able to evoke a response.

Facilitation and effect

The Wedensky phenomena are probably basic properties of most excitable tissue and are closely related. The specific distinction is that the enhancement of Wedensky facilitation occurs distal to a blocked maximum impulse, whereas the enhancement of Wedensky effect follows a propagated or conducted maximum impulse within the same tissue. Based on Wedensky phenomena, a far-field electrical bias (electrotonic current) will allow a previously sub-threshold pulse to stimulate.

Wedensky facilitation was first observed in nerve tissue. Many years later, it was established that it can also occur in cardiac tissue. Hodgkin[8] showed in nerve that the increase in excitability caused by a blocked impulse below the zone of block is due to spread of electrotonic current, producing an extrinsic potential beyond the block.

The importance of electronic spread was documented by Hoffman and Cranefield[9] who reported that the summation of a decrementally conducted impulse through the AV node with electrotonic spread of a His bundle potential resulted in a fairly normal action potential. Alanis and Benitez[10,11] studied the action potential of AV node transitional cells in rabbits. They concluded that the transitional potentials are composed of two independent components: an active response plus an electrotonic potential generated by the contiguous tissues. The interpretation of one component being due to electrotonic activation was supported by the marked latency between the initiation of the fast and slow components of the transitional potential, as the distance separating two contiguous cells was "probably" too small to explain the magnitude of the observed delay. Electrotonic spread was also considered to account for the different duration of action potentials in AV nodal cells of rabbits as reported by Mendez and Moe.[12] They observed a block at different levels inside the AV node during propagation of premature impulses and suggested that, when block occurs, local circuits between active and inactive regions provide repolarising current to the distal active region, which will shorten the action potentials of these cells. By contrast, when propagation is successful, the impulse may stop, only resuming conduction after a delay. While the impulse is arrested, depolarising current will tend to shorten the action potential of the active region, but when propagation restarts, the newly excited tissue will provide depolarising current to the previously active region, causing delay in repolarisation.

Investigations discussed so far concerned mainly transmission through the AV node. However, similar observations were also reported in other cardiac tissues. Mendez et al.[13] demonstrated that, in canine junctions between Purkinje fibre and ventricular muscle, conditions prevailed, which in many respects resemble those in the AV node. Determination of action potentials in various portions of specialised conducting fibres, from "central Purkinje" fibres (false tendon) to peripheral (ramification over the surface of the basal area of papillary muscle) and in ventricular (papillary) muscle fibres, showed that the changes in the action potential were not abrupt but continuous. The continuous gradation of the action potential duration between specialised and muscular fibres was attributed to electrotonic interactions, and low resistance of intercellular connections to current flow, rather than to inherent characteristics of the cells.

Wedensky facilitation in human electrocardiograms was proposed where sub-threshold impulses of electrotonic pacemakers became suprathreshold when the impulse fell at the top of or shortly after the P wave.[1,14] In 1968, Fisch et al.[14] reported an instance of multifunctioning cardiac pacemaker in which pacemaker stimulus elicited a response when:

● falling during the supernormal period of ventricular recovery, or
● being synchronous with or closely following the P wave.

They suggested that the excitation of the ventricle by a sub-threshold stimulus could be, at least partly, explained by Wedensky facilitation.

Schamroth et al.[1] observed relatively prolonged temporary enhancement of conductivity during high grade AV block in a 50-year-old man with moderate essential hypertension and calcific aortic valve disease. There was no evidence of coronary disease or cardiac failure. They suggested that this observation must be related to some effect of the preceding ventricular activation, and was best explained by both Wedensky phenomena. Wedensky facilitation was used to explain the initiation of AV conduction. An impulse from a ventricular escape beat, an AV nodal escape beat, or an electrical pacemaker enters the AV node, and reaches the area of block. This lowers the threshold beyond the block and allows a subsequent anterograde impulse to be conducted. Conduction of the second and later sinus impulse (maintenance of AV conduction) was most likely due to Wedensky effect. Each conducted sinus impulse was equivalent to the experimental maximum induction shock and temporarily lowered the threshold of the depressed area within the AV node. If a succeeding impulse fell within this period of enhancement, conduction succeeded. If it was too late, conduction failed. Schamroth et al. viewed the Wedensky phenomena as belonging to a series of safety mechanisms. The advent of AV block permitted an escape beat (the first mechanism). This temporarily improved conduction by Wedensky facilitation (the second safety mechanism). The facilitated conduction was maintained by the Wedensky effect (the third mechanism). These three mechanisms created a self-perpetuating series, which is consistent with clinical observations of spontaneous recovery from many bouts of ventricular asystole.

Wedensky inhibition

The third mechanism described by Wedensky is the so-called Wedensky inhibition.[7] It refers to the frequency-dependent impairment of impulse transmission across a segmental block in nerve, ultimately ending in complete block of all impulses at high stimulation frequencies. In 1983, Antzelevitch et al.[15] reported this mechanism in isolated cardiac tissues. They found this to result from influences exerted not only by impulses transmitted across the area of block but also by impulses blocked at the proximal border of the inexcitable zone. The electrotonic image of a non-conducted response was observed to exert an important inhibitory effect on the electronically mediated transmission of a subsequent impulse, thus causing block or delay. The phenomenon (frequently also termed "electrotonic inhibition") showed both time and voltage dependence.

Potential clinical use of Wedensky modulation

The concepts of Wedensky facilitation were recently used to develop an external test for the risk of ventricular tachycardia (VT). The technical set-up of such a test was introduced by Hoium *et al.*[16] They assumed that VT patients have a region of the ventricle with slow conduction. Thus, a sub-threshold electric impulse influencing field across the heart should accelerate conduction through this region. This might slightly modulate the QRS complex.

A slight transcutaneous biasing current was applied through the patient chest synchronous with the QRS complex of odd numbered (1, 3, 5, etc.) normal sinus beats. The resulting QRS complexes were then compared to the even numbered (2, 4, 6, etc.) unbiased beats. Sub-threshold stimulated and non-stimulated QRS complexes were recorded during the same experimental session and signal averaged separately. The electrographic recordings were obtained with standard orthogonal leads. They investigated the different waveform between stimulated and non-stimulated complexes. That allowed the visualisation of a possible analogue of late potentials throughout the QRS complex rather than only in the early ST segment. The difference area was computed and reported as a microinduction response.

The data obtained using this approach were used later in a study aimed to investigate whether Wedensky facilitation induced in this way differentiates between normal subjects and VT patients. Study population consisted of 47 patients with EP documented VT (mean age 63 ± 13 years, 83% male) and 30 healthy controls (mean age 44 ± 16 years, 60% male). Patients were subjected to a sub-threshold external stimulation between precordial and left subscapular patches. Stimuli of 5, 10, 20, and 40 mA were delivered for 2 ms either simultaneously with R wave detection or 20 ms after R wave detection.

In order to detect even minor changes within the QRS complex, each lead of both stimulated and non-stimulated averaged complexes was decomposed using wavelet analysis (Morlet analysing wavelet[17] with 53 scales covering the range of 40–250 Hz). The wavelet residuum (WR) corresponding to Wedensky facilitation was obtained by subtracting the vector magnitude of wavelet decomposition of non-stimulated QRS from the vector magnitude decomposition of the sub-threshold stimulated QRS complexes. Figure 16.3 shows the surface of WR in a window ± 5 ms from the R peak (stimulation moment) and in surrounding windows when the external stimulation of 20 mA was delivered synchronously with the R wave detection. WR showed an increase of the three–dimensional envelope surface at and after the stimulation, which was more marked in healthy volunteers than in VT patients. The maximum changes in wavelet residuum increased with

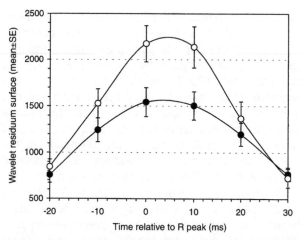

Figure 16.3 Results of experimental setting when external stimuli of 20 mA were delivered synchronously with R peak detection. The differences between wavelet three-dimensional envelope of stimulated and non-stimulated QRS complexes in a window ± 5 ms around the stimulation moment and in surrounding 10 ms windows were calculated. They characterised Wedensky facilitation. These differences are significantly more expressed in healthy volunteers (empty circles) compared to VT patients (filled circles).

stimulation sub-threshold energy as follows: 5 mA: control 1993 ± 181 technical units, VT patients 1488 ± 159 ($P < 0.04$); 10 mA: control 2151 ± 200, VT patients 1822 ± 131 ($P < 0.05$); 20 mA: control 2171 ± 198, VT patients 1543 ± 154 ($P < 0.01$); 40 mA: control 2746 ± 332, VT patients 1842 ± 177 ($P < 0.02$).[18]

A similar trend is shown in Fig. 16.4. The WR showed a sharp increase in the spectral power of the stimulated complex that was more marked in healthy controls ($P < 0.01$) than in VT patients.[19] Figure 16.5 demonstrates the changes in surface area of WR when measured in a window centred around the stimulation moment and the subsequent 10 ms window when the external stimulation was delivered 20 ms after R peak detection. All differences between VT patients and healthy controls were highly statistically significant (up to $P < 0.00005$). The separation of the groups was more significant in the window around the stimulation moment than in the subsequent window. The significance decreased with increasing sub-threshold stimulation energy.[20]

To investigate the reproducibility of WR under different energy of stimulation, stimulated and non-stimulated recordings of 79 healthy controls and 91 VT patients were divided into two halves of 76 ± 35 cardiac cycles.[21] WR was computed for each half of each recording separately. Reproducibility of WR was assessed using the relative errors of repeated measurement and correlated with number of averaged QRS complexes. Figure 16.6 shows the correlation coefficient between the number of averaged

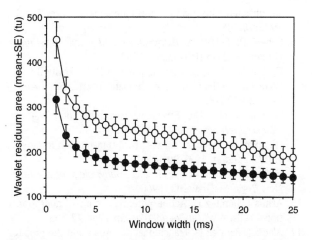

Figure 16.4 Results of experimental settings when external stimuli of 20 mA were delivered synchronously with R wave detection. The surface area of the wavelet residuum was investigated in windows of 1–25 ms following the stimulation (horizontal axis). Vertical axis shows mean ± standard error of wavelet residuum area. VT patients and healthy controls are shown with filled and empty circles. tu = technical units.

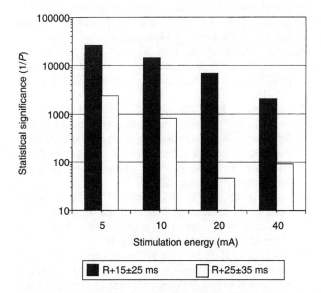

Figure 16.5 Results of experimental settings when external stimuli were delivered for 2 ms after a 20 ms delay following a real-time R wave detection. The surface area of the three-dimensional envelope of the wavelet residuum is measured in a window 20±5 ms after the R peak (i.e. a window centred round the stimulation moment – dark bars) and the subsequent 10 ms window (30±5 ms after the R peak – open bars). Energy of external stimulus is shows on horizontal axis. Vertical axis shows logarithmic scale of invert *P* value of the statistical comparison between VT patient and healthy controls.

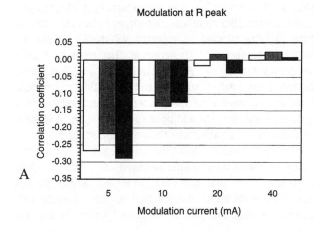

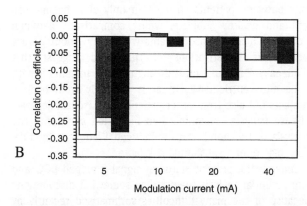

Figure 16.6 Correlation coefficient between the number of averaged cycles and the wavelet residuum of a window of 0–5, 0–25, and –5 – +5 ms (open, light and dark bars, respectively) for modulations synchronous with R peak (panel A) and delayed for 20 ms (panel B).

cycles and WR that was decreasing with increased stimulation energy.

All these studies demonstrated that:

- wavelet decomposition of signal averaged ECG is a suitable tool to analyse Wedensky modulation;
- Wedensky modulation in the late QRS complex is short;
- VT patients are less sensitive to the Wedensky modulation especially at very low sub-threshold energies, and
- when higher stimulation energies are used, prolonged experiments are not necessary.

Conclusion

The mechanisms contributing to the non-invasively induced Wedensky phenomenon are poorly understood. The fact that the differences between the externally modulated and unmodulated QRS complexes are larger in healthy subjects than in patients with documented VT speaks against the original hypothesis of the concept that tried to induce Wedensky facilitation. At the same time, the differences between the healthy subjects and VT patients are indisputable as already confirmed in separate and independent groups of subjects. In addition, the separation of healthy subjects from VT patients by the wavelet-decomposed modulated and unmodulated QRS complexes is statistically independent of other signal averaged ECG factors.[22] It is therefore likely that not only Wedensky facilitation but also Wedensky effect plays a role in this non-invasively induced modulation, hence the term "Wedensky modulation".

So far, however, the comparisons have been performed only between patients with VT (mainly of ischaemic origin) and healthy subjects, whilst comparisons between ischaemic heart disease patients with and without VT are lacking. If investigations of this kind suggest that Wedensky modulation distinguishes patients with ischaemic ventricular tachycardia not only from healthy subjects but also from other patients with ischaemic heart disease (such as uncomplicated infarction survivors), the analysis of the non-invasively induced Wedensky modulation, may offer a substantial risk factor.

Indeed, the present status of signal averaged ECG and late potential analysis seems to be somewhat discouraging because of the many difficulties summarised recently by Kulakowski.[23] Whilst the other factors used for tachycardia and sudden death risk assessment (e.g. the autonomic, repolarisation, functional, etc. markers) have been advanced to a level of practical applicability, the markers investigating the abnormalities of myocardial depolarisation need a substantial advance to reach the hopes originally put into signal-averaged ECG. The dynamic aspect of Wedensky modulation seems to be an elegant possibility of such an advance. Nevertheless, further studies are still needed before this technology can be recommended for practical clinical use.

References

1. Schamroth L, Friedberg HD. Wedensky facilitation and the Wedensky effect during high grade A-V block in the human heart. *Am J Cardiol* 1969;**23**:893–97.
2. Wedensky NE. Über die Beziehung zwischen Reizung und Erregung im Tetanus. *Ber Acad Wiss (St Petersburg)* 1887;**54**:96, App. 3.
3. Samojloff A. Die Aktivierung der für den Muskel unterschwelligen indirekten Reize durch einen maximalen Nerveneinzelreiz. *Pflügers Arch ges Physiol* 1930;**225**:482.
4. Goldenberg M, Rothberger CJ. Untersuchungen an der spezifischen Muskulatur des Hundeherzens. *Z ges Exp Me* 1933;**90**:508.
5. Scherf D, Schott A. *Extrasystoles and allied arrhythmias*. London: William Heinemann, 1953.
6. Castellanos A, Jr, Lemberg L, Johnson D, Berkovitz BV. The Wedensky effect in the human heart. *Br Heart J* 1966;**28**:276–83.
7. Wedensky NE. Die Erregung, Hemmung und Narkose. *Pflügers Arch ges Physiol* 1903;**100**:1–9.
8. Hodgkin AL. Evidence for electrical transmission in nerve. *J Physiol London*, 1937;**90**:183–232.
9. Hoffman BF, Cranefield PF. *Electrophysiology of the heart*. New York: McGraw-Hill, 1960.
10. Alanis J, Benitez D. Action potential from A-V node transitional cells. *Arch Int Physiol Biochim* 1964;**72**:765
11. Alanis J, Benitez D. Transitional potentials and the propagation of impulses through different cardiac cells. In: *Electrophysiology and ultrastructure of the heart*. New York: Grune & Stratton, 1967, p. 153.
12. Mendez C, Moe GK. Some characteristics of transmembrane potentials of A-V nodal cells during propagation of premature beats. *Circ Res* 1966;**19**:993.
13. Mendez C, Mueller WJ, Merideth J, Moe GK. Interaction of transmembrane potentials in canine Purkinje fibers and at Purkinje fiber–muscle junctions. *Circulation Res* 1969;**24**:361.
14. Fisch C, Knoebel SB. 'Wedensky facilitation' in the human heart. *Am Heart J* 1966;**76**:90–2.
15. Antzelevitch C, Moe GK. Electrotonic inhibition and summation of impulse conduction in mammalian Purkinje fibers. *Am J Physiol* 1983;**14**:H42–H53.
16. Hoium HH, Brewer JE, Kroll KC, Kroll MW, Kroll KJ. Use of sub-threshold transcutaneous biasing as a possible prognostic test for ventricular tachycardia. *RBM* 1994;**16**:111–15.
17. Hnatkova K, Kroll MW, Ryan SJ *et al*. Wavelet decomposition of Wedensky modulated electrocardiograms: Differences between patients with ventricular tachycardia and healthy volunteers. In: Murray A, Arzbaecher R eds. *Computers in cardiology 1999*. Hanover: IEEE Computer Society Press, 1999, pp. 157–60.
18. Hnatkova K, Benditt DG, Malik M *et al*. Wedensky transthoracic stimulation: Dose response in healthy volunteers and ventricular tachycardia patients. *Pacing Clin Electrophysiol* 1999;**22**:836(Abstr. 543).
19. Hnatkova K, Malik M, Kroll MW *et al*. QRS complex alternans detected by wavelet decomposition of signal averaged electrocardiograms: Differences between patients with ventricular tachycardia and normal healthy volunteers. *Pacing Clin Electrophysiol* 1999;**22**:864(Abstr. 655).
20. Hnatkova K, Stanton MS, Ryan SJ *et al*. Wedensky phenomenon within the late potential region: Dose related separation of patients with ventricular tachycardia from healthy controls. *Pacing Clin Electrophysiol* 1999;**22**:748(Abstr. 194).
21. Hnatkova K, Ryan SJ, Benditt DG *et al*. Reproducibility of non-invasive Wedensky modulation in man is dependent on number of averaged cardiac cycles. p.461 & *Pacing Clin Electrophysiol* 2000;**23**:668 (Abstr. 461).

22. Hnatkova K, Kroll MW, Ryan SJ *et al*. Wedensky modulated signal averaged electrocardiograms – combination of time-domain and wavelet decomposition parameters for identification of ventricular tachycardia patients. *Circulation* 1999;**100**(Suppl. 1):1052 (Abstr. 833).

23. Kulakowski P. Ventricular signal averaging: Is it completely dead? *Cardiac Electrophysiol Rev* 1999;**3**:264–8.

17 Ambulatory electrocardiography: use in arrhythmia risk assessment

Morrison Hodges and James J Bailey

It is almost 40 years since Norman Holter published his classic paper describing the first clinical use of ambulatory electrocardiography (AECG).[1] Significant advances in recording techniques, playback methods, and diagnostic algorithms have occurred during those years. AECG is still used primarily for its original purpose – monitoring cardiac rhythm – but is now also used for evaluating ST-segment deviations, abnormalities in the QT interval, RR interval changes (heart rate variability), QRST morphology including late potentials, and beat-to-beat T wave changes (T wave alternans). In this chapter we review the role of AECG in stratifying risk for serious ventricular arrhythmias. We also briefly review the current and future states of AECG technology.

State of the art of AECG technology

In 2000, the typical AECG recorder is a small and light-weight device that records an analogue signal of two or three bipolar leads. The usual recording format has been magnetic tape cassettes, and this is still the most common type in use. After recording, the tape must be converted to digital format for subsequent analysis by computer programs and human observers. However, most new versions of AECG recorders record directly in digital format, with storage on solid-state devices, either small hard disks or on memory chips. Many of the newer digital AECG recorders have analysis algorithms built into the device, so that some form of "on-the-fly" analysis can occur. The amount of memory in solid-state devices has increased recently, so that all data for 24 hours can be recovered for later analysis and review ("full disclosure"). Digital recorders obviate many of the technical problems associated with analogue tape recorders, such as variations in tape speed, and problems with equipment maintenance. The only important disadvantage of digital recorders is the increased cost of equipment.

Clinical value of AECG for risk stratification

Early studies with AECG showed clearly that frequent ventricular ectopy was associated with subsequent mortality[2] and

sudden cardiac death.[3] Studies such as these led to the "VPC hypothesis," which assumed that a premature ventricular beat was the trigger for initiation of ventricular tachycardia and fibrillation. It seemed logical to assume that suppression of the trigger would reduce the likelihood of fatal arrhythmias, but multiple clinical trials showed that this was not the case; indeed, mortality was increased in most trials.[4,5]

Despite the disappointing results of the CAST, SWORD, and other trials, interest in using AECG for risk stratification continues, because recent trials have clearly shown that the implantable cardioverter–defibrillator (ICD) is highly effective at treating otherwise-fatal ventricular arrhythmias. With such an effective treatment available, it is important to be able to identify those individual patients most likely to benefit from it.[6] Guidelines have recently been published for the use of the ICD.[7] AECG has only a partial and non-essential role in the selection of patients with Class I (beneficial, useful, and effective) indications. One of the four Class I indications does include patients with non-sustained ventricular tachycardia (NSVT), which can of course be detected with AECG. Patients with NSVT must also have a prior myocardial infarction, left ventricular dysfunction, and an inducible severe ventricular arrhythmia at electrophysiological study not suppressible by a Class I antiarrhythmic drug in order to qualify for an ICD. Thus, it is possible that AECG could be used as a screening tool to identify patients with NSVT who should undergo further testing.

For a screening tool to be useful, it must have three features: simplicity, inexpensiveness, and adequate accuracy.[8] It is debatable whether or not AECG is sufficiently simple and inexpensive to be performed in, say, everyone with coronary heart disease but, if it were accurate enough to identify individuals with a very high likelihood of needing an ICD, the difficulty and cost of the test would likely be tolerable. Thus, the accuracy of AECG for predicting SCD is worth examining in detail.

The AECG as a screening tool

The usefulness of a screening tool is best examined from the standpoint of Bayesian analysis: sensitivity, specificity, positive predictive value, and negative predictive value.[8] Ideally, one would like a test with a high sensitivity (a high rate of positive results in those with the condition) and a very high positive predictive value (a very high rate of the condition in those with a positive test), so that few patients would be exposed unnecessarily to treatment (an ICD in the case of sudden cardiac death). A test with a very high negative predictive value (NPV) is also desirable, since it allows the clinician to reassure a patient that his or her risk of a serious arrhythmia is very low. On the other hand, if the prevalence of serious arrhythmias is low in the population to which the patient belongs, the prior probability is low already, and a NPV would have to be very high indeed to be clinically useful.

One of the problems with SCD is that only about one-third of patients who have SCD are in groups currently thought to be at high risk for SCD.[9] In order to detect the large number of patients who will have SCD despite being in the "lower-risk" group, one would have to examine a very large number of patients. In this situation a very high specificity (a very high rate of negative tests in those without the condition) as well as a very high positive predictive value are essential. This almost always results in a lower sensitivity but, since some patients can potentially be detected in a situation in which almost no patients are presently being detected, a higher sensitivity, whilst desirable, is not necessarily required in order to do some good. It is a situation in which a quarter-full glass is better than an empty glass.

Many investigators have evaluated the usefulness of AECG for the prediction of arrhythmic events and SCD. In Tables 17.1 and 17.2 we list studies that used AECG for risk stratification. These papers were identified by a search of MEDLINE for papers with "ambulatory ECG" and "risk stratification" as keywords. Papers were selected for inclusion if they had data for actual numbers of patients in the four categories needed for calculation of Bayesian statistics (i.e. numbers of true and false positives, and true and false negatives). In some situations the number of patients was obtained by translating bar height in a graph to a percentage or a number. The studies were divided into three categories of disease: post-myocardial infarction (post-MI), congestive heart failure (CHF), and hypertrophic cardiomyopathy (HCM). The post-MI group was further divided into those that looked at the frequency of ventricular premature contractions (VPC), and those that looked at NSVT and complex ventricular arrhythmias (VA). Complex VA was usually defined as Class 4 or higher using the Lown classification.[10] This latter grouping usually included NSVT. All of the post-MI studies enrolled consecutive patients with myocardial infarction.

In order to compare the various studies, and to get an overall estimate of the test accuracy, we used the tech-

niques of Littenberg, Moses, and Shapiro.[11,12] Their technique uses a logistic transform to generate a curve that is weighted by the number of patients in a given study. Summary weight-fitted receiver-operating characteristic (ROC) curves were constructed for selected categories. Subsequently, weighted composite mean values for sensitivity and specificity and 95% confidence intervals were calculated and placed on the summary ROC curves.

Post-myocardial infarction studies

In Table 17.1A and Fig.17.1 are shown data from eight studies that looked at the prognostic value of frequent VPCs on the AECG after a myocardial infarction. The overall event rate was 2.1% per year, and the positive predictive value (PPV) was 4% per year (sensitivity and specificity are not time dependent, but PPV is). The very low PPV means that if one uses VPCs on an AECG as a screening tool, 24 patients would be needlessly treated each year in order to successfully treat one patient during that year. Furthermore, this approach would only pick up just over one-third of the patients who would have an event. These data are heavily weighted by one study, that of Maggioni *et al.*,[13] but the data of the other studies are not markedly different. Clearly, it would seem that using frequent VPCs on an AECG is not a good screening tool, and is of very limited use in individual patients for predicting future events.

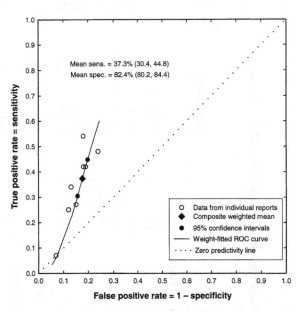

Figure 17.1 Weight-fitted receiver-operating characteristic (ROC) curve for eight post-MI studies. The mean sensitivity and specificity are shown, along with their 95% confidence limits. The diagonal line of identity indicates a useless test; any points below this line would represent misleading data.

Table 17.1 Bayesian data from post-MI AECG studies

Author	Test	End-point	No. of patients	TP	FN	FP	TN	Sens	Spec	PPV	Average follow-up (months)	PPV per year
A. Post-MI VPC studies												
Bigger[18]	≥3 VPCs/h	All deaths	715	54	58	147	456	0.48	0.76	0.27	30.0	0.11
Farrell[19]	>10 VPCs/h	Arrhythmic events	416	13	11	71	321	0.54	0.82	0.16	20.0	0.09
Kostis[20]	≥10 VPCs/h	SCD	1 640	19	57	192	1 372	0.25	0.88	0.09	25.0	0.04
Kuchar[16]	≥10 VPCs/h	Arrhythmic events	206	1	14	14	177	0.07	0.93	0.07	14.0	0.06
Maggioni[13]	>10 VPCs/h	SCD	8 552	35	49	1 652	6 816	0.42	0.81	0.02	6.0	0.04
Mukarji[21]	>10 VPCs/h	SCD	533	10	19	68	436	0.34	0.87	0.13	18.0	0.09
Pedretti[17]	>6 VPCs/h	Arrhythmic events	303	8	11	48	236	0.42	0.82	0.14	15.0	0.11
Rouleau[22]	>10 VPCs/h	Cardiac deaths	1 600	20	54	231	1 295	0.27	0.85	0.08	12.0	0.08
PVC totals/averages			*13 965*	*160*	*273*	*2 423*	*11 109*	*0.37*	*0.82*	*0.06*	*17.5*	*0.04*
B. Post-MI NSVT/complex VA studies												
El-Sherif[23]	Complex VA	Arrhythmic events	1 158	27	18	345	768	0.60	0.69	0.07	12.0	0.07
Farrell[19]	NSVT	Arrhythmic events	416	13	11	73	319	0.54	0.82	0.15	20.0	0.09
Gomes[24]	Couplets	Arrhythmic events	76	7	3	22	44	0.70	0.67	0.33	14.0	0.21
Gomes[24]	NSVT	Arrhythmic events	94	6	10	12	66	0.38	0.85	0.33	14.0	0.29
Hermosillo[25]	Complex VA	Arrhythmic events	200	8	13	14	165	0.38	0.92	0.36	12.0	0.36
Kostis[20]	Couplets or NSVT	SCD	1 640	26	50	301	1 263	0.34	0.81	0.08	25.0	0.04
Kuchar[16]	Complex VA	Arrhythmic events	206	11	4	62	129	0.73	0.68	0.15	14.0	0.13
Maggioni[13]	NSVT	SCD	8 552	11	73	565	7 903	0.13	0.93	0.02	6.0	0.04
McClements[26]	Complex VA	Arrhythmic events	301	5	8	74	214	0.39	0.74	0.06	13.0	0.06
Olson[27]	Complex VA	Cardiac death	115	8	4	30	73	0.67	0.71	0.21	12.0	0.21
Pedretti[17]	NSVT	Arrhythmic events	303	9	10	72	212	0.47	0.75	0.11	15.0	0.09
Richards[28]	Complex VA	Arrhythmic events	358	14	3	205	136	0.82	0.40	0.06	12.0	0.06
Ruberman[3]	Complex VA	SCD	1 739	68	71	394	1 206	0.49	0.75	0.15	60.0	0.03
Steinberg[29]	Complex VA	Arrhythmic events	181	7	9	45	120	0.44	0.73	0.14	14.0	0.12
Verzoni[30]	Complex VA	Arrhythmic events	208	4	2	58	144	0.67	0.71	0.07	12.0	0.07
Zhang[31]	Complex VA	SCD	60	6	3	15	36	0.67	0.71	0.29	10.0	0.34
NSVT totals/averages			*15 607*	*230*	*292*	*2 287*	*12 798*	*0.44*	*0.85*	*0.09*	*16.6*	*0.07*

Abbreviations: FN = false negative; FP = false positive; MI = myocardial infarct; NSVT = non-sustained ventricular tachycardia; Sens = sensitivity; Spec = specificity; TN = true negative; TP = true positive; VA = ventricular arrhythmias; VPC = ventricular premature contractions.

Table 17.2 Bayesian data for AECG studies in CHF and HCM patients

Author	Test	End-point	No. of patients	TP	FN	FP	TN	Sens	Spec	PPV	Average follow-up (months)	PPV per year
A. CHF VPC studies												
Teerlink[32]	>30 VPCs/h	SCD	1080	105	34	542	399	0.76	0.42	0.16	NA	NA
B. CHF NSVT studies												
Doval[33]	NSVT	SCD	516	41	30	132	313	0.58	0.70	0.24	24.0	0.12
Szabó[34]	NSVT	SCD	204	10	13	62	119	0.43	0.66	0.14	21.0	0.08
Teerlink[32]	NSVT	SCD	1080	105	34	558	383	0.76	0.41	0.16	NA	NA
CHF NSVT totals/averages			*1800*	*156*	*77*	*752*	*815*	*0.67*	*0.52*	*0.17*	*N/A*	*N/A*
C. HCM studies												
Hodges[35]	NSVT	SCD	103	2	1	33	67	0.67	0.67	0.06	33.0	0.02
Maron[36]	NSVT	SCD	83	4	2	13	64	0.83	0.24	0.24	36.0	0.08
McKenna[37]	NSVT	SCD	86	5	2	19	60	0.71	0.76	0.21	31.0	0.02
Spirito[38]	NSVT	SCD	151	3	3	39	106	0.50	0.73	0.07	46.0	0.02
HCM totals/averages			*423*	*14*	*8*	*104*	*297*	*0.64*	*0.74*	*0.12*	*35.5*	*0.04*

Abbreviations: NA = not available; N/A = not applicable; other abbreviations as in Table 17.1.

The same statements can be made about the use of findings of non-sustained ventricular tachycardia (NSVT) or complex ventricular arrhythmias (VA) on the AECG. These data are shown in Table 17.1B and Fig. 17.2. While the PPV is almost twice as high, it is still very low, and sensitivities, whilst in general higher than for VPCs alone, are still not high enough to make screening for NSVT/complex VA worthwhile. In addition, it seems that an overall PPV of 7% is too low to use as an indication for a therapy such as an ICD.

Whilst it is true that the NPVs for the post-MI studies are very high, these high values are only marginally useful because the event rate in this population is low. For example, the NPV for NSVT/complex VA is 97.8%, but the prevalence (prior probability) of SCD and serious arrhythmic events is only 3.3%, which means that the average patient had a 96.7% chance of survival *before* the AECG was performed.

Thus, it seems fair to conclude that AECG alone has a very limited role in stratifying risk after a myocardial infarction. As noted below, however, it is possible that AECG can be a valuable clinical tool when used in conjunction with other tests and indications.

Studies in congestive heart failure patients

Although ventricular arrhythmias and sudden cardiac death are common in patients with congestive heart fail-

ure, fewer studies of AECG as a prognostic method are available in this group. Tables 17.2A and 17.2B and Fig. 17.3 show results for CHF patients. Sensitivity and PPV are higher in all studies than they are in post-MI patients. Nevertheless, the values are still low enough that it seems unlikely that AECG alone can be used to decide to implement even a very efficacious therapy such as an ICD.

Studies in patients with hypertrophic cardiomyopathy

Table 17.2C and Fig. 17.3 show results for patients with hypertrophic cardiomyopathy, another condition in which sudden death is possible and ICDs have the potential to markedly prolong life.[14] Results for HCM patients are similar to those in CHF patients, namely, while sensitivities and PPVs are higher than those for post-MI patients, they are still not high enough to justify routinely using AECG VA data alone to make clinical decisions.

Studies combining AECG with other tests

In general, the use of multiple tests will improve prediction when compared with single tests alone.[15] In Table 17.3 and Fig. 17.4 are shown the results from seven studies in which AECG was evaluated alone, and in combination with one or two other studies. In two studies[16,17] the numbers of events and of patients studied differ from earlier tables, because all patients did not have multiple tests

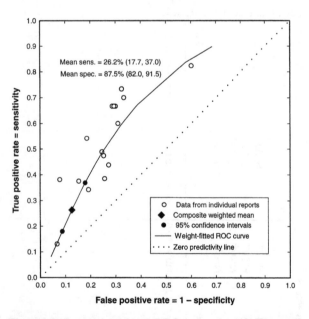

Figure 17.2 Weight-fitted ROC curve for NSVT/complex VA post-MI studies. These mean values are heavily weighted by the study of Maggioni *et al.*[13] which has more than half the patients. Note that the confidence intervals are not symmetric. The mean values differ from those given in Table 17.1B because of the weighting used by the techniques for calculation.[11,12]

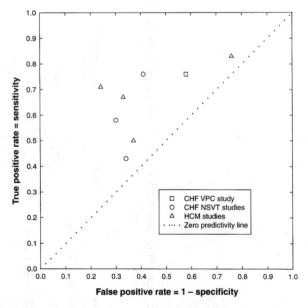

Figure 17.3 Plot of true- and false-positive rates for CHF and HCM studies.

Table 17.3 Studies combining ventricular arrhythmia on AECG with other tests for predicting risk of arrhythmic events after myocardial infarction

Author	Number of patients in study	Number of events	Test(s) combined with ventricular arrhythmia	Sensitivity		Specificity		Positive predictive value	
				VA only	VA combined	VA only	VA combined	VA only	VA combined
Bigger[18]	715	112	EF, HRV	0.48	0.10	0.76	0.98	0.27	0.46
El-Sherif[23]	1158	45	SAECG	0.60	0.36	0.69	0.95	0.07	0.24
Farrell[19]	416	24	SAECG, HRV	0.54	0.29	0.82	0.99	0.15	0.58
Kuchar[16]	200	15	SAECG	0.73	0.65	0.68	0.89	0.15	0.31
Mukharji[21]	533	29	EF	0.35	0.24	0.87	0.93	0.13	0.18
Olson[27]	115	12	EF	0.67	0.50	0.71	0.91	0.21	0.40
Pedretti[17]	292	18	SAECG, EF	0.47	0.17	0.75	0.99	0.11	0.50
Totals/averages	*3429*	*255*		*0.55*	*0.33*	*0.75*	*0.95*	*0.16*	*0.38*

Abbreviations: AECG = ambulatory ECG; VA = significant ventricular arrhythmia on AECG exam; EF = ejection fraction; HRV = heart rate variability; SAECG = signal-averaged ECG.

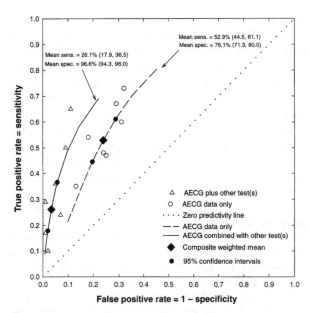

Figure 17.4 Weight-fitted ROC curves for selected studies that had data for combining AECG data with other tests. Note that where the curves overlap on an axis, the combination of tests is clearly superior.

performed. The combined tests were considered "positive" only when all of the individual tests were positive. The combined tests were "negative" when one or more of the individual tests were negative.

In general, the results of combining tests are much better than for the AECG alone. Specificities increase significantly, and, as expected, sensitivities decrease somewhat. The average PPV of nearly 40% means that three patients would be needlessly treated for every two that benefit. While the overall sensitivity is low, it is still above zero, and as noted above that could be advantageous when the alternative is not detecting anyone. The false-positive rate is low (≈ 3%) and could possibly be decreased even lower by using different cutpoints for abnormality for tests such as ejection fraction, signal-averaged ECG, and heart rate variability, without lowering sensitivity to a useless level.

Thus, it appears that AECG data alone cannot be used to make crucial positive clinical decisions in an individual patient, such as deciding whether or not to implant an ICD. The AECG may be very useful in this regard, however, when used in conjunction with other tests, such as those listed in Table 17.3. Given the demonstrated efficacy of the ICD, it is very important that additional studies in this area be carried out.

Future technical developments of the AECG

The AECG is still widely used as a clinical tool, and it is likely that future technical developments will occur that will increase its use. For example, more accurate real-time computer algorithms may eliminate the need for technical or professional over-reading, which would lower the cost significantly for an AECG. If ventricular arrhythmia, heart rate variability, and signal-averaged ECG data could be accurately and automatically generated by a very small steady-state AECG device, that could immediately be used in conjunction with other information relatively easily obtained, such as clinical data (age, gender, prior disease, etc.) and ejection fraction, then the 40–year-old AECG may experience an impressive rejuvenation.

References

1. Holter NJ. New method for heart studies. Continuous electrocardiography of active subjects over long periods is now practical. *Science* 1961;**134**:1214–20.
2. Ruberman W, Weinblatt E, Goldberg JD, Frank CW, Shapiro S. Ventricular premature beats and mortality after myocardial infarction. *New Engl J Med* 1977;**297**:750–7.
3. Ruberman W, Weinblatt E, Goldberg JD, Frank CW, Chaudhary BS, Shapiro S. Ventricular premature complexes and sudden death after myocardial infarction. *Circulation* 1981;**64**:297–305.
4. Echt DS, Liebson PR, Mitchell LB *et al*. Mortality and morbidity in patients receiving encainide, flecainide, or placebo – The Cardiac Arrhythmia Suppression Trial. *New Engl J Med* 1991;**324**:781–8.
5. Waldo AL, Camm AJ, DeRuyter H *et al*. Effect of *d*-sotalol on mortality in patients with left ventricular dysfunction after recent and remote myocardial infarction. *Lancet* 1996;**348**:7–12.
6. Domanski MJ, Zipes DP, Schron E. Treatment of sudden cardiac death. Current understandings from randomised trials and future research directions. *Circulation* 1997;**95**: 2694–9.
7. Gregoratos G, Cheitlin MD, Conill A *et al*. ACC/AHA guidelines for implantation of cardiac pacemakers and anti-arrhythmia devices: executive summary – a report of the American College of Cardiology/American Heart Association Task Force on Practice Guidelines (Committee on Pacemaker Implantation). *Circulation* 1998;**97**:1325–35.
8. Morrison AS. Screening. In Rothman KJ, Greenland S eds. *Modern epidemiology*. Philadelphia: Lipponcott-Raven, 1998, pp. 499–518.
9. Hodges M, Church, TR. Identifying individual patients with coronary heart disease who are at risk of sudden cardiac death. (Submitted for publication, 2000.)
10. Lown B, Wolf M. Approaches to sudden death from coronary heart disease. *Circulation* 1971;**44**:130–42.
11. Littenberg B,.Moses LE. Estimating diagnostic accuracy from multiple conflicting reports: a new meta-analytic method. *Med Decis Making* 1993;**13**:313–21.
12. Moses LE, Shapiro D, Littenberg B. Combining independent studies of a diagnostic test into a summary ROC curve: data-analytic approaches and some additional considerations. *Stat Med* 1993;**12**:1293–316.
13. Maggioni AP, Zuanetti G, Franzosi MG *et al*. Prevalence and prognostic significance of ventricular arrhythmias after acute myocardial infarction in the fibrinolytic era. GISSI-2 results. *Circulation* 1993;**87**:312–22.
14. Maron BJ, Shen WK, Link MS *et al*. Efficacy of implantable cardioverter–defibrillators for the prevention of sudden death in patients with hypertrophic cardiomyopathy. *New Engl J Med* 2000;**342**:365–73.
15. Church TR. Risk assessment and risk stratification in sudden cardiac death: a biostatistician's view. *Pacing Clin Electrophysiol* 1997;**20**:2520–32.
16. Kuchar DL, Thorburn CW, Sammel NL. Prediction of serious arrhythmic events after myocardial infarction: signal-averaged electrocardiogram, Holter monitoring and radionuclide ventriculography. *J Am Coll Cardiol* 1987;**9**: 531–8.
17. Pedretti R, Etro MD, Laporta A, Braga SS, Caru B. Prediction of late arrhythmic events after acute myocardial infarction from combined use of non-invasive prognostic variables and inducibility of sustained monomorphic ventricular tachycardia. *Am J Cardiol* 1993;**71**:1131–41.
18. Bigger JT Jr, Fleiss JL, Steinman RC, Rolnitzky LM, Kleiger RE, Rottman JN. Frequency domain measures of heart period variability and mortality after myocardial infarction. *Circulation* 1992;**85**:164–71.
19. Farrell TG, Bashir Y, Cripps T *et al*. Risk stratification for arrhythmic events in postinfarction patients based on heart rate variability, ambulatory electrocardiographic variables and the signal-averaged electrocardiogram. *J Am Coll Cardiol* 1991;**18**:687–97.
20. Kostis JB, Byington R, Friedman LM, Goldstein S, Furberg C. Prognostic significance of ventricular ectopic activity in survivors of acute myocardial infarction. *J Am Coll Cardiol* 1987;**10**:231–42.
21. Mukharji J, Rude RE, Poole WK *et al*. Risk factors for sudden death after acute myocardial infarction: 2-year follow-up. *Am J Cardiol* 1984;**54**:31–6.
22. Rouleau JL, Talajic M, Sussex B *et al*. Myocardial infarction patients in the 1990s – their risk factors, stratification and survival in Canada: the Canadian Assessment of Myocardial Infarction (CAMI) Study. *J Am Coll Cardiol* 1996;**27**: 1119–27.
23. El-Sherif N, Denes P, Katz R *et al*. Definition of the best prediction criteria of the time domain signal-averaged electrocardiogram for serious arrhythmic events in the postinfarction period. *J Am Coll Cardiol* 1995;**25**:908–14.
24. Gomes JA, Winters SL, Martinson M, Machac J, Stewart D, Targonski A. The prognostic significance of quantitative signal-averaged variables relative to clinical variables, site of myocardial infarction, ejection fraction and ventricular premature beats: A prospective study. *J Am Coll Cardiol* 1989;**13**:377–84.
25. Hermosillo AG, Araya V, Casanova JM. Risk stratification for malignant arrhythmic events in patients with an acute myocardial infarction: role of an open infarct-related artery and the signal-averaged ECG. *Coron Artery Dis* 1995;**6**: 973–83.
26. McClements BM,.Adgey AA. Value of signal-averaged electrocardiography, radionuclide ventriculography, Holter

monitoring and clinical variables for prediction of arrhythmic events in survivors of acute myocardial infarction in the thrombolytic era. *J Am Coll Cardiol* 1993;**21**:1419–27.

27. Olson HG, Lyons KP, Troop P, Butman S, Piters KM. The high-risk acute myocardial infarction patient at 1-year follow-up: identification at hospital discharge by ambulatory electrocardiography and radionuclide ventriculography. *Am Heart J* 1984;**107**:358–66.

28. Richards DA, Byth K, Ross DL, Uther JB. What is the best predictor of spontaneous ventricular tachycardia and sudden death after myocardial infarction? *Circulation* 1991;**83**:756–63.

29. Steinberg JS, Regan A, Sciacca RR, Bigger JT Jr, Fleiss JL. Predicting arrhythmic events after acute myocardial infarction using the signal-averaged electrocardiogram. *Am J Cardiol* 1992;**69**:13–21.

30. Verzoni A, Romano S, Pozzoni L, Tarricone D, Sangiorgio S, Croce L. Prognostic significance and evolution of late ventricular potentials in the first year after myocardial infarction: a prospective study. *Pacing Clin Electrophysiol* 1989;**12**:41–51.

31. Zhang YZ, Wang SW, Hu DY, Zhu GY. Prediction of life-threatening arrhythmia in patients after myocardial infarction by late potentials, ejection fraction and Holter monitoring. *Jap Heart J* 1992;**33**:15–23.

32. Teerlink JR, Jalaluddin M, Anderson S *et al*. Ambulatory ventricular arrhythmias in patients with heart failure do not specifically predict an increased risk of sudden death. *Circulation* 2000;**101**:40–6.

33. Doval HC, Nul DR, Grancelli HO *et al*. Non-sustained ventricular tachycardia in severe heart failure. Independent marker of increased mortality due to sudden death. *Circulation* 1996;**94**:3198–203.

34. Szabó BM, van Veldhuisen DJ, Crijns HJ, Wiesfeld AC, Hillege HL, Lie KI. Value of ambulatory electrocardiographic monitoring to identify increased risk of sudden death in patients with left ventricular dysfunction and heart failure. *Eur Heart J* 1994;**15**:928–33.

35. Hodges M, Poliac LC, Casey S, Maron BJ. Patterns and prognostic significance of ventricular ectopy in an unselected and unreferred patient population with hypertrophic cardiomyopathy. *J Am Coll Cardiol* 1997;**29**(Suppl. A):511A.

36. Maron BJ, Savage DD, Wolfson JK, Epstein SE. Prognostic significance of 24 hour ambulatory electrocardiographic monitoring in patients with hypertrophic cardiomyopathy: a prospective study. *Am J Cardiol* 1981;**48**:252–7.

37. McKenna WJ, England D, Doi YL, Deanfield JE, Oakley C, Goodwin JF. Arrhythmia in hypertrophic cardiomyopathy. I: Influence on prognosis. *Br Heart J* 1981;**46**:168–72.

38. Spirito P, Rapezzi C, Autore C *et al*. Prognosis of asymptomatic patients with hypertrophic cardiomyopathy and non-sustained ventricular tachycardia. *Circulation* 1994;**90**: 2743–7.

18 Event loop recorders and implantable monitors

Mark L Brown

Ambulatory ECG recording devices have been used to assist in the diagnosis and documentation of symptoms caused by arrhythmias and conduction abnormalities for many years.[1] Increased emphasis on outpatient monitoring and improvements in device technology have expanded the indications for ambulatory ECG. Primary indications for ambulatory ECG monitoring include palpitations, syncope and near syncope, assessment of antiarrhythmic drug therapy and arrhythmia screening in patients at high risk. Analysis of ST-segment elevation from ambulatory ECG in patients with coronary artery disease has been shown to be clinically useful in assessment of myocardial ischaemia. Several other direct and indirect measures of cardiac performance from ambulatory recordings with external and implanted devices are being studied to determine their clinical value.

The principal use of ambulatory ECGs remains arrhythmia monitoring. An arrhythmic origin of symptoms is confirmed by consistent temporal association of symptoms with arrhythmia or conduction abnormalities. Likewise, a consistent absence of ECG abnormality correlated with recurrent symptoms excludes an arrhythmic aetiology. The prevalence of abnormal ECG in otherwise healthy individuals is not well known, so there is considerable debate regarding therapeutic options of patients with arrhythmia in the absence of symptoms. In addition to providing initial diagnosis and documentation of an arrhythmic aetiology for symptomatic episodes, ambulatory recording also serves as a tool for monitoring efficacy of arrhythmia therapy and for confirming correct operation of pacemakers and cardioverter/defibrillators (ICDs).

Description of ambulatory ECG devices

Holter monitors

Holter monitoring has been available for many years and is the standard against which other recording systems are evaluated. Holter monitoring provides high quality multi-electrode recording for up to 72 hours of continuous recording. During recording patients are instructed to press an event button and write an entry in a diary during specific activities, such as eating or lying down or when symptoms occur. Recently, Holter recorders have been developed, which in addition to recording ECG also record data telemetered from implanted ICDs and pacemakers for diagnostic purposes. These data include intracardiac electrograms and sensing and detection information. The primary advantages of Holter recording are relative ease of use, low cost, and historical acceptance. It is ideal for recording asymptomatic ECG or ECG during symptoms that occur frequently. Holter recording is limited by the relative short recording duration and the lack of definite correlation between symptoms and ECG recording.

Event recorders

Event recorders are available in hand-held or wristwatch format devices (Fig.18.1) capable of recording several minutes of ECG when the patient presses a button. The hand-held unit is placed on the chest while a button is pressed. When the button is released, the recording stops. In this manner, several short recordings or a single longer recording are possible. Once recorded, the ECG can be transmitted to a physician's office or monitoring service transtelephonically so that it may be analysed. These event recorders can record ECG only after the onset of symptoms, which may be adequate when symptoms are relatively long in duration and symptoms are not debilitating.

For short, infrequent symptomatic episodes or syncopal episodes, continuous loop recorders (Fig. 18.2) are more appropriate. These differ from event recorders in that ECG electrodes are worn continuously and the recorder continuously records until the patient or another person presses a button causing the recording to stop a few seconds or minutes later. The pre- and post-trigger recording duration is programmable from several seconds to several minutes depending on device. As with event recorders, the recorded ECG can be transmitted transtelephonically

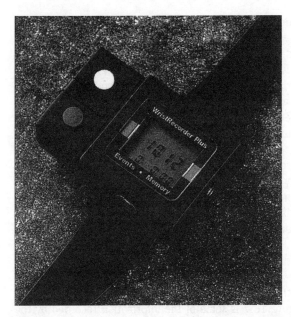

Figure 18.1 The WristRecorder^{SM} "Plus" external event recorder manufactured by Ralin Medical can store up to 5 minutes of ECG.

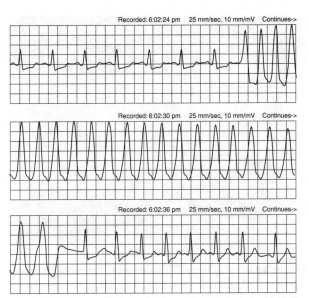

Figure 18.3 A sample recording from an external loop recorder in which a short non-sustain ventricular tachycardia was captured.

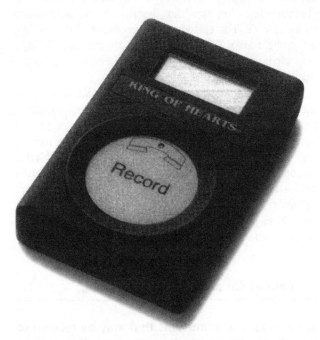

Figure 18.2 The King of Hearts Express® external loop recorder manufactured by ALARIS Medical Systems, Inc. can store up to 5 minutes of ECG.

to a physician or monitoring service. Loop recorders are typically used in monitoring applications lasting 2–4 weeks.

Figure 18.3 is an example of a recording made with an external ECG monitor and transmitted to a monitoring service. In this figure, the patient has a brief non-sustained episode of ventricular tachycardia.

Implantable loop recorders

Implantable devices provide loop recording capability with a monitoring period of months to years. The Reveal® insertable loop recorder (Medtronic, Inc.)[2] was created to provide ambulatory ECG monitoring for syncope. Syncopal events can go undiagnosed for years because of the difficulty in recording these very infrequent symptoms that disable the patient. The Reveal® is implanted subcutaneously and event recording is triggered with a hand-held activator. Implantable pacemakers and cardioverter/defibrillators also provide valuable long-term monitoring features that can be used to document arrhythmias and/or arrhythmia-free periods, which can help assess the efficacy of device and drug therapy.

The Reveal® implantable loop recorder (ILR) is a small, leadless device that is easily implanted subcutaneously in minutes. Typically, the ILR is placed in the left pectoral region. Two electrodes 37 mm apart on the surface of the can are used to record a subcutaneous ECG. The ILR has memory capacity to store up to 42 minutes of ECG that can be used for one long recording or several shorter ones (Fig. 18.4). Events are stored when the ILR is triggered by placing a hand-held patient activator over the implanted device and pushing a button on the activator. An audible and visual notification on the activator confirms that the recording has been accomplished. Recordings are

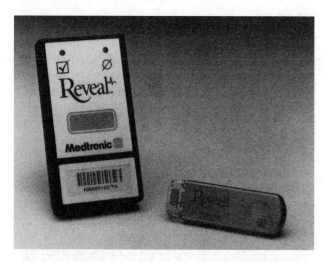

Figure 18.4 The Reveal® implantable loop recorder manufactured by Medtronic, Inc. can store up to 42 minutes of subcutaneous ECG.

retrieved with a device programmer via telemetry and can be displayed, printed and/or saved to disk. Primary indication for the device is infrequent syncope/pre-syncope that has failed diagnosis by other clinical and laboratory methods (Fig. 18.5). Recent ACC/AHA guidelines also list palpitations as a Class I indication for ambulatory ECG monitoring. Recent reports[3] indicate that the ILR has been used to identify an underlying cardiovascular cause of atypical seizures in patients previously diagnosed as having treatment resistant epilepsy. The ILR has also been used to monitor the mechanism of onset of symptomatic episodes of atrial fibrillation.[4] Future versions of the device will include automatic triggers for ventricular and supraventricular arrhythmias and will allow transtelephonic transmission of recordings.

Implantable pacemakers and defibrillators

Implantable pacemakers and ICDs, in addition to their indicated function, contain large memories (32 K for pacemakers and 512 K for ICDs) devoted to storing "diagnostic" information. These data provide several clinically relevant functions. Originally included to verify correct device operation and lead function and to assist physicians in patient-dependent programming of devices, these diagnostics have expanded to collecting long-term trend data and detailed episode data for both treated and untreated arrhythmias to assist in patient monitoring. These data may be used to monitor patient status or determine drug and device therapeutic effectiveness. Diagnostics can be categorised as trend data, consisting of counts of events over time, or episode data, which may contain detailed

information regarding treated arrhythmias or summary data, such as time of occurrence and duration of episode. Trend data stored by pacemakers and ICDs include heart rate, frequency of APCs and VPCs, frequency and duration of atrial arrhythmias (mode-switch episodes in pacemakers), and patient activity levels. These data are displayed as event counts, trend plots, or histograms. Figure 18.6 is a histogram report from a dual-chamber pacemaker with atrial antitachycardia pacing capability that is currently undergoing clinical trial. The histogram displays the time of day that AF/AT episodes started over a 6-week follow-up period. Detailed episode data may include electrograms (EGMs), markers and intervals, therapy sequence, programmed therapy and detection options, and therapy outcome. Some devices store detailed episode data for arrhythmias not treated by the device to confirm correct device operation and validate the occurrence of the arrhythmia.

Figure 18.7 is some of the information recorded by the Gem DR® (Medtronic, Inc) dual chamber ICD from an episode of AF/AT that conducted rapidly to the ventricle. The episode was recorded when ventricular detection and therapy was appropriately withheld by PR Logic®, the dual chamber detection algorithm, because it was determined to be an SVT. The episode display consists of two EGMs, a near-field atrial EGM and a far-field ventricular EGM, a dual chamber marker channel, and an interval plot showing atrial and ventricular intervals.

Additional monitoring features of ICDs and pacemakers include audible patient alerts that can notify the patient of potential device problems, such as battery depletion or suspected lead problems. Future atrial arrhythmia devices may alert the patient that they are experiencing an atrial episode for which they may want to deliver drug and/or device therapy. In conjunction with a hand-held patient activator, these devices will allow the patient to mark an episode as symptomatic and/or confirm that patient symptoms are due to an atrial arrhythmia.

Indications for ambulatory monitoring

Assessment of symptoms that may be related to arrhythmias or conduction abnormalities

Palpitations

Palpitations are a common presenting symptom. Though most often benign, palpitations can indicate a significant arrhythmia. Arrhythmic causes of palpitations include atrial or ventricular premature beats, and supraventricular or ventricular tachycardia. First- or second-degree heart block may also cause palpitations. Patients with structural heart disease such as previous myocardial infarction or

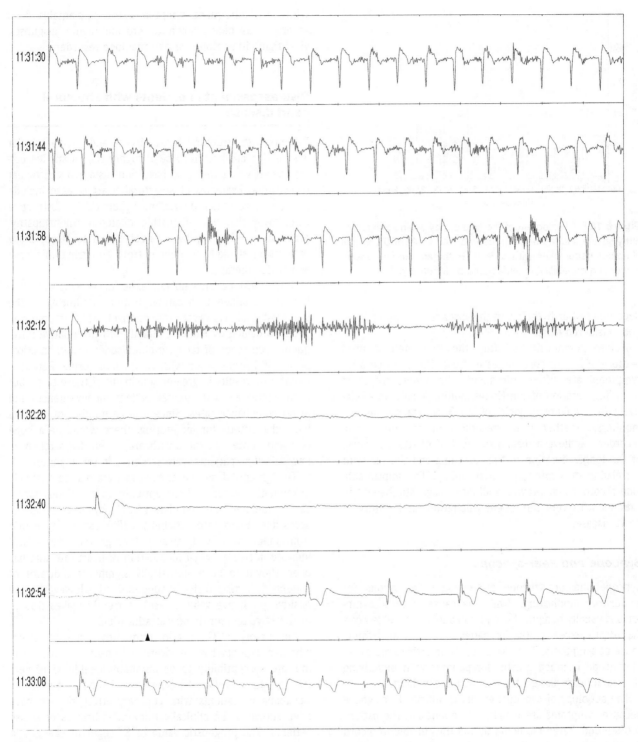

Figure 18.5 A sample recording from Reveal® in which complete heart block in conjunction with a long ventricular escape interval was identified as the cause of syncope.

dilated or hypertrophic cardiomyopathy have a substantially greater likelihood of serious arrhythmia. Symptoms often are infrequent and sustain for only a short time. Diagnosis of an arrhythymic cause of symptoms requires that the patient sustain symptoms while the ECG is being recorded and temporal association of ECG with symptoms can be made. When this is achieved, arrhythmia is either diagnosed or ruled out as the cause of symptoms.

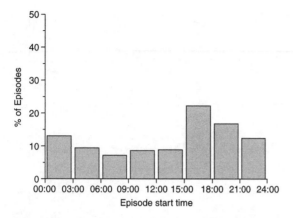

Figure 18.6 Histogram of the time of day when atrial tachyarrhythmia episodes began recorded with an AT500®, a dual chamber pacemaker with atrial ATP therapy and extensive monitoring capability, manufactured by Medtronic, Inc.

Recordings of arrhythmias in the absence of symptoms are not considered diagnostic.

Holter monitoring is often the first method used because of its low cost and ease of use. However, because symptoms are often infrequent, the inherently short recording duration of the Holter monitor results in a relatively low diagnostic yield of 30–35%. Transtelephonic monitors, whether event recorders or continuous-loop recorders, achieve a diagnostic yield of 65–85%, because of the longer duration of the recording and the inherent correlation of symptoms and recording. The implantable loop recorder may provide additional diagnostic benefit in patients with very infrequent palpitations and history of heart disease.

Syncope and near-syncope

Syncope and pre-syncope are common indications for ambulatory monitoring. While the cause of these symptoms is usually benign, the 1-year incidence of sudden cardiac death exceeds 20% for patients with an arrhythmic cause of symptoms. The likelihood of an arrhythmic cause of syncope is much greater for patients with underlying structural heart disease than for patients without.

The aetiology of syncopal events is difficult to diagnose because symptoms are usually infrequent and the patient is often debilitated momentarily and thus unable to record the event promptly. Holter monitoring is often the first diagnostic tool used for patients in whom the likelihood of an arrhythmic cause of syncope is high on the basis of history. However, the diagnostic yield of Holter monitoring is less than 20% because of the relatively short recording period and the infrequency of events. External loop recorders have been shown to achieve approximately double the diagnostic yield of Holter monitors. For patients

with very infrequent symptoms, the implantable loop recorder has been shown to provide higher diagnostic yield than either Holter or external loop recorders.

Risk assessment in patients with structural heart disease

Patients with structural heart disease and left ventricular dysfunction are known to be at higher risk of sudden cardiac death when they also have non-sustained ventricular tachycardia. Examples of structural heart disease include previous myocardial infarction, hypertrophic obstructive cardiomyopathy, and idiopathic dilated cardiomyopathy. Ambulatory ECG may be a valuable tool to select those patients most likely to benefit from antiarrhythmic drug and device therapy.

Since most patients do not experience symptoms during non-sustained tachycardia, Holter monitoring is the indicated tool. However, the relatively short monitoring period provided by Holter coupled with the relative infrequent occurrence of tachycardia episodes results in a low power of discrimination with Holter monitoring. Repeated monitoring results in greater sensitivity of these tests, but at an increased cost, greater patient inconvenience, and lower compliance rates. Since a large number of patients meet the criteria for monitoring, there would be a huge cost and burden on the healthcare system for a relatively low yield if all patients were screened in this manner.

Though episodes of ventricular tachycardia are relatively infrequent, measures of susceptibility to ventricular tachycardia evaluated from ambulatory ECG may more temporally accessible. Heart rate variability (HRV) can be measured from ambulatory ECG. Low values for high frequency of HRV indicate decreased vagal modulation of heart rate that has been shown to be a statistically significant indicator of patients at increased risk of sudden death. However, a low positive predictive value of HRV currently makes this an unattractive tool for therapy stratification.

Ambulatory ECG is also frequently used to assess whether patients have myocardial ischaemia, which may indicate susceptibility to or imminent likelihood of ventricular tachycardia. ST-segment changes caused by ischaemia in patients with coronary artery disease have been shown to be clinically relevant indicators of at-risk patients. The prognostic value of ST-segment changes in patients without coronary artery disease has not been shown. In the future, implantable devices will provide continuous long-term monitoring of ischaemia, which may prove to be much more sensitive and specific than current measures based on Holter recording. Exercise testing is still the standard technique for assessing myocardial ischaemia, unless the patient is unable to perform the test in which case ambulatory monitoring is used.

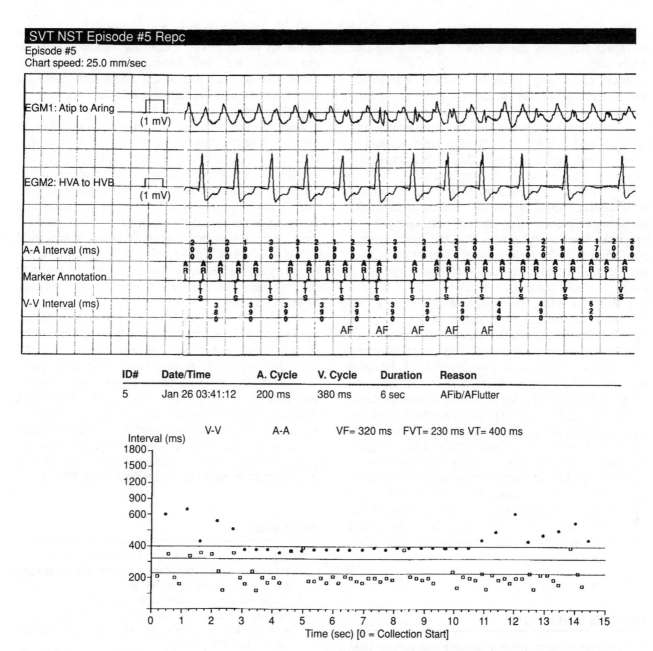

Figure 18.7 Episode recording of an atrial fibrillation/flutter episode recorded by a Gem DR® dual-chamber defibrillator manufactured by Medtronic, Inc. The top panel displays a near-field atrial electrogram, far-field ventricular electrogram, and dual chamber Marker® channel with annotation indicating the beat on which rate-based ventricular detection would have detected and treated the patient for ventricular tachycardia if not for the atrial information. The bottom panel shows the atrial and ventricular intervals for this episode.

Assessment of safety and efficacy of antiarrhythmic therapy

Some modern Holter recorders have the capability to receive telemetry from implanted devices and record these data, consisting of intracardiac electrogram and device-specific status information, in addition to the surface ECG typically stored with Holters. These recordings are a powerful tool for analysing the operation of implanted devices, from determining the appropriateness of sensing and detection to the effectiveness and safety of device therapy. Coupled with the implanted device's internal episode storage, a very accurate assessment of device operation can be derived. Even without the additional telemetry information from the device, Holter recordings are useful for assessing proper implantable device operation. Holters capable of recording telemetered device data are usually proprietary and may not be generally available to physicians.

Antiarrhythmic drug therapy for ventricular arrhythmias can be titrated on an outpatient basis in patients implanted with an ICD. The ICD can provide therapy when antiarrhythmic drugs fail or are pro-arrhythmic and provide a stored record of the frequency and duration of episodes along with electrogram data to help assess the therapeutic effect of the antiarrhythmic drugs.

The effectiveness of antiarrhythmic drugs for symptomatic supraventricular tachycardia including atrial fibrillation is often assessed on the basis of patient reporting of symptoms. There is concern regarding this approach especially when antiarrhythmic drugs are supplemented with rate controlling drugs that may mask the symptoms of arrhythmia. With the increased risk of stroke associated with atrial fibrillation, the masking of symptoms may be hazardous to the patient unless antithrombolytic drugs are also used. One means of assessing whether asymptomatic arrhythmia has been suppressed by drugs is periodic monitoring either with Holter or event recorders. Daily transmissions of ECG recordings with event monitors are commonly used. Patients implanted with atrial or ventricular defibrillators or pacemakers have the benefit of continuous arrhythmia monitoring provided by the device. While the count of modeswitch episodes was used as a surrogate for episodes of atrial fibrillation in older pacemakers, newer models have the ability to detect and record atrial fibrillation and other supraventricular tachycardias. They also are able to maintain daily counts of ventricular and atrial ectopy and non-sustained runs of tachycardia. Atrial and ventricular ICDs also have these monitoring capabilities.

Emerging technologies

An implantable haemodynamic monitor that records right ventricular pressure, heart rate, activity, mixed venous oxygen saturation, and estimated pulmonary artery diastolic pressure has been reported.[5] The device has been used to provide continuous ambulatory haemodynamic monitoring in patients with severe cardiopulmonary disease. This device is similar in size to an ICD and uses a single lead incorporating biosensors to measure pressure and oxygen saturation placed in the right ventricle. The device has a memory capacity for 3 weeks of data storage

at low resolution. Clinical utility of this device is being evaluated. In the future, monitoring functions found in this device will be incorporated into therapeutic implantable devices providing a powerful combination for closed loop therapy and patient notification of changes in physiologic status.

Automatic detection and discrimination of supraventricular and ventricular tachyarrhythmias and bradyarrhythmias is being incorporated into both external and implantable ambulatory ECG devices. It is expected that these devices will be able to detect and log asymptomatic as well as symptomatic episodes by sensing R waves at a minimum. Some devices are expected to sense P waves, T waves and ST segment changes indicative of myocardial ischaemia. Current dual chamber ICDs and pacemakers have very high sensitivity and specificity for the detection of arrhythmias. Some are now sensing T waves and measuring QT intervals

Ambulatory ECG monitoring has become a primary diagnostic tool for the evaluation of symptoms suggestive of arrhythmias and conduction abnormalities. External event and loop recorders have been shown to be useful for diagnosing brief, infrequent symptomatic episodes, and for monitoring therapy effectiveness. Implantable devices provide for long-term monitoring over months or years that would be impractical or impossible with external monitors. Increased storage capacity, improved displays, and experience in the use of this data will result in improved patient care for patients with these devices.

References

1. Zimetbaum PJ, Josephson, ME. The evolving role of ambulatory arrhythmia monitoring in general clinical practice. *Ann Intern Med* 1999;**130**:848–56.
2. *Reveal® Reference Manual*, Medtronic, Inc.
3. Zaidi A, Crampton S, Clugh P *et al.* Misdiagnosis of epilepsy – many seizure-like episodes have a cardiovascular cause. *PACE* 1999;**22**:814.
4. Schwartzman D, Wackowski C, Brown ML, Mehra R. Electrocardiographic events preceding atrial fibrillation captured by an implantable loop recorder: observations and potential utility. *J Am Coll Cardiol* 1999;**33**:103A.
5. Ohlsson Å, Nordlander R, Bennett T *et al.* Continuous ambulatory haemodynamic monitoring with an implantable system. *Eur Heart J* 1998;**19**:174–84.
6. Crawford MH, Bernstein SJ. ACC/AHA guidelines for ambulatory electrocardiography: executive summary and recommendations. *Circulation* 1999;**100**:886–93.

19 Basic autonomic tests

Federico Lombardi

In spite of the consistency of experimental and clinical observations indicating a determinant role of autonomic nervous system in initiating, maintaining and terminating supraventricular and ventricular arrhythmias, an exhaustive autonomic evaluation is rarely performed in patients with arrhythmias.[1-4] The main explanation of this finding is the fact that most of the techniques used to evaluate autonomic function are either too simple to provide consistent results or too complex to be used in the normal clinical practice. Before the introduction of techniques like analysis of hear rate variability[5] or of baroreflex sensitivity[6] that will be discussed later in this book, evaluation of autonomic nervous system has been limited to the analysis of instantaneous heart rate and arterial blood pressure changes during intervention likely to produce reflex changes in sympathetic and vagal activity directed to the cardiovascular system. Postural changes, alteration in respiratory pattern, painful stimulation, and sustained muscular contraction are only a few examples of the different types of stimuli used to activated different reflexogenic areas and to produce changes in autonomic control of sinus node pacemaker activity, stroke volume, and vascular resistance.

For example, analysis of changes in instantaneous heart rate has been consistently used to detect a sympathetic activation when tachycardia was observed or a vagal activation when bradycardia occurred. Despite the simplicity of the measure and the introduction of new and more sophisticated techniques, the analysis of instantaneous heart rate is regaining, in these last years, an important role in clinical cardiology after the reappraisal that this parameter may be successfully used to identify patients at risk after myocardial infarction.[7]

On the contrary, manoeuvres like the Valsalva or carotid sinus massage are nowadays more commonly used to make a correct diagnosis or to interrupt supraventricular arrhythmias rather than to characterise the autonomic profile and hence the pro-arrhythmic risk of a patient. The complexity of the mechanisms involved in autonomic control of cardiovascular function and in particular of sinus node pacemaker activity and the necessary involvement of patient cooperation may explain the progressive abandon of these manoeuvres in the routine clinical practice in favour of more recent techniques such as heart rate variability and baroreflex sensitivity analysis.[5,6]

Nevertheless, these simple and inexpensive tests are probably underused and must be reconsidered, in our opinion, within the attempt of obtaining a rapid, although incomplete, preliminary bedside information on the presence of alteration in neural control mechanisms before performing more expensive and time consuming procedures.

In the following pages the most relevant basic autonomic test will be briefly discussed in relation to their use in the management of patients with arrhythmias with particular emphasis on risk stratification.

The Valsalva manoeuvre

It consists of a forced exhalation against a close glottis or, more rarely, blowing into a manometer to reach and maintain a level of 40 mmHg for at least 15 seconds. Four phases characterise this manoeuvre:

- During phase 1, there is a rise in intrathoracic pressure with a transient increase in cardiac output.
- During phase 2 (straining), systemic venous return diminishes and stroke volume and pulse pressure decrease. As a result instantaneous heart rate increases.
- During phase 3, which corresponds to the cessation of straining, there is an abrupt decline in arterial pressure.
- At the release of straining (phase 4), within a few beats there is a marked increase in arterial pressure and a reflex bradycardia.

Thus, vagal tone is activated in response to the short lasting sympathetic activation of phase 2 and as a result of arterial baroreceptor activation occurring during the increase in arterial blood pressure of phase 4.

In the past, particularly in the evaluation of autonomic neuropathy in patients with diabetes, a ratio between RR intervals of phase 4 and 2 less than 1.2 was considered abnormal.[8] Despite the simplicity of the manoeuvre, which has been frequently used in the pre-echocardiographic era to differentiate cardiac murmurs, this test is nowadays mainly, if not exclusively, used for the diagnosis and termination of supraventricular arrhythmias.

It was the work of Waxman, Cameron, and Waldo[9] that has contributed to our understanding of the critical role of autonomic nervous system in initiating, maintaining and terminating supraventricular tachycardias. These authors were the first to compare the spontaneous termination and Valsalva-induced termination of paroxysmal supraventricular tachycardia (PSVT). In the first case, they noticed that the tachycardia terminated spontaneously when an induced episode of PSVT resulted in a marked hypotension. Recovery of sinus rhythm was associated with an overshoot of blood pressure and reflex bradycardia. Alternatively, the Valsalva manoeuvre interrupted the induced PSVT as a consequence of the vagal activation secondary to the phase 4 overshoot in blood pressure. These authors also provided unequivocal evidence for the value of autonomic tests to differentiate the different types of supraventricular tachycardias.

The electrophysiological mechanisms and determinants of vagal manoeuvres for termination of PSVT were recently analysed by Wen and co-workers.[10] They studied 133 patients with PSVT, and assessed the effects of different vagal manoeuvres on arrhythmia termination. Baroreflex sensitivity and beta-adrenergic sensitivity of PSVT patients and controls were also analysed. Vagal manoeuvres were effective in 53% of patients with atrioventricular reciprocating and in 33% of patients with atrioventricular nodal re-entrant tachycardia. The anti-arrhythmic effect of Valsalva manoeuvre was related to termination of retrograde conduction in atrioventricular nodal re-entrant tachycardia.

Lim and co-workers[11] also reported the efficacy of Valsalva manoeuvre and carotid sinus massage in terminating PSVT in the Emergency Room. All patients presented with regular and narrow QRS tachycardia and were randomised to either Valsalva manoeuvre or carotid massage. If the tachycardia was not terminated by the first method, the alternative vagal manoeuvre was performed and, if it was still ineffective, electrical cardioversion or pharmacological interventions were used. The overall efficacy of Valsalva manoeuvre was about 20% and was similar to that of carotid massage. Both vagal manoeuvres were effective in at least a quarter of patients admitted to the Emergency Room.

Deep breath test

Instantaneous heart rate is markedly influenced by breathing (see Chapter 21 on heart rate variability): inspiration leads to a rise in heart rate whereas expiration prolongs heart period. In the deep breath test, the subject is asked to breathe deeply and regularly six times for 5 seconds each. For each of the six breathing phases the shortest heart period during inspiration and longer one during expiration are measured. The difference between the two measures provides an index of respiratory sinus arrhythmia and of its vagal modulation.[12]

The predictive value of deep breath test and Valsalva manoeuvre was recently examined in a group of post-myocardial infarction patients by Andresen and colleagues.[12] These authors observed that an abnormal Valsalva and deep breath test were present in, respectively, 32 and 37% of subjects. Patients with an abnormal test were characterised by a significant older age and by a greater incidence of hypertension, whereas left ventricular function and arrhythmias during Holter monitoring were similar in both groups. During a 2-year follow-up, 21 patients died, 16 of cardiac causes. In patients with an abnormal deep breath test the mortality was 26% in comparison to 11% observed in patients with a normal test. In patients with an abnormal Valsalva manoeuvre the mortality rate was greater (31 versus 13%) than in patients with a normal test. These data seem therefore to indicate that patients with an abnormal vagal modulation of sinus node as indicated by the altered heart rate response to these autonomic tests, have an increased risk of cardiac events.[12]

Orthostatic (tilt) test

During the last 15 years head-up and less frequently head-down tilt have become a common procedure in the evaluation of patients with unexplained syncope[13] as well as a useful tool to evaluate in the clinical setting the integrity of autonomic control mechanisms.[14,15]

Despite the lack of consensus[16] on the precise modality of execution of the test in relation to tilt angle (ranging from 60 to 90°) and duration of orthostatism (from 15 to 60 minutes), this manoeuvre is associated with a reflex increase in sympathetic tone and a reduction in vagal modulation of sinus node. The change in autonomic balance is reflected by an increase in heart rate and in peripheral vascular resistance as well as by a specific pattern in short-term heart rate variability analysis characterised by a predominance of low frequency (LF) component in comparison to the high frequency (HF) one and by a LF/HF ratio greater than 2.[5,14,15]

The clinical use of the test in the evaluation of autonomic control mechanisms is indicated by two major findings. In normal subjects it is possible to determine progressive levels of sympathetic activation by gradually increase the tilt angle. It was observed that tilt angle was significantly correlated with heart rate (RR interval) and with the power in normalised units of LF component.[17]

In patients after myocardial infarction, the tilt test was used[18,19] to evaluate the presence of alterations in autonomic control mechanisms as well as the recovery toward a more physiological sympathovagal balance. It is worthwhile to recall that, after an acute myocardial infarction, two distinct heart rate variability patterns can be detected.[18–20] In patients with an uncomplicated myocardial infarction and with preserved heart rate variability, spectral analysis of short-term recordings is characterised by a predominant LF. In these subjects, tilt did not further alter the spectral pattern observed in the acute phase of myocardial infarction, whereas, after a few months, when signs of sympathetic activation were no longer present, tilt manoeuvre was associated with a physiological response of spectral components to orthostatic stimulation: an increase in LF and a reduction in HF.

In high-risk post-myocardial infarction patients, who are characterised by depressed heart rate variability and by a marked reduction or even absence of LF component, tilt manoeuvre exerts negligible effect on the spectral profile. In these subjects, the persistent alteration in neural control mechanisms induced by myocardial infarction not only represents a determinant component of their susceptibility to ventricular arrhythmias and sudden cardiac death, but also prevents a physiological response to the orthostatic stimulus as indicated by the absence of changes in the LF spectral component. These observations suggest that head-up tilt might be usefully used to better define the alterations in sympathovagal balance and their pattern of recovery in the convalescent phase of a myocardial infarction rather than directly contributing to the identification of patients at risk.

Head-up tilt has been used to evaluate, in the laboratory, the effects of sympathetic activation on ventricular arrhythmias and in particular on their rate dependence. It was found[21] that a 90° tilt was associated with opposite effects on the number of spontaneous ventricular ectopic beats in relation to the presence or absence of organic heart disease. A significant reduction was observed in apparently healthy subject, whereas a significant increase was noticed in patients with organic heart disease.

This manoeuvre could also be used to evaluate the effect of sympathetic activation on parameters such as QT dispersion[22] or T wave alternans[23] known to indirectly reflect cardiac electrical instability.

Finally, it must be recalled that tilting may produce an opposite effect on autonomic control mechanisms by downward rotating patient position. Head-down tilt is commonly used to increase arterial pressure during hypotension secondary to ventricular and supraventricular arrhythmias. This manoeuvre determines an increase in venous return and a pressure-dependent vagal activation that may be further potentiated by carotid sinus massage.

Cold pressor test

Immersion of a limb in icy water is associated with severe pain that induces a reflex sympathetic activation. As result of the rise in arterial blood pressure and heart rate, there is an increase in oxygen demand that is matched, in normal subjects, by coronary vasodilatation. This manoeuvre has been extensively used to evaluate coronary vasomotion in patients with ischaemic heart disease with normal or stenotic coronary arteries and in patients with unexplained chest pain.[24]

In a recent study, for example, it was hypothesised[25] that an increased cardiovascular reactivity to a cold pressor test might characterise patients admitted to the hospital with chest pain in comparison to patients with chest pain with suspected, but not later confirmed, coronary artery disease. The percentage increase in heart rate and arterial blood pressure induced by a cold pressor test was significantly larger in patients with coronary artery disease than in patients with normal coronary artery, thus confirming the important role of cardiovascular hyper-reactivity in the genesis of transient myocardial ischaemia.

The use of a cold pressor test in the evaluation of arrhythmic risk is a rare procedure. It is, however, possible that, in selected groups of patients with abnormal coronary vasomotion, this test might provide information on the effects of transient myocardial ischaemia on cardiac electrical properties and arrhythmogenesis.

Isometric handgrip

An isometric muscle contraction is accompanied by an increase in heart rate, arterial blood pressure, and cardiac output. The cardiovascular response is initially mainly elicited from the central nervous system and maintained by the effects of persistent activation of receptors located within the active musculature. This manoeuvre is therefore associated with a reflex inhibition of vagal tone and activation of sympathetic mechanisms. The difficulty of an appropriate and sustained execution of this manoeuvre has prevented its use in the study and management of patients with supraventricular and ventricular arrhythmias.

Conclusions

Basic autonomic tests are only rarely used in clinical cardiology as a consequence of the fact that determination of left ventricular ejection fraction and analysis of 24-h Holter recordings have demonstrated unequivocally their value in the assessment of arrhythmic risk after myocardial infarction. Nevertheless these tests, with their simplicity of execution and very limited cost, may provide important information on two aspects of relevant interest.

They may furnish a bedside and immediately available assessment of the capability of sinus pacemaker activity to respond to changes in sympathetic or vagal modulation of sinus node.

They may allow a direct and repeatable appraisal of the effects of a vagal or sympathetic activation on cardiac electrical properties and in particular on conduction system.

A future and more extensive use of basic autonomic tests will require, however, a standardisation of the manoeuvre and of the interpretation of the observed results in order to facilitate our understanding of autonomic control of cardiovascular function.

References

1. Lown B, Verrier RL. Neural activity and ventricular fibrillation. *New Engl J Med* 1976;**294**:1165–76.
2. Lombardi F, Verrier RL, Lown B. Relationship between sympathetic neural activity, coronary dynamics, and vulnerability to ventricular fibrillation during myocardial ischaemia and reperfusion. *Am Heart J* 1983;**105**:958–65.
3. SchwartzPJ, La Rovere MT, Vanoli E. Autonomic nervous system and sudden cardiac death: experimental basis and clinical observations for post-myocardial infarction risk stratification. *Circulation* 1992;**85**:I77–91.
4. Zipes DP. Autonomic modulation of cardiac arrhythmias. In: Zipes DP, Jalifwe J, eds. *Cardiac electrophysiology – from cell to bedside*. Philadelphia: WB Saunders Co., 1995, pp. 441–53.
5. Task Force of the European Society of Cardiology and the North American Society of Pacing and Electrophysiology. Heart rate variability. Standards of measurement, physiological interpretation, and clinical use. *Circulation* 1996;**93**:1043–65.
6. Smyth HS, Sleight P, Pickering GW. A quantitative method of assessing baroreflex sensitivity. *Circ Res* 1969;**24**:109–21.
7. Ferrari R, Lombardi F, Rapezzi C. The revival of heart rate. *Eur Heart J* 1999;**20**:853–4.
8. Ewing DJ, Martyn CN, Young RJ, Clarke BF. The value of autonomic function tests: 10 years experience in diabetes. *Diab Care* 1985;**8**:491–8.
9. Waxman MB, Cameron DA, Wald RB. Interactions between the autonomic nervous system and supraventricular tachycardia in humans. In: Zipes DP, Jalifwe J, eds. *Cardiac electrophysiology – from cell to bedside*. Philadelphia: WB Saunders Co., 1995, pp. 699–722.
10. Wen ZC, Chen SA, Tai CT, Chiang CE, Chiou CW, Chang MS. Electrophysiological mechanisms and determinants of vagal maneuvers for termination of paroxysmal supraventricular tachycardia. *Circulation* 1998;**24**:2716–23.
11. Lim SH, Anantharaman V, Teo WS, Goh PP, Tan AT. Comparison of treatment of supraventricular tachycardia by Valsalva maneuver and carotid sinus massage. *Ann Emerg Med* 1998;**31**:30–5.
12. Andresen D, Bruggemann T, Behrens S, Ehlers C. Heart rate response to provocative maneuvers. In: Malik M, Camm AJ, eds. *Heart rate variability*, Armonk, NY: Futura Publishing Company, Inc.,1995, pp. 267–74.
13. Benditt D, Ferguson D, Grubb B *et al.* ACC expert consensus document: tilt table testing for assessing syncope. *J Am Coll Cardiol* 1996;**28**:263–75.
14. Pagani M, Lombardi F, Guzzetti S *et al.* Power spectral analysis of heart rate and arterial pressure variabilities as a marker of sympathovagal interaction in man and conscious dog. *Circ Res* 1986;**59**:178–93.
15. Malliani A, Pagani M, Lombardi F, Cerutti S. Cardiovascular neural regulation explored in the frequency domain. *Circulation* 1991;**84**:482–92.
16. Robotis DA, Huang DT, Daubert JP. Head-up tilt-table testing: an overview. *Ann Non-Invas Electrocardiol* 1999;**4**:212–18.
17. Montano N, Gnecchi Ruscone T, Porta A *et al.* Power spectrum analysis of heart rate variability to assess the changes in sympathovagal balance during graded orthostatic tilt. *Circulation* 1994;**90**:1826–31.
18. Lombardi F, Sandrone G, Perpruner S *et al.* Heart rate variability as an index of sympathovagal interaction after acute myocardial infarction. *Am J Cardiol* 1987;**60**:1239–45.
19. Lombardi F, Malliani A, Pagani M, Cerutti S. Heart rate variability and its sympatho-vagal modulation. *Cardiovasc Res* 1996;**32**:208–16.
20. Lombardi F. Chaos heart rate variability and arrhythmic mortality. *Circulation* 2000;**101**:8–10.
21. Lombardi F, Malfatto G, Belloni A, Garimoldi M. Effects of sympathetic activation on ventricular ectopic beats in subjects with and without evidence of organic heart disease. *Eur Heart J* 1987;**8**:1065–74.
22. Kern MJ, Horowitz JD, Ganz P *et al.* Attenuation of coronary vascular resistance by selective alpha1-adrenergic blockade in patients with coronary artery disease. *J Am Coll Cardiol* 1985;**5**:840–7.
23. Statters DB, Malik M, Ward D, Camm AJ. QT dispersion: problems of methodology and clinical significance. *J Cardiovasc Electrophysiol* 1994;**5**:672–85.
24. Rosenbaum DS, Jackson LE, Smith JM, Garan H, Ruskin JN, Cohen RJ. Electrical alternans and vulnerability to ventricular arrhythmias. *New Engl J Med* 1994;**330**:235–41.
25. Sevre K, Rostrup M. Blood pressure and heart rate response to cold pressor test in patients admitted to hospital due to chest pain. *Blood Press* 1999;**8**:110–13.

Acknowledgements

Partially supported by 40% Research Grant from Ministero Università e Ricerca Scientifica e Tecnologica.

20 Heart rate assessment and monitoring

Xavier Copie, Olivier Piot, Thomas Lavergne, Louis Guize and Jean-Yves Le Heuzey

Heart rate is probably the easiest cardiovascular parameter to assess, and yet its regulation is complex and incompletely understood, as is its physiological and pathophysiological significance. More attention has been dedicated in the past to the study of blood pressure and its prognostic significance than to heart rate. Recently, the recognition of heart rate variability as a mean to study the effect of the autonomic nervous system on the heart has sometimes overshadowed the importance of heart rate itself.[1] Nevertheless heart rate may provide important information on the clinical status and the life expectancy of many mammals, including humans.[2]

Heart rate is recognised as a health indicator from two points of view:

- Heart rate is often regarded as the effect of the autonomic nervous system on intrinsic heart rate[3] and, as such, represents an approach to the evaluation of the sympathovagal balance.
- Heart rate is also taken into account from a mechanistic point of view. Higher heart rates may increase atherogenesis through an increase in oscillations in shear stress and are also often associated with early stages of hypertension.

However, despite an extensive literature on its prognostic value, heart rate is not often used in clinical practice where the analysis of heart rate variability for assessing the autonomic nervous system receives more attention.[4] Similarly more studies are devoted to the understanding and treatment of high blood pressure than to fast heart rate, despite much evidence of the major pathophysiological contribution of heart rate to global morbidity and mortality.[5]

Measurement of heart rate

Heart rate represents the number of heart beats per minute and should be easy to measure. The measure of heart rate is easier than the measure of heart rate variability. For instance, when heart rate is being measured from a 24-h Holter recording, the only requirements are to identify all RR intervals and the duration of the recording. Heart rate will simply be calculated as the ratio between the number of RR intervals and the duration of the recording in minutes. The precise duration of each RR interval is not required. On the contrary, when measuring heart rate variability, each RR interval should be determined as precisely as possible. Variations in the fiducial point, that is the reference point of the QRS complex, will modify (and increase) heart rate variability with no effect on heart rate.

Different methods are used to measure the so-called "heart rate". The heart rate is often assumed to be identical to the pulse rate measured at the level of the radial artery. This assumption may be valid in most patients. However, the pulse rate may fail to detect premature ventricular or atrial beats and may underestimate heart rate in patients with fast and irregular heart rates such as in atrial fibrillation. Cardiac auscultation is a more accurate mean of measuring heart rate and should be preferred in patients with known or suspected irregular heart beats. Rarely, heart rate is derived from intra-arterial blood pressure waveforms obtained over either short or long periods of time.

Finally, heart rate is often measured from ECG recordings of various duration. This method has several advantages and is favoured by many investigators. First, the ECG recording allows discrimination between normal sinus beats and ectopic beats. Second, heart rate can be measured from ECG samples long after the recording, a practical advantage of major importance in large cooperative studies. Finally, ambulatory ECG recordings allow determination of heart rate over prolonged periods of time, which is of major importance to study the effect of the autonomic nervous system on the heart.

Besides those technical requirements, clinical conditions and duration of the measure of heart rate may influence the result. Heart rate is sometimes assessed from an ECG on a single RR interval, as the ratio between 60 000 and the RR interval in milliseconds. The method should be referred as instantaneous heart rate and may not represent the true heart rate of the subject, especially if a high heart rate variability is present. This method is preferred in studies using a standard 12-lead ECG to measure heart rate. In some studies, heart rate is calculated over a 30-s period,[6] but some authors use a 15-s [7] and others 1-min period.[8] Surprisingly, the duration of recording is not reported in the vast majority of studies.

Heart rate can also be measured accurately from 24-h Holter recordings. Recently, a lot of attention was dedicated to prolonged ECG recordings to assess both heart rate and heart rate variability. In a study by van Hoogenhuyze and co-workers, it was shown that the reproducibility of heart rate measurements obtained from 24-h Holter recordings in healthy volunteers and patients with heart failure exceeded that of heart rate variability.[9] However, the prognostic significance of heart rate as compared to heart rate variability is controversial and will be discussed below. Similarly, although the duration of ECG recordings for assessing heart rate variability has been discussed in several studies,[10–12] little is known of the optimal duration of recording to enhance the predictive value of heart rate.

Finally, the conditions of recording should be stated. When heart rate is being measured at the bedside, the type of observer should be stated (whether it was a physician, a nurse, or a technician), and whether the heart rate was measured using automatic instrumentation. A greater reaction has been demonstrated when heart rate is measured by a physician rather than a nurse.[13] The position of the body should also be taken into account: measures of heart rate over a short period of time will differ if the patient is supine or sitting. The duration of resting time before heart rate measurement is also important. Most authors allow patients to rest for 5 min before measurement but some authors use a longer time,[14] or do not allow patients to rest before heart rate measurement.[15]

Univariate association between heart rate and mortality and morbidity

A number of studies have assessed heart rate as a possible risk stratifier, yielding sometimes conflicting results. The points important to consider before admitting conflicting results are:

- the type of the population studied;
- the risk supposedly stratified by heart rate (whether it is total, a specific cause of mortality, or morbidity);
- the incidence of the risk stratified (to be able to compare different predictive values of heart rate); and
- the way heart rate was measured.

Another important point, which will be discussed below, is the comparison of heart rate with other risk stratifiers, and the method used to compare them.

Several studies have assessed the predictive value of

heart rate in the general population.[16–25] The first study to report an association between increased heart rate and mortality in the general population was published as early as 1945.[16] Since then, large epidemiological studies have confirmed this finding. Resting heart rate is definitely accepted as a strong prognostic factor of all-cause mortality, but there are still controversies concerning the predictive value of heart rate for specific cardiovascular causes of mortality. A strong association between elevated heart rate and non-cardiovascular death (specifically cancer) was found in several studies.[18,19,26] This association between heart rate and cancer remained significant even after data for the first 2 years of follow-up had been eliminated.[26]

As compared with total mortality, the association between heart rate and cardiovascular mortality is more controversial.[5] However, this association was demonstrated in a number of studies.[16–19,21] A recent study by Benetos *et al.* based on 19 386 subjects followed-up for more than 18 years demonstrated a positive association between heart rate and both all-cause and cardiovascular death in men, whereas the association with heart rate was only statistically significant for non-cardiovascular death in women.[21] Mean heart rate measured on the first two hours of ambulatory ECG was significantly associated with all-cause mortality in an elderly cohort of the Framingham heart study[24] and with the risk of cardiac events.[25]

The specific relation between heart rate and sudden death in the general population was the subject of fewer reports. However, a univariate association between heart rate and sudden death has been demonstrated in different studies.[20,22,23] Resting heart rate measured from a standard ECG was positively associated with sudden cardiac death in two large prospective studies, examining specifically the risk of sudden death in men.[20,22] In a study of 7735 British men followed up for 8 years, Wannamethee *et al.* found a 4.8 relative risk (age-adjusted) for sudden cardiac death between subjects with a resting heart rate above 90/min and below 60/min. An increased resting heart rate was associated with a 1.42 relative risk in univariate analysis in the Paris Prospective Study.[22] In the study by Algra and co-workers, 24-hour mean heart rate was assessed as a predictor of sudden death in a large population.[23] There was no clear relation between 24-hour mean heart rate and the subsequent risk of sudden cardiac death. Patients with a mean heart rate below 70 or above 80 had a non-significant increase in the relative risk of sudden death as compared to patients between these two values. However, patients in whom the minimum heart rate was above 65/min had a significant increase in the risk of sudden death as compared to patients with a minimum heart rate below 65/min.

After myocardial infarction an elevated resting heart rate has long been recognised as an important predictor of mortality.[27–32] A resting heart rate above 90/min was associated with both an increased risk of all-cause mortality and sudden death.[28] More recently, in the thrombolytic era, heart rate was shown to be a significant predictor of 30-day mortality in the GUSTO Trial.[32]

The prognostic value of heart rate measured from 24-hour ambulatory ECG monitoring after myocardial infarction has been assessed more recently. Several studies have found a univariate association between mean heart rate and mortality after myocardial infarction.[33–36] In the study by Copie and co-workers, patients in the lowest heart rate quartile had a 2.1% all-cause mortality, as compared to 22.2% in the highest quartile. These figures were respectively 1.4 and 11.1% for sudden death. Patients with a mean 24-hour RR interval below 700 ms (i.e. a mean heart rate above 85/min) had a 2-year risk of cardiac death of 20%.[4]

In patients with heart failure, an elevated heart rate has been associated with worsened prognosis in some studies,[37–39] whereas others did not find a significant relation between prognosis and heart rate.[4]

Multivariate association between heart rate and prognosis: influence of therapeutic interventions

As explained above, heart rate has been found to be associated with prognosis in various populations in a number of studies. However, heart rate is not an independent factor and may both be influenced and influence other known risk stratifiers. For example, heart rate may increase in patients with depressed left ventricular ejection fraction after myocardial infarction. A univariate analysis could obviate the fact that heart rate may only represent a surrogate for overt signs of heart failure or, on the contrary, that sophisticated measures of left ventricular ejection fraction could easily be replaced by a measure of heart rate over a few heart beats. Therefore a multivariate approach is paramount to assess the clinical value of heart rate in a different patient population.

In the general population, resting heart rate was shown to be independently associated with prognosis and that it provided prognosis information beyond other clinical variables. In the Framingham Study, a multivariate analysis demonstrated that all-cause mortality, coronary deaths, and sudden cardiac death were all independently related to heart rate after adjustment for a number of clinical variables, such as systolic blood pressure, serum cholesterol, glucose intolerance, smoking, ECG-left ventricular hypertrophy, and age.[18] This independent predictive value of heart rate was further confirmed in patients with hypertension in the same population (Fig. 20.1).[41] These data are in accordance with other population-based studies, such as the Paris Prospective Study where resting heart rate was specifically associated with sudden death,[22] and the three Chicago epidemiological studies (Fig. 20.2).[17] In

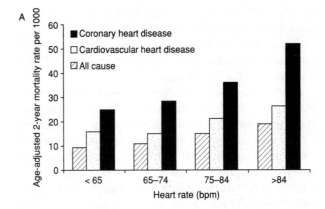

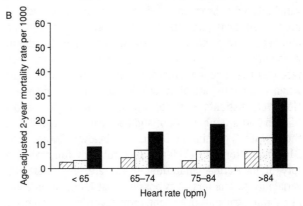

Figure 20.1 Association of heart rate with mortality rate among men (A) and women (B) with hypertension. Data from 36-year follow-up of the Framingham study. (Adapted from reference 41.)

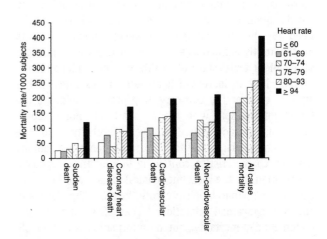

Figure 20.2 All-cause mortality at 15 years, coronary heart disease mortality, cardiovascular mortality, and non-cardiovascular mortality, versus heart rate among 1233 men, in the Chicago People Gas Company study. (Adapted from reference 17.)

the IPC study, heart rate was shown to be an independent predictor of non-cardiovascular mortality in both sexes, and of cardiovascular mortality in men.[21] However, heart rate was not an independent significant predictor of cardiovascular mortality in women.

In the general population, mean heart rate measured from long-term ECG recordings was not shown to be associated with prognosis independently of heart rate variability.[23–25] Age and heart rate are two major determinants of heart rate variability and should be taken into account when assessing it.[42] However, in the Framingham study where heart rate variability was studied from 2-hour ambulatory ECG recordings, little was added to heart rate variability with heart rate.[24] In a multivariate analysis, 2-hour mean heart rate was shown to predict cardiac events independently of clinical variables, but not of heart rate variability.[25] In the study by Algra and co-workers, heart rate was not independently associated with sudden death when heart rate variability was included in the analysis.[23] However, patients with a minimum heart rate above 65/min had a double risk of sudden death compared with those with a minimum heart rate below 65/min, after adjustment for age, evidence of cardiac dysfunction, history of myocardial infarction, heart rate, and heart rate variability parameters. It is possible that information about heart rate available from long-term recordings should not be limited to the mean RR interval, but could include other parameters such as diurnal and nocturnal heart rate, maximum and minimum heart rate, and differences between diurnal and nocturnal heart rate.

After myocardial infarction, resting heart rate is associated with mortality independently of other clinical variables. In the study by Ruberman and co-workers, a resting heart rate above 90/min was associated with all-cause mortality, independently of the presence of complex ventricular premature beats, congestive heart failure, and the need for diuretic therapy.[28] However, sudden coronary death, strictly defined as a death occurring within minutes of a patient usual state of health, was not independently predicted by an increased heart rate in this study. Other studies, such as the coronary drug project, yielded a different information, with resting heart rate not independently associated with the 3-year mortality.[27] In the GUSTO megatrial, elevated heart rate at entry was among the five characteristics containing 90% of the prognostic information in the baseline clinical data, together with age, lower systolic blood pressure, higher Killip class, and anterior myocardial infarction.[32] These five variables predicted 30-day mortality, but no information was available concerning the long-term and sudden death mortality of these 41 021 patients.

Mean heart rate computed from ambulatory ECG recording is also of prognostic significance after myocardial infarction.[4] However, controversies arose from the comparison between heart rate variability and heart rate itself. In the landmark study by Kleiger and co-workers, a SDNN (standard deviation of all normal to normal RR intervals) below 50 ms was shown to predict mortality independently of an average RR interval below 750 ms.[33] This analysis was further emphasised by the same team in a thorough study stating that mean RR interval did not provide prognosis information beyond heart rate variability.[43] In the study by Farrell and co-workers from the St George's group, a mean RR interval below 750 ms was significantly associated with arrhythmic events in the univariate analysis, but heart rate added little if any further information to heart rate variability.[34] However, the relation between heart rate and heart rate variability is far from simple[1] and their comparative predictive values were further studied in the St George's group by Copie and co-workers.[4] A total of 579 patients followed up for 2 years were included in the analysis. The end-points considered were all-cause mortality, cardiac mortality, sudden death, and non-sudden cardiac death, and the three risk stratifiers studied were 24-hour mean RR interval, heart rate variability, and left ventricular ejection fraction. The receiver operating characteristics curves of the three variables for the four end-points considered are displayed in Fig. 20.3. Mean RR interval and heart rate variability performed better than ejection fraction in predicting all-cause mortality, cardiac death, and sudden death. For the prediction of non-sudden cardiac death, the differences between the three variables were negligible. For prediction of end-points of all categories, heart rate variability performed slightly better than mean RR interval in the low sensitivity range, whereas mean RR interval outperformed heart rate variability slightly in the high sensitivity range.

This topic was further analysed by the same authors studying gender differences in risk stratification after myocardial infarction.[35] It was shown that heart rate variability outperformed both heart rate and left ventricular ejection fraction in the prediction of cardiac mortality in men. However, the reverse was true in women, with heart rate being more powerful than heart rate variability and ejection fraction in the prediction of cardiac death (Fig. 20.4). However, owing to the small number of women included in post-myocardial infarction populations, the difference between heart rate and heart rate variability did not reach statistical significance. This intriguing finding deserves confirmation in a different post-myocardial infarction population.

More recently, the analysis of a new Holter based parameter for risk stratification after myocardial infarction led to a reappraisal of the value of mean RR interval.[36] With a dichotomy limit set at 800 ms (that is 75 beats per minute), 24-hour mean heart rate was found to be independently associated with mortality in a multivariate analysis of the EMIAT database. This was not the case in

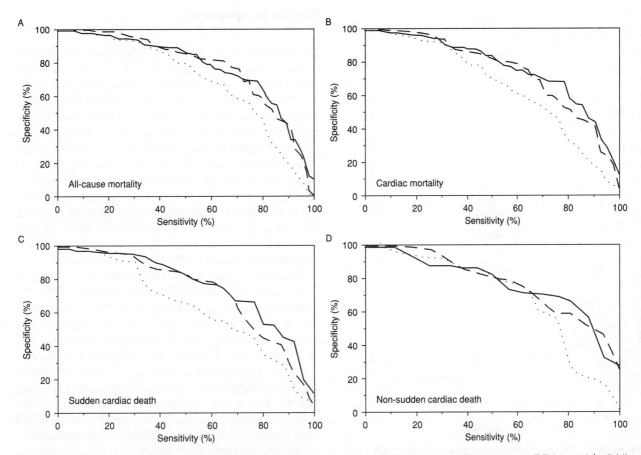

Figure 20.3 Receiver operating characteristics curves showing the sensitivity and specificity of mean RR interval (solid lines), heart rate variability (dashed lines) and left ventricular ejection fraction (dotted lines) for the prediction of all-cause mortality (A), cardiac mortality (B), sudden cardiac death (C), and non-sudden cardiac death (D). Data from 2-year follow-up of the St George's post-myocardial infarction database (Adapted from reference 4.)

heart rate variability. However, in the MPIP database, only a left ventricular ejection fraction below 30% and the new parameter turbulence slope were independent predictors of mortality. This recent study highlights the importance of the *a priori* choice of a dichotomy limit. From the study by Copie and co-workers, it could have been suspected that a mean RR interval at 750 ms did not compare favourably with heart rate variability, and that choosing a mean RR interval at 800 ms could have enhanced the sensitivity to specificity ratio. Also, large post-myocardial infarction databases with 24-h Holter available are scarce and may differ because of temporal and geographical differences in the management of myocardial infarction. Therefore it is of paramount importance that indices and hypotheses validated on a specific database are confirmed on other databases, with acknowledgement of their possible differences.

In patients with heart failure, the prognostic value of heart rate has been studied less extensively. Resting heart rate was found to be associated with mortality or heart transplant in univariate analysis in the study by Wijbenga and co-workers, but its prognostic value was not independent of other variables such as heart rate variability and left ventricular ejection fraction.[39] Mean heart rate dichotomised at 750 ms was not significantly associated with either cardiac death or sudden death in the study by Brouwer and co-workers in univariate analysis.[38] Similarly, mean RR interval did not differ significantly between survivors and heart failure patients who died of cardiac causes in the study by Ponikowski and co-workers.[40] In these populations, heart rate variability was a significant and independent predictor of mortality, adding information to previously known prognostic factors.[44]

Cardiovascular as well as non-cardiovascular treatments can modify heart rate significantly. However, the influence of drug therapy on the predictive value of heart rate has not been studied extensively. To do so, one could compare the predictive value of heart rate between a placebo arm and an active treatment arm of a study with a drug known to influence heart rate. However, it is likely that

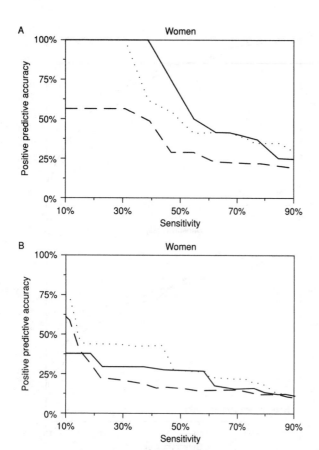

Figure 20.4 Positive predictive characteristics of left ventricular ejection fraction (dashed line), mean RR interval (full line), and heart rate variability (dotted line) in women (A) and men (B). Data from 3-year follow-up of the St George's post-myocardial infarction database. (Adapted from reference 35.)

drugs able to modify heart rate may strongly influence the prognosis. Therefore one would be left with the comparison of two groups with different heart rates, different treatments, and different prognosis. The statistical approach for such a comparison is clearly complex.

Nevertheless, treatments known to decrease heart rate, such as beta-blocking agents have often been shown to improve prognosis, and conversely heart rate increasing treatments such as positive inotropic agents may worsen prognosis. Therefore, it is possible that the predictive value of heart rate may not be decreased by treatments influencing heart rate, but could very well be increased. Before a comprehensive study is performed, this remains speculative.

Clinical perspectives

Several trials have shown the clinical benefit of heart rate lowering drugs such as beta-blockers.[45] Numerous treatments influence the autonomic nervous system and consequently may modify heart rate.[46,47] Recent experiments have shown that heart rate may be the most reliable parameter to assess modifications in autonomic tone.[48] Therefore heart rate could represent a useful marker to assess the likelihood of a supposed benefit of a new treatment. For instance, before a large trial with a new treatment is begun in heart failure, the effect of this treatment on ejection fraction, exercise capabilities, and peak VO_2 are generally assessed. Measuring the effect of this new treatment on 24-hour mean heart rate could provide hints on whether this new treatment will prove beneficial or not in these patients.

Furthermore positive outcome in large trials are a statistical result on a population with the net effect being the result of a majority of patients improved by the treatment, patients experiencing a neutral effect of the treatment, and patients having their condition potentially worsened by the treatment. The net effect is positive but this cannot rule out deleterious effects in some individuals. Identifying subgroups of patients who could potentially benefit more or, on the contrary, be harmed by a new treatment would be clinically relevant. In the first CIBIS trial assessing the effect of bisoprolol on mortality in patients with severe heart failure, the statistical analysis did not show a significant benefit of the treatment.[49] However, further analyses showed that patients with a high baseline heart rate, who decreased it significantly with active treatment, had an improved prognosis.[50]

Heart rate could also in itself be a target to improve survival in different populations. Although a considerable amount of work concerns patients with high blood pressure or high cholesterol, virtually no study was performed to improve the prognosis of patients with elevated heart rate. Several treatments could be studied in this indication, not only beta-blockers, but also non-dihydropyridine calcium channel blockers, or a specific sinus node inhibitor such as zatebradine.[51]

Heart rate is easy to measure and yields important prognostic information. Although it is clear that heart rate is a potent and independent variable for assessing the risk of all-cause mortality, data on the specific risk of sudden death are scarce and more controversial. It would also be important to determine whether heart rate measured during ambulatory ECG recordings provides more prognostic information as compared to heart rate measured over short resting periods. Finally, more work is needed to assess the potential benefit of targeting increased heart rate in different patient populations.

References

1. Coumel P, Maison-Blanche P, Catuli D. Heart rate and heart rate variability in normal young adults. *J Cardiovasc Electrophysiol* 1994;**5**:899–911.

2. Levine HJ. Rest heart rate and life expectancy. *J Am Coll Cardiol* 1997;**30**:1104–6.

3. Jose AD, Collison D. The normal and determinants of the intrinsic heart rate in man. *Cardiovasc Res* 1970;**4**:160–7.

4. Copie X, Hnatkova K, Staunton A, Lü Fei, Camm AJ, Malik M. Predictive power of increased heart rate versus depressed left ventricular ejection fraction and heart rate variability for risk stratification after myocardial infarction. A two-year follow-up study. *J Am Coll Cardiol* 1996;**27**:270–6.

5. Palatini P, Julius S. Heart rate and the cardiovascular risk. *J Hypertens* 1997;**15**:3–17.

6. Gillum RF, Makuk DM, Feldman JJ. Pulse rate, coronary heart disease, and death: the NHANES I epidemiologic follow-up study. *Am Heart J* 1991;**121**:172–7.

7. Stern MP, Morales PA, Haffner SM, Valdez RA. Hyperdynamic circulation and the insulin resistance syndrome (syndrome X). *Hypertension* 1992;**20**:802–8.

8. Erikssen J, Rodhal K. Resting heart rate in apparently healthy middle-aged men. *Eur J Appl Physiol* 1979;**42**:61–9.

9. van Hoogenhuyze D, Weistein N, Martin *et al.* Reproducibility and relation to mean heart rate of heart rate variability in normal subjects and in patients with congestive heart failure secondary to coronary artery disease. *Am J Cardiol* 1991;**68**:1668–76.

10. Malik M, Farrell T, Camm AJ. Circadian rhythm of heart rate variability after myocardial infarction and its influence on the prognostic value of heart rate variability. *Am J Cardiol* 1990;**66**:1049–54.

11. Lü Fei, Copie X, Malik M, Camm AJ. Short- and long-term assessment of heart rate variability for risk stratification after acute myocardial infarction. *Am J Cardiol* 1996;**77**:681–4.

12. Bigger JT, Fleiss JL, Rolnitzky LM, Steinman RC. The ability of several short-term measures of RR variability to predict mortality after myocardial infarction. *Circulation* 1993;**88**:927–34.

13. Mancia G, Parati G, Pomidossi G, Grassi G, Gagodei R, Zanchetti A. Alerting reaction and rise in blood pressure during measurement by physician and nurse. *Hypertension* 1987;**9**:209–15.

14. Feskens EJM, Kromhout D. Hyperinsulinemia. Risk factors, and coronary heart disease. *Arterioscler Thromb* 1994;**14**:1641–7.

15. Selby JV, Friedman GD, Quesenberry CP Jr. Precursors of essential hypertension: pulmonary function, heart rate, uric acid, serum cholesterol, and other serum chemistries. *Am J Epidemiol* 1990;**131**:1017–27.

16. Levy RL, White PD, Stroud WD, Hillman CC. Transient tachycardia: prognostic significance alone and in association with transient hypertension. *JAMA* 1945;**129**:585–8.

17. Dyer AR, Persky V, Stamler J *et al.* Heart rate as a prognostic factor for coronary heart disease and mortality: findings in three Chicago epidemiologic studies. *Am J Epidemiol* 1980;**112**:736–49.

18. Kannel WB, Kannel C, Paffenbarger RS *et al.* Heart rate and cardiovascular mortality: the Framingham study. *Am Heart J* 1987;**113**:1489–94.

19. Filipovsky J, Ducimetière P, Safar M. Prognostic significance of exercise blood pressure and heart rate in middle-aged men. *Hypertension* 1992;**20**:333–9.

20. Wannamethee G, Shaper AG, Macfarlane PW *et al.* Risk factors for sudden cardiac death in middle-aged British men. *Circulation* 1995;**91**:1749–56.

21. Benetos A, Rudnichi A, Thomas F, Safar M, Guize L. Influence of heart rate on mortality in a French population. Role of age, gender, and blood pressure. *Hypertension* 1999;**33**:44–52.

22. Jouven X, Desnos M, Guerot C, Ducimetière P. Predicting sudden death in the population. The Paris prospective study I. *Circulation* 1999;**99**:1978–83.

23. Algra A, Tijssen JGP, Roetlandt JRTC, Pool J, Lubsen J. Heart rate variability fom 24-hour electrocardiography and the 2-year risk of sudden death. *Circulation* 1993;**88**:180–5.

24. Tsuji H, Venditti FJ, Manders ES *et al.* Reduced heart rate variability and mortality risk in an elderly cohort. The Framingham heart study. *Circulation* 1994;**90**:878–83.

25. Tsuji H, Larson MG, Venditti FJ *et al.* Impact of reduced heart rate variability on risk for cardiac events. The Framingham heart study. *Circulation* 1996;**94**:2850–5.

26. Persky V, Dyer AR, Leonas J, Stamler J, Berkson DM, Lindberg HA. Heart rate: a risk factor for cancer? *Am J Epidemiol* 1981;**114**:477–87.

27. The Coronary Drug Project Research Group. The prognostic importance of the electrocardiogram after myocardial infarction. experience in the coronary drug project. *Ann Int Med* 1972;**77**:677–89.

28. Ruberman W, Weinblatt E, Goldberg JD, Frank CW, Shapiro S. Ventricular premature beats and mortality after myocardial infarction. *New Engl J Med* 1977;**297**:750–7.

29. The Multicenter Postinfarction Research Group. Risk stratification and survival after myocardial infarction. *New Engl J Med* 1983;**309**:331–6.

30. Crimm A, Severance HW, Coffey K, McKinnis R, Wagner GS, Califf RM. Prognostic significance of isolated sinus tachycardia during the first three days of acute myocardial infarction. *Am J Med* 1984;**73**:983–8.

31. Fioretti P, Brower R, Simoons ML *et al.* Relative value of clinical variables, bicycle ergometry, rest radionuclide ventriculography, and 24-hour ambulatory electrocardiographic monitoring at discharge to predict 1 year survival after myocardial infarction. *J Am Coll Cardiol* 1986;**8**:40–9.

32. Lee KL, Woodlief LH, Topol EJ *et al.* Predictors of 30-day mortality in the era of reperfusion for acute myocardial infarction. Results from an international trial of 41 021 patients. *Circulation* 1995;**91**:1659–68.

33. Kleiger RE, Miller JP, Bigger JT Jr, Moss AJ. Decreased heart rate variability and its association with increased mortality after acute myocardial infarction. *Am J Cardiol* 1987;**59**:256–62.

34. Farrell TG, Bashir Y, Cripps T *et al.* Risk stratification for

arrhythmic events in postinfarction patients based on heart rate variability, ambulatory electrocardiographic variables and the signal-averaged electrocardiogram. *J Am Coll Cardiol* 1991;**18**:687–97.

35. Copie X, Hnatkova K, Lü Fei, Staunton A, Camm AJ, Malik M. Gender specificities in risk stratification after myocardial infarction. *Ann Noninvasiv Electrocardiol* 1997;**2**:59–68.

36. Schmidt G, Malik M, Barthel P *et al.* Heart rate turbulence after ventricular premature beats as a predictor of mortality after acute myocardial infarction. *Lancet* 1999;**353**:1390–6.

37. Binder T, Frey B, Porenta G *et al.* Prognostic value of heart rate variability in patients awaiting cardiac transplantation. *PACE* 1992;**15** (part II):2215–20.

38. Brouwer J, van Veldhuisen DJ, Man in't Veld AJ *et al.* Prognostic value of heart rate variability during long-term follow-up in patients with mild to moderate heart failure. *J Am Coll Cardiol* 1996;**28**:1183–9.

39. Wijbenga JAM, Balk AHMM, Meij SH, Simoons ML, Malik M. Heart rate variability index in congestive heart failure: relation to clinical variables and prognosis. *Eur Heart J* 1998;**19**:1719–24.

40. Ponikowski P, Anker SD, Chua TP *et al.* Depressed heart rate variability as an independent predictor of death in chronic congestive heart failure secondary to ischemic or idiopathic dilated cardiomyopathy. *Am J Cardiol* 1997;**79**:1645–50.

41. Gillman MW, Kannel WB, Belanger A, D'Agostino RB. Influence of heart rate on mortality among persons with hypertension: the Framingham study. *Am Heart J* 1993;**125**:1148–54.

42. Tsuji H, Venditti FJ, Manders ES *et al.* Determinants of heart rate variability. *J Am Coll Cardiol* 1996;**28**:1539–46.

43. Fleiss JL, Bigger JT, Rolnitzky LM. The correlation between heart period variability and mean period length. *Statistics Med* 1992;**11**:125–9.

44. Copie X, Guize L, Le Heuzey JY. Heart rate variability in heart failure. *Heart Failure* 1998;**14**:185–91.

45. Laperche T, Logeart D, Cohen-Solal A, Gourgon R. Potential interest of heart rate lowering drugs. *Heart* 1999;**81**:336–41.

46. Copie X, Guize L, Le Heuzey JY. Concomitant therapy and autonomic tests. In: Malik M, ed. *Clinical guide to cardiac autonomic tests.* Dordrecht: Kluwer 1998, pp.301–30.

47. Copie X, Pousset F, Lechat Ph, Jaillon P, Guize L, Le Heuzey JY, and CIBIS investigators. Effects of beta-blockade with bisoprolol on heart rate variability in patients with advanced heart failure: analysis of scatterplots of RR intervals at selected heart rates. *Am Heart J* 1996;**132**:369–75.

48. Goldberger JJ. How do you identify an index of sympathovagal balance ? *PACE* 1999;**22**:838.

49. CIBIS Investigators and Committees. A randomized trial of beta-blockade in heart failure. The Cardiac Insufficiency Bisoprolol Study (CIBIS). *Circulation* 1994;**90**:1765–73.

50. Lechat P, Escolano S, Golmard JL *et al.* on behalf of CIBIS investigators. Prognosis value of bisoprolol-induced hemodynamic effects in heart failure during the Cardiac Insufficiency Bisoprolol Study. *Circulation* 1997;**96**:2197–205.

51. Frishman WH, Pepine CJ, Weiss R *et al.* The addition of direct sinus node inhibitor (zatebradine) provides no greater exercise tolerance benefit to patients with angina pectoris treated with extended-release nifedipine: results of a multicenter, randomised, double-blind, placebo controlled, parallel group study. *J Am Coll Cardiol* 1995;**26**:305–12.

21 Heart rate variability

Robert E Kleiger and Phyllis K Stein

As has become abundantly clear to readers of this book, considerable scientific effort has focused on arrhythmia risk stratification and management. Measurement of heart rate variability (HRV) has been an important part of this picture, because analysis of HRV provides information about the functioning of the autonomic nervous system, a central player in arrhythmogenesis. Clinically, HRV can be obtained via routine Holter monitoring and is expressed in the time and/or frequency domain. Both time and frequency domain HRV are usually reported. They are closely related[1] and are calculated from *normal-to-normal (NN) interbeat intervals* only. Ectopic beats do not affect HRV, but if there are more than 10–20% ectopic beats, frequency domain HRV cannot reliably be determined. Time domain HRV is based on statistical calculations. Table 21.1 lists standard time domain HRV and their definitions and synonyms. SDNN and SDANN both primarily reflect long-term or circadian rhythms.[2] SDNNIDX, an intermediate between long- and short-term variability reflects both sympathetic and parasympathetic influences on the heart rate. Time domain variables, which reflect short-term

changes in HRV, include pNN50 and rMSSD. Under normal circumstances, these indices predominantly reflect vagal modulation of the SA node;[3] however, if calculated over 24 hours, they are also influenced by long-term and circadian changes. Time domain HRV indices that adjust for heart rate, e.g. the coefficient of variance and pNN6.25% are also found in the literature.

HRV analysis in the frequency domain requires fast Fourier or autoregressive techniques and provides information about the amount of the variance (power) in the heart's rhythm, explained by periodic oscillations of heart rate at different frequencies. This can be thought of as similar to the process of decomposing a complex musical sound into individual underlying notes. The underlying frequencies of the heart rate signal, when grouped together in bands, provide a more detailed view of autonomic modulation of the heart. The Task Force of the European Society of Cardiology and the North American Society of Pacing and Electrophysiology recommended that, when frequency domain HRV is determined for clinical purposes, it should be calculated in four bands.[3] Table 21.2 provides

Table 21.1 Commonly used time domain indices of heart rate variability, usually computed over 24 hours unless otherwise stated

HRV Index	Synonyms	Definition
AVGNN (ms)	(AVGRR, mean NN)	Average of N–Ns
SDNN (ms)	(SDRR)	Standard deviation of all NN intervals
SDANN (ms)		Standard deviation of the average of NN intervals for each 5-min period
SDNNIDX (ms)	(SD, SDNN$_i$)	Average of the standard deviations of NN intervals for each 5-min period
rMSSD (ms)		Root mean square of successive differences of times between adjacent cycles
pNN50 (%)		Proportion of times between adjacent cycles that are different by >50 ms
pNN6.25 (%)		Proportion of times between adjacent cycles that are different by >6.25% of AVGNN
Counts		Number of beats where the difference in NN from the previous beat is >50 ms
Coefficient of variance	(CV)	(SDNN/AVGNN) averaged for every 5 min

Table 21.2 Standard frequency domain indices of heart rate variability

HRV index	Abbreviation	Frequency range	Cycle length
Total power	TP	1.15×10^{-5}–0.4 Hz	24 cycles/min to 1 cycle/24 h
Ultra low frequency power	ULF	1.15×10^{-5}–0.0033 Hz	5 min to 24 h/cycle
Very low frequency power	VLF	0.0033–0.04 Hz	25 s to 5 min/cycle
Low frequency power	LF	0.04–0.15 Hz	6.7 s to 25 s/cycle
High frequency power	HF	0.15–0.4 Hz	9 to 24 per cycle/min

definitions for the components of frequency domain HRV. High-frequency (HF) power is the highest frequency band quantified. It is parasympathetically mediated, abolished by atropine infusion[4,5] and reflects primarily respiration-mediated HRV. The group of frequencies just below HF is the low-frequency (LF) band, modulated by both the sympathetic and parasympathetic nervous systems.[4,5] LF is virtually abolished by total autonomic blockade[5,6] and is strongly affected by the oscillatory rhythm of the baroreceptor system.[7] Short-term estimates of both LF and HF power are sometimes obtained during measurements of signal-averaged ECGs. Even slower modulations of heart rate are reflected in the very low frequency (VLF) band. VLF may represent the influence of the peripheral vasomotor and renin–angiotensin systems.[8] The remainder of the power spectrum is quantified as ultra low-frequency power (ULF). ULF encompasses all variations in HR with a period of more than 5 min to 24 hours, and reflects primarily circadian but also neuroendocrine and other rhythms.[9] These indices may be combined in total power (TP), which, because it reflects the total variance, should be similar to SDNN.[2] While LF and HF can reliably be obtained with commercial Holter scanners, ULF and TP values are not comparable to those reported in the literature, because commercial scanners are usually limited to analysing data in 10-min segments or shorter.[10]

It has been clearly established that HF power normally reflects vagal modulation of the heart rate. It has also been claimed that LF power, especially LF power normalised to TP, primarily reflects sympathetic modulation of heart rate,[11] and that the LF/HF ratio reflects "sympathovagal balance".[12] Although there is supporting experimental evidence derived from the association between manoeuvres that both increase sympathetic tone and LF power,[11,12] there is a large body of contradictory data as well.[4,13–15] The majority consensus is that LF power reflects a mixture of sympathetic and parasympathetic effects on heart rate which can under certain circumstances reflect sympathetic tone.[16] The same can be said for the LF/HF ratio as a marker of sympathovagal balance.

Another index of HRV seen in the literature but not routinely available for clinical use is the HRV index, a geo-metric measure used in many of the studies from the group at St George's Hospital in London. This index was developed to make accurate HRV measurement less dependent on detailed, meticulous scanning techniques. The HRV index is computed from the histogram of all RR intervals by dividing the total number of NN intervals by the number of NN intervals at the peak of the histogram (i.e. the number with modal duration).[17] HRV index measures longer-term HRV and correlates with SDNN or SDANN. Vagal modulation of heart rate cannot be assessed by this method, and accuracy is limited with bimodally distributed RR-interval histograms.

The "first generation" of HRV research in cardiology was largely based on time and frequency domain analysis. Currently, there is an explosion of newer methods, based on more sophisticated non-linear mathematical techniques. Although these measures are not yet available clinically, there is evidence that they may have better predictive value,[18] or that a combination of standard and non-linear techniques could provide optimal risk stratification.[19] These techniques are described elsewhere in this book.

In general, conditions that change autonomic tone will change heart rate and HRV, but *heart rate and HRV are not surrogates for one another.* Examples of conditions that change both heart rate and HRV include exercise, fever, mental stimulation, emotions, tilt table testing etc., as well as medications and surgery. An increase in parasympathetic (vagal) tone results in decreased heart rate and usually increased HRV, but maximal vagal stimulation will actually *reduce* HRV. Vagal withdrawal or sympathetic stimulation results in increased heart rate and usually decreased HRV. However, it must be emphasised that, although it is often stated that HRV reflects autonomic tone, HRV reflects phasic cardiac autonomic modulation only, and longer-term indices of HRV, which are often the best predictors of outcome, may reflect other, unknown influences.[20] Thus, low values for HRV, while clearly associated with adverse outcomes, could reflect a marked reduction in central modulation of heart rate or a marked lack of response of the sinus node, either of which could even be due to saturation from very elevated tonic levels of autonomic tone or other factors. Despite these limitations, under most circumstances, measurement of HRV provides a useful assessment of cardiac autonomic balance.

Autonomic function and arrhythmia risk

The link between autonomic modulation and arrhythmic risk is well established. A variety of experimental and clinical data support the hypothesis that increased vagal tone reduces the risk of malignant ventricular arrhythmias, whereas sympathetic stimulation enhances it.[21–23] Changes in HRV immediately prior to the onset of ventricular arrhythmias have been documented.[24–26] The molecular mechanistic means by which alteration in autonomic tone affects the risk of arrhythmias is not yet clear. Various manoeuvres, including:

- drug therapy with scopolamine or low dose atropine;
- stimulation of the cholinergic receptors with oxotremorine;
- cervical ganglion stellectomy, and
- beta-blockade can decrease sympathetic and/or increase parasympathetic modulation of heart rate in animal models.[27]

Each of these measures can increase HRV and most have been found to be protective against lethal arrhythmias. Scopolamine, however, despite the increase in vagally-modulated HRV with treatment, has been found to have minimal antifibrillatory effects.[1] This result suggests that increased HRV does not always translate to decreased risk of arrhythmic events.

Because of the strong relationship of autonomic tone and vulnerability to arrhythmias, measurement of autonomic tone would be expected to be integral to risk stratification. Autonomic tone in human studies and in animal models can be assessed by pharmacologic autonomic blockade, baroreceptor sensitivity, and HRV measurements. In clinical practice, HRV measurements can be easily and non-invasively obtained while the patient goes about normal activities or, in experimental studies, under carefully controlled conditions in the laboratory. Clinical studies have indicated that many interventions associated with better survival are also associated with increased HRV. For example, patients receiving thrombolysis post-myocardial (MI) infarction have higher HRV[29] and the degree of infarct-related coronary artery patency strongly influences HRV.[30] Pharmacological interventions associated with increased HRV and better survival include:

- beta-blockers without ISA post-MI;[31,32]
- ACE inhibitors[33,34] and carvedilol[35] in CHF;
- sotalol in patients with ventricular arrhythmias,[36,37] and
- oestrogen replacement therapy in post-menopausal women.[38]

Lifestyle changes associated with better survival post-MI, such as exercise training,[39] major weight loss,[40] and smoking cessation[41] also result in improved HRV. Reduced dietary fat intake has recently been reported to increase vagally-modulated HRV in healthy women.[42] There is even limited evidence that biofeedback training can improve HRV in at-risk patients.[43] However, the relationship between increased HRV and better survival has not been conclusively established because, for example, in stable CHF patients, while digoxin increases HRV,[44] it does not reduce mortality.

Relationship of HRV and arrhythmia risk

As will be discussed in greater detail below, there is considerable evidence that HRV is altered in patients at risk for arrhythmic events. In cross-sectional studies, significant HRV differences have been found between high- and low-risk patients. HRV has been shown to be a powerful risk stratifier for overall mortality, cardiac mortality, and arrhythmic events, and HRV in combination with other risk factors has identified post-MI patients at risk for mortality with a positive predictive accuracy of as much as 50%. Although the relationship between HRV and arrhythmic outcome has been investigated for a number of cardiac pathologies including:

- dilated cardiomyopathy ● Chagas' disease ● cardiac transplantation ● congestive heart failure, and ● hypertrophic cardiomyopathy;

as well as in non-cardiac disease states such as:

- diabetes ● chronic alcoholism ● COPD, and ● end-stage renal disease;

the post-MI population has been the most extensively studied and will be the primary focus of this chapter.

Representative cross-sectional studies comparing HRV in high- and low-risk patients are shown in Table 21.3. As can be seen on this table, comparisons of patients with sustained ventricular arrhythmias and similar patients without sustained arrhythmias, and of patients with and without a history of VF or sudden death have found reduced HRV in at risk patients. Three studies (not shown on the table), each involving a slightly different patient population, have compared patients who were and were not inducible on EPS. In one, reduced HRV from an 11-beat strip recorded immediately prior to EPS was found in 92% of inducible patients and only 3% of controls.[45] In contrast, whilst a trend to significant differences in 24-h HRV was found in another study,[46] the third failed to find differences in 24-h HRV.[47] Perkiomiaki *et al.* have suggested that decreased HRV identifies patients at risk for VF or unstable VT, but not patients with inducible or clinically stable monomor-

Table 21.3 Representative cross-sectional comparisons of heart rate variability (HRV) in patients with and without arrhythmic events

Source (study)	Number of patients	HRV measure	Population	Comparisons	HRV differences
[1] Anderson et al., 1996 (ESVEM)	360	24 h	Patients with sustained ventricular arrhythmias	ESVEM vs CAPS and MPIP patients	Time and frequency domain HRV more similar to MPIP (recent MI) than CAPS (chronic CAD)
[2] Counihan et al., 1993 (St. George's)	104	24 h	Patients with hypertropic cardiomyopathy in sinus rhythm, off medications	26 with NSVT on Holter vs none	SDNNIDX, pNN50, LF, HF less in patients with NSVT
[3] Dougherty and Burr, 1992	21	24 h	Sudden death patients	Survivors (N = 16), non-survivors of SCD (N = 5), controls (N = 5)	SDNN, SDANN, SDNNIDX, TP, VLF, LF lowest in non-survivors. No difference in rMSSD or HF
[4] Perkiomaki et al., 1997	90	24 h	Post-MI	N = 30 survivors of VF with previous MI and inducible unstable VT vs N = 30 POMI with clinical and inducible stable monomorphic VT vs N = 30 matched controls without history of arrhythmia for >2 years POMI	SDNN, HRV from Poincaré plots reduced in VF patients but not in VT patients compared with post-MI controls. Decreased HRV better than increased QT dispersion in identifying VF
[5] Poinkowski et al., 1996	50	24 h	Advanced CHF	Patients with (N = 25) and without (N = 25) VT on Holter	Markedly lower HRV in patients with VT. HF power only independent predictor
[6] van Boven et al., 1995 (REGRES)	312	24 h	Significant CAD and LVEF ≥30%	Patients with VT but no silent ischaemia vs patients with transient ischaemia but no VT vs patients with both ischaemia and ventricular arrhythmias vs patients with no abnormalities	Highest rMSSD and HF in group with VT but no silent ischaemia. Lowest rMSSD and HF in group with both

Abbreviations: CAD = coronary artery disease; CHF = congestive heart failure; NSVT = non-sustained ventricular tachycardia; SCD = sudden cardiac death; see also Tables 21.1 and 21.2.
[1] Anderson KP, Bigger JT Jr, Freedman RA. Electrocardiographic predictors in the ESVEM trial: unsustained ventricular tachycardia, heart period variability, and the signal-averaged electrocardiogram. *Prog Cardiovasc Dis* 1996;**38**:463–88.
[2] Counihan PJ, Fei L, Bashir Y, Farrell TG, Haywood GA, McKenna WJ. Assessment of heart rate variability in hypertrophic cardiomyopathy. Association with clinical and prognostic features. *Circulation* 1993;**88**:1682–90.
[3] Dougherty CM, Burr RL. Comparison of heart rate variability in survivors and nonsurvivors of sudden cardiac arrest. *Am J Cardiol* 1992;**70**:441–8.
[4] Perkiomaki JS, Huikuri HV, Koistinen JM, Makikallio T, Castellanos A, Myerburg RJ. Heart rate variability and dispersion of QT interval in patients with vulnerability to ventricular tachycardia and ventricular fibrillation after previous myocardial infarction. *J Am Coll Cardiol* 1997;**30**:1331–8.
[5] Ponikowski P, Anker SD, Amadi A et al. Heart rhythms, ventricular arrhythmias, and death in chronic heart failure. *J Card Fail* 1996;**2**:177–83.
[6] van Boven AJ, Jukema JW, Crijns HJ, Lie KI. Heart rate variability profiles in symptomatic coronary artery disease and preserved left ventricular function: relation to ventricular tachycardia and transient myocardial ischaemia. Regression Growth Evaluation Statin Study (REGRESS). *Am Heart J* 1995;**130**:1020–5.

phic VT.[48] Further results from larger investigations, like the ESVEM and MUSTT trails, will more clearly characterise differences in between patients at high and low risk of arrhythmic events. However, it has become clear from the studies on ICDs that patients at risk of sudden death, because of severe systolic dysfunction and episodes of NSVT, are at high risk of arrhythmic death irrespective of whether they demonstrate inducible VT. It is also clear that the population suitable for electrophysiological study using the criteria of depressed LVEF and NSVT or positive late potentials is very large and probably exceeds the practical limits of such studies. Thus, a risk stratifier that predicts sudden death as well as the electrophysiological study or could define subgroups at risk with either high or very low VT inducibility would be highly desirable.

Table 21.4 lists representative prospective studies of the relationship between HRV and all-cause or cardiac mortality in post-MI patients. Because arrhythmic death is the most common fatal outcome post-MI, risk factors for overall mortality are considered reasonable surrogates for risk factors for arrhythmic events. The first large study of HRV in post-MI patients who survived hospitalisation was the MPIP (Multicenter Postinfarction Project) study.[49] Over 800 patients had 24-hour ambulatory monitoring and SDNN was measured. SDNN less than 50 ms was associated with a relative risk of 5.3 of mortality compared to patients with SDNN of or greater than 100 ms. The striking relationship between SDNN and mortality in MPIP is shown in Fig. 21.1.

Although SDNN was significantly correlated with heart rate, ejection fraction, and VPC frequency, it remained an independent predictor of mortality over the 31-month mean follow-up period. Further analyses of MPIP data also documented the use of 24-hour spectral analysis of HRV[50] to risk stratify post-MI populations. The results of MPIP were validated in numerous studies (Table 21.4). MPIP, however, took place prior to the thrombolytic era and did not specify the mechanism of mortality. Both issues have been subsequently been addressed. Recent studies involving patients who received thrombolysis for acute MI showed that in the thrombolytic era, low HRV continues to predict mortality.[51,52] It is important to keep in mind that in almost all of these studies, HRV was measured in the peri-infarction period and cut points are applicable only to such patients. Studies suggest, however, that HRV continues to risk stratify after MI. Bigger *et al.* in the CAPS (Cardiac Arrhythmia Pilot Study) measured HRV 1 year post-MI. Although the cut points were higher, decreased HRV remained a strong predictor of mortality over a 3-year follow-up. Also, a recent re-analysis of the tapes from the CAST (Cardiac Arrhythmia Suppression Trial) has shown that HRV remains a predictor of mortality in patients recorded over a broad range of times (71 ± 119 days) post-MI and followed for 363 ± 243 days, although reduced HRV due to CABG surgery post-MI or diabetes appears to confound HRV-based risk stratification.[53]

Table 21.5 shows representative prospective studies of predictive value of HRV for arrhythmic versus non-arrhythmic death. HRV predicted sudden death independent of, and sometimes better than, any other non-invasive measure. For example, the group at St George's London Hospital have used HRV (usually HRV index) to stratify post-MI patients. In one such study of over 400 patients, ejection fraction, VPC frequency and repetitiveness, late potentials, and ejection fraction were measured as well as HRV, and deaths were characterised as cardiac, arrhythmic, or sudden. All cases of resuscitated ventricular fibrillation and sustained ventricular tachycardia were determined.[54] Depressed HRV predicted both total cardiac mortality and, even more strongly, arrhythmic events. Such studies have been criticised on the grounds that all sudden deaths, usually defined as death occurring within 1 hour of symptom onset or unexpectedly during sleep, are not necessarily arrhythmic. Moreover, analyses of data from stored ECGs in AICDs suggest that arrhythmia was the mechanism in only two-thirds of sudden deaths.[55] Results, however, clearly indicate that the relationship between decreased HRV and risk of arrhythmic events is robust.

Depressed HRV has also been found to predict both mortality and arrhythmic events in other cardiac populations, including dilated cardiomyopathy and congestive heart failure. In this context, it is possible that HRV may play a role in stratifying patients for cardiac transplanta-

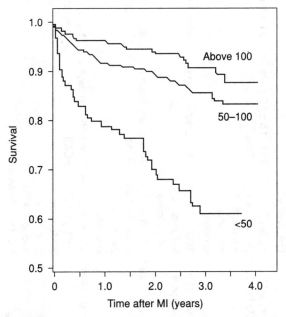

Figure 21.1 Kaplan–Meier survival curves for survival over total follow-up period as a function of heart rate variability in the MPIP study. SDNN <50 ms significant by log-rank test from both other groups ($P < 0.0001$).

Table 21.4 Heart rate variability (HRV) predictors of all-cause or cardiac mortality in post-myocardial infarction (POMI) patients

Source (study)	Number of patients (events)	HRV* measure, when obtained	Follow-up	End-points	HRV predictors
[1]Bigger et al., 1992 (MPIP)	715 (119 deaths)	24 h, 2 weeks POMI	up to 4 years	All-cause mortality	All frequency domain HRV univariate predictors. Decreased ULF + decreased VLF best predictor
[2]Bigger et al., 1993b (CAPS)	331 (30 deaths)	24 h, 1 year after enrolling in CAPS and 1 week after stopping medications	3 years	All-cause mortality from National Death Index	ULF, VLF, LF, HF all significant, univariate predictors. After adjustment for covariates, VLF strongest predictor
[3]Kleiger et al., 1987 (MPIP)	808 (127 deaths)	24 h, 11 ± 3 days POMI	4 years	All-cause mortality	SDNN <50 ms vs SDNN >100 ms (RR = 5.3)
[4]Kleiger et al., 1999 (CAST)	497 without diabetes or CABG POMI (39 deaths)	24 h, 71 ± 119 days POMI	363 ± 243 days	All-cause mortality	Decreased ln SDANN and increased ln rMSSD independent predictors of mortality
[5]La Rovere et al., 1998 (ATRAMI)	1284 (44 cardiac deaths, 5 non-fatal sudden)	24 h, 15 ± 10 days POMI	21 ± 8 months	Cardiac mortality	SDNN <70 ms vs SDNN >70 ms (RR = 3.2)
[6]Odemuyiwa et al., 1991 (St George's Hospital)	385 (44 deaths, 14 sudden)	24 h, predischarge	151–1618 days	All-cause mortality	HRV index ≤39 sens 75%, spec 52% compared with LVEF ≤40 which had spec of 40%. HRV + LVEF better spec for sens <60%
[7]Quintana et al., 1997	74 (18 deaths 9 non-fatal MI), 24 normal controls	24 h, mean 4 days POMI	36 ± 15 months	Mortality, mortality or non-fatal infarction	Ln VLF <5.99 independent predictor of mortality (RR = 1.9) or mortality/non-fatal infarction (RR = 2.2)
[8]Touboul et al., 1997 (GREPI)	471 (26 deaths for/1 year FU, 39 for long term FU, 9 sudden) 45% had thrombolysis	24 h HRV, 10 days POMI	1 year, long term (median 31.4 months)	All-cause mortality	Night-time AVGNN <750 ms (RR = 3.2), daytime SDNN <100 ms (RR = 2.6). Same predictors for 1 year and long-term mortality

Study	n	Follow-up	Recording	Endpoint	Results
[9]Viashnav et al., 1994	226 (19 cardiac deaths)	mean 8 months	24 h, mean 83 hours POMI	Mortality	Cox regression not performed. Decreased SDNN, SDANN, SDNNIDX, LF, HF, LF/HF among non-survivors, but rMSSD and pNN50 not different
[10]Zabel et al., 1998	250	mean 32 months	24 h HRV, stable, before discharge	Mortality, VT or resuscitated VF	SDNN significantly higher in event-free patients
[11]Zuanetti et al., 1996 (GISSI)	567 males treated with thrombolysis (52 deaths, 44 cardiac)	1000 days	24 h at discharge (median 13 days)	All-cause mortality	Independent predictors: NN50+ (RR = 3.5), SDNN (RR = 3.0), rMSSD (RR = 2.8)

Abbreviations: spec = specificity; sens = sensitivity; see also Tables 21.1 and 21.2.
*HRV combined with other risk stratifiers shown on Table 21.6.

[1]Bigger JT Jr, Fleiss JL, Steinman RC, Rolnitzky LM, Kleiger RE, Rottman JN. Frequency domain measures of heart period variability and mortality after myocardial infarction. Circulation 1992;85:164–71.

[2]Bigger JT Jr, Fleiss JL, Rolnitzky LM, Steinman RC. Frequency domain measures of heart period variability to assess risk late after myocardial infarction J Am Coll Cardiol 1993;21:729–36.

[3]Kleiger RE, Miller JP, Bigger JT, Moss AJ and the Multicenter Post-Infarction Research Group. Decreased heart rate variability and its association with increased mortality after acute myocardial infarction. Am J Cardiol 1987;59:256.

[4]Kleiger RE, Stein PK, Domitrovich PP, Rottman JN. CABG and diabetes confound HRV prediction of mortality post-MI (abs). PACE 1999;22(part II).

[5]La Rovere MT, Bigger JT Jr, Marcus FI, Mortara A, Schwartz PJ for the ATRAMI Investigators. Baroreflex sensitivity and heart rate variability in prediction of total cardiac mortality after myocardial infarction. Lancet 1998;351:478–84.

[6]Odemuyiwa O, Malik M, Farrell T, Bashir Y, Poloniecki J, Camm J. Comparison of the predictive characteristics of heart rate variability index and left ventricular ejection fraction for all-cause mortality, arrhythmic events and sudden death after acute myocardial infarction. Am J Cardiol 1991;68:434–9.

[7]Quintana M, Storck N, Lindblad LE, Lindvall K, Ericson M. Heart rate variability as a means of assessing prognosis after acute myocardial infarction. A 3-year follow-up study. Eur Heart J 1997;18:789–97.

[8]Touboul P, Andre-Fouet X, Leizorovicz A et al. Risk stratification after myocardial infarction. A reappraisal in the era of thrombolysis. The Groupe d'Etude du Pronostic de l'Infarctus du Myocarde (GREPI). Eur Heart J 1997;18:99–107.

[9]Vaishnav S, Stevenson R, Marchant B, Lagi K, Ranjadayalan K, Timmis AD. Relation between heart rate variability early after acute myocardial infarction and long-term mortality. Am J Cardiol 1994;73:653–7.

[10]Zabel M, Klingenheben T, Franz MR, Hohnloser SH. Assessment of QT dispersion of prediction of mortality or arrhythmic events after myocardial infarction. Results of a prospective, long-term follow up study. Circulation 1998;97:2543–50.

[11]Zuanetti G, Neilson James MM, Latini R, Santoro E, Maggioni AP, Ewing DJ. Prognostic significance of heart rate variability in post-myocardial infarction patients in the fibrinolytic ear. The GISSI-2 results. Circulation 1996;94:432–6.

Table 21.5 Selected studies of heart rate variability (HRV) predictors of arrhythmic events or sudden death post-myocardial infarction (POMI)

Source (study)	Number of patients (events)	HRV measure, when obtained	Follow-up	End-points	HRV predictors
[1]Bigger et al., 1992 (MPIP)	715 (68 arrhythmic deaths)	24 h, 11 ± 3 days POMI	up to 4 years	Arrhythmic death	VLF <180 ms^2 strongest independent predictor (RR = 2.5) but all frequency domain HRV significant
[2]Cripps et al., 1991 (St George's)	177 (17 end-points)	24 h, median 7 days POMI	median 16 months	Sudden death, sustained VT	HRV index 16.8 ± 8.0 in those with end-points vs 29.0 ± 11.2 in those without. HRV index <25 vs HRV index >25 (RR = 7.0). HRV single most powerful predictor
[3]Farrell et al., 1991 (St George's)	416 (24 end-points)	24 h, day 6 or 7 POMI	mean 612 days	Sudden death, life-threatening ventricular arrhythmia	HRV index <20 best univariate predictor (RR = 6.67) but PPA 17%
[4]Lanza et al., 1998	239 (26 deaths, 19 cardiac, 12 sudden)	24 h, predischarge	median 28 months	Total cardiac mortality, sudden death, all-cause mortality	HRV cut-points chosen for sudden death SDNNIDX <20 ms (RR = 6.7) SDANN <50 ms (RR = 7.4) and VLF <18 ms, (RR = 6.7) (best univariate) HRV not independent predictor
[5]Oedemuyiwa et al., 1991 (St George's)	385 (26 arrhythmic events including 14 sudden deaths)	24h, median 7 days POMI	≥5 months	Arrhythmic death, sudden death	For arrhythmic events. HRV index ≤30 sens 75%, spec 76%. For same sensitivity, LVEF had specificity of 45%. LVEF + HRV index had better specificity for sensitivity between 25 and 75%. HRV index better predictor than LVEF for arrhythmic events and sudden death

Abbreviations: LVEF = left ventricular ejection fraction; POMI = post-myocardial infarction; PPA = positive predictive accuracy; VT = ventricular tachycardia; see also Tables 21.1 and 21.2.

[1]Bigger JT, Fleiss JL, Steinman RC, Rolnitzky LM, Kleiger RE, Rottman JN. Frequency domain measures of heart period variability and mortality after myocardial infarction. *Circulation* 1992;**85**:164–71.

[2]Cripps TR, Malik M, Farrell TG, Camm AJ. Prognostic value of reduced heart rate variability after myocardial infarction: clinical evaluation of a new analysis method. *Br Heart J* 1991;**65**:14–19.

[3]Farrell TG, Bashir Y, Cripps T et al. Risk stratification for arrhythmic events in postinfarction patients based on heart rate variability, ambulatory electrocardiographic variables and the signal-averaged electrocardiogram. *J Am Coll Cardiol* 1991;**18**:687–97.

[4]Lanza GA, Guido V, Galeazzi M et al. Prognostic role of heart rate variability in patients with a recent acute myocardial infarction. *Am J Cardiol* 1998;**82**:1323–8.

[5]Odemuyiwa O, Malik M, Farrell T et al. Comparison of the predictive characteristics of heart rate variability index and left ventricular ejection fraction for all-cause mortality, arrhythmic events and sudden death after acute myocardial infarction. *Am J Cardiol* 1991;**68**:434.

tion. For example, Binder *et al.* found that SDANN less than 55 ms identified patients awaiting cardiac transplantation whose risk of mortality was 20 times that of patients with higher HRV.[56]

Although, as can be appreciated from the discussion above, decreased HRV is a risk factor for arrhythmic events, HRV by itself lacks the positive predictive accuracy to risk stratify in a clinical setting. It must be noted, however, that normal HRV, in the absence of other major risk factors, is associated with a very low risk of events. Also, combining decreased HRV with other risk factors substantially improves power to risk stratify. As can be seen on Table 21.6, combining depressed HRV and positive late potentials or repetitive or high frequency of VPCs identified subgroups with high sensitivity (greater than 50%) for arrhythmic events with positive predictive accuracies of over 35%. Figure 21.2 from the original MPIP paper clearly demonstrates the combined effect of HRV and another risk factor, in this case over 10 VPCs/h on mortality. Note that in patients with SDNN over 100 ms, frequent VPCs have *no* effect on mortality.

Recently, in ATRAMI (Autonomic Tone and Reflexes After Myocardial Infarction), the predictive value of combining HRV with baroreceptor sensitivity (BRS) was tested.[51] Although BRS will be discussed in detail in the following chapter, it bears mentioning that there is a significant body of literature supporting the value of BRS, another method for assessing autonomic control of the heart, for risk stratification, especially for arrhythmic events.[57] Furthermore, the relatively modest correlation between BRS and HRV (r = ~0.60) means that each is measuring a different aspect of cardiac autonomic modulation.[58] As shown on Table 21.6, the primary finding of ATRAMI was that either decreased HRV *or* decreased BRS carries similar

prognostic value, but the combination of decreased values for *both* identifies a group with a 17% 2-year mortality in a population whose overall 2-year mortality was 4%. Interestingly, low BRS was predictive of outcome only in patients less than 65 years old, but low SDNN had greater predictive value in patients over 65 years old. Low BRS plus low LVEF in younger patients identified those with a relative risk for mortality of 11.5. Low HRV plus low LVEF in older patients identified those with relative risk of mortality of 5.9. ATRAMI will likely result in an increased interest in measurement of BRS as a complement to HRV for risk stratification.

Another study which suggested a potential way that HRV will be used in combination with other risk factors was EMIAT.[59] In EMIAT, even though overall mortality was not reduced with amiodarone treatment, patients with both depressed HRV and low LVEF benefited significantly in terms of reduction in both arrhythmic events and total cardiac mortality.

Clinical implications

How can the clinician apply these research results to routine practice? Although it may be premature to recommend routine Holter monitoring for measurement of HRV, in many settings indices of HRV are found on routine Holter reports obtained for another purpose. While, in general, decreased HRV by itself has lacked sufficient positive predictive value, HRV can make important contributions to risk stratification and treatment decisions. What is often overlooked is that normal HRV, e.g. SDNN over 100 ms in a patient with a recent MI, is a powerful *negative* risk stratifier, i.e. patients with normal HRV, in the absence of other significant risk factors, can be considered low-risk individuals. In addition, as previously mentioned, various studies have shown that the combination of decreased HRV and other risk stratifiers can identify higher risk patients.

To summarise, measurement of autonomic function appears to provide important information for stratification of cardiac patients for risk of malignant arrhythmias. Currently, decreased HRV in combination with other risk factors provides the best method for identifying high-risk patients, although the high-risk subgroups identified with good sensitivity and specificity are relatively small. Normal HRV is a negative risk stratifier. It appears that the combination of decreased HRV and decreased BRS may provide improved risk stratification post-MI. Non-linear indices of HRV may potentially be used to further refine HRV as a clinical tool.

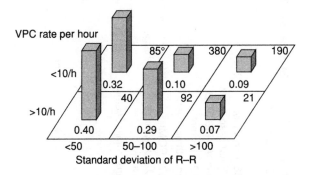

Figure 21.2 Heart rate variability and ventricular premature complex (VPC) frequency versus mortality in the MPIP study. The number of patients in each group is given in the upper right corner. The proportion dying is shown by the height of the bar and the number below each bar.

Table 21.6 Selected studies of heart rate variability (HRV) in combination with other risk factors as a predictor of outcome in post-myocardial infarction (POMI) patients

Source (study)	Number of patients (events)	HRV measure, when obtained	Follow-up	End-points	HRV + other predictors
[1]Bigger et al., 1992 (MPIP)	715 (119 deaths)	24 h, 2 weeks POMI	up to 4 years	All-cause mortality	Decreased ULF or VLF + >3 VPC/h (40–44% mortality) Decreased ULF or VLF + LVEF <40% (48–49% mortality) Decreased ULF and VLF + >3 VPC/h (53% mortality) Decreased ULF and VLF + LVEF <40% (56% mortality)
[2]Farrell et al., 1991 (St George's)	416 (24 end-points)	24 h, day 6 or 7 POMI	mean 612 days	Sudden death, life-threatening ventricular arrhythmia	HRV index <20 ms + repetitive ventricular forms + late potential: 20% sens, 99% spec, 58% PPA, 95% NPA
[3]Filipecki et al., 1996	56 with VT or VF not associated with AMI (8 SCD, 12 recurrent arrhythmic events)	24 h	24 months	Sudden death, recurrence of malignant arrhythmias or ICD discharges	Best model LVEF <40% + either SDNNIDX <43 ms or LF power <16 ms Sens 58%, spec 97%, PPA 82%
[4]Hartikainen et al., 1996 (St George's)	575 POMI (29 arrhythmic, 18 non-arrhythmic deaths)	24h HRV, before discharge	>2 years	Arrhythmic and non-arrhythmic death	HRV index <20 + runs of VT predicted arrhythmic death HRV index <20 + frequent ectopic beats + LVEF <40% predicted non-arrhythmic death If selected patients with decreased HRV, long QRS duration or ventricular arrhythmias and excluded lowest EF, 75% of deaths were arrhythmic If selected patients with low LVEF and excluded lowest HRV, 75% of deaths were non-arrhythmic

	n		Endpoint	Follow-up	Results
[5]Kleiger et al., 1987 (MPIP)	808 (127 deaths)	24 h, 11 ± 3 days POMI	All-cause mortality	4 years	SDNN <50 ms + AVGRR <750 (37% mortality) SDNN <50 ms + LVEF <30% (49% mortality) SDNN <50 ms + >10 VPC/h (40% mortality) SDNN <50 ms + runs or couplets (50% mortality)
[6]La Rovere et al., 1998 (ATRAMI)	1284 (44 cardiac deaths, 5 non-fatal sudden)	24h, 15 ± 10 days POMI	Cardiac mortality	21 ± 8 months	SDNN <70 ms + BRS <3.0 ms (17% mortality) vs SDNN >105 ms + BRS >6.1 ms (2% mortality)
[7]Reinhardt et al., 1996 (Post-Infarction Late Potential Study)	553 men <66 yrs with Q-wave MI (25 arrhythmic events)	24h HRV 2–4 weeks POMI	Sustained VT, VF, sudden death	6 months	rMSSD <36 ms + QRS duration >103 ms 14% events vs no events for rMSSD ≥36 ms + QRS duration ≤103 ms

Abbreviations: BRS = baroreceptor sensitivity; EF = ejection fraction; LVEF = left ventricular ejection fraction; NPA = negative predictive accuracy; PPA = positive predictive accuracy; VF = ventricular fibrillation; VT = ventricular tachycardia; see also Tables 21.1 and 21.2.

[1]Bigger JT Jr, Fleiss JL, Steinman RC, Rolnitzky LM, Kleiger RE, Rottman JN. Frequency domain measures of heart period variability and mortality after myocardial infarction. Circulation 1992;**85**:164–71.

[2]Farrell TG, Bashir Y, Cripps T et al. Risk stratification for arrhythmic events in postinfarction patients based on heart rate variability, ambulatory electrocardiographic variables and the signal-averaged electrocardiogram. J Am Coll Cardiol 1991;**18**:687–97.

[3]Filipecki A, Trusz-Gluza M, Szydlo K, Giec L. Value of heart rate variability parameters for prediction of serious arrhythmic events in patients with malignant ventricular arrhythmias. Pacing Clin Electrophysiol 1996;**19**:1852–6

[4]Hartikainen JE, Malik M, Staunton A, Poloniecki J, Camm AJ. Distinction between arrhythmic and non arrhythmic death after acute myocardial infarction based on heart rate variability, signal-averaged electrocardiogram, ventricular arrhythmias and left ventricular ejection fraction. J Am Coll Cardiol 1996;**28**:296–304.

[5]Kleiger RE, Miller JP, Bigger JT, Moss AJ and the Multicenter Post-Infarction Research Group. Decreased heart rate variability and its association with increased mortality after acute myocardial infarction. Am J Cardiol 1987;**59**:256.

[6]La Rovere MT, Bigger JT Jr, Marcus FI, Mortara A, Schwartz PJ for the ATRAMI Investigators. Baroreflex sensitivity and heart rate variability in prediction of total cardiac mortality after myocardial infarction. Lancet 1998;**351**:478–84.

[7]Reinhardt L, Makijarvi M, Fetsch T et al. Noninvasive risk modeling after myocardial infarction. Am J Cardiol 1996;**78**:627–32.

References

1. Kleiger RE, Bigger JT, Bosner MS *et al*. Stability over time of variables measuring heart rate variability in normal subjects. *Am J Cardiol* 1991;**68**:626.

2. Kleiger RE, Stein PK, Bosner, MS, Rottman, JN. Time domain measurements of heart rate variability. *Cardiol Clin N Amer* 1992;**10**:487–98.

3. Task Force of the European Society of Cardiology and the North American Society of Pacing and Electrophysiology. Heart rate variability. Standards of Measurement, physiological interpretation and clinical use. *Circulation* 1996;**93**: 1043–65.

4. Akselrod S, Gordon D, Madwed JB, Snidman NC, Shannon DC, Cohen RJ. Hemodynamic regulation: investigation by spectral analysis. *Am J Physiol* (*Heart Circ Physiol*) 1985;**249**:H867–H875.

5. Pomeranz B, Macaulay RJB, Caudill MA *et al*. Assessment of autonomic function in humans by heart rate spectral analysis. *Am J Physiol* (*Heart Circ Physiol*) 1985;**17**:H151–H153.

6. Ahmed MW, Kadish AH, Parker MA, Goldberger JJ. Effect of physiologic and pharmacologic adrenergic stimulation on heart rate variability. *J Am Coll Cardiol* 1994;**24**:1082–90.

7. Fallen EL, Kamath MV, Ghista DN. Power spectrum of heart rate variability: A non-invasive test of integrated neuro-cardiac function. *Clin Invest Med* 1988;**11**:331–40.

8. Akselrod S, Gordon D, Ubel FA, Shannon DC, Barger AC, Cohen RJ. Power spectrum analysis of heart rate fluctuation: A quantitative probe of beat-to-beat cardiovascular control. *Science* 1981;**213**:220–2.

9. Saul JP. Beat-to-beat variations of heart rate reflect modulation of cardiac autonomic outflow. *Neural Inform Process Sys* 1990;**5**:32–7.

10. Bilge AR, Stein PK, Domitrovich PP *et al*. Alternative methods for assessing the ultra-low frequency component of heart rate variability: Application to clinical recordings. *Int J Cardiol* 1999;**71**:1–6.

11. Malliani A, Pagani M, Lombardi F, Cerutti S. Cardiovascular neural regulation explored in the frequency domain. *Circulation* 1991;**84**:482–92.

12. Malliani A, Pagani M, Lombardi F. Physiology and clinical implications of variability of cardiovascular parameters with focus on heart rate and blood pressure. *Am J Cardiol* 1994;**73**:3C–9C.

13. Cacioppo JT, Berntson GG, Binkley PF, Quigley KS, Uchine BN, Fieldstone A. Autonomic cardiac control. II. Noninvasive indices and basal response as revealed by autonomic blockade. *Psychophysiology* 1994;**31**:586–98.

14. Hopf H-B, Skyschally A, Heusch G, Peters J. Low -frequency spectral power of heart rate variability in not a specific marker of cardiac sympathetic modulation. *Anaesthesiology* 1995;**82**:609–19.

15. Arai Y, Saul JP, Albrecht P *et al*. Modulation of cardiac autonomic activity during and immediately after exercise. *Am J Physiol* 1989;**256**:H132–H141.

16. Berntson GG, Bigger JT Jr, Eckberg DL *et al*. Heart rate variability: Origins, methods, and interpretive caveats. *Psychophysiology* 1997;**34**:623–48.

17. Malik M, Farrell T, Cripps T, Camm AJ. Heart rate variability in relation to prognosis after myocardial infarction: selection of optimal processing techniques. *Eur Heart J* 1989;**10**:1060–74.

18. Huikuri HV, Mäkikallio TH, Airaksinen KE *et al*. Power-law relationship of heart rate variability as a predictor of mortality in the elderly. *Circulation* 1998; **97**:2031–6.

19. Voss A, Hnatkova K, Wessel N *et al*. Multiparametric analysis of heart rate variability used for risk stratification among survivors of acute myocardial infarction. *Pacing Clin Electrophysiol* 1998; **21**(1 Pt 2):186–92.

20. Malik M, Camm AJ. Components of heart rate variability – what they really mean and what we really measure. *Am J Cardiol* 1993;**72**:821–2.

21. Billman GE, Hoskins RS. Time-series analysis of heart rate variability during submaximal exercise. Evidence for reduced cardiac vagal tone in animals susceptible to ventricular fibrillation. *Circulation* 1986; **80**:146–57.

22. Corr PB, Yamada KA, Witkowski FX. Mechanisms controlling cardiac autonomic function and their relation to arrhythmogenesis. In: Fozzard HA, Haber E, Jenning RB, Katz AM, eds. *The heart and cardiovascular system*. NY: Raven Press. 1986, p.1343ff.

23. Hull SS Jr, Evans AR, Vanoli E *et al*. Heart rate variability before and after myocardial infarction in conscious dogs at high and low risk of sudden death. *J Am Coll Cardiol* 1990;**16**:978–85.

24. Huikuri HV. Heart rate dynamics and vulnerability to ventricular tachyarrhythmias. *Ann Med* 1997;**29**:321–5.

25. Fei L, Statters DJ, Hnatkova K *et al*. Change of autonomic influence on the heart immediately before the onset of spontaneous idiopathic ventricular tachycardia. *J Am Coll Cardiol* 1994;**24**:1515–22.

26. Valkama JO, Huikuri HV, Airaksinen KE, Linnaluoto MK, Takkunen JT. Changes in frequency domain measures of heart rate variability in relation to the onset of ventricular tachycardia in acute myocardial infarction. *Int J Cardiol* 1993;**38**:177–82.

27. Vanoli E, Cerati D, Pedretti RF. Autonomic control of heart rate: pharmacological and nonpharmacological modulation. *Basic Res Cardiol* 1998;Suppl. 1:133–42.

28. Hull SS Jr, Vanoli E, Adamson PB, De Ferrari GM, Foreman RD, Schwartz PJ. Do increases in markers of vagal activity imply protection from sudden death? The case of scopolamine. *Circulation* 1995:**91**:2516–19.

29. Chen CK, Liou YM, Lee WL *et al*. The effect of thrombolytic therapy on short- and long-term cardiac autonomic activity in patients with acute myocardial infarction. *Chin Med J* 1996;**58**:392–9.

30. Hermosillo AG, Dorado M, Casanova JM *et al*. Influence of infarct-related artery patency on the indexes of parasympathetic activity and prevalence of late potentials in survivors of acute myocardial infarction. *J Am Coll Cardiol* 1993;**22**:695–706.

31. Sandrone G, Mortara A, Torzillo D, La Rovere MT, Malliani A, Lombardi, F. Effects of beta blockers (atenolol or metoprolol) on heart rate variability after acute myocardial infarction. *Am J Cardiol* 1994;**74**:340–5.

32. Yusuf S, Peto R, Lewis J, Collins R, Sleight P. Beta blockade

during and after myocardial infarction: *Progr Cardiovasc Dis* 1985;**XXVII**:335–71.

33. SOLVD Investigators. Effect of enalapril on survival in patients with reduced left ventricular ejection fraction and congestive heart failure. *N Engl J Med* 1991;**325**:293–302.

34. Binkley PF, Haas GJ, Starling RC *et al.* Sustained augmentation of parasympathetic tone with angiotensin-converting enzyme inhibition in patients with congestive heart failure. *J Am Col Cardiol* 1993;**21**:655–61.

35. Goldsmith RL, Bigger JT Jr, Bloomfield DM *et al.* Long-term carvedilol therapy increases parasympathetic nervous system activity in chronic congestive heart failure. *Am J Cardiol* 1997;**80**:1101–4.

36. Hohnloser SH, Klingenheben T, Zabel M, Just H. Effect of sotalol on heart rate variability assessed by Holter monitoring in patients with ventricular arrhythmias. *Am J Cardiol* 1993;**72**:67A–71A.

37. Lazzara. Results of Holter ECG-guided therapy for ventricular arrhythmias: the ESVEM trial. *PACE* 1994:**17**:473–7.

38. Rosano GMC, Patrizi R, Leonardo F *et al.* Effect of estrogen replacement therapy on heart rate variability and heart rate in healthy postmenopausal women. *Am J Cardiol* 1997;**80**:815–17.

39. Stein PK, Rottman JN, Kleiger RE, Ehsani AA. Exercise training increases heart rate variability in normal older adults. *J Am Col Cardiol* 1996;**27**(2) Suppl. A:146A.

40. Karason K, Molgaard H, Wikstrand J, Sjostrom L. Heart rate variability in obesity and the effect of weight loss. *Am J Cardiol* 1999;**83**:1242–7.

41. Stein PK, Rottman JN, Kleiger RE. Effect of 21 mg transdermal nicotine patches and smoking cessation on heart rate variability. *Am J Cardiol* 1996; **77**:701–5.

42. Pellizzer Am, Straznicky NE, Lim S, Kamen PW, Krum H. Reduced dietary fat intake increases parasympathetic activity in premenopausal women. *Clin Exp Pharmacol Physiol* 1999;**26**:656–60.

43. Cowan MJ, Kogan H, Burr R *et al.* Power spectral analysis of heart rate variability after biofeedback training. *J Electrocardiol* 1990;**23** Suppl.:85–94.

44. Flapan AD, Goodfield NE, Wright RA, Francis CM, Neilson MH. Effects of digoxin on time domain measures of heart rate variability in patients with stable chronic cardiac failure: withdrawal and comparison group studies. *Int J Cardiol* 1997;**59**:29–36.

45. Bikkina M, Alpert MA, Mukerji R, Mulekar M, Cheng BY, Mukerji V. Diminished short-term heart rate variability predicts inducible ventricular tachycardia. *Chest* 1998;**113**:312–16.

46. Pedretti RF, Colombo E, Sarzi Braga S, Caru B. Effect of thrombolysis on heart rate variability and life-threatening ventricular arrhythmias in survivors of acute myocardial infarction. *J Am Coll Cardiol* 1994;**23**:19–26.

47. Valkama JO, Huikuri HV, Koistinen MJ, Yli-Mayry S, Airaksinen KE, Myerburg RJ. Relation between heart rate variability and spontaneous and induced ventricular

arrhythmias in patients with coronary artery disease. *J Am Coll Cardiol* 1995;**25**:437–43.

48. Perkiomaki JS, Huikuri HV, Koistinen JM, Makikallio T, Castellanos A, Myerburg RJ. Heart rate variability and dispersion of QT interval in patients with vulnerability to ventricular tachycardia and ventricular fibrillation after previous myocardial infarction. *J Am Coll Cardiol* 1997;**30**:1331–8.

49. Kleiger RE, Miller JP, Bigger JT, Moss AJ and the Multicenter Post-Infarction Research Group. Decreased heart rate variability and its association with increased mortality after acute myocardial infarction. *Am J Cardiol* 1987;**59**:256.

50. Bigger JT, Fleiss JL, Steinman RC, Rolnitzky LM, Kleiger RE, Rottman JN. Frequency domain measures of heart period variability and mortality after myocardial infarction. *Circulation* 1992;**85**:164–71.

51. La Rovere MT, Bigger, JT Jr, Marcus FI, Mortara A, Schwartz PJ for the ATRAMI Investigators. Baroreflex sensitivity and heart rate variability in prediction of total cardiac mortality after myocardial infarction. *Lancet* 1998;**351**:478–84.

52. Zuanetti G, Neilson James MM, Latini R, Santoro E, Maggioni AP, Ewing DJ. Prognostic significance of heart rate variability in post-myocardial infarction patients in the fibrinolytic ear. The GISSI-2 results. *Circulation* 1996;**94**:432–6.

53. Kleiger RE, Stein PK, Domitrovich PP, Rottman, JN. CABG and diabetes confound HRV prediction of mortality post-MI (abs). *PACE* 1999;**22**(Part II).

54. Farrell TG, Bashir Y, Cripps T *et al.* Risk stratification for arrhythmic events in postinfarction patients based on heart rate variability, ambulatory electrocardiographic variables and the signal-averaged electrocardiogram. *J Am Coll Cardiol* 1991;**18**:687–97.

55. Pires LA, Hull ML, Nino CL, May LM, Ganji JR. Sudden death in recipients of transvenous implantable cardioverter defibrillator systems: Terminal events, predictors, and potential mechanisms. *J Cardiovasc Electrophysiol* 1999;**10**:1049–56.

56. Binder T, Frey B, Porenta G *et al.* Prognostic value of heart rate variability in patients awaiting cardiac transplantation. *Pacing Clin Electrophysiol* 1992;**15**:2215–20.

57. Farrell TG, Odemuyiwa O, Bashir Y *et al.* Prognostic value of baroreflex sensitivity testing after acute myocardial infarction. *Br Heart J* 1992;**67**:129–37.

58. Bigger JT Jr, La Rovere MT, Steinman RC *et al.* Comparison of baroreflex sensitivity and heart period variability after myocardial infarction. *J Am Coll Cardiol* 1989;**14**:1511–18.

59. Malik M, Camm JA, Julian DG *et al.,* on behalf of the EMIAT investigators. Depressed heart rate variability identifies postinfarction patients who might benefit from prophylactic treatment with amiodarone. A substudy of EMIAT (The European Myocardial Infarct Amiodarone Trial). *J Am Coll Cardiol* 2000;**35**:1263–75.

22 Baroreflex sensitivity

Maria Teresa La Rovere, Andrea Mortara and Gian Domenico Pinna

The autonomic nervous system regulates cardiac electrophysiology by complex interactions between catecholamines and acetylcholine release and their effects on specific receptors at the cell membrane. It has been known for many years that sympathetic stimulation may be arrhythmogenic, particularly in conditions of acute myocardial ischaemia, while vagal stimulation may reduce the potential for lethal arrhythmias. The large amount of available information about the role exerted by the autonomic nervous system on the development of cardiac arrhythmias has been recently reviewed.[1] As a consequence, increasing interest has been placed on measurements that might inform on physiological and pathophysiological mechanisms governing sympathetic and vagal outflow to the heart.

The arterial baroreceptors play a major role in controlling the activity of cardiac autonomic nerves through which they provide quick adaptations to changes in pressure and tissue perfusion in response to daily activities. The importance of arterial baroreceptors in the regulation of the cardiovascular system and in the maintenance of circulatory homeostasis has been widely recognised in human physiology. More recently evaluation of baroreflex sensitivity (BRS) has become a clinical tool, as it has been recognised that vagal and sympathetic control is deranged profoundly in a variety of cardiac diseases[2] and that alterations in the sensitivity of baroreflex control of the heart may be highly relevant for the outcome of such patients.

This chapter will outline:

- the physiological basis for the baroreflex control of heart rate and its evaluation in clinical practice;
- the interaction between baroreceptor reflexes and cardiac electrophysiology;
- the clinical value of the analysis of baroreceptor abnormalities in the identification of high-risk patients.

The arterial baroreceptor reflex

The afferent portion of the arterial baroreceptor reflex involves changes in the arterial blood pressure, detected by stretch receptors mainly located in the wall of the carotid sinus and in the wall of the aortic arch. The efferent portion of the arc carries autonomic signals from the central nervous system: sympathetic and parasympathetic outputs interact to compensate for changes in arterial blood pressure. In response to an arterial pressure increase, a reflex decrease in sympathetic activity reduces heart rate, cardiac contractility, and peripheral resistance, whereas a reflex increase in vagal activity increases tonic cardiac slowing. Opposite changes are associated with an arterial pressure decrease.

Arterial baroreflex responses, however, are much more complex then described, as they are modulated by the interaction between high brain centres and afferent inputs from multiple reflexogenic areas in the heart, lungs, and in the vessels. One example is represented by the interaction between the baroreceptor reflex and respiratory activity that contributes to the origin of respiratory sinus arrhythmia. Firing in the cardiac vagal efferent fibres is enhanced in the expiratory phase of respiration, whilst there is a reduction during the inspiratory phase, which is associated with tachycardia. This autonomic modulation is mediated both by the direct effect of the oscillatory activity of the respiratory centres and by reflex activity from the lungs, and from arterial baroreceptors, which are sensitive to respiratory-related changes in stroke volume and cardiac output.

The slowing in heart rate following increased frequency of discharge of cardiac vagal efferent fibres is achieved by hyperpolarising the pacemaker cells and slowing the rate of spontaneous depolarisation. At the experimental level the latency of the chronotropic response evoked by vagal stimulation is very short (about 150 ms) owing to direct coupling of muscarinic receptors to ACh-regulated K^+ channels in the pacemaker cells membranes, and the effect of the stimulus depends on its timing relative to the cardiac cycle. The increases in heart rate are achieved by the effect of the neurally released noradrenaline on various ionic currents that augment the rate of diastolic depolarisation of pacemaker cells. The latent period for the response to sympathetic stimulation is about 1–2 s, and the response does not reach a plateau until about 30–60 s after the beginning of neural stimulation. The slower response of sympathetic activity as compared to the vagal ones may be principally related to the slow release of noradrenaline from the sympathetic nerve endings in the heart. As sympathetic responses are slower than vagal ones, the fastest baroreflex control involves changes in heart rate, which are vagally mediated. The time relation between the rise of arterial pressure and the resulting reflex bradycardia has been examined in young healthy subjects,[3] and it has been estimated to be approximately only 475 ms, thus indicating that heart rate can be reflexly regulated on a beat-to-beat basis.

The relative contribution of vagal and sympathetic mechanisms in the control of the sinus node depends on their tonic levels of activity in various conditions. Resting healthy people have relatively strong vagal inhibition and only weak sympathetic stimulation. During circumstances, such as exercise, vagal activity is low and heart rate control is mediated principally by sympathetic mechanisms. Abnormalities in baroreceptor mechanisms occurring in a variety of pathological conditions, could compromise their tonic restraining influence on the heart and circulation leading to sympatho-excitation and parasympathetic withdrawal.

The phenylephrine test

Among the various quantitative approaches developed for evaluating BRS,[4] the technique most widely used to test baroreflexes in human subjects has been to measure heart rate responses to injection of pressor and depressor drugs free of cardiac action. Loading of the baroreceptors owing to vasopressor agents, such as phenylephrine, has become the reference for the clinical use of BRS. Generally, an increase in systolic arterial pressure by 20–40 mmHg activates baroreceptors to operate in the linear portion of their reflex response. In normal subjects RR intervals have shown an average lengthening of 14 ms per millimeter of mercury rise in systolic arterial pressure following bolus infusion of small doses (25–100 micrograms) of the drug.[5] Given the rapidity of vagal responses (within one or two beats), it is commonly assumed that each heart period value is mainly related on a cause–effect basis to the previous systolic pressure peak, and that this relation is linear. Accordingly, heart rate and blood pressure need to be recorded on a beat-to-beat basis, and prolongations of RR intervals are plotted as a function of the previous systolic peak. The slope of the regression line between changes in systolic arterial pressure and the attendant increase in RR interval provides the quantitative estimation of the arterial baroreflex control of heart rate (Fig. 22.1). The development of devices for non-invasive recording of blood pressure has overcome the need for arterial cannulation[6,7] and facilitated a more widespread use of the technique.

In the evaluation of a BRS test, the goodness of the linear association between systolic arterial pressure and RR interval changes is assessed by Pearson's correlation coefficient. When the observed correlation coefficient is not statistically significant (i.e. when there is no evidence of a linear relation between pressure and RR changes), the test result should be disregarded. However, when baroreflex gain is near zero – thus describing the absence of any response between pressure elevation and RR interval (as it is commonly observed among patients with severe heart

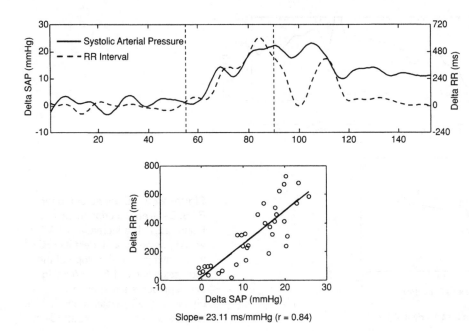

Figure 22.1 Example of a normal BRS. On the top, beat-to-beat changes in systolic blood pressure (SAP) (continuous line) and in RR interval (dotted line) with respect to baseline values are reported. Analysis is limited to the first major increase in systolic arterial pressure with the attendant changes in RR interval (points included between dotted lines). These points are used for calculation of the regression line (on the bottom). The increase in SAP is >20 mmHg and is accompanied by a consistent increase in RR interval. Accordingly the slope of the regression line is 23.11 ms/mmHg and represents a response primarily characterised by an increase in efferent vagus nerve activity to the sinus node.

Slope= 23.11 ms/mmHg (r = 0.84)

failure)[8] – the correlation coefficient is obviously not significant. These results should not be disregarded provided an adequate increase in systolic arterial pressure has been obtained.

Several injections are generally repeated at intervals of a few minutes and the corresponding slopes are averaged in order to reduce measurement variability between tests. This variability is mainly due to the rate of injection, steepness of arterial pressure increase, and selection of the time window used for analysis. The final slope is generally obtained by averaging at least three slopes with the highest correlation coefficients. Sometimes such variability is best handled by performing weighted averages of slopes, with those slopes displaying the least variance given the greatest weight.

BRS is severely reduced in patients with heart disease of different aetiology.[9] In patients after myocardial infarction (MI) the average RR intervals lengthening was 7 ms/mmHg,[10–12] and even greater reductions have been reported in patients with severe heart failure.[8] Accordingly, a depressed BRS slope is interpreted as a reduced capability of vagal reflexes which may also be associated with the presence of elevated sympathetic activity (Fig. 22.2).

The dosage of phenylephrine and time of injection may vary widely according to the patients under evaluation. In patients after a recent MI,[10] phenylephrine has been injected over 30 s, and boluses of 150–350 microgram (2–4 microgram/kg) have been administered. In patients with congestive heart failure,[8] even higher doses (up to 10 microgram/kg) have been used to elicit baroreceptor responses, and the rate of injection has been increased.

The major criticism that the phenylephrine test has been subjected to is that the phenylephrine injection, by acutely increasing left ventricular afterload, may activate other receptors, such as cardiac mechanoreceptors. However, when BRS is used to draw inferences on the amount of autonomic mediators (acetylcholine, norepinephrine) released at cardiac level, a most important question for cardiac electrophysiology, this is no longer a limitation. Indeed, the fact that vasoactive drugs induce a simultaneous activation of multiple reflexogenic areas is actually an advantage for the purpose of using BRS as a measure of net autonomic balance to the heart. On the other hand, when compared to other techniques such as the neck chamber,[4] it has the advantage that the subject is unaware of the stimulus, and this avoids the influence of emotional factors which, by increasing sympathetic activity, could reduce heart rate response.

BRS and ventricular arrhythmias

Two aspects of the complex relationship between baroreceptor reflexes and cardiac electrophysiology are now addressed:

- the role of baroreceptor reflexes in the susceptibility to ventricular arrhythmias, and
- their importance in the clinical response to sustained rhythm disorders.

Cardiovascular disease may alter baroreceptor function, primarily because of a decreased capability to activate vagal reflexes.[9] A case in point is represented by MI,

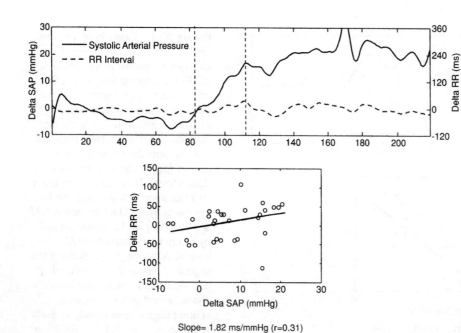

Slope= 1.82 ms/mmHg (r=0.31)

Figure 22.2 Example of a poor BRS. Detailed description as in Figure 22.1. The increase in SAP is accompanied by a modest increase in RR interval and the slope of the regression line is 1.82 ms/mmHg and represents a response characterised by weak vagal reflexes.

which often significantly impairs BRS. The first evidence that MI reduces BRS came from a prospective study in 55 conscious dogs, in whom BRS was measured before and 1 month after MI.[13] It was observed that, in over 70% of the animals, BRS had a marked decrease, whilst in almost 20% there was no change. This pattern appeared to be confirmed in man.[14] Thus, it can be expected that most post-MI patients will have a reduced ability to activate vagal reflexes and, in general, a loss in adequate responses to blood pressure changes. The underlying mechanism has not yet been demonstrated; however, a tenable hypothesis has been advanced.[13,15] It was specifically proposed that MI could often augment sympathetic afferent traffic and that this, in turn, would reduce vagal efferent activity. The presence of a necrotic and non-contracting segment may indeed alter the geometry of the beating heart and increase beyond normal the firing of sympathetic and vagal afferent fibres by mechanical distortion of their sensory endings.[16] Excitation of cardiac sympathetic afferent fibres inhibits tonic vagal efferent activity and blunts the baroreceptor-mediated reflex increase in vagal activity elicited by a blood pressure rise.

There is an important part of the concept that MI alters baroreceptor reflexes[17,18] that, interestingly, has largely escaped general appreciation: this alteration does not appear to affect equally the vagal and sympathetic components of the baroreceptor reflex. As shown in Fig. 22.3, whereas the loss in the capability of reflexly increasing vagal activity, quantified by the heart rate reduction in response to a blood pressure increase, is lost to a major extent, the capability to increase sympathetic activity reflexly, quantified by the heart rate increase in response to a blood pressure decrease, is impaired by a lesser degree. The practical, and clinically relevant, implication is that, in most cases of MI, the impairment in baroreceptor reflexes will affect vagal more than sympathetic responses. The consequence will be a shift toward autonomic responses, characterised by a sympathetic dominance. As electrical stability is concerned, this is a detrimental change.

The most impressive counterpart of this concept is represented by the increased risk for ventricular fibrillation during acute myocardial ischaemia observed in those post-MI dogs who also have a marked reduction in BRS.[13,17] This finding, which proved critical for all the related developments culminating in the clinical use of BRS as a risk stratifier after MI, came from an established canine preparation for sudden cardiac death based on a brief episode of acute myocardial ischaemia produced in conditions of physiologically elevated sympathetic activity in conscious dogs with a healed MI.[18] As shown in Fig. 22.4, the animals with a more depressed BRS had a much higher probability to be in the group that developed ventricular fibrillation during the ischaemic episode, whereas those

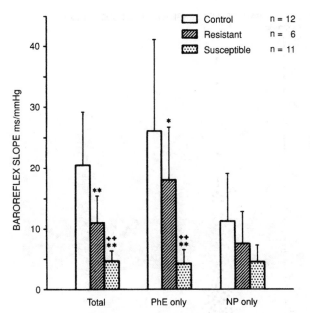

Figure 22.3 Composite slopes for all dogs under study. Total = RR interval response to both an increase and a decrease in pressure. Plotted as mean ± SD. (Reproduced with permission from ref. 17.)
Abbreviations: Phe = phenylephrine response, NP = nitroprusside response. * $P <0.05$ versus control dogs; ** $P <0.01$ versus control dogs; ++ $P <0.01$ versus resistant dogs.

with a better preserved BRS were more likely to be in the group that survived the test without major arrhythmias.

The mechanism relating a loss in BRS to increased propensity toward ventricular fibrillation is likely to involve, to a major extent, the vagal component of the baroreflex. Several lines of evidence support this argument. There is an impressive correlation between the occurrence of reductions in heart rate during acute myocardial ischaemia, which is associated with a greater probability of survival,[18] and a well-preserved BRS and, conversely, between further increases in heart rate and depressed BRS. This suggests that the animals with high BRS slopes are also those more likely to respond to acute ischaemia with powerful vagal reflexes. Protection from ventricular fibrillation, among the high-risk animals, has been conferred by a variety of interventions all resulting in augmented cardiac-bound vagal activity. These include direct vagal stimulation (Fig. 22.5),[19] exercise training,[20] and muscarinic agonists.[21]

The potential for an antifibrillatory effect of vagal activity has been recently demonstrated at the clinical level. In the study by Mitrani *et al.*,[22] patients with previously implanted cardioverter defibrillators had induction of ventricular fibrillation both in the control state and after infusion of phenylephrine. As they did not perform assessment

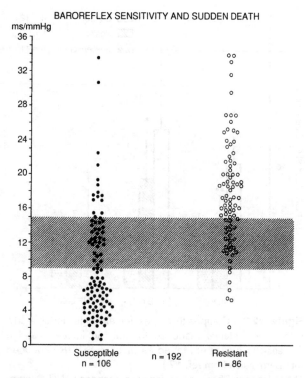

BAROREFLEX SENSITIVITY AND SUDDEN DEATH

Figure 22.4 Plot of baroreflex sensitivity in 192 dogs after infarction and its relation with susceptibility to sudden death. Dashed areas is an arbitrary grey zone. At <9 ms/mmHg, 91% of the dogs were susceptible to sudden death, whereas at >15 ms/mmHg, 80% of the dogs survived during the exercise and ischaemia test. (Reproduced with permission from ref. 13.)

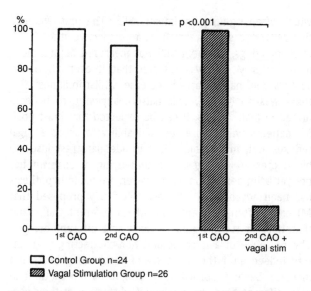

☐ Control Group n=24
▨ Vagal Stimulation Group n=26

Figure 22.5 Incidence of ventricular fibrillation in two consecutive exercise and ischaemia tests in the control group and in the group in which vagal stimulation (stim) was performed during the second coronary occlusion (CAO). In this latter group only those dogs who had ventricular fibrillation in the final exercise and ischaemia test in control conditions were considered for the analysis. (Reproduced with permission from ref. 19.)

of BRS, vagal activation following phenylephrine injection was defined as an increase in sinus cycle length of at least 10% of the baseline value. It was observed that, in the majority of patients who had such vagal response, there was an increase in the energy required to induce ventricular fibrillation, whilst this was observed in only 20% of patients who did not show signs of vagal activation.

Clinical responses to sustained ventricular arrhythmias are highly variable. Although factors, such as the extent of left ventricular dysfunction and the ventricular rate, are major determinants of the haemodynamic impact of the arrhythmia, blood pressure responses and symptoms may be very different, in spite of similar degree of ventricular function and similar rate. Indeed, given the exquisite sensitivity of baroreceptors to changes in arterial pressure, ongoing autonomic responses play a primary role in the haemodynamic adjustments to rapid ventricular rhythms. The attendant blood pressure decrease unloads arterial baroreceptors, thus leading to a vagal withdrawal and to a generalised increase in sympathetic activity aimed at restoring arterial pressure.

The clinical relevance of the baroreflex-mediated responses to the support of arterial pressure has been addressed by Landolina *et al.*[23] In their study, patients with a healed MI, who had sustained monomorphic ventricular tachycardia (VT), were divided into two groups according to whether the VT was well or poorly tolerated: the group presenting with syncope or signs of shock during VT had a significantly lower BRS in response to phenylephrine injection. Only BRS, not age, left ventricular ejection fraction or VT cycle length correlated with the tolerability of the VT. Several observations point to inadequate baroreflex-mediated sympatho-excitation during the arrhythmia as the leading cause of the unfavourable haemodynamic profile of patients with poorly tolerated VT. During sustained ventricular tachycardia, Smith *et al.*[24] have demonstrated that the sympatho-excitatory response was directly related to the estimated arterial baroreflex gain. Moreover, in a recent study, Hamdam *et al.*[25] have evaluated the relationship between arterial baroreflex sympathetic gain and blood pressure recovery during rapid ventricular pacing in patients referred for electrophysiological study. Sympathetic gain was assessed as the slope of the regression between changes in efferent post-ganglionic muscle sympathetic neural activity recorded at the peroneal nerve and changes in diastolic blood pressure during nitroprusside infusion; it was found that recovery of arterial pressure during rapid ventricular pacing was positively related to baroreflex gain.

Baroreceptor responses in risk stratification

Following the experimental background previously discussed,[13,17,18] a large body of clinical evidence has now been accumulated showing that, among patients with a previous MI, the information provided by the analysis of BRS significantly adds to the well-recognised measures of cardiovascular outcome.[10–12] Specifically, the most recent results of the ATRAMI study,[12] in 1284 patients below 80 years of age who were followed for an average follow-up of 21 months, have demonstrated that cardiac mortality was higher among patients with a depressed BRS (<3 ms/mmHg, by the phenylephrine method) than among patients with more preserved vagal reflexes (BRS >6.1 ms/mmHg) (9% versus 2% respectively, P <0.001) (Fig. 22.6). In a multivariate model, in which left ventricular ejection fraction and ventricular premature contractions ≥10/h were included, low BRS was significantly associated with an increased mortality risk of 2.8 (95% CI 1.40–6.16).

In the clinical perspective, the most relevant result of the ATRAMI study is the demonstration of the meaningful value for risk stratification of the combination of haemodynamic and autonomic information. As shown in Fig. 22.7, among patients with reduced LVEF, the 2-year mortality rose from 8 to 18% (P <0.01) in the presence of a depressed BRS. Importantly, mortality did not differ significantly among patients with reduced LVEF and BRS >3 ms/mmHg and patients with preserved LVEF but BRS <3 ms/mmHg. These findings suggest that, within patients with a similar substrate (i.e. depressed LVEF), what significantly influences their survival appears to be the pre-

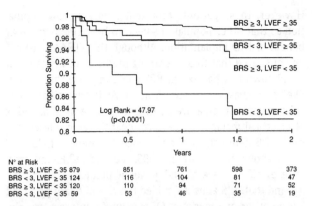

Figure 22.7 Kaplan–Meier survival curves for total cardiac mortality according to the association of LVEF and BRS. The total population has been divided into four groups after dichotomisation of the variables below and above the lowest 15th percentile (LVEF = 35%; BRS = 3 ms/mmHg). The P value refers to differences in events rate between subgroups. In patients with LVEF <35% cardiac mortality rate at 2 years is affected by the association with BRS <3 ms/mmHg). (Reproduced with permission from ref. 12.)

served ability to increase vagal activity reflexly and strengthen the importance of restoring autonomic imbalance in patients with depressed LVEF. The observation that, among patients with similarly low ejection fraction values, mortality was greatly influenced by BRS, highlights the importance of factors that modulate a vulnerable substrate. The relationship between the autonomic balance and arrhythmic propensity has been addressed by the use of programmed ventricular stimulation to evaluate the inducibility of sustained monomorphic ventricular tachycardia 7–10 days after MI.[26] Although "inducible" patients had a BRS markedly lower than "non-inducible" patients (1.85 ± 1.5 versus 7.8 ± 4.5 ms/mmHg, P <0.001), a markedly depressed BRS was also found among patients developing polymorphic ventricular tachycardia, thus showing a lack of correlation between the autonomic balance and the re-entrant arrhythmogenic substrate. Five major arrhythmic events were observed during the follow-up period, all of which were correctly identified by depressed BRS (<3 ms/mmHg) and programmed electrical stimulation. If electrical testing had been limited to those patients with a depressed BRS (<3 ms/mmHg), then only 16% of the patients would have required an electrophysiological study and 87% of the patients who developed sustained monomorphic ventricular tachycardia would have been identified.

It has been recently emphasised that post-MI survivors with systolic ventricular dysfunction and non-sustained ventricular tachycardia (NSVT) should be considered for implantation of a cardioverter defibrillator (ICD) in the presence of a positive programmed electrical stimulation.[27]

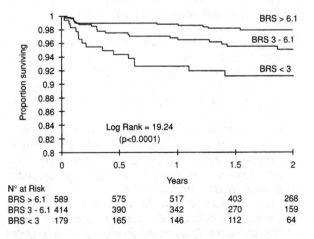

Figure 22.6 Kaplan–Meier survival curves for total cardiac mortality according to BRS stratified at three cut-off values: below the lowest 15th percentile (BRS <3 ms/mmHg), from the 15th percentile to the median value (BRS 3–6.1 ms/mmHg), above the median value (BRS >6.1 ms/mmHg). (Reproduced with permission from ref. 12.)

However, these patients represent a very narrow population so that other populations need to be defined who may benefit of ICD implantation. Although the ATRAMI study[12] demonstrated that BRS is a strong predictor of mortality, it is unknown to what extent BRS could improve the "Madit-like" non-invasive risk stratification. As in the initial analysis ventricular premature contractions were used as index of electrical instability, we have recently reconsidered the value of BRS in light of the presence or absence of NSVT.[28] It was shown that depressed BRS, reduced LVEF, and presence of NSVT were all independent predictors of mortality, and that BRS almost doubled the risk of death provided by the other two markers. Of meaningful interest was the observation that among patients with reduced LVEF but without NSVT, mortality differed significantly according to the presence or absence of a depressed BRS. Therefore the analysis of vagal reflexes could contribute to identify other than "Madit-like" patients at a similarly increased risk of death.

Summary

The analysis of BRS – an indirect measure of human sympathetic and vagus nerve traffic – has gained considerable attention as a tool that might inform on physiological and pathophysiological mechanisms, and might represent a new approach for identifying patients at higher risk. These data should be taken as a clear message signalling that the time is ripe for the inclusion of autonomic markers in the risk stratification of patients with ischaemic heart disease and that, given the significant technical evolution of implantable devices, this may lead to a better tailored therapy for the individual patient.

References

1. Schwartz PJ, Zipes DP. Autonomic modulation of cardiac arrhythmias. In: Zipes DP, Jalife J, eds. *Cardiac electrophysiology. From cell to bedside*. 3rd edn. Philadelphia: WB Saunders Co, 1999, pp.300–14.
2. Eckberg DL, Sleight P. *Human baroreflexes in heart and disease*. Oxford: Clarendon Press, 1992.
3. Pickering TG, Davies J. Estimation of the conduction time of the baroreceptor cardiac reflex in man. *Cardiovasc Res* 1973;**7**:213–19.
4. La Rovere MT, Pinna GD, Mortara A. Assessment of baroreflex sensitivity. In: Malik M, ed. *Clinical guide to cardiac autonomic tests*. Dordrecht: Kluwer Academic Publishers, 1998, 257–81.
5. Bristow JD, Honour AJ, Pickering TG, Sleight P. Cardiovascular and respiratory changes during sleep in normal and hypertensive subjects. *Cardiovasc Res* 1969;**3**:476–85.
6. Parati G, Casadei R, Groppelli A, Di Rienzo M, Mancia G. Comparison of finger and intra-arterial blood pressure monitoring at rest and during laboratory testing. *Hypertension* 1989;**13**:647-55.
7. Pinna GD, La Rovere MT, Maestri R, Mortara A, Bigger JT Jr, Schwartz PJ. Comparison between invasive and noninvasive measurements of baroreflex sensitivity: implications from studies on risk stratification after a myocardial infarction. *Eur Heart J* 2000; (Aug).
8. Maestri R, Mortara A, Bigger JT, Schwartz PJ. Comparison between invasive and non-invasive measurements of baroreflex sensitivity. Implications for studies on risk stratification after a myocardial infarction. *Eur Heart J* 2000;**18**:1522–9.
9. Eckberg DL, Drabinsky M, Braunwald E. Defective cardiac parasympathetic control in patients with heart disease. *New Engl J Med* 1971;**285**:877–83.
10. La Rovere MT, Specchia G, Mortara A, Schwartz PJ. Baroreflex sensitivity, clinical correlates and cardiovascular mortality among patients with a first myocardial infarction. A prospective study. *Circulation* 1988;**78**:816–24.
11. Farrell TG, Odemuyiwa O, Bashir Y *et al*. Prognostic value of baroreflex sensitivity testing after acute myocardial infarction. *Br Heart J* 1992;**67**:129–37.
12. La Rovere MT, Bigger JT Jr, Marcus FI, Mortara A, Schwartz PJ for the ATRAMI (Autonomic Tone and Reflexes After Myocardial Infarction) Investigators. Baroreflex sensitivity and heart rate variability in prediction of total cardiac mortality after myocardial infarction. *Lancet* 1998;**351**:478–84.
13. Schwartz PJ, Vanoli E, Stramba-Badiale M, De Ferrari GM, Billman GE, Foreman RD. Autonomic mechanisms and sudden death. New insights from analysis of baroreceptor reflexes in conscious dogs with and without a myocardial infarction. *Circulation* 1988;**78**:969–79.
14. Schwartz PJ, Zaza A, Pala M, Locati E, Beria G, Zanchetti A. Baroreflex sensitivity and its evolution during the first year after myocardial infarction. *J Am Coll Cardiol* 1988;**12**:629–36.
15. Cerati D, Schwartz PJ. Single cardiac vagal fiber activity, acute myocardial ischemia, and risk for sudden death. *Circ Res* 1991;**69**:1389–401.
16. Malliani A, Recordati G, Schwartz PJ. Nervous activity of afferent cardiac sympathetic fibres with atrial and ventricular endings. *J Physiol (London)* 1973;**229**:457–69.
17. Billman GE, Schwartz PJ, Stone HL. Baroreceptor control of heart rate: a predictor of sudden cardiac death. *Circulation* 1982;**66**:874–80.
18. Schwartz PJ, Billman GE, Stone HL. Autonomic mechanisms in ventricular fibrillation induced by myocardial ischemia during exercise in dogs with a healed myocardial infarction: An experimental preparation for sudden cardiac death. *Circulation* 1984;**69**:780–90.
19. Vanoli E, De Ferrari GM, Stramba-Badiale M, Hull SS Jr, Foreman RD, Schwartz PJ. Vagal stimulation and prevention of sudden death in conscious dogs with a healed myocardial infarction. *Circ Res* 1991;**68**:1471–81.
20. Billman GE, Schwartz PJ, Stone HL. The effects of daily exercise on susceptibility to sudden cardiac death. *Circulation* 1984;**69**:1182–9.
21. De Ferrari GM, Salvati P, Grossoni M *et al*. Pharmacologic modulation of the autonomic nervous system in the pre-

vention of sudden cardiac death. A study with propranolol, methacholine and oxotremorine in conscious dogs with a healed myocardial infarction. *J Am Coll Cardiol* 1993;**22**: 283–90.

22. Mitrani RD, Miles WM, Klein LS, Zipes DP. Phenylephrine increases T wave shock energy required to induce ventricular fibrillation. *J Cardiovasc Electrophysiol* 1998;**9**:34–40.

23. Landolina M, Mantica M, Pessano P *et al.* Impaired baroreflex sensitivity is correlated with hemodynamic deterioration of sustained ventricular tachycardia. *J Am Coll Cardiol* 1997;**29**:568–75.

24. Smith ML, Carlson MD, Thames MD. Reflex control of the heart and circulation: implications for cardiovascular electrophysiology. *J Cardiovasc Electrophysiol* 1992;**2**:441–9.

25. Hamdan MH, Joglar JA, Page RL *et al.* Baroreflex gain pre-

dicts blood pressure recovery during simulated ventricular tachycardia in humans. *Circulation* 1999;**100**:381–6.

26. Farrell TG, Paul V, Cripps TR *et al.*: Baroreflex sensitivity and electrophysiological correlates in patients after acute myocardial infarction. *Circulation* 1991;**83**:945–52.

27. Moss AJ, Hall WJ, Cannon DS *et al.* for the Multicenter Automatic Defibrillator Implantation Trial Investigators. Improved survival with an implanted defibrillator in patients with coronary disease at high risk for ventricular arrhythmia. *New Engl J Med* 1996;**335**:1933–40.

28. La Rovere MT, Pinna GD, Bigger JT Jr *et al.* for the ATRAMI Investigators. Baroreceptor sensitivity improves the prediction of mortality after myocardial infarction when added to noninvasive MADIT criteria. *Circulation* 1999;**100** (Suppl. I):I–571.

23 Heart rate turbulence

Georg Schmidt

Identification of high-risk patients after acute myocardial infarction is essential for successful prophylactic therapy. Establishing a new powerful method for risk prediction independent of the available stratifiers is therefore of considerable practical value. The following chapter describes a new method for risk stratification based on fluctuations of sinus rhythm cycle length after a single ventricular premature contraction (VPC). We termed such fluctuations "heart rate turbulence".[1] In low-risk patients, sinus rhythm exhibits a characteristic biphasic pattern of early acceleration and subsequent deceleration after a VPC (Fig. 23.1). In postinfarction patients at high risk of subsequent death, heart rate turbulence is attenuated or missing.

Quantification of heart rate turbulence

Various numerical descriptors characterising both phases of heart rate turbulence were investigated in a pilot study.[2] The aim was to identify descriptors that:

● were independent of each other;

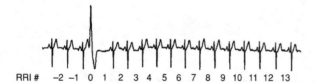

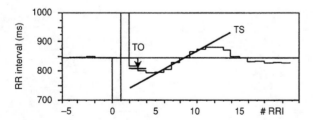

Figure 23.1 The upper diagram shows an ECG with a PVC embedded in a sequence of normal beats. The bottom diagram shows the corresponding HRT tachogram as the typical pattern of a long-term survivor.

● separated patients who did and did not die during the follow-up; and
● were predictors of mortality independent of age, LVEF, and other Holter-based risk factors.

The *initial acceleration* was quantified by the relative change of RR intervals immediately after and before a VPC and was termed "turbulence onset" (TO). In precise numerical terms we used the following formula:

TO is the difference between the mean of the first two sinus RR intervals following a VPC and the last two sinus RR intervals before the VPC divided by the mean of the last two sinus RR intervals before the VPC,

$$TO = \frac{(RR_1 + RR_2) - (RR_{-2} + RR_{-1})}{(RR_{-2} + RR_{-1})} \times 100$$

with RR_i being the i-th sinus rhythm following ($i > 0$) the compensatory pause of the VPC or preceding ($i < 0$) the coupling interval of the VPC. These measurements were first performed for each single VPC and subsequently averaged to obtain the value characterising the patient. TO >0% corresponds to sinus rhythm deceleration after a VPC and TO <0% to sinus rhythm acceleration after a VPC. The optimal dichotomy for TO was 0%.

The *subsequent deceleration* rate was quantified by the steepest regression line between the RR interval count and duration. The corresponding parameter was termed "turbulence slope" (TS). In precise numerical terms we used the following formula:

TS is the maximum positive slope of a regression line assessed over any sequence of five subsequent sinus rhythm RR intervals within the first 20 sinus rhythm RR intervals after a VPC. The value of TS is expressed in milliseconds per RR interval. It was obtained from the tachogram:

$$\overline{RR}_1, \overline{RR}_2, \overline{RR}_3, \ldots, \overline{RR}_{20} \text{ for each recording}$$

with $\overline{RR}_i$ being the average of i-th sinus rhythm RR intervals after the compensatory pause of a singular VPC. The optimal dichotomy for TS was 2.5 ms per RR interval.

The algorithm for heart rate turbulence quantification can only deliver usable results if the triggering event is a true VPC (and not an artefact, T-wave, or similar). In addition, it must be ensured that the sinus rhythm immediately preceding and following the VPC is free from arrhythmia, artefacts, and false classifications of QRS complexes. These preconditions can be fulfilled by using filter algorithms. The heart rate turbulence source code and the filter algorithm can be downloaded under http://www.h-r-t.com.

Clinical value for risk prediction

The heart rate turbulence quantification method was developed in an open study and blindly validated in two large independent populations of myocardial infarction survivors, namely the population of the Multicenter Postinfarction Program (MPIP) study[3] and in the placebo arm of the European Myocardial Infarction Amiodarone Trial (EMIAT).[4]

In both, MPIP and EMIAT populations, a strong and significant association of TO and TS with total mortality was noticed. In EMIAT, TS was the strongest *univariate* mortality predictor; in MPIP it was the second powerful *univariate* mortality predictor after reduced LVEF (Table 23.1). Simultaneous use of TO and TS provided highest relative risks in both, the MPIP population (5.0, CI 2.8–8.8) and the EMIAT population (4.4, CI 2.6–7.5, Table 23.1).

Figure 23.2 shows Kaplan–Meier cumulative survival curves for combined use of TO and TS in MPIP and EMIAT. In the MPIP population the 2-year mortality rate of 9, 15, and 32% was noted in patients with TO <0% and TS >2.5 (both factors normal), patients with either TO ≥0% or TS ≤2.5 (one factor abnormal), and patients with TO ≥0% and TS ≤2.5 (both factors abnormal), respectively. In EMIAT these figures were 9, 18 and 34, respectively. All differences were highly significant (*P* <0.0001).

In both MPIP and EMIAT populations the combination of abnormal TO (≥0%) and abnormal TS (≤2.5 ms per RR interval) was the most powerful *multivariate* mortality predictor (Table 23.2). In the MPIP population LVEF and the combination of TO and TS were the only independent mortality predictors (*P* <0.001 and *P* <0.0001, respectively). The relative risk for LVEF (≥30% versus <30%) was 2.9; the relative risk of the TO/TS combination (TS >2.5 and TO <0% versus TS ≤2.5 and TO ≥0%) was 3.2. In EMIAT four variables were independent predictors: the strongest predictor was the combination of TO and TS with a relative risk of 3.2, while the other significant predictors were: history of previous myocardial infarction, LVEF, and mean heart rate, with relative risks between 1.7 and 1.8.

The additive value of heart rate turbulence in combination with other risk predictors has been studied by Malik *et al.* in 912 post-MI patients enrolled in the ATRAMI study.[5] In the practically relevant range of 30–50% sensitivity, TS was the strongest univariate predictor (Table 23.3). TS was additive to every other risk predictor

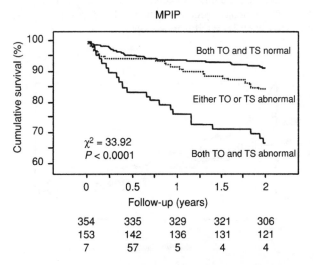

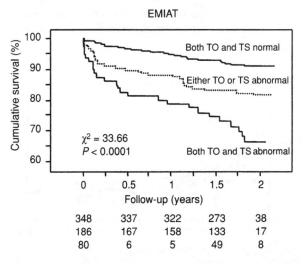

Figure 23.2 Kaplan–Meier survival curves in MPIP and EMIAT patients stratified in three groups: TO <0% and TS >2.5 ms/RRI (both factors normal); either TO ≥0% or TS ≤2.5 ms/RRI (one of the factors abnormal); TO ≥0% and TS ≤2.5 ms/RRI (both factors abnormal).

Table 23.1   Association of risk variables with total mortality in a univariate analysis

Variable	MPIP population		EMIAT population	
	Relative hazard (95% CI)	P	Relative hazard (95% CI)	P
Age >65 years	1.8 (1.1–3.0)	0.02	1.6 (1.1–2.5)	0.02
Previous MI	1.9 (1.2–3.0)	0.008	1.9 (1.2–2.8)	0.004
Mean RR <800 ms	1.5 (0.9–2.3)	0.1	2.6 (1.7–4.1)	<0.0001
HRV index ≤20 units	2.4 (1.5–3.8)	0.0002	2.5 (1.7–3.9)	<0.0001
Arrhythmia on Holter	2.2 (1.4–3.5)	0.0008	2.2 (1.4–3.4)	0.0003
LVEF <30%	4.0 (2.5–6.4)	<0.0001	2.2 (1.4–3.5)	0.0004
TO ≥0%	2.1 (1.3–3.4)	0.002	2.4 (1.5–3.6)	0.0001
TS ≤2.5 ms/RR	3.5 (2.2–5.5)	<0.0001	2.7 (1.8–4.2)	<0.0001
Combined TO and TS*	5.0 (2.8–8.8)	<0.0001	4.4 (2.6–7.5)	<0.0001

*TO ≥0% and TS ≤2.5 ms/RR interval versus TO <0% and TS >2.5 ms/RR interval.
Abbreviations: HRV = heart rate variability; LVEF = left ventricular ejection fraction; MI = myocardial infarction; RR = RR interval; TO = turbulence onset; TS = turbulence slope.

Table 23.2   Relative hazards of individuals variables in a multivariate analysis

Variable	MPIP population		EMIAT population	
	Relative hazard (95% CI)	P	Relative hazard (95% CI)	P
Age >65 years	–	–	–	–
Previous MI	–	–	1.8 (1.2–2.7)	0.01
Mean RR <800 ms	–	–	1.8 (1.1–2.9)	0.01
HRV index ≤20 units	–	–	–	–
Arrhythmia on Holter	–	–	–	–
LVEF <30%	2.9 (1.8–4.9)	0.0001	1.7 (1.1–2.7)	0.03
Combined TO and TS*	3.2 (1.7–6.0)	0.0002	3.2 (1.8–5.6)	<0.0001

*TO ≥0% and TS ≤2.5 ms/RR interval versus TO <0% and TS >2.5 ms/RR interval.
Abbreviations: HRV = heart rate variability; LVEF = left ventricular ejection fraction; MI = myocardial infarction; RR = RR interval; TO = turbulence onset; TS = turbulence slope.

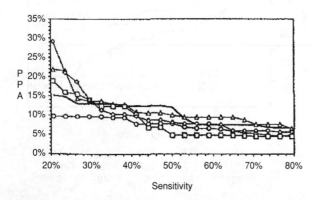 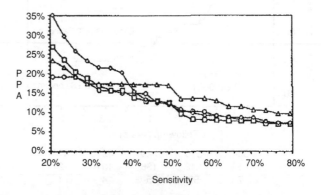

Figure 23.3   Positive predictive accuracies (PPA) of various risk predictors at different sensitivity levels. Left panel: single stratifiers (turbulence slope: bold line; baroreflex sensitivity: circles; left ventricular ejection fraction: triangles; mean heart-rate: squares; heart rate variability index; diamonds). Right panel: stratifiers combined with turbulence slope.

Table 23.3 Positive predictive accuracies of various risk predictors at a sensitivity level of 40%

Variable	PPA (%)
TS	12.5
BRS	7.8
LVEF	10.9
Mean HR	10.4
HRV index	9.9

Abbreviations: BRS = baroreflex sensitivity; HR = heart rate; HRV = heart rate variability; LVEF = left ventricular ejection fraction; PPA = positive predictive accuracy; TS = turbulence slope.

(Figure 23.3). At 40% sensitivity, TS showed best results when combined with heart rate variability and left ventricular ejection fraction.[6]

Impact of clinical covariants on heart rate turbulence

In the entire EMIAT population, i.e. the placebo arm and the amiodarone arm, we performed subgroup analyses to investigate the impact of clinical covariants on heart rate turbulence.[7] These included age of the patient at date of study enrolment, the presence or absence of diabetes mellitus, mean heart rate, HRV index as well as VPC count in the 24-h Holter ECG and left ventricular ejection fraction.

All covariants had a significant impact on heart rate turbulence. Heart rate turbulence was significantly reduced with higher age of the patient, presence of diabetes mellitus, higher mean heart rate, lower HRV index, higher number of VPCs and lower LVEF (Figs 23.4–23.9). As far as age, diabetes mellitus, mean heart rate, and HRV index are concerned (all of which are known markers of autonomic function or associated with autonomic dysfunction), *both* measures of heart rate turbulence, i.e. TO and

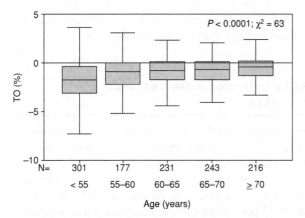 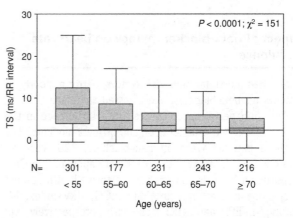

Figure 23.4 Heart rate turbulence and age of the patient at study enrolment (age). Both, turbulence onset (TO) and turbulence slope (TS) are significantly reduced at a higher age.

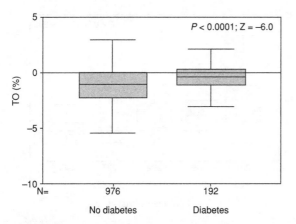 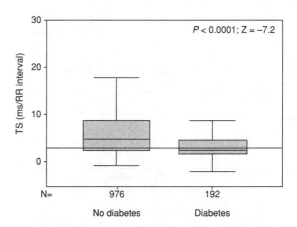

Figure 23.5 Heart rate turbulence in non-diabetic and diabetic patients. Both, turbulence onset (TO) and turbulence slope (TS) are significantly reduced in diabetic patients.

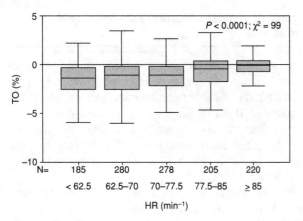

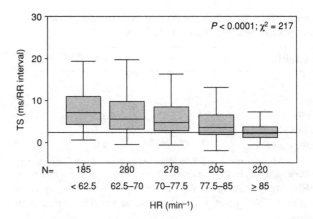

Figure 23.6 Heart rate turbulence and mean heart rate (HR) in the 24-hour Holter ECG. Both, turbulence onset (TO) and turbulence slope (TS) are significantly reduced at lower HR.

TS, were affected to a comparable extent. This applied also to the VPC count. The impact of LVEF on heart rate turbulence was smaller with only slight but significant effects on TO and TS.

Impact of beta-blocker therapy on heart rate turbulence

Established postinfarction risk factors perform poorly in patients on beta-blockers. We assessed therefore the risk stratification performance of heart rate turbulence in the EMIAT placebo arm patients on and off beta-blockers. 271 of these patients were on beta-blockers, 320 were off beta-blockers. In analogy to our primary approach,[1] a Cox-proportional hazards analysis was performed with respect to age, mean heart rate in Holter ECG, HRV index, MI history, LVEF, and HRT, all with prospectively set

dichotomy limits. In patients on and off beta-blockers, 2-year mortality was 12.9% and 14.7%, respectively. In patients off beta-blockers, HRT, history of previous infarction, LVEF, and mean heart rate were independent predictors of mortality, whilst in patients on beta-blockers, HRT was the only independent predictor (see Table 23.4 for the results of the multivariate analysis).

Physiologic mechanisms of heart rate turbulence

The underlying mechanisms of heart rate turbulence have not been fully identified. However, it has been known for decades that a ventricular systole can influence the rate of sinus nodal discharge, even in the absence of retrograde atrioventricular conduction. As early as 1909, first observations of the so-called ventriculophasic sinus arrhythmia

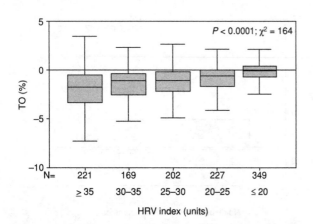

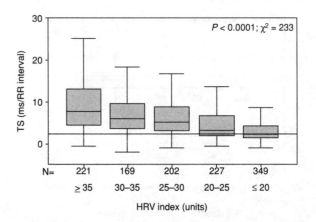

Figure 23.7 Heart rate turbulence and heart rate variability index (HRV index) in the 24-hour Holter ECG. Both, turbulence onset (TO) and turbulence slope (TS) are significantly reduced at lower HRV indices.

Table 23.4   Relative hazards of individual variables in patients on and off beta-blockers (multivariate analysis)

Variable	Off beta-blockers		On beta-blockers	
	Relative hazard	*P*	Relative hazard	*P*
Previous MI	2.2	0.02	–	–
Mean RR <800 ms	1.9	0.02	–	–
LVEF <30%	2.4	0.01	–	–
Combined TO and TS*	3.7	0.0005	3.8	0.004

*TO ≥0% and TS ≤2.5 ms/RR interval versus TO <0% and TS >2.5 ms/RR interval.
Abbreviations: LVEF = left ventricular ejection fraction; MI = myocardial infarction; RR = RR interval; TO = turbulence onset; TS = turbulence slope.

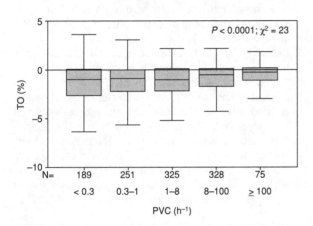
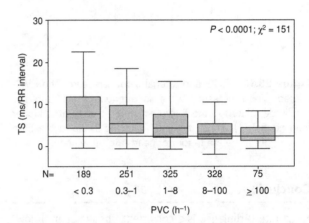

Figure 23.8   Heart rate turbulence and heart count of premature ventricular contractions (PVC) (HRV index) in the 24-hour Holter ECG. Both, turbulence onset (TO) and turbulence slope (TS) are significantly reduced at higher PVC counts.

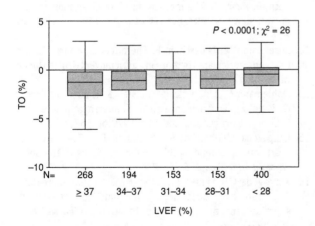
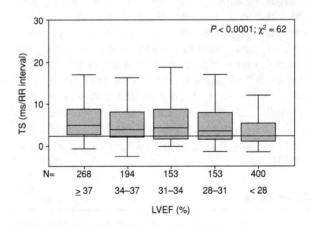

Figure 23.9   Heart rate turbulence and left ventricular ejection fraction (LVEF). Turbulence onset (TO) and turbulence slope (TS) are only slightly reduced at lower LVEF. Owing to the large number of observations, these differences reach the level of significance.

were made in experimental atrioventricular block.[8] Various pathophysiological mechanisms have been discussed to explain the ventriculophasic mechanisms, including changes in autonomic tone,[9–13] traction on the atrium as well as atrial appendages, atrioventricular junc-

tion, the sinus nodal region,[9,14–16] and transient improvement of the blood supply to the sinus node.[9,17,18]

We presume that heart rate turbulence is initiated by a baroreflex: the slight perturbation in arterial blood pressure caused by the VPC (i.e. a lower blood pressure amplitude of the premature beat and a higher blood pressure amplitude of the ensuing normal beat; Fig. 23.10) may be considered the triggering event. When the autonomic control system is intact, this fleeting change is registered immediately with an instantaneous response of the sinus node in the form of heart rate turbulence. If the autonomic control system is impaired, this reaction is either weakened or entirely missing. Our findings concerning the impact of clinical covariants related to autonomic function like age of the patient, presence of diabetes mellitus, mean heart rate, and HRV index in the 24-h Holter ECG support this hypothesis.

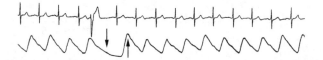

Figure 23.10   ECG and arterial blood pressure. The PVC-related blood pressure wave is attenuated (↓), and the amplitude related to the first postextrasystolic beat is higher than normal (↑). These fleeting variations in blood pressure are thought to be the trigger of heart rate turbulence.

Conclusion

Heart rate turbulence is a consistent phenomenon in low-risk patients with ischaemic heart disease. The absence of this phenomenon indicates a significantly increased risk of subsequent mortality. The measures for quantifying heart rate turbulence, TO, and TS are independent of each other and independent of other conventional risk predictors. The combination of TO and TS is a very strong risk predictor, even when adjusted for other established mortality predictors, such as LVEF, arrhythmia count, heart rate variability, mean heart rate, and history of previous myocardial infarction. Moreover, heart rate turbulence is predictive even in patients on beta-blockers. The combination of TO and TS is by far the strongest Holter-based risk predictor.

References

1. Schmidt G, Malik M, Barthel P *et al.* Heart rate turbulence after ventricular premature beats as a predictor of mortality after acute myocardial infarction. *Lancet* 1999;**353**:1390–6.
2. Schneider R, Barthel P, Schmidt G. Methods for the assessment of heart rate turbulence in Holter-ECGs. *J Am Coll Cardiol* 1999;**33**(Suppl. A):351A.
3. Multicenter Postinfarction Research Group. Risk stratification and survival after myocardial infarction. *New Engl J Med* 1983;**309**:331–6.
4. Julian DG, Camm AJ, Frangin G *et al.* Randomised trial of effect of amiodarone on mortality in patients with left-ventricular dysfunction after recent myocardial infarction: EMIAT. European Myocardial Infarct Amiodarone Trial Investigators. *Lancet* 1997;**349**:667–74.
5. La Rovere MT, Bigger JT, Jr, Marcus FI, Mortara A, Schwartz PJ. Baroreflex sensitivity and heart rate variability in prediction of total cardiac mortality after myocardial infarction. ATRAMI (Autonomic Tone and Reflexes After Myocardial Infarction) Investigators. *Lancet* 1998;**351**: 478–84.
6. Malik M, Schmidt G, Barthel P *et al.* Heart rate turbulence is a post-infarction mortality predictor which is independent of and additive to other recognised risk factors. *PACE* 1999;**22**(Part II):741.
7. Barthel P, Schmidt G, Schneider R *et al.* Heart rate turbulence in patients with and without autonomic dysfunction. *J Am Coll Cardiol* 1999;**33**(Suppl. A):136A.
8. Erlanger J, Blackman JR. Further studies in the physiology of heart block in mammals. Chronic auriculo-ventricular heart-block in the dog. *Heart* 1909:177.
9. Parsonnet AE, Miller R. Heart block. The influence of ventricular systole upon the auricular rhythm in complete and incomplete heart block. *Am Heart J* 1944:676–87.
10. Jedlicka J, Martin P. Time course of vagal effects studied in clinical electrocardiograms. *Eur Heart J* 1987;**8**:762–72.
11. Skanes AC, Tang AS. Ventriculophasic modulation of atrioventricular nodal conduction in humans. *Circulation* 1998;**97**:2245–51.
12. Roth IR, Kirsch B. The mechanism of irregular sinus rhythm in auriculoventricular heart block. *Am Heart J* 1948;**36**: 257–76.
13. Rosenbaum M, Lepeschkin E. The effect of ventricular systole on auricular rhythm in auriculoventricular block. *Circulation* 1955;**11**:240–61.
14. Döhlemann C, Murawski P, Theissen K, Haider M, Forster C, Poppl SJ. Ventriculophasische Sinusarrhythmie bei ventrikulärer Extrasystolie. *Z Kardiol* 1979;**68**:557–65.
15. Kappagoda CT, Linden RJ, Saunders DA. The effect on heart rate of distending the atrial appendages in the dog. *J Physiol Lond* 1972;**225**:705–19.
16. Kappagoda CT, Linden RJ, Snow HM. A reflex increase in heart rate from distension of the junction between the superior vena cava and the right atrium. *J Physiol Lond* 1972;**220**:177–97.
17. Wenckebach KF, Winterberg H. *Die unregelmäßige Herztätigkeit*. 1st edn. Leipzig: Verlag von Wilhelm Engelmann, 1927.
18. Hashimoto K, Tanaka S, Hirata M, Chiba S. Responses of the sino-atrial node to change in pressure in the sinus node artery. *Circ Res* 1967;**21**:297–304.

24 T wave dynamicity

Pierre Maison Blanche and Philippe Coumel

Our understanding of sudden cardiac death and how to prevent it remains limited. There is compelling data suggesting that abnormalities in the ventricular repolarisation process may be an important marker of potential malignant arrhythmias. In clinical practice, the only repolarisation feature considered in the past years was the duration of the QT interval from surface 12-lead ECG recordings.[1-4] However, controversy persists regarding the significance of the heart rate-adjusted QT interval as a risk factor for sudden cardiac arrest.

More recently, the capability to characterise various facets of ventricular repolarisation was made available in many commercial machines. This mainly includes automatic measurement of QT dispersion from resting ECGs (interlead variability of the QT duration), determination of the presence of a microvolt T-wave alternans (beat-to-beat variability of the ECG waveform) and calculation of the rate-dependence of the QT interval, from exercise tests or from ambulatory 24-hour ECG recordings.

What is T-wave dynamicity ?

A thorough review of previously published works suggests the following definition: QT dynamicity puts together all the pathophysiological influences known to modulate the QT interval. The critical point is that it combines *rate and rate-independent factors*, such as the autonomic nervous system, gender, age, pharmacological and metabolite influences.

What is the reason of the persisting confusion regarding QT dynamicity? In our opinion, it results partly from the lack of interest in rate-independent factors, but also there are some as yet unsolved issues regarding the *appropriate rate environment* for evaluating QT dynamicity. Everybody agrees that there is a time delay between a change in heart rate and the subsequent change in QT interval. The mean time to reach steady state has been repeatedly found to be about 2 minutes, and this time constant is often referred to as "QT adaptation". Consequently, if the relation between QT and RR intervals is not considered in steady state, it will be modulated by the current degree of

"QT adaptation", as shown in Fig. 24.1. To make a distinction between QT dynamicity and QT adaptation is not purely semantic: it is tightly associated with some methodological issues in clinical research.

If the dynamic variation of QT interval to heart rate is evaluated on a *beat-to-beat* basis, as is the case in many published reports,[5-8] the QT/RR relation will probably mix up the two phenomena, since steady state cannot be reached after a single RR interval (Fig. 24.1). On the other hand, a strict steady state environment can only be obtained with *artificial pacing protocols*,[9] which cannot be considered as reliable surrogates of the spontaneous heart rate variations in daily ambulatory conditions.

Actually, the lack of standardisation regarding the heart rate environment in the *non-invasive evaluation* of QT dynamicity considerably jeopardises the clinical use of QT dynamicity for assessment of the arrhythmic risk.

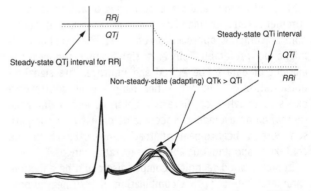

Figure 24.1 Effect of heart rate environment on QT interval. Superimposed cardiac beats in the lower part of the figure are preceded by the same RR interval (RRi) but a different heart rate environment. Some complexes are preceded by a stable heart rate whereas other complexes are preceded either by an accelerating trend (longer QT intervals) or by a decelerating trend (shorter QT intervals). In the upper part of the figure, a sudden heart rate change is shown (RR decreases from RRj to RRi). Away from steady state, the QT interval (QTk) has not yet reached full adaptation and is longer than its corresponding steady state value QTi. (See Reference 21 for more details.)

In this report, we will successively examine updated technical concepts of QT dynamicity, and thereafter its pathophysiological aspects.

Methodological aspects of QT dynamicity

The availability of QT dynamicity softwares from commercial systems should not mask some yet unsolved issues regarding the exact definition of the T wave! If most studies consider the return to the isoelectric line or the nadir between the T wave and the U wave, others claim that the method of Surawicz (intersection between the isoelectric line and the tangent to descending limb of the T wave) is more reliable.[10] What is true for resting ECG machines, although working on high-quality data, is even more critical for thousands of cardiac beats often collected in ambulatory conditions, and corrupted by some background noise. In addition, computerised methods work well in the presence of good quality ECG and monophasic T waves, since most algorithms have been validated using normal electrocardiograms, but unfortunately this is not true for abnormal electrocardiograms with the T wave not clearly defined morphologically or characterised by irregular shapes. It is generally accepted that, below 0.25 mV of T wave amplitude, automatic QT interval measurement performed inaccurately and lack of agreement between manual and automatic measurements have been repeatedly reported.[11,12]

Therefore, editing tools offered by the manufacturers are probably as important as the signal processing algorithm itself: a computerised analysis cannot be performed blindly, and visual reviewing of automatic measurement remains mandatory. From a technical standpoint, averaging approaches, on a 15–30 second basis might be preferable, since it significantly reduces the amount of data to be edited and improves the signal-to-noise ratio.[13–16] On the other hand, some controversy exists as to whether there is a potential loss of information when an averaging process is being used, in comparison with a beat-to-beat approach, in particular in the context of spontaneous abrupt heart rate changes.[5,8,17]

In fact, a good technical compromise could be a flexible parameter set-up, with a combination of *both* beat-to-beat and averaging analyses, depending on conditions such as heart rate patterns or ECG data quality. As discussed above, the dispute about which method is superior (averaging or beat-to-beat) ignores that full adaptation of QT interval is achieved only after 1 or 2 minutes. To the best of our knowledge, only two groups of researchers tried to introduce an alternative approach to take QT adaptation into account: Kligfield and co-workers in the USA and our group in Paris. Kligfield uses a gently graded treadmill protocol (the "Cornell protocol"), which produces small heart rate increments in 2-minutes stages.[18,19] Then, this group performs an averaging of the *final 20 seconds* of each exercise stage, i.e in relative steady heart rate conditions. In our method described in detail elsewhere, we use a selective beat averaged from 24-hour ECG recordings, to obtain cardiac complexes that are *preceded by the same stable heart rate*[20,21] defined by equal RR intervals within an observation period (say of 1 minute). However, today these alternative approaches are not recognised as gold standards.

Physiology of QT dynamicity

So, it is not surprising that literature remains extremely confusing regarding the nature of the relation between the ventricular repolarisation duration and the cardiac cycle length. This brief review cannot definitely answer such a critical issue. As said earlier, an attractive explanation of the discrepancies could be the rate environment in which the QT/RR relation is evaluated: schematically, most studies based on *dynamic* tests, such as exercise or tilting work, and on a beat-to-beat basis report a curvilinear QT/RR relation (the recovery phase being different from the intitial phase of the test), whereas others, mainly using 24-hour ECG data probably with more *smoothed* heart rate changes, found a linear relation.[6–8,13–20]

In addition to the choice of the clinical protocol, a thorough review of each published study allows us to recognise some specific patterns of the ECG analysis, which can significantly influence the results (such as the dilemma of averaging or not, or the use of the heart rate expressed in beats per minute versus the use of the RR interval in milliseconds). Therefore, it is often difficult to compare two studies with apparently similar aims.

One of the most important clinical messages provided by recent studies is the importance of rate-independent influences on the QT interval duration. The relationship between the QT interval and heart rate is steeper in females when compared to males, and the differences in QT duration between gender are more marked at long cycle lengths. This could explain the female prevalence among patients developing torsade de pointes.[20,22] Studies in which the QT interval was measured at different ages, including children, demonstrated that the gender effects appear only after puberty. Recent findings suggest that these ECG differences are directly related to sex hormones, which modulate potassium channel proteins.[23]

Autonomic influences on the repolarisation process have also been extensively investigated. Using the concept of the "slope" of the QT/RR relation, it has been shown that it shows a circadian modulation, with a larger dynamicity (slope) at daytime,[14,16,17,20,23,24] in particular during morning hours. Within a single subject, the mean heart rate of the circadian period is consistently correlated with the corresponding individual QT/RR slope, as shown in Figure 24.2.[20] Heart rate effects match well with both the circadian modulation and the gender differences of QT/RR slopes. In fact, the stronger rate-dependence found during the day and in females is associated with a faster heart rate. Indirect evaluation of the autonomic influences has also been performed after beta-blocker administration.[24–27] Sympathetic blockade strongly modifies the rate-dependence of the QT interval, with a resulting "biphasic effect" on the QT interval duration (prolonged or shortened by beta-blockers when compared to baseline), depending on the level of the heart rate considered.[25,26] Autonomic dysfunction is an interesting clinical model, in particular the parasympathetic activity impairment associated with diabetic neuropathy.[28,29] The slope of the QT/RR relationship is greater in patients with parasympathetic neuropathy. Finally, one study reported that the amplitude of the circadian modulation of QT dynamicity decreases with increasing age.[20]

Surprisingly, these large rate-independent sources of variations are often ignored in statistical analyses, therefore limiting the clinical implications of the reported findings.

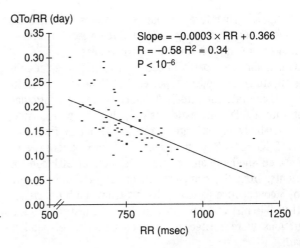

Figure 24.2 QT rate dependence and heart rate influences. This figure shows the regression analysis between the individual mean RR interval and individual slope of the QTo/RR relation, in a group of healthy subjects, during the diurnal period. In this example, RR interval may explain 34% (R^2) of the diurnal QTo/RR slope. QTo: interval between QRS onset and QT offset. (See Reference 20 for more details.)

The role of QT dynamicity in ischaemic and non-ischaemic cardiomyopathies

Regardless of these technical and pathophysiological issues, QT dynamicity has been consistently found to be a strong *discriminator* between cardiac pathologies.

After myocardial infarction, many studies using different systems reported that QT dynamicity is impaired in patients with spontaneous ventricular arrhythmias.[17,24,25,30–34] An *increased* QT/RR slope is observed in patients at risk, in particular at daytime and following awakening. Physicians still have to be cautious about these preliminary encouraging results. The number of patients included in retrospective studies remains relatively small, with the noticeable exception of the study reported by Chevalier in 391 patients, during a follow-up of 80 months, unfortunately only available in abstract form.[34]

Table 24.1 shows the values of the QT/RR slopes from three different studies in post-myocardial infarction

patients.[17,32,33] The slopes are strongly influenced by the methodological approach, QT dynamicity being larger from averaging techniques (Milliez and co-workers) when compared with a beat-to-beat analysis (Yi and co-workers).

Also, although it has been suggested that the individual value of the QT/RR relation could bear a prognostic information after myocardial infarction, this repolarisation marker has not yet been applied in a large prospective trial. The pathophysiological implications of an *increased* QT/RR slope in sudden cardiac death victims is poorly understood. It is generally accepted that a *prolonged* action potential duration is a potential trigger for ventricular tachyarrhythmias. However, we found that at shortened cycle lengths (i.e. at 600 ms RR interval), frequently observed immediately before spontaneous tachycardia onset, the QT interval was *shorter* in patients with ventricular arrhythmias after myocardial infarction, as shown

Table 24.1 QT/RR slope values in post-MI

Author	Group	QT 600 ms	QT 1000 ms	QT/RR day	QT/RR night	QT/RR morning
Yi	SCD	–	409 ms	0.162	0.141	–
N = 14	survivors	–	379 ms	0.102	0.109	–
Milliez	SCD	–	458 ms	0.253	0.236	0.273
N = 60	survivors	–	446 ms	0.201	0.172	0.243
Extramiana	VT	353 ms	453 ms	0.190	0.180	0.251
N = 23	No VT	379 ms	444 ms	0.153	0.138	0.179

SCD = sudden cardiac death; VT = ventricular tachycardia.

in Table 1.[32] Therefore, it could be hypothesised that an *increase in QT shortening* could induce a *lack of protection* againt re-entrant ventricular arrhythmias.

Our findings are partly in accordance with an epidemiological study previously reported by Algra and co-workers.[35] Using rate-corrected QT intervals (Bazett's formula) but with a fully automatic analysis, this group calculated the variability of the rate-corrected QT (QTc) from 24-hour ECG recordings in a cohort of 305 patients, 104 who died suddenly and a random sample of 201 control patients, from the complete Rotterdam QT study cohort (6693 consecutive patients). In this study, both *prolonged* (QTc >440 ms) and *shortened* (QTc <400 ms) mean QTc durations were related to an increased risk of sudden death.

To the best of our knowledge, the prognostic value of QT dynamicity in idiopathic dilated cardiomyopathy has been evaluated in a single study only, reported in Abstract form.[36] Using a commercial system, Fauchier and co-workers found that QT dynamicity, expressed as QT/RR slopes, is related to haemodynamic status and bears some prognostic value: in this study, an increased QTend/RR slope during the daytime period was an independent predictor of cardiac events (cardiac death or heart transplantation).

QT dynamicity and the risk of developing drug-induced torsade de pointes

The pro-arrhythmic potential of class IA antiarrhythmic agents (quinidine, disopyramide) is well recognised and attributed to their potential of provoking torsade de pointes. The negative results of the CAST study have also outlined that class IC drugs may occasionally exacerbate or induce ventricular arrhythmias. The evident failure of class I agents to prevent sudden death has increased interest in class III drugs. For some time the only available agents were sotalol and amiodarone, but recently a large number of selective class III agents (*d*-sotalol, ibutilide, dofetilide, azimilide) have been extensively evaluated. Drugs that have been associated with the development of torsade not only include antiarrhythmic agents, but also antibacterial and psychotropic agents and antihistamines. Most of these non-cardiovascular drugs depress cardiac ion channels, particularly the repolarising potassium currents. Overdosage of these drugs or co-administration with another compound that inhibits their metabolism (such as inhibition of the cytochrome P450 3A4 hepatic enzyme) can induce torsade de pointes.

Therefore, the clinical value of non-invasive ECG tests to recognise patients at an increased risk of arrhythmias is important. Strikingly, few data are available on an appropriate strategy to quantitate that risk.[37] Indeed, plasma drug levels and absolute QTc interval prolongation have not been found to be good predictors of torsade (no upper limit of acceptable QT prolongation has been identified).

Spontaneous sequences of onset of torsade

A consistent reported feature in torsade de pointes associated with acquired prolonged repolarisation is the presence of a pause determining a "short-long" sequence.[38,39] We found that stereotyped oscillatory patterns preceded not only the torsade, but also salvos and isolated ventricular premature beats. Actually, the entire initiating sequence can be defined as "short-long-short" (SLS) sequences since the long cycle is generally a post extrasystolic pause.[39]

The finding that specific heart rate sequences *and* QT variability are both involved in the initiation of torsade agrees well with many experimental studies. Vos *et al.* developed a canine model with a high incidence of reproducible torsade by mimicking the SLS intervals with specific pacing modes. He confirmed that in order to induce torsade, the pacing interval and the QT duration have to be sufficiently long, but a sudden rate change and the simultaneous presence of early after-depolarisations on the monophasic action potential recordings are also required.[40]

In humans, QT dynamicity patterns preceding the onset of drug-induced torsade have been investigated in a limited number of reports. Gilmour and co-workers measured RR and QT intervals in Holter recordings (on a beat-to-beat basis) obtained from seven patients referred to Lariboisière University Hospital for syncope associated with documented torsade.[41] He found that, keeping in mind the limitation of the beat-to beat approach, the slope of the linear relation between the RR and the QT intervals was less steep for the 10 intervals that preceded an episode of ventricular arrhythmia than for earlier intervals. Consequently, the QT interval was longer for any given RR interval than immediately after an episode of arrhythmias. In a case control study, Svernhage and co-workers tried to identify early ECG signs of torsade following intravenous administration of almokalant, a Class II antiarrhythmic compound.[42] Continuous precordial ECG recordings were examined before and after drug infusion. She reported that changes in T wave *morphology* were commonly seen during the administration of almokalant (T wave flattening), but the changes were more pronounced in patients with torsade. In this study, the most striking early predictor of torsade was the prolongation of Q-T apex interval.

The role of the drug rate-dependent effects on QT intervals

Most cardiovascular and non-cardiovascular drugs that prolong repolarisation exhibit "reverse rate-dependence", i.e.

the magnitude of the increase in the repolarisation duration is less pronounced at fast heart rates. In other terms, the QT prolongation is more marked at slow heart rates. Quinidine, *d*-sotalol, dofetilide, and sematilide induce a reverse rate-dependence of the QT prolongation, as shown by data from many experimental studies,[43,44] which used either Holter monitoring or exercise testing in humans.

The increase of the QT interval at slow heart rate suggests that it could contribute to the occurrence of bradycardia-dependent torsade. However, it has never been demonstrated that the degree of the QT rate-adaptation under antiarrhythmic agents was directly related to the risk of torsade,. Nevertheless, the lack of reverse rate dependency of QT interval under a drug is currently associated with a "safe" profile of the drug, as it is the case for amiodarone.[45]

QT dynamicity in the long QT syndrome

The congenital long QT syndrome was one of the first pathology investigated using QT dynamicity.[7] Notably, it has been found that QT interval rate adaptation, calculated from exercise tests or from Holter recordings, was *larger* in mutation carriers when compared to non-affected family members or normal controls, at least in the LQT1 form (i.e mutation on chromosome 11, with IKs potassium channel impairment).[7,8,14] The hypothesis of a lack of QT shortening in the long QT syndrome, which was the rationale to conduct such studies, was not confirmed. However, QT dynamicity as a diagnosis tool to identify mutation carriers within a family is not yet recommended by the Long QT Syndrome Registry members

To evaluate the *risk of cardiac events in family members* of probands with the long QT syndrome, the role of the resting ECG variables has been evidenced from this registry.[46] In addition to other clinical variables such as gender (in first-degree relatives only), and closeness of the relationship to the proband, the strong prognostic importance of repolarisation duration has been confirmed (the incidence of cardiac events in the group of family members presenting a QTc interval of >500 ms is as high as 30–45%). It has also been hypothesised that the dynamics of the QT interval might contain information in terms of both diagnosis and prognosis. Using a ventricular pacing protocol, Linker reported a considerable variation in the rate-related QT interval shortening between patients (eight patients with either Romano–Ward or Jervell syndrome, free of any medication). Most of the patients tended to shorten their QT interval with increasing pacing rates. However, QT dynamics was abnormal in a few cases with a total loss of QT adaptation and these abnormalities were exaggerated by isoproterenol and lessened by pro-

pranolol. In this very selected population, Linker could not identify any QT dynamics abnormalities associated with the tendency to develop torsade de pointes.[47]

Recent preliminary data from our group suggest that separate analysis of diurnal and nocturnal QT rate-dependence (using 24-hour ambulatory ECG) could give some prognostic information. When compared to asymptomatic KVLQT1 carriers, symptomatic KVLQT1 patients exhibited lower diurnal QT rate adaptation.[48] However, there are very limited data about the potential interest of QT dynamicity as a "prognostic" criterion in the long QT syndrome.

Conclusions

Since the relatively widespread availability of commercial softwares for automatic or semi-automatic measurement of the QT interval, data on QT dynamicity are rapidly increasing. However, the modes of analysis of these data remain confusing and we have discussed in this chapter the critical role of the heart rate environment. Nevertheless, we consider that there is a growing evidence suggesting the important clinical role of QT dynamicity.

Definitive answers should be provided sooner or later from retrospective analysis of specific databases, such as ancillary studies with the EMIAT Holter database, the International Long QT Syndrome Registry, or databases constituted by patients exhibiting drug-induced torsade de pointes while under cardiovascular or non-cardiovascular agent.

References

1. Goldberg RJ, Bengston J, Chen Z *et al.* Duration of the QT interval and total and cardiovascular mortality in healthy persons (The Framingham Study Experience). *Am J Cardiol* 1991; **67**:55–8.
2. Algra A, Tijssen JGP, Roelandt JRTC *et al.* QTc prolongation measured by standard 12 lead electrocardiography is an independent risk factor for sudden death due to cardiac arrest. *Circulation* 1991; **83**:1888–94.
3. Elming H, Holm E, Torp-Pedersen C *et al.* The prognostic value of the QT interval and QT interval dispersion in all-cause and cardiac mortality and morbidity in a population of Danish citizens. *Eur Heart J* 1998;**19**:1391–400.
4. Brooksby P, Batin PD, Nolan J *et al.* The relationship between QT intervals and mortality in ambulant patients with chronic heart failure. The United Kingdom heart failure evaluation and assessment of risk trial (UK-HEART). *Eur Heart J* 1999;**20**:1335–41.
5. Marti V, Guindo J, Homs E *et al.* Peaks of QTc lengthening measured in Holter recordings as a marker of life-threatening arrhythmias in postmyocardial patients. *Am Heart J* 1992;**124**:234–5.

6. Sarma JSM, Sarma RJ, Bilitch M *et al.* An exponential formula for heart rate dependence of QT interval during exercise and cardiac pacing in humans: reevaluation of Bazett's formula. *Am J Cardiol* 1984;**54**:103–8.

7. Merri M, Moss AJ, Benhorin J *et al.* Relation between ventricular repolarisation duration and cardiac cycle length during 24-hour Holter recordings. Findings in normal patients and patients with long QT syndrome. *Circulation* 1992;**85**:1816–21.

8. Swan H, Viitasalo M, Piipo K *et al.* Sinus node function and ventricular repolarization during exercise stress test in long QT syndrome patients with KvLQT1 and HERG potassium channel defects. *J Am Coll Cardiol* 1999;**4**:823–9.

9. Franz MR, Swerdlow CD, Liem BL *et al.* Cycle-length dependence of human action potential duration in vivo: effects of single extrastimuli, sudden sustained rate acceleration and deceleration, and different steady-state frequencies. *J Clin Invest* 1988;**82**:972–9.

10. Lepeschkin E, Surawicz B. The measurement of the Q-T interval of the electrocardiogram. *Circulation* 1952;**51**:378–88

11. Savelieva I, Gang Y, Guo X *et al.* Agreement and reproducibility of automatic versus manual measurement of QT interval and QT dispersion. *Am J Cardiol* 1998;**81**:471–7.

12. McLaughlin NB, Campbell RWF, Murray A. Comparison of automatic QT measurement techniques in the normal 12 lead electrocardiogram. *Br Heart J* 1995;**74**:84–9.

13. Singh JP, Musialek P, Sleight P *et al.* Effect of atenolol or metoprolol on waking hour dynamics of the QT interval in myocardial infarction. *Am J Cardiol* 1998;**81**:924–6.

14. Neyroud N, Maison Blanche P, Denjoy I *et al.* Diagnostic performance of QT interval variables from 24-hour electrocardiography in the long QT syndrome. *Eur Heart J* 1998;**19**:158–65.

15. Molnar J, Zhang F, Weiss J *et al.* Diurnal pattern of QTc interval: how long is prolonged? Possible relation to triggers of cardiovascular events. *J Am Coll Cardiol* 1996;**27**:76.

16. Tavernier R, Joardens L, Haerynck F *et al.* Changes in the QT interval and its adaptation to rate, assessed with continuous electrocardiographic recordings in patients with ventricular fibrillation, as compared to normal individuals without arrhythmias. *Eur Heart J* 1997;**18**:994–9.

17. Yi G, Hua Guo X, Gallagher MM *et al.* Circadian pattern of QT/RR adaptation in patients with and without sudden cardiac death after myocardial infarction. *Ann Noninvas Electrocardiol* 1999;**4**:286–94.

18. Lax KG, Okin PM, Kligfield P. Electrocardiographic repolarization measurements at rest and during exercise in normal subjects and in patients with coronary artery disease. *Am Heart J* 1994;**128**:271–80.

19. Kligfield P, Lax KG, Okin PM. QT interval–heart rate relation during exercise in normal men and women: definition by linear regression analysis. *J Am Coll Cardiol* 1996;**28**:1547–55.

20. Extramiana F, Maison Blanche P, Badilini F *et al.* Circadian modulation of QT rate dependence in healthy volunteers. Gender and age differences. *J Electrocardiol* 1999;**32**:33–43.

21. Badilini F, Maison Blanche P, Childers R *et al.* QT interval analysis on ambulatory ECG recordings: a selective beat averaging approach. *Med Biol Eng Comput* 1999;**37**:71–9.

22. Stramba-Badiale M, Locati EH, Courville J *et al.* Gender and the relationship between ventricular repolarization and cardiac cycle length during 24-hour Holter recordings. *Eur Heart J* 1997;**18**:1000–6.

23. Drici MD, Burklow TR, Haridasse V *et al.* Sex hormones prolong the QT interval and downregulate potassium channel expression in the rabbit heart. *Circulation* 1996;**94**:1471–4.

23. Browne KF, Prystowsky E, Heger JJ *et al.* Modulation of the QT interval by the autonomic nervous system. *PACE* 1983;**6**:1050–6.

24. Singh JP, Musialek P, Sleight P *et al.* Effect of atenolol or metoprolol on waking hour dynamics of the QT interval in myocardial infarction. *Am J Cardiol* 1998;**81**:924–6.

25. Hintze U, Wupper F, Mickley H *et al.* Effects of beta-blockers on the relation between QT interval and heart rate in survivors of acute myocardial infarction. *Ann Noninvas Electrocardiol* 1998;**3**:319–26.

26. Sarma JSM, Venkataraman K, Samant DR *et al.* Effect of propranolol on the QT intervals of normal individuals during exercise: a new method for studying interventions. *Br Heart J* 1988;**60**:434–9.

27. Viitasalo M, Karjalainen J. QT interval at heart rates from 50 to 120 beats per minutes during 24-hour electrocardiographic recordings in 100 healthy men. Effects of atenolol. *Circulation* 1992;**86**:1439–42.

28. Ong JJC, Sarma JSM, Venkataraman K *et al.* Circadian rhythmicity of heart rate and QTc interval in diabetic autonomic neuropathy: implications for the mechanism of sudden death. *Am Heart J* 1993;**125**:744–52.

29. Shimono M, Fujiki A, Asahi T *et al.* Alteration in QT-RR relationship in diabetic patients with autonomic dysfunction. *Ann Noninvas Electrocardiol* 1999;**4**:176–83.

30. Viitasalo M, Karjalainen J, Makijarvi M *et al.* Autonomic modulation of QT intervals in post-myocardial infarction patients with and without ventricular fibrillation. *Am J Cardiol* 1998;**82**:154–9.

31. Kluge P, Walter T, Neugebauer A. Comparison of QT/RR relationship using two algorithms of QT interval analysis for identification of high risk patients for life-threatening ventricular arrhythmias. *Ann Noninvas Electrocardiol* 1997;**2**:3–8.

32. Extramiana F, Neyroud N, Huikuri H *et al.* QT interval and arrhythmic risk assessment after myocardial infarction. *Am J Cardiol* 1999;**83**:266–9.

33. Milliez P, Leenhardt A, Maison Blanche P *et al.* Arrhythmic death in the EMIAT trial: role of ventricular repolarization dynamicity as a new discriminant risk factor. *Circulation* 1999;**100**:1–159 (A).

34. Chevalier P, Codreanu A, Kirkorian G *et al.* Automatic Holter analysis of rate-dependent changes of the QT interval: new markers to predict long-term mortality after myocardial infarction. *Circulation* 1998;**98**:1–81(A).

35. Algra A, Tijssen JGP, Roelandt JRTC *et al.* QT interval variables from 24-hour electrocardiography and the two year risk of sudden death. *Br Heart J* 1993;**70**:43–8.

36. Fauchier L, Babuty D, Autret ML *et al.* QT interval dynamicity in idiopathic dilated cardiomyopathy: relationship with haemodynamic status and prognostic value. *Eur Heart J* 1999;**7** (A).

37. Roden DM, Woosley RL, Primm RK. Incidence and clinical features of the quinidine-associated long QT syndrome: implications for patient care. *Am Heart J* 1986;**111**:1088–93

38. Kay GN, Plumb VJ, Arciniegas JG *et al.* Torsade de pointes: the long–short initiating sequence and other clinical features: observation in 32 patients. *J Am Coll Cardiol* 1983;**2**:806–17.

39. Locati EH, Maison-Blanche P, Dejode P *et al.* Spontaneous sequences of onset of torsade de pointes in patients with acquired prolonged repolarization: quantitative analysis of Holter recordings. *J Am Coll Cardiol.* 1995;**25**:1564–75.

40. Vos MA, Verduyn C, Gorgels APM *et al.* Reproducible induction of early after-depolarizations and torsade de pointes arrhythmias by *d*-sotalol and pacing in dogs with chronic atrioventricular block. *Circulation* 1995;**91**:864–72.

41. Gilmour RF, Riccio ML, Locati EH *et al.* Time- and rate-dependent alterations of the QT interval precede the onset of torsade de pointes in patients with acquired QT prolongation. *J Am Coll Cardiol* 1997;**30**:209–17.

42. Svernhage E, Houltz B, Blomstrom P *et al.* Early electrocardiographic signs of drug-induced torsade de pointes. *Ann Noninvas Electrocardiol* 1998;**3**:252–60.

43. Funck-Brentano C, Kibleur Y, Le Coz F *et al.* Rate dependence of sotalol-induced prolongation of ventricular repolarization during exercise in humans. *Circulation* 1991;**8B3**:536–45.

44. Lande G, Maison Blanche P, Fayn J *et al.* Dynamic analysis of dofetilide-induced changes in ventricular repolarization. *Clin Pharmacol Ther* 1998;**64**:312–21.

45. Bril A, Forest MC, Cheval B *et al.* Combined potassium and calcium channel antagonistic activities as a basis for neutral frequency dependent increase in action potential duration: comparison between BRL-32872 and azimilide. *Cardiovasc Res* 1998;**37**:130–40.

46. Zareba W, Moss AJ, Le Cessie S *et al.* Risk of cardiac events in family members of patients with long QT syndrome. *J Am Coll Cardiol.* 1995;**26**:1685–91.

47. Linker NJ, Camm AJ, Ward DE. Dynamics of ventricular repolarization in the congenital long QT syndromes. *Br Heart J* 1991;**66**:230–7.

48. Neyroud N, Denjoy I, Maison-Blanche P *et al.* Characteristics of the day–night behavior of ventricular repolarization in the long QT syndrome. *Eur Heart J* 1996;**17**:375 (A).

25 Repolarisation alternans

Daniel M Bloomfield and Richard J Cohen

The measurement of microvolt level repolarisation alternans, better known as T wave alternans (TWA), is increasingly being used as a measure of susceptibility to ventricular tachyarrhythmias and sudden cardiac death. In this chapter we briefly review the history of TWA, the techniques for its measurement, the clinical data establishing its value as a predictor of arrhythmia risk, and its role in clinical risk stratification.

Electrical alternans represents an alteration in the morphology of an electrocardiographic waveform on an every other beat basis (Fig. 25.1). *True electrical alternans* represents alternation in intrinsic cardiac electrical processes. *Mechanical alternans* may occur in the setting of pericardial effusion in which the entire heart moves in an alternating pattern in successive beats. Mechanical alternans may give rise to *apparent electrical alternans* because of the rotation of the cardiac electrical axis on an every other beat basis. Here we will discuss only true electrical alternans. Electrical alternans was described as early as 1909.[1–3] Historically, electrical alternans has been associated with a variety of conditions such as Prinzmetal's angina,[4] electrolyte abnormalities,[5,6] acute ischaemia,[7] and the long QT syndrome.[8] Each of these conditions is in turn associated with an increased risk of ventricular arrhythmias. In particular, in the case of the long QT syndrome, sudden death may occur in the teenage or pre-teenage years. TWA visible on the surface ECG is quite common in the long QT syndrome, particularly during emotional or exercise stress (Fig. 25.2).

However, TWA visible on the surface ECG, is quite a rare phenomenon. In 1948, Kalter and Schwartz[9] reviewed the world's literature on TWA and reported a total of 46 cases including five new cases that they reported from a review of 8084 clinical electrocardiograms (ECGs) taken on 6059 patients. Thus the incidence of TWA was approximately 1 in 1212 patients. Interestingly, Kalter and Schwartz reported a mortality of 61% in the reported cases. However, because visible TWA is so rare, it had been generally considered in the literature to be essentially an electrocardiographic curiosity, and was not specifically associated with arrhythmic risk.

Smith and Cohen[10] in 1984 reported, in a finite element model of cardiac conduction, that electrical alternans was a marker of increased susceptibility to re-entrant arrhythmias. The mechanism underlying the association of electrical alternans with susceptibility to re-entrant arrhythmias in this model, was that dispersion of refractoriness led, on the one hand, to wave front fractionation and re-entry and, on the other hand, to some regions of the myocardium being capable of only conducting on an every other beat basis. This alternation in conduction in turn was reflected in the simulated ECG as electrical alternans.

Another mechanism that can lead to the development of TWA, is alternation in the duration of the action potential. Action potential alternans is a well recognised phenomenon that can occur in diseased tissue and the cellular and ionic basis for which has been investigated.[11,12] Mathematically one would expect action potential alternans (Fig. 25.3a) to be initiated when the slope of the restitution curve (dependence of action potential duration on preceding diastolic interval, see Fig. 25.3b) exceeds unity at the current value of the diastolic interval. Recent experimental studies[13,14] suggest that localised

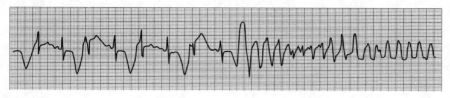

Figure 25.1 Visible T wave alternans preceding the onset of ventricular fibrillation. (Reproduced with permission from Raeder EA, Rosenbaum DS, Bhasin R, Cohen RJ. Letters to the Editor: Alternating morphology of the qrst complex preceding sudden death. *N Engl J Med* 1992;**326**:271–2, figure 2.)

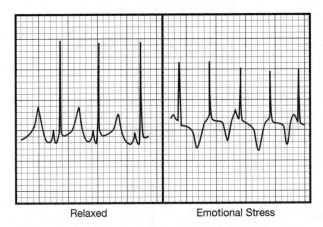

Figure 25.2 Emotional excitement inducing T wave alternans in a patient with the long QT syndrome. (Adapted with permission from reference 8, figure 1.)

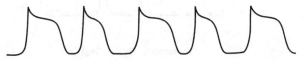

Figure 25.3a Example of action potential alternans. (Reproduced with permission from Cohen RJ. T wave alternans and Laplacian imaging. In: Zipes DP, Jalife J, eds. *Cardiac electrophysiology: from cell to bedside.* Philadelphia: Saunders, 1999, pp. 781–9, figure 87-6.)

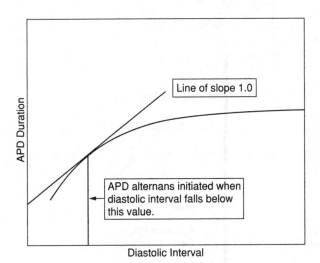

Figure 25.3b Restitution curve illustrating that action potential alternans is initiated when the diastolic interval falls to a value where the slope of the curve exceeds unity.

reflected in the surface ECG as repolarisation alternans. Favouring this mechanism is the observation that clinically, in the surface ECG, repolarisation alternans tends to be larger in magnitude and more prevalent than depolarisation alternans. This would be expected if action potential alternans was the cause of TWA but not if alternans was due to a localised 2:1 conduction block. The data of Pastore *et al.*[13] and Chinushi *et al.*[14] suggest that TWA is not just a marker for increased susceptibility to ventricular arrhythmias, but that it is mechanistically involved in the development of re-entrant arrhythmias.

Technique for measurement of microvolt level TWA

From the observations of Smith and Cohen[10] the hypothesis was developed that TWA might be commonly associated with susceptibility to ventricular arrhythmias, but that its amplitude was generally too small to be detected by visual inspection of the surface ECG. The hypothesis was that TWA was present in patients susceptible to ventricular arrhythmias, but that the alternation involved only microvolt level changes in T wave morphology. This led to the development of the Spectral Method[16] for the detection of microvolt level TWA.

In this method (Fig. 25.4), the T wave in each beat is sampled at corresponding points with the same offset with respect to a fiducial point. A series of amplitudes of the T waves at these points is constructed, usually for 128 beats. The power spectrum of this beat series is then constructed using Fourier analysis techniques. Alternans appears as a peak at the last point in the spectrum at a frequency of 0.5 cycles per beat, corresponding to a period of two beats. Separate power spectra are computed for different points in the T wave corresponding to different offsets from a fiducial point. These spectra are then averaged to generate a composite power spectrum. Two numerical indices of alternans are obtained. One is V_{alt}, the alternans voltage. This corresponds to the square root of the amplitude of the alternans peak above the background noise level. V_{alt} represents the magnitude of the alternating variation in T wave morphology compared to the mean T wave. The second index is k, the alternans ratio, which is the amplitude of the alternans peak above the background noise level measured in units of the standard deviation of the noise. Generally, the alternans index is required to be greater than or equal to 3.0 in order for the alternans peak to be considered statistically significant.

The spectral method is effective in detecting microvolt level TWA, even in the presence of ECG noise which is significantly greater in magnitude than V_{alt}. The reason for this effectiveness is that all fluctuations in T wave morphology that do not occur on an every-other-beat basis are

alternation in action potential duration may cause TWA and lead to the development of re-entrant arrhythmias. The action potential alternans, which may occur discordantly in different regions of the myocardium,[15] not only causes dynamic dispersion of recovery but also may be

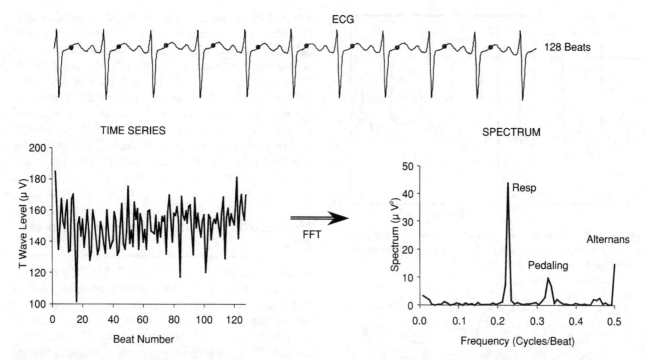

Figure 25.4a Spectral method for assessing T wave alternans. The amplitudes of corresponding points on the T wave are measured for 128 beats. A time series consisting of these 128 amplitudes is created. The power spectrum of this time series is computed using fast Fourier transform methods. In the power spectrum obtained from recordings during bicycle exercise, peaks corresponding to frequencies of respiration, pedalling, and alternans are illustrated. (Reproduced with permission from Cohen RJ. T wave alternans and Laplacian imaging. In: Zipes DP, Jalife J, eds. *Cardiac electrophysiology: from cell to bedside*. Philadelphia: Saunders, 1999, pp. 781–9, figure 87-2.)

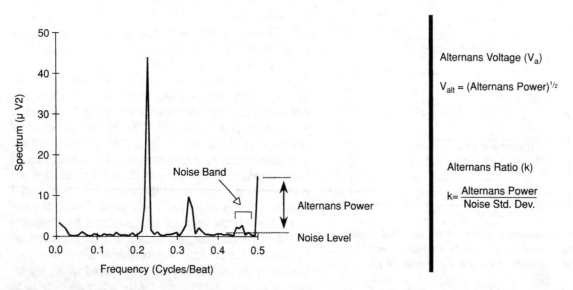

Figure 25.4b Computation of spectral measures of T wave alternans. An average power spectrum, consisting of the average of power spectra from points spanning the T wave, is computed. Using this average power spectrum, the alternans voltage (V_{alt}) is computed as the square root of the of the alternans power, which is the amplitude of the last point in the power spectrum above the mean noise level in the reference noise band. The alternans ratio (k) is the ratio of the alternans power to the standard deviation of the noise measured in the reference noise band in the average power spectrum. (Reproduced with permission from Cohen RJ. T wave alternans and Laplacian imaging. In: Zipes DP, Jalife J, eds. *Cardiac electrophysiology: from cell to bedside*. Philadelphia: Saunders, 1999, pp. 781–9, figure 87-3A.)

shifted away from the alternans peak in the power spectrum. In addition, the fact that the spectral method incorporates a measure of statistical significance permits one to distinguish between true alternans and artefact resulting from the presence of noise. Other methods (for example, see Nearing et al.[17]) have been proposed for the measurement of TWA, but generally their effectiveness has not been demonstrated for the measurement of alternans at a microvolt level under clinical conditions.

Studies of T measured during cardiac pacing

The spectral method was applied in animal studies[16] to detect TWA under a variety of conditions, which alter susceptibility to ventricular arrhythmias – hypothermia, coronary artery ligation, and rapid pacing. The level of TWA was compared with the ventricular fibrillation threshold (VFT) as an invasive measure of cardiac electrical stability. The level of TWA was inversely related to the magnitude of the VFT across each intervention and combinations of interventions (Fig. 25.5). This study led to a clinical investigation.[18] In this study, 83 consecutive patients undergoing invasive electrophysiological testing (EP) had TWA measured using the spectral method during atrial pacing at 100 bpm prior to programmed ventricular stimulation. The presence of TWA was compared with the outcome of EP and with arrhythmia-free survival during a 20-month follow-up. TWA predicted EP outcome with a sensitivity of 81% and specificity of 84%. More significantly, Kaplan–Meier analysis revealed that at 20 months of follow-up only 6% of patients who tested negative for TWA had arrhythmic events as compared to 81% of patients who tested positive (Fig. 25.6). EP was an equivalent predictor of arrhythmic events in this study. In these studies TWA performed substantially better as predictor of arrhythmic events than either signal-averaged electrocardiogram (SAECG) or QT dispersion.[19,20]

Measurement of T-wave alternans during exercise or pharmacologic stress

The limitation of the Rosenbaum et al.[18] study was that TWA was measured during atrial pacing and thus did not truly represent a non-invasive test. Previous animal data[16] had demonstrated that TWA is highly dependent on heart rate. Thus, in order to measure TWA with adequate sensitivity, it is necessary to elevate the heart rate. Non-invasive measurement of TWA during exercise testing was a technical challenge in that one needed to detect microvolt level fluctuations in T wave morphology in the presence of artefact resulting from the exercise. These challenges were overcome by the use of multicontact electrodes in combination with sophisticated signal processing techniques.[21] The multicontact electrodes can be used to increase the signal-to-noise ratio in the following way. Since each of the contacts of one electrode are located in proximity to each other, the electrocardiographic signal detected by each should be nearly identical. However, the noise recorded by each electrode may be quite different depending on the impedance of the contact–skin connection, local muscle noise, and motion artefact. Thus the signals from each of the electrodes can be combined to increase the signal and reduce the noise. By using advanced signal processing in combination with multicontact electrodes it is now possible to measure TWA routinely during bicycle or treadmill exercise stress with commercially available equipment (CH 2000 system, Cambridge Heart Inc, Bedford, Massachusetts, USA).

In addition to the noise problems associated with measuring TWA during exercise stress, the interpretation of the TWA test now must take into account the dynamic variation of heart rate with exercise. Patients susceptible to ventricular tachyarrhythmias tend to develop sustained alternans during exercise stress (Fig. 25.7). Sustained alternans is alternans that is consistently present above a patient-specific onset heart rate. Alternans that occurs episodically and does bear a consistent relationship to heart rate has not been associated with increased arrhythmic risk.

Some standard criteria used for the interpretation of TWA tests are listed below.

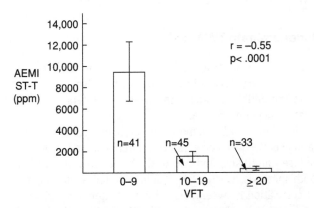

Figure 25.5 Relationship between the level of repolarisation alternans and the ventricular fibrillation threshold (measured in milliamperes) in 119 paired measurements made in 20 dogs during different interventions: hypothermia, coronary artery ligation, and pacing induced tachycardia. (Reproduced with permission from reference 16, figure 8.)

Positive TWA test

The usual criteria used to define a positive TWA test indicative of arrhythmic risk is the presence of sustained alter-

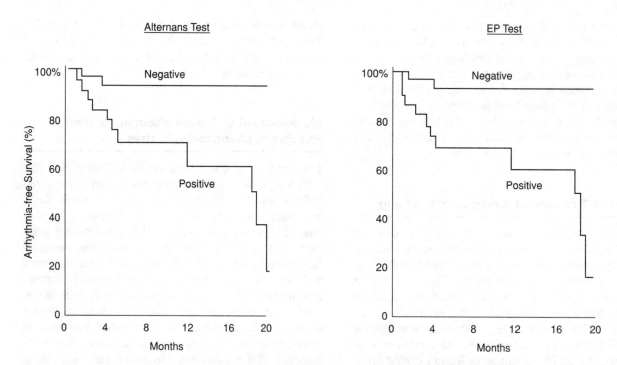

Figure 25.6 *Left*: the relation between T wave alternans and arrhythmia-free survival in 66 patients. Kaplan–Meier life table arrhythmia-free survival is compared in patients with and without significant T wave alternans. Note that the presence of T wave alternans strongly identifies those patients who are at risk for reduced arrhythmia-free survival. *Right*: arrhythmia-free survival in patients with positive electrophysiologic tests (+EP) is compared with survival in patients in whom ventricular arrhythmias were not induced at electrophysiologic testing (–EP). Note that the predictive value of both electrophysiologic testing and T wave alternans is essentially indistinguishable in these plots. (Reprinted with permission from reference 18, figure 5, Copyright 1994, Massachusetts Medical Society.)

nans of amplitude at least 1.9 µV, with $k \geq 3.0$, and at least 1 minute in duration, including some period of artefact-free data, in a vector lead, or two adjacent precordial leads ($k \geq 3.0$ required in only one of the two precordial leads) with onset either at the resting heart rate or at a heart rate less than or equal to 110 bpm. A period of artefact-free data is a period during which the frequency of of ectopic beats $\leq 10\%$, the rate of stepping or pedalling is not at half the heart rate, respiration rate is not at one-fourth of the heart rate, the heart rate is not changing more rapidly than 30 bpm over a 128 beat interval, and RR interval alternans ≥ 2 ms is not present.

Negative TWA test

A test is usually defined as negative if it does not meet the criteria for a positive test and the maximum negative heart rate (MaxNegHR) ≥ 105 bpm (A rules). The MaxNegHR is defined to be the highest heart rate at which at least 1 minute of data is present without significant alternans, with a noise level ≤ 1.8 µV in the vector magnitude lead and with fewer than 10% ectopic beats. An alternative definition of a

negative test also allows, in patients who stop exercise due to fatigue or symptoms, for a MaxNegHR <105 bpm provided that the MaxNegHR is within 5 bpm of the maximum heart rate, which in turn is ≥ 80 bpm (B rules).

Indeterminate TWA test

An indeterminate test is a test that does not meet the criteria for being classified as positive or negative.

In the definitions above the heart rate refers to a 128-beat averaged heart rate.

Hohnloser *et al.*[22] demonstrated a high degree of correlation between pacing-induced alternans and exercise-induced alternans, and the onset heart rates obtained in both methods. Coch *et al.*[23] demonstrated a high degree of correlation between pacing-induced alternans and alternans-induced pharmacologically by adminstration of atropine. Ritvo *et al.*[24] demonstrated high concordance between exercise and pharmacologic testing using dobutamine and atropine. It appears that, for the onset of TWA, the key variable is the heart rate and not the means used to raise the heart rate.

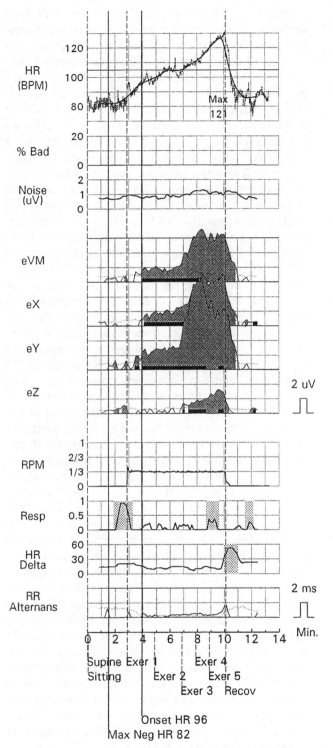

Clinical studies of exercise-induced TWA

Caref *et al.*[25] demonstrated that, in patients without a history of cardiac disease, exercise-induced TWA is very rare (incidence on the order of 1%). In a pilot study Estes *et al.*[26] demonstrated that TWA was highly predictive of the outcome of EP testing.

Klingenheben *et al.*[27] tested TWA as a predictor of appropriate discharge of an implantable cardioverter/defibrillator (ICD) during an 18-month follow-up in 95 patients who received ICDs for standard clinical indications (primarily resuscitated cardiac arrest). In addition to TWA testing, patients were evaluated by means of EP, left ventricular ejection fraction (LVEF), baroreceptor sensitivity (BRS), SAECG, QT dispersion (QTD), and from 24-hour ECG monitoring: presence of non-sustained ventricular tachycardia (NSVT), mean interbeat interval, and SDNN measure of heart rate variability. Of all the arrhythmic risk stratifiers, only TWA ($P = 0.006$; RR = 2.5), and LVEF ($P = 0.04$; RR = 1.4) were statistically significant univariate predictors of appropriate ICD discharge. On multivariate analysis only TWA was a statistically significant independent predictor.

During a 12-month follow-up in 102 patients tested for TWA predischarge after acute myocardial infarction,[28] 28% of TWA-positive patients had sustained ventricular tachycardia or fibrillation (positive predictive value), whereas 98% of the TWA-negative patients did not have such an event (negative predictive value). The sensitivity was 93%, RR 16.8, and $P = 0.006$ (Fig. 25.8). In this study, LVEF and SAECG had substantially lower relative risks, and negative predictive values and sensitivities, but somewhat higher positive predictive values. In another study in patients after acute myocardial infarction,[29] it was reported that TWA evolves during the 4–6 weeks postinfarction, thus indicating that risk stratification for late arrhythmic events should be performed 4–6 weeks after infarction.

Gold *et al.*[30] reported preliminary results from a multicentre trial in patients undergoing EP study that TWA predicted arrhythmic events or death during 1 year follow-up with a positive predictive value of 18.3%, negative predictive value of 98.3%, and RR of 10.6 ($P <0.011$) compared to a positive predictive value of 22.9%, negative predictive value of 93.9% and relative risk of 3.7 ($P <0.029$) for EP. Importantly, TWA predicted arrhythmic events in patients with and without reduced LVEF, and in patients with both ischaemic and non-ischaemic heart disease.[31] In a sub-study of this trial[32] of

Figure 25.7 Trend plot of bicycle exercise TWA test in a patient with sustained alternans. Tracings from top to bottom: Heart rate, percent ectopic beats, noise level (mV) in vector magnitude lead, V_{alt} (µV) in vector magnitude and orthogonal leads X, Y, Z (precordial leads not shown) – shading indicates alternans ratio exceeds 3.0, pedalling rate (rpm), respiratory activity at one-fourth of the heart rate, maximum heart rate change over 128 beats, RR alternans magnitude (ms). The beginning of the MaxNegHR interval and time of onset of sustained alternans are shown together with their associated heart rates. Because the onset heart rate is less than or equal to 110 bpm, this is a positive test.

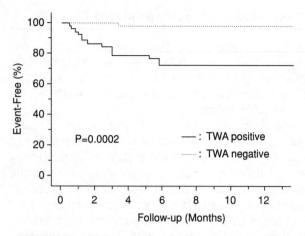

Figure 25.8 Arrhythmia-free survival in 102 post-myocardial infarction patients based on TWA classification. (Reproduced with permission from reference 28, figure 4A.)

130 patients with syncope of unkown origin during a 12-month follow-up, TWA was a significant predictor of ventricular tachyarrhythmic events or death, with positive predictive value of 0.19 and a negative predictive value of 0.97, RR 7.1, and *P* <0.01, whereas as EP was not a significant predictor of end-point events. In a study[33] of 107 patients with congestive heart failure, of seven non-invasive measures of arrhythmic risk only TWA was a statistically significant predictor of ventricular tachyarrhythmic events. During 18 months of follow-up, 21% of TWA positive patients had endpoint events whereas nine of the TWA negative patients had such events (negative predictive value = 100%). In another study[34] of patients with dilated cardiomyopathy, TWA was a highly accurate predictor (*P* = 0.003) of ventricular tachycardia (sustained or non-sustained). Another report showed that, in dilated cardiomyopathy patients, TWA also identified all patients with a subsequent sustained ventricular tachyarrhythmia.[35] Several studies suggest that TWA measures alterations in arrhythmic substrate induced pharmacologically by administration of procainamide,[36] flecainide,[37] amiodarone,[38] or beta-blockers.[39] Procainamide, amiodarone, and beta-blockers were reported on average to reduce the level of TWA whereas flecainide tended to induce alternans.

Clinical use of TWA

TWA can now be conveniently measured non-invasively during exercise stress (or during pharmacologic stress or during pacing). A growing body of clinical data has now been accumulated in a variety of patient populations that suggests that TWA is a powerful predictor of arrhythmic risk. Patients who are TWA positive have a substantial risk of ventricular tachyarrhythmic events and, equally important, TWA-negative patients are at quite low risk. In direct comparisons, TWA has compared favourably to other non-invasive risk stratifiers. The data suggest that TWA has a similar positive predictive value to EP but a better negative predictive value.[18,27,30–32] Further, data suggest that TWA status changes with pharmacologically-induced alterations in myocardial electrical stability. However, at the present time there are no completed randomised trials that demonstrate that prophylactic treatment with ICDs or drugs, in patients identified to be at risk on the basis of a positive TWA test, results in a reduction in mortality or arrhythmic events. Such trials are only now being organised and will require a number of years to complete.

The current clinical use of TWA in risk stratification can be guided by the existing clinical data, which indicate that TWA identifies patients both at high risk of ventricular arrhythmias and a second group at quite low risk. However, in the absence of definitive clinical data demonstrating a clinical benefit of treatment based on TWA status, decisions regarding whether and how to treat high-risk patients must rely on clinical judgement. Figure 25.9 illustrates possible ways TWA may be integrated into clinical strategies for identifying high-risk patients. These clinical algorithms are to be considered only as tentative proposals until the needed prospective clinical trials are conducted – ultimately prospective clinical trials should be used to guide patient management.

These figures incorporate the following rationales. In these algorithms, a negative TWA test identifies a patient who can now be considered low risk for sudden death. The negative predictive value of TWA is sufficiently high that patients who test TWA negative may not need invasive EP testing (the negative predictive value of TWA appears to be consistently superior to that of EP[18,27,30–32]). In patients with unexplained syncope, patients with a negative TWA test may not need an EP study to determine if they have inducible VT, and further diagnostic testing can be directed at other causes of syncope. Patients with reduced LVEF being screened for risk of sudden death who have a negative TWA test, probably do not require a further evaluation with an EP study. Patients with a positive TWA test, especially if they have reduced LVEF, are at high risk of sudden death and may be considered for EP (if they have ischaemic heart disease – EP is not generally thought to be of use in patients with non-ischaemic heart disease) and prophylactic antiarrhythmic therapy (ICD or possibly sotalol or amiodarone). Patients with syncope of unknown origin, TWA, and reduced LVEF can be considered to be at very high risk and merit consideration for ICD therapy (with or without an additional EP study depending on the patient).

Future directions in repolarisation alternans testing

Measurement of TWA is currently a robust technology. However, there is still room for technical advances. Some

A

Proposed Protocol for Prophylactic
Management to Prevent Sudden Cardiac
Death in Patients with Known Heart Disease
and Unexplained Syncope

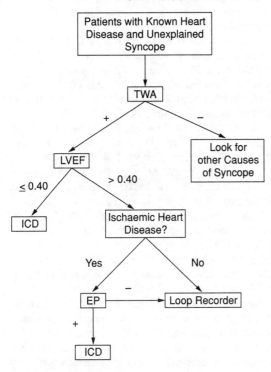

B

Proposed Protocol for Prophylactic
Management to Prevent Sudden Cardiac
Death in Patients with Non-Ischaemic Heart
Disease and LV Dysfunction but Without a
History of Syncope

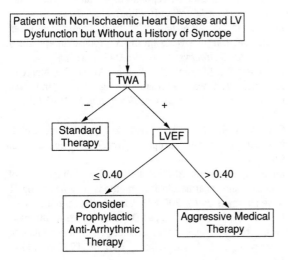

C

Proposed Protocol for Prophylactic
Management to Prevent Sudden Cardiac
Death in Patients with Ischaemic Heart
Disease and LV Dysfunction but Without a
History of Syncope

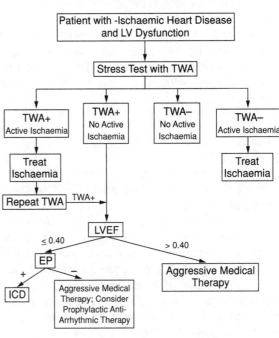

Figure 25.9 Possible clinical algorithms for the incorporation of TWA and LVEF into clinical risk stratification and patient management to reduce risk of sudden cardiac death. *Panel A.* Patients with known heart disease and unexplained syncope. *Panel B.* Patients with non-ischaemic heart disease and LV dysfunction but without a history of syncope. *Panel C.* Patients with ischaemic heart disease and LV dysfunction.

technical improvements in TWA testing are already in the process of being implemented. Improvements in the signal processing techniques are reducing the incidence of false positive TWA tests from noise or motion artefact. These improvements should further increase the positive predictive value of the test. In addition, a computer algorithm for automatic classification of the TWA test result will assist physicians in the interpretation of the test and help ensure a greater degree of uniformity in the interpretation of the test at different centres. Analysis of data from clinical trials in different patient populations will be used to optimise the rules and cut-off values used for interpretation of the test.

Perhaps the most important advances with respect to TWA will come from prospective clinical trials, in particular treatment trials, which will test the clinical benefit deriving from the clinical use of TWA to identify high- and low-risk patients for arrhythmic risk. More work also remains to be done in evaluating how TWA can be best used in conjunction with other measures of arrhythmic risk.

Conclusion

The measurement of microvolt level TWA has been demonstrated to be an effective non-invasive predictor of ventricular tachyarrhythmic events and sudden cardiac death in a variety of patient populations. TWA can be conveniently measured during exercise stress with the use of commercial equipment. There is a role for the clinical use of TWA in arrhythmic risk stratification in conjunction with clinical history and other risk stratifiers. There is a need for prospective clinical treatment trials to demonstrate that prophylactic therapy of patients with TWA results in a clinical benefit.

References

1. Hering HE. Experimentelle studien an Saugethieren über das Elektrocardiogram. *Z Exper Pathol Therap* 1909;**7**:363.
2. Lewis T. Notes upon alternation of the heart. *Q J Med* 1910;**4**:141–4.
3. Mines GR. On functional analysis by the action of electrolytes. *J Physiol* 1913;**46**:188–235.
4. Kleinfeld MJ, Rozanski JJ. Alternans of the ST segment in Prinzmetal's angina. *Circulation* 1977;**55**:574–7.
5. Reddy CVR, Kiok JP, Khan RG, El-Sherif N. Repolarization alternans associated with alcoholism and hypomagnesemia. *Am J Cardiol* 1984;**53**:390–1.
6. Shimoni Z, Flatau E, Schiller D, Barzilay E, Kohn D. Electrical alternans of giant U waves with multiple electrolyte deficits. *Am J Cardiol* 1984;**54**:920–1.
7. Salerno JA, Previtali M, Panciroli C *et al*. Ventricular arrhythmias during acute myocardial ischaemia in man. The role and significance of R-ST-T alternans and the prevention of ischaemic sudden death by medical treatment. *Eur Heart J* 1986;**7** (Suppl. A):63–75.
8. Schwartz P, Malliani A. Electrical alternation of the T wave: clinical and experimental evidence of its relationship with the sympathetic nervous system and with the long Q-T syndrome. *Am Heart J* 1975;**89**:45–50.
9. Kalter HH, Schwartz ML. Electrical alternans. *NY State J Med* 1948;**1**:1164–6.
10. Smith JM, Cohen RJ. Simple finite-element model accounts for wide range of cardiac dysrhythmias. *PNAS* 1984;**81**:233–7.
11. Shimizu W, Antelevitch C. Cellular and ionic basis for T-wave alternans under long-QT conditions. *Circulation* 1999;**99**:1499–507.
12. Verrier RL, Nearing BD. Electrophysiologic basis for T wave alternans as an index of vulnerability to ventricular fibrillation. *J Cardiovasc Electrophys* 1994;**5**:445–61.
13. Pastore JM, Girouard SD, Laurita KR, Akar FG, Rosenbaum DS. Mechanism linking T-wave alternans to the genesis of cardiac fibrillation. *Circulation* 1999;**99**:1385–94.
14. Chinushi M, Restivo M, Caref EB, and El-Sherif N. Electrophysiological Basis of arrhythmogenicity of QT/T alternans in the long QT syndrome. *Circ Res* 1998;**83**:614–28.
15. Konta T, Ikeda K, Yamaki M *et al*. Significance of discordant ST alternans in ventricular fibrillation. *Circulation* 1990;**82**:2185–9.
16. Smith JM, Clancy EA, Valeri CR, Ruskin JN, Cohen RJ. Electrical alternans and cardiac electrical instability. *Circulation* 1988;**77**:110–21.
17. Nearing DN, Huang AH, Verrier RL. Dynamic tracking of cardiac vulnerability by complex demodulation of the T-wave. *Science* 1991;**252**:437–40.
18. Rosenbaum DS, Jackson LE, Smith JM, Garan H, Ruskin JN, Cohen RJ. Electrical alternans and vulnerability to ventricular arrhythmias. *New Engl J Med* 1994;**330**:235–41.
19. Armoundas A, Rosenbaum DS, Ruskin JN, Garan H, Cohen RJ. Prognostic significance of electrical alternans versus signal averaged electrocardiography in predicting the outcome of electrophysiological testing and arrhythmia-free survival. *Heart* 1998:**80**:251–6.
20. Armoundas AA, Osaka M, Mela T *et al*. T-wave alternans and dispersion of the QT interval as risk stratification markers in patients susceptible to sustained ventricular arrhythmias. *Am J Cardiol* 1998;**82**: 1127–9.
21. Rosenbaum DS, Albrecht P, Cohen RJ. Predicting sudden cardiac death from T wave alternans: promise and pitfalls. *J Cardiovasc Electrophysiol* 1996;**7**:1095–111.
22. Hohnloser SH, Klingenheben T, Zabel M, Li, YG, Albrecht, P, Cohen RJ. T Wave alternans during exercise and atrial pacing in humans. *J Cardiovasc Electrophysiol* 1997;**8**:987–93.
23. Coch M, Weber S, Buck L, Waldecker B. Assessment of T-wave alternation using atropine. *Circulation* (Suppl.) 1998; **98**:I-442.
24. Ritvo BS, Magnano AR, Bloomfield DM. Comparison of exercise and pharmacological methods of measuring T wave alternans. *PACE* 2000;**23**:Abstract 541, p 688.
25. Estes MNA, Michaud G, Zipes DP *et al*. Electrical alternans during rest and exercise as predictors of vulnerability to ventricular arrhythmias. *Am J Cardiol* 1997;**80**:1314–18.
26. Caref E, Stoyanovsky V, Cohen RJ, El-Sherif N. Incidence of T-wave alternans in normal subjects, and effect of heart rate on onset. *Circulation* 1997;**96**:Abstract 3256.
27. Hohnloser SH, Klingenheben T, Yi-Gang L, Zabel M, Peetermans J, Cohen RJ. T wave alternans as a predictor of recurrent ventricular tachyarrhythmias in ICD recipients:

prospective comparison with conventional risk markers. *J Cardiovasc Electrophysiol* 1998;**9**:1258–68.

28. Ikeda T, Takami M, Kondo N *et al*. Combined assessment of T-wave alternans and late potentials used to predict arrhythmic events after myocardial infarction. *J Am Coll Cardiol* 2000;**35**:722–30.

29. Hohnloser SH, Huikiri H. Schwartz PJ *et al*. T-wave alternans in post myocardial infarction patients. *J Am Coll Cardiol* 1999;**33** (Suppl. A):144A.

30. Gold MR, Bloomfield DM, Anderson KP *et al*. T wave alternans predicts arrhythmia vulnerability in patients undergoing electrophysiology study. *Circulation* (Suppl.) 1998;**98**: I-647–8.

31. Bloomfield DM, Gold MR, Anderson KP, *et al*. T Wave alternans predicts events independent of ejection fraction and etiology of heart disease in patients undergoing electrophysiologic testing for evaluation of known or suspected ventricular arrhythmias. *PACE* (abstract for 2000 NASPE conference, accepted for publication).

32. Bloomfield DM, Gold MR, Anderson KP *et al*. T wave alternans predicts events in patients with syncope undergoing electrophysiologic testing. *Circulation* (Suppl.) 1999;**22**: I–508.

33. Klingenheben T, Zabel M, D'Agostino RB *et al*. Predictive value of T wave alternans for arrhythmic events in patients with congestive heart failure. *The Lancet* 2000;**356**:651–2.

34. Adachi K, Ohnishi Y, Shima T *et al*. Determinant of microvolt-level T-wave alternans in patients with dilated cardiomyopathy. *J Am Coll Cardiol* 1999;**34**:374–80.

35. Klingenheben T, Credner SC, Bender B, Cohen RJ, Hohnloser SH. Exercise induced microvolt level T-wave alternans identifies patients with non-ischemic dilated cardiomyopathy at high risk of ventricular tachyarrhythmic events. *PACE* 1999;**22**(Suppl. II):860.

36. Kavesh NG, Shorofsky SR, Sarang SE, Gold MR. The effect of procainamide on T wave alternans. *J Cardiovasc Electrophysiol* 1999;**10**:649–54.

37. Tachibana H, Yamaki M, Kubota I, Watanabe T, Yamauchi S, Tomoike H. Intracoronary flecainide induces ST alternans and reentrant arrhythmia on intact canine heart. *Circulation* 1999;**99**:1637–43.

38. Groh WJ, Shinn TS, Englestein EE, Zipes DP. Amiodarone reduces the prevalence of T wave alternans in a population with ventricular tachyarrhythmias. *J Cardiovasc Electrophysiol* 1999;**10**:1335–9.

39. Kirk MK, Cooklin M, Shorofsky SR, Gold MR. Beta adrenergic blockade decreases T-wave alternans. *J Am Coll Cardiol* 1999:**33**(Suppl. A): 108A.

26 Social and psychosocial influences on sudden cardiac death, ventricular arrhythmia and cardiac autonomic function

Harry Hemingway

Introduction and model

The importance of better understanding of arrhythmic risk lies, in public health terms, in the prevention of sudden cardiac death (SCD). Approximately 50% of all coronary deaths are sudden, occurring within 1 hour of the onset of symptoms.[1] Most cases of SCD have coronary artery disease present at autopsy,[2,3] although in approximately 50% this will not have been clinically apparent prior to death.[4] SCD is most often due to ventricular fibrillation, and cardiac autonomic function may play an important role in setting arrhythmic threshold.[5,6] Figure 26.1 illustrates this simple model of arrhythmic risk and gives the structure for this review.

SCD is not, however, distributed equally in society. In one study of 1608 cases of SCD, the age-adjusted rates of SCD were higher among those with less education, an effect that was stronger than for people dying of non-sudden cardiac death.[1] Educational level and other markers of socioeconomic status (SES), such as occupation and income, consistently show inverse associations with the

incidence of cardiovascular disease.[7] Social status may influence coronary risk via the behavioural coronary risk factors of smoking, exercise, diet, and alcohol. However, the finding that SES gradients in heart disease are observed among non-smokers and are independent of the classical risk factors of cholesterol and blood pressure[8] suggests another possibility, that aspects of the psychosocial environment related to SES may be involved.[9]

Recently reviewed evidence from prospective epidemiological studies,[10] supported by non-human primate data,[11] suggests that psychosocial factors – such as anxiety, depression, hostility/Type A behaviour, social supports, and work characteristics – may play a direct causal role in coronary heart disease. The majority of these studies relate a single questionnaire measurement of a psychosocial factor to incident coronary events many years later. Such measurements may reflect chronic exposure to an adverse psychosocial environment that is relatively stable over time. Furthermore, the risk is distributed in a dose–response fashion and is not confined to the extremes of the distribution. Since SCD is a common mode of coronary death, such assessments of psychosocial factors may predict SCD simply because they predict the presence of coronary artery disease (CHD).

Acute psychosocial stressors – defined as events producing demands likely to tax or exceed an individual's adaptive responses over minutes, hours, and days – may represent more proximate "triggers" of sudden cardiac events. Such acute psychosocial stressors may trigger ischaemia or infarction.[12] Whilst laboratory-based measures of acute psychological stress have been extensively studied, the challenge lies in determining the effects of real-life acute stressors.

Determining the causality of putative psychosocial factors in arrhythmic risk may yield important insights into the pathogenesis of arrhythmic risk itself; mechanisms by which psychosocial factors might cause CHD (in which electrophysiological pathways are one of a number under

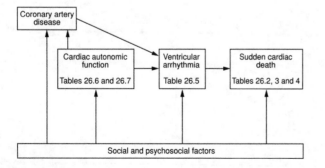

Figure 26.1 Possible pathways by which social and psychosocial factors may influence sudden cardiac death, ventricular arrhythmia, and cardiac autonomic function. (Tables where evidence is reviewed.)

consideration) and, ultimately, strategies for prevention of SCD. As numerous reviews demonstrate, the clinical and biological plausibility for social and psychosocial factors being associated with arrhythmic risk is not at issue. The question lies in the quality of the evidence that psychosocial factors play a causal role. Previous reviews of this area have not been systematic in the identification of literature for review, the method of describing individual study results, or in the method of summarising findings from diverse types of study. For these reasons, gaps in current understanding are not clearly defined and non-contributory studies continue to be published. It is the objective therefore of this chapter *to determine the strength of evidence for associations between social and psychosocial factors and SCD, ventricular arrhythmia, and cardiac autonomic function.* The structure of this review (outlined in Fig. 26.1) is based on each of the measured outcomes: SCD, ventricular arrhythmia, and cardiac autonomic function.

Method

Identification of relevant articles in New English language peer-reviewed journals was carried out using PubMed from 1970–October 1999 (www.ncbi.nlm.nih.gov/). As well as the use of MESH headings (psychosocial, social, sudden death, ANS, and arrhythmia), articles were also identified by searching on any author who had contributed one relevant article and by using the artificial intelligence "Related Articles" function in PubMed. The bibliographies of all retrieved articles were hand searched for further relevant articles. It is acknowledged that the reproducibility of these methods for reviewing non-randomised trial literature spanning widely different types of studies has not been well described. Each study was categorised as positive if one or more measure of SES or psychosocial factors showed a significant ($P < 0.05$) association with SCD, ventricular arrhythmia, or cardiac autonomic function. The methodological quality of studies, the direction of associations and issues of multiple comparisons are considered in individual studies. In the absence of any previous systematic review in this area, a deliberately relaxed definition of positive studies was used that did not take account of methodological quality.

Animal studies

Animal studies, unlike human studies, offer the important advantages of direct study of arrhythmia precipitation; manipulation of psychosocial stressors that are observable, and not relying on language-based self-reports, which have a potential for bias. However, in animals and humans, ventricular fibrillation and sudden death remain rare events, and most animal models have chosen to concentrate on proxies, such as the threshold for repetitive ventricular activity. All of the identified studies (Table 26.1) were positive and all examined acute psychosocial stressors. Taken as a whole these studies provide important evidence for the model of causation of SCD, i.e. that there are central and autonomic (sympathetic and parasympathetic) influences on ventricular arrhythmias, which may be mediated by environmental, presumed psychosocial, stressors. Studies in pigs with coronary occlusion in an unfamiliar laboratory setting found that latency to ventricular fibrillation was lengthened by adaptation, beta-blockade, or blockade of frontal cortical brain stem pathways.[13,14] A study of male rats faced with aggressive lactating female rats found that 12/12 rats developed VT, preceded by periods of low R-R variability (using telemetrically recorded ECGs).

There is a role for further animal work, particularly where the animal is observed in its natural environment, for example using telemetrically recorded ECGs, and social factors that are real life (such as dominance) or long term can be studied. For example Eisermann[15] studied rabbits in a seminatural environment and found that a measure of SES (dominance) was associated with radiotelemetric heart rate recordings over 1500 days; subordinate rabbits had chronically elevated heart rate not explained by limited access to burrow shelter. Similar findings have been made in squirrel monkeys,[16] macaques and baboons,[17] and tree shrews.[18]

Sudden cardiac death

Death occurring within 1 hour of the onset of symptoms, in the absence of a non-cardiac cause may be termed "sudden cardiac death". Compared with non-sudden cardiac death, SCD is less frequently associated with acute coronary thrombosis, plaque rupture, or acute myocardial infarction.[2] This observation has stimulated enquiry into differences in the risk factors for acute myocardial infarction and SCD, and supports the importance of electrical events which leave no postmortem clues.

Methodological issues

There are major methodological problems facing studies of SCD. Definition of SCD remains problematic. More recent studies have termed death sudden that is less than 1 hour from the onset of symptoms, but earlier studies included deaths up to 24 hours from symptom onset. Since up to one-third of sudden unexplained deaths have a non-cardiac cause

Table 26.1 SES and psychosocial factors: associations with sudden cardiac death, ventricular arrhythmia, and cardiac autonomic function in experimental animal studies

Author, year	Animal	Experimental setting	Acute psychosocial factor	Relieving factor	Outcome	Results	Summary
Lown 1973[54]	Dog	Conscious	Pavlovian sling: tension on leash and sound of switch preceding electrical shock	Cage in sound-attenuated room	Threshold for repetitive ventricular response	Lowered in sling dogs	+
Corbalan 1974[55]	Dog	Conscious; coronary occlusion	Ditto	Ditto	Threshold for repetitive ventricular responses VPB, VT	Lowered before coronary occlusion in the sling group 7/8 dogs placed in sling developed VPB or VT; none in cage group	+
Johansson 1974[56]	Pig	Conscious	Psychological		Ventricular arrhythmias Cardiomyopathy	Cardiomyopathy consistent with reflex catecholamine release	+
Skinner 1975[13]	Pig	Conscious farm pigs; coronary occlusion	Unfamiliar (laboratory) vs familiar surroundings	Adaptation to laboratory Propranolol	Latency to VF	VF delayed or prevented by adaptation or beta blockade	+
Corley 1977[57]	Squirrel Monkey	11 pairs (1 avoidance, 1 yoked)	Electrical shock: yoked monkey had no control	Avoidance monkey could make a lever response	Autopsy findings Sudden death	Avoidance monkeys showed more myofibrillar degeneration and 3 died suddenly after bradycardia	+
Liang 1979[58]	Dog	Conscious	Pavlovian sling	Cage	Threshold for repetitive ventricular response	Associated with circulating catecholamines	+
Natelson 1979[59]	Guinea pig		Restraint stress	Unrestrained	VPB, VT	Ventricular arrhythmias occurred in 7/7 restrained guinea pigs; couplets and VT in 3; no arrhythmia in unrestrained guinea pigs	+
Skinner 1981[14]	Pig	Coronary occlusion	Unfamiliar laboratory electrical shock	Adaptation to laboratory Cryoblockade of frontal cortical brain-stem pathways Central administration of propranolol	VT	Reduced risk of VF by frontal blockade of frontal cortical brain-stem pathways	+
Verrier 1982[60]	Dog	Coronary occlusion	Pavlovian sling	Cage Atropine Beta-blockade Stellectomy	Threshold for repetitive ventricular response	Vagal blockade with atropine reduced threshold in sling; propranolol prevented the decrease; bilateral stellectomy afforded only partial protection	+
Sgoifo 1994[61]	Rat (Wistar male)		Aggressive lactating female rats		Telemetric ECG for HRV (time domain) and VPB, VT	12/12 rats developed VT, preceded by periods of low R-R variability	+
Sgoifo 1997[62]	Rat (wild type)		Social stressor (defeat) Non-social stressor (restraint)		Ditto	Social stressor associated with more sympathetic changes and VPB than the non-social stressor	+
Sgoifo 1998[63]	Rat (Wistar and wild type)		Defeat		Ditto	Higher sympathetic tone, low parasympathetic antagonism and more VPB in wild type rats	+

Abbreviations: HRV = heart rate variability; VF = ventricular fibrillation; VPB = ventricular premature beats; VT = ventricular tachycardia.

revealed at autopsy (such as cerebral haemorrhage or pulmonary embolus[2]), studies without autopsy confirmation of presumed cardiac cause are subject to considerable misclassification, which will tend to bias results to the null. Despite the assumption that SCD is arrhythmic in origin, none of the identified studies directly measured arrhythmias. The largest number of SCD events in prospective studies was 98,[19] and some were considerably smaller leading to wide confidence intervals[20,21] and the possibility of Type II error. Studies of SCD share a bias of differing access to community resuscitation. Retrospective studies in seeking to determine the recent antecedents of SCD are subject to recall bias, since next of kin may give differing accounts from the decadent and may be inclined to amplify explanations more for a sudden than a non-sudden death. Conversely prospective studies are not subject to recall bias but, with long periods of follow-up, are able to examine the effects only of chronic measures of psychosocial stress.

Retrospective and post-mortem studies (Table 26.2)

All 14 of the identified retrospective studies of SCD were positive. Cebelin studied the autopsies of 497 homicide victims in 15 of whom there were no internal injuries or blood loss to explain death.[22] Among 10 of these 15 there was myofibrillar degeneration, which was not present among 15 people who had been killed in road traffic accidents. The authors inferred that this was consistent with the fear of imminent injury (absent in the road traffic accidents) leading to a catecholamine-induced stress cardiomyopathy and SCD. Talbott et al.[23] compared 80 female SCDs with live age-, race-, and sex-matched neighbourhood controls and found an excess of psychiatric history and death of a significant other among the cases. Community-wide stressors offer the opportunity to study the impact on SCD in the absence of next-of-kin questionnaires, thus removing the potential for recall bias, but raising the problem of ecological fallacy, since the psychosocial stressor for the individual who died is inferred not measured. Increases in the number of SCDs on the day of an earthquake[24] or during the threat of missile attack[25,26] have been reported.

Prospective studies in healthy populations (Table 26.3)

Distinguishing psychosocial effects on SCD in patients with established coronary disease separately from healthy populations is important. If effects are seen in healthy populations where prolonged periods of follow-up are required to accrue sufficient events, then this argues against psychosocial factors acting purely as triggers. Of all the cardiovascu-

lar disease cohort studies, only a proportion has incorporated psychosocial questionnaires in their risk factor measurements, and only a proportion of the latter studies has obtained data on the suddenness of cardiac death. The effect of psychosocial factors on cardiac death separately in healthy and patient populations has been systematically reviewed.[10] Since approximately 50% of cardiac deaths are sudden it is likely that psychosocial factors will in addition predict SCD; 5/6 identified studies were positive. No prospective studies of SCD in women were identified. The two studies by Kawachi et al. are particularly important. Anxiety measured in men in the Health Professionals study[27] and in the Normative Aging Study[20] using two different validated instruments was associated with SCD. Although the number of SCD events was small, the effects were large, specific for SCD, independent of other risk factors, and demonstrated dose response effects.

The chronobiology of SCD has been interpreted as being consistent with a psychosocial mechanism. Thus some[28] but not all[29] studies find a Monday excess of SCD, consistent with the threat of returning to a stressful work environment. SCD and non-fatal MI show a marked circadian rhythm, being more common in the morning. This circadian rhythm may be masked by treatment with beta-blockers suggesting the possibility that the morning excess may be mediated by the sympathetic nervous system.[30]

Prospective studies in CHD patient populations (Table 26.4)

Five of the six identified studies were positive. All studies were in post-MI populations, rather than other patient groups at high risk of SCD (e.g. patients resuscitated from near sudden death, undergoing electrophysiological studies or with implantable defibrillators). All the studies made assessments of chronic psychosocial factors; there were no diary studies with prospective records of a patient's acute and chronic psychosocial state. Ruberman found effects of low education and low social supports on SCD in a post-MI population, although in a retrospective study none of the four factors identified on interview with the patient's wife accounted for the education differences in survival. Brackett 1988[31] examined 1012 post-MI survivors in the Recurrent Coronary Prevention Project and found an effect for Type A and other psychosocial factors on SCD but not non-sudden cardiac death.

Ventricular arrhythmia

Ventricular arrhythmias are important because they are the most common proximate cause of SCD; they are elec-

Table 26.2 SES and psychosocial factors: associations with sudden cardiac death in retrospective studies

Author, year	Sudden deaths				Comparison group	Psychosocial factor (A = acute, C = chronic)	Results	Summary
	Number (% women)	% autopsy	Age	Source and definition				
Greene 1972[64]	25 (0)	NS	55.6	NS	None	A, C	Acute anger or anxiety superimposed on a background of depression	+
Rahe 1973[65]	126 (18)	NS	56	<1 h from symptom onset	279 AMI survivors	A/C: 42 life-change questions	Increase in magnitude of life changes 6 months prior to event particularly apparent for SCD	+
Myers 1975[66]	100 (0)	100	NS	<24 h	Proven AMI; autopsy and living	A	23 had intense stress 30 min	+
Talbott 1977[67]	64 (100)	NS	55.6	<24 h, out of hospital, not infirm before death	64 live age-related neighbourhood controls	C	Fewer married, more educational incongruity with spouses, fewer children: 12/64 (vs 0) had definite psychiatric history	+
Rissanen 1978[68]	118 (20)	100	31–83	<24 h, witnessed	None	A, C: long-standing stress including troubles at work, family; acute stress (emotional + physical)	30 had long-standing stress, leading to death with 2–24 h from symptom onset, with definite AMI; 23 patients had acute stress, death occurred less than 2 h from symptom onset and uncommonly had AMI	+
Cebelin 1980[22]	15 (40)	100	1–82	Murder victims	15 road traffic accident deaths	A: inferred	15/497 had no evidence of internal injury in whom 10 had myofibrillar degeneration (vs 0/15 of comparison group)	+
Talbott 1981[23,69]	80 (100)	52.5	25–64	<24 h from symptom onset; not infirm before death	80 live age, race, sex matched controls	A, C: 28 recent life events, SES (education)	SCD cases had more psychiatric history, smoking, death of significant other within last 6 months and less education compared with controls	+
Beard 1982[70]	1054	NS	NS	<24 h from symptom onset	None	A: inferred	SCD peak on Saturday: in men decreasing trend from Sat through to Friday regardless of baseline disease; no seasonal variation	+
Kirschner 1986[71]	18 (0)	100	19–51	Unexplained nocturnal deaths	None	C: inferred, refugees from S.E. Asia		+
Meisel 1991[25]	41 (NS)	NS	NS	NS	January 1990 (not under missile threat)	A: inferred, threat of war	41 sudden deaths in January 1991 vs 22 in January 1990	+
Sexton 1993[72]	155 (0)	72	30–69	<1 h from symptom onset	Expected numbers based on all CHD deaths in men aged 30–69	C: SES (occupation)	Observed vs expected cases of SCD among those not working was 56 vs 30 ($P <0.0001$). No differences in observed/expected in non-manual or manual occupations	+
Escobedo 1996[1]	1608 (43)	NS	25–>85	<1 h	1585 non-sudden CHD deaths and 1053 CHD deaths unknown timing	C: SES (education)	Aged-adjusted rates for SCD by the educational categories were 88.9, 95.2, 129.2 per 100 000 (16, 26, 54% of SCD) respectively, vs 99.4, 111.2 and 123.8 for non-sudden cardiac death	+
Leor 1996[24]	24 (24)	100	38–92	<1 h	Mean daily rate of SCD prior to earthquake	A: inferred, Northridge earthquake	24 cases of SCD on day of earthquake vs daily mean of 4.6 prior to earthquake	+
Weisenberg 1996[26]	68 (44)	NS	76.3	NS	213 cases in 5 control periods	A: inferred in relation to threat of war	Higher rate of SCD during threat of war but not significant; no association with degree of threat in different geographical regions	+

Source of psychosocial data was next of kin interviews, except where psychosocial factor was inferred.
Abbreviations: AMI = acute myocardial infarction; CHD = coronary heart disease; NS = not stated; SCD = sudden cardiac death; SES = socioeconomic status.

Table 26.3 SES and psychosocial factors: associations with sudden cardiac death in prospective studies in healthy populations

Author, year	Total sample (% women)	Age at entry	Psychosocial factor (A = acute, C = chronic)	Follow-up (years)	SCD: number	Time of SCD	Results	Summary
Rabkin 1980[28]	3983 (0)	25–34 (69%)	A: inferred from day of week	29	152	<24 h	Excess of SCD on Mondays; only in those without previous CHD	+
Salonen 1982[73]	2455 (0)	25–59	C: SES (education ≤7 years) and continuous psychosocial stress ≥1 year	6.5	27	NS	5.0 for the effect of education; no significant effect of psychosocial stress	+
Hinkle 1988[74]	301 (0)	54–62	C: SES (education), Type A, Type B, hostility	20	65	Direct observation of sudden loss of consciousness	Low education was and psychosocial factors were not associated	+
Kagan 1989[19]	7591 (0)	46–68	C: SES (occupation)	18	131 98	1–24 h <1 h	Blue collar protective	–
Kawachi 1994[20]	33 999 (0)	42–77	C: anxiety (Crown–Crisp)	2	16	<1 h	Phobic anxiety associated with SCD (RR 6.08 (95% CI 2.35–15.73) not non-fatal MI	+
Kawachi 1994[21]	2280 (0)	21–80	C: anxiety (Cornell Medical Index)	32	26	<1 h	RR 5.73 (95% CI 1.26–26.1)	+

Abbreviations: CHD = coronary heart disease; NS = not stated; MI = myocardial infarction; SCD = sudden cardiac death; SES = socioeconomic status.

Table 26.4 SES and psychosocial factors: associations with sudden cardiac death in prospective studies in CHD patient populations

Author, year	Total sample (% women)	Age at entry	Patient group	Psychosocial factor (A = acute, C = chronic)	Follow-up (years)	SCD: number	SCD timing	Results	Summary
Bruhn 1974[75]	67 (21)	25–80	MI survivors and 67 healthy age, sex, type of job matched controls	C: Sisyphus pattern, Type A, depression	10	23	NS	Sisyphus pattern and Type A more frequent among cases than controls and predicted SCD	+
Weinblatt 1978[76]	1739 (0)	30–69	MI survivors	C: SES (education), life stress, social isolation, Type A, depression	3	NS	<1 h	Among those with complex VOB, low education had 33% mortality vs 9% in better educated; not present among those without complex VPB	+
Ruberman 1983[77]	1684 (0)	35–74	MI survivors	C: wife assessed mood, communication, anxiety/ worry, striving	3.5		<1 h	None of the four factors explained the large SES (education) differences in SCD rates	–
Ruberman 1984[78]	2062 (0)	30–69	MI survivors	C: SES (education), life stress, social isolation, Type A, depression	3	68	<1 h	Isolation and stress combined to predict SCD in both those with and without VPB	+
Brackett 1988[31]	1012 (8)	53	MI survivors: mean 42 months	C: SES (education) Type A (videotaped interview)	4.5	23	<1 h	Low education, Type A, and other psychosocial factors predicted SCD but not non-sudden cardiac death	+
Ahern 1990[79,80]	331		≥10 VPB per hour or ≥5 non-sustained VT 6–60 days post-MI	C: anxiety, depression, Type A, B, social support and desirability			Cardiac arrest	Depression, Type B	+

Abbreviations: NS = not stated; MI = myocardial infarction; SCD = sudden cardiac death; SES = socioeconomic status; VPB = ventricular premature beats.

trical "accidents", which, with appropriate treatment, may be terminated and the risk of recurrence lowered. The morbidity associated with non-fatal ventricular arrhythmias is also considerable. Better understanding the role of psychosocial factors in the ventricular arrhythmias may therefore offer insights into prevention and treatment.

Methodological issues

Because of the rarity and seriousness of VT or VF, many studies use proxy measures of arrhythmic risk, such as ventricular premature beats or QT interval. Whilst this may offer advantages in terms of statistical power and practicability, negative results[32] may simply question the adequacy of the proxy rather than test the psychosocial-arrhythmia hypothesis. There is a lack of population based studies, and (in common with SCD studies) there is a lack of studies examining real-life acute psychosocial stressors measured in patient populations (0/21 studies) using prospective designs.

QT interval (Table 26.5)

All identified studies were positive. Prolongation of the QT interval has been shown in prospective cohort studies to predict CHD mortality and SCD in healthy populations. Among the rare genetic "long QT syndrome", ventricular arrhythmias are common and lead to premature death; among 328 families, acute emotional stress is reported as the most common single precipitant of syncope or arrhythmia. Toivonen found among 30 healthy physicians subjected to the naturalistic acute stressor of an emergency call waking them from sleep, the QT interval was between 59–67 ms longer than under equivalent heart rates during stable conditions.[33]

VPB (Table 26.5)

Ten of 12 identified studies were positive but the negative studies are important. In one of the few prospective studies designed to test the psychosocial-arrhythmia hypothesis, Follick et al. found no associations between a battery of carefully measured psychosocial factors (including depression, anxiety, Type A, anger) measured in state and trait form and VPB on 24-h ECG carried out at 3, 6 and 12 month follow-up.[32] One of the reasons for this may lie in the highly selected nature of the population; all participants were MI survivors with ventricular arrhythmias and, in such a setting, psychosocial factors may not further predict risk. However, the one population-based study, among healthy civil servants, found no evidence that

VPB were related to SES.[34] Thus the marker of ventricular arrhythmia, VPB, may not be an appropriate proxy for ventricular arrhythmia.

VT and VF (Table 26.5)

Eleven of 12 identified studies were positive. Reich et al. found that 25/117 patients referred for antiarrhythmic management were experiencing acute emotional disturbances during the 24 hours preceding the arrhythmias. Eighteen had two or more episodes associated with psychological disturbances. These 25 patients were distinguished from the rest of the series in having generally less severe structural heart disease.[35] Brodsky et al.[36] selected 6 patients with life-threatening ventricular tachyarrhythmia without underlying structural heart disease. Five of these six patients experienced marked psychological stress. Each of these five patients had recurrent rapid monomorphic ventricular tachycardia related to changes in tone of the sympathetic nervous system. Kennedy et al.[37] prospectively examined 88 patients undergoing programmed electrical stimulation for the diagnosis and treatment of supraventricular and ventricular tachyarrhythmias, or syncope of unknown origin. Whilst depression and cognitive impairment were related to mortality, they were not related to arrhythmia severity or treatment efficacy.

Cardiac autonomic function

Cardiac autonomic function is one of the most important predictors of SCD and serious ventricular arrhythmia in patients with myocardial infarction.[38,39] But what in turn sets cardiac autonomic tone? One possibility is that social and psychosocial phenomena play an important role. The autonomic nervous system has for decades been considered a key putative pathway linking psychosocial to pathological processes. Social and psychosocial factors related to tonic and reflex sympathetic:parasympathetic balance may affect arrhythmic risk directly by lowering threshold for ventricular arrhythmia or indirectly by causing coronary artery disease (see Fig. 26.1). Autonomic function is implicated in CHD aetiology via effects on the endothelium and platelet adhesiveness, and on the risk factors that cluster together in the metabolic syndrome (systolic blood pressure, HDL, triglycerides, glucose, and waist hip ratio).[40] SES may be related to features of the metabolic syndrome.[41] The central nervous system is involved both in the conscious experience of psychosocial stressors and in mediating arrhythmic threshold.

Heart rate, a crude marker of autonomic function, is an independent predictor of CHD events and is higher in those with low SES[42] or low social support at work.[43]

Heart rate variability (HRV) measured in short (5 min) or long (24 h) electrocardiographic recordings offers potential advantages over simple measurements of heart rate at rest or in response to a laboratory stressor. Power spectral analysis of HRV gives a valid measure of parasympathetic tone and parasympathetic:sympathetic balance; increasingly it is this balance, rather than a single arm of the autonomic nervous system, which is considered important. HRV is clinically relevant, predicting prognosis post-myocardial infarction,[44] CHD aetiology,[45] all-cause mortality,[46] and ventricular tachycardia.[39] The "reactivity" of heart rate and blood pressure to psychosocial stress is outside the scope of this review because these measures have less clear relations with arrhythmic risk, do not measure vagal influences and, until recently at least, were not used in the study of real life psychosocial stressors.

Methodological issues

There was an important lack of standardised[47] measurement protocols and complete reporting of HRV measures. Only five studies had more than 100 participants. Only two studies were population based and the remainder gave sparse details of the means of selection of their patients. There is thus a serious potential for selection bias. There was a lack of studies examining psychosocial stressors in a continuous or dose–response fashion, the majority treating the psychosocial factor as a qualitative (present or absent) variable. No studies were identified that considered acute real-life stressors applicable to a general population. Although there were seven studies that examined HRV over a 24-h period during "normal daily activities" none of these reported psychosocial stressors within these, using diary or other methods. None of the four studies in patients with CAD included measures of sympathetic:parasympathetic balance.

Cardiac autonomic function in healthy samples (Table 26.6)

Seventeen of 18 identified studies were positive. Both of the negative studies involved aspects of the psychosocial work environment.[48,49] The study by Kawachi is important because it is one of the few studies that was population based and analysed a continuously distributed anxiety score finding an inverse linear relationship with HRV; for Crown Crisp scores 0–1 (low anxiety), 2, 3, ≥4, SDNN was respectively 3.54, 3.37, 3.35, 3.11 when adjustment was made for age, heart rate, and body mass index. De Meersman[50] examined the effects of a real-life stressor – research students giving a presentation in the setting of a (critical) audience and without an audience. There was

lower LF and higher HF in the no-audience recordings. Among the only population-based study of healthy women, Horsten found that social isolation and inability to relieve anger by talking to others were associated with low HRV.[51] In the ARIC study there is an association between educational attainment and low heart rate variability.[45]

Cardiac autonomic function in patients with psychiatric morbidity of coronary disease (Table 26.7)

Eleven of the 12 identified studies were positive; seven studies examined anxiety/panic disorder, and a mixed pattern emerged with some studies finding reduced LF, increased LF, or reduced HF; eight studies examined depression, four of these being among patients with CAD, and all showed higher depression to be associated with lower SDNN or other vagally mediated measures. Baroreflex control (BRC) of heart rate reflects largely reflex control of heart rate, rather than the tonic vagal activity reflected in heart rate variability. Non-invasive measurements of BRC among 56 men and women with major depression showed that state anxiety (measured using the Spielberger scale) was negatively correlated with levels of BRC(SPEC) (r = −0.32, $P < 0.05$), whereas depression severity was not related to either respiratory sinus arrhythmia or BRC.[52] Amongst 66 patients with CAD, high scores on the Beck Depression Inventory were associated with lower age-adjusted BRS compared with low depressive symptomatology (4.5 ± 2.7 vs 6.5 ± 2.8 ms/mmHg).[53]

Summary of strength of evidence

There are no studies in healthy populations that have combined measures of psychosocial factors, autonomic function, ventricular arrhythmia, and SCD. Chronic psychosocial factors, such as anxiety, depression, and social supports measured at a single time-point predict CHD events years later.[10]

There were major methodological weaknesses with many studies paying inadequate attention to: study design; hypothesis specification; standardised measurement and reporting of outcomes; statistical power; selection of population-based samples; examining the psychosocial factors most consistently related to CHD; measurement of psychosocial factors on continuous scales, using acute real-life and chronic stressors. The only prospective study that was designed to test directly the psychosocial-arrhythmic risk hypothesis was negative. The proportions of positive studies were: animal studies for all three outcomes (12/12); human studies of SCD, retrospective (14/14), prospective healthy (5/6) and prospective patient populations (5/6);

Table 26.5 SES and psychosocial factors: associations with ventricular premature beats, ventricular tachycardia, ventricular fibrillation and QT interval

Author, year	Total sample (% women)	Age	Patient group	Design	Psychosocial factor (A = acute, C = chronic)	Ventricular arrhythmia: type (n patients)	Results	Summary
Healthy populations								
Taggard 1973[81]	23 (91)	21–58	Healthy (17 hospital doctors)	Real life stressor	A: public speaking	VPB, catecholamines	VPB >6 min occurred in 6/23 subjects, but in 0/8 when treated with oxprenolol	+
Cook 1982[82]	14		Ships' pilots	Real life stressor	C: Eysenck neuroticism	VPB >1 (n = 8) on ambulatory ECG	8 pilots with VPB were more neurotic than those without; aberrant beats occurred mainly at times of manoeuvring ships in hazardous conditions	+
Rainey 1982[83]			Depressed and drug-free	Healthy controls	C: depression	QT interval	Prolonged QT interval was more frequent and more severe among depressed than controls	+
Hijzen 1985[84]				Emotional and physical stress		QT interval	Shorter in physical rather than emotional stress	+
Katz 1985[85]	102 (37)	19–69	38 arrhythmia, 30 with >30 VPB per hour and no MI	34 age- and sex-matched general medical or surgical controls	C: personality inventories: 72 scales	VPB >30 h and no MI	Depression more common than among controls	+
Huang 1989[86]	17	26–74		Laboratory stressor	A: inactivity, neutral discussion, stressful discussion, reassurance	QT interval	Shortened in most who responded with anger to the stressful situation; lengthened in 2 who reacted with despondency	+
Toivonen 1997[33]	30 (30)		Healthy physicians	Real life stressor	A: awakening from emergency calls	QT interval, cycle length before and first 30 s after emergency call	QT interval 59–67 ms longer than at same heart rate during stable conditions	+
Hemingway 1999[34]	17 000 (0)	40–69	Population based, civil servants	Cross-sectional	C: SES (civil service employment grade)	VPB on resting ECG	Not related to employment grade	–
Patient populations								
Lown 1973[54]				Clinical stressor	A: psychological stress	Threshold for repetitive ventricular response	Increased sympathetic activity associated with ventricular arrhythmia	+
Lown 1976[87]	1		Patient with VF	Clinical stressor	A: recall of intense emotion	VF (2)	VF precipitated by recall of emotional stress	+
Lynch 1977[88]	225 (42)		Patients in CCU	Clinical stressor	A: pulse palpation on ward round	Ventricular arrhythmia	Reduced as a result of the ward round	+
Lown 1978[89]	19 (10)		Ventricular arrhythmia	Laboratory stressor	A: mental arithmetic, reading task, emotional recall	VPB	11/19 showed an increase in VPB activity	+
Weinblatt 1978[90]			MI survivors	Cross-sectional	C: SES (education) low social support	VPB on 3 h ECG		+
Donlon 1979[91]	1 (0)	38	MI	Laboratory stressor (62 minute filmed psychiatric interview)	A: 2 independent ratings each minute of degree of stress the patient showed	VPB measured for each of 62 min	VPB >4 min were significantly more common during stress	+

Study	N (events)	Age	Population	Design	Psychological measure	Arrhythmia outcome	Comments	Association
Orth-Gomer 1980[92]	150 (0)	58	50 CHD 50 high risk 50 healthy	Cross-sectional	Emotions profile index depression; Type A	VPB on 24 h ECG	Depression in healthy men was associated with prognostically severe ventricular arrhythmia	+
Graboys 1981[93]					Celtic play-offs	VPB, ventricular arrhythmia		+
Reich 1981[35]	117	17–79	62 cardiac arrest survivors 55 symptomatic VT	Retrospective	Interviewed by cardiologist and psychiatrist for triggers	Cardiac arrests symptomatic VT	25 patients were experiencing acute emotional disturbances during 24 hours preceding arrhythmia	+
Krantz 1982[94]	26 (0)		CABG	Clinical stressor	Type A	VT or VF	4/12 Type A and 0/6 non-Type A	+
Freeman 1984[95]	104 (0)		CABG	Clinical stressor	Type A, depression, anxiety, competitive behaviour	Ventricular arrhythmia	Only competitive behaviour-associated	+
Jennings 1984[96]	22 (0)		11 CHD 11 healthy volunteers	Laboratory stressor	Type A and performance tasks	VPB	Type A was associated with higher prevalence of ectopy	+
Tavazzi 1986[97]	19		MI mean 37 days	Laboratory stressor	Mental arithmetic stressor	Mean ventricular refractory period, unsustained VT, VF	7 patients developed VT during stress; VF provoked in 2 patients with extrastimuli during stress	+
Brodsky 1987[36]	6 (100)	22–60	Ventricular tachyarrhythmia without structural disease	Prospective, 38 month follow-up	Psychological stress	VT	5/6 had marked psychological stress; VT related to sympathetic activity and improved by beta-blocker during 38 month follow-up	+
Kennedy 1987[37]	88	52.2	Programmed electrical stimulation for ventricular (66), supraventricular (12) arrhythmias or syncope (10)	Prospective	Depression and cognitive impairment	Programmed electrical stimulation of arrhythmia	Neither related to arrhythmia severity or treatment efficacy	–
Follick 1988[98]	125 (26)	54.5	MI survivors	Prospective, 12 m follow-up	Depression, SCL-90 sum of 9 scales	VPB over 1 year follow-up (N = 59) by transtelephonic ECG	Distress showed direct relation to VPB on follow-up independent of cardiac risk and prescription of beta-blockers	+
Hatton 1989[99]	17 (12)	27–74	Electrophysiological studies for VF (4) or VT (13)		Desire for control, locus of control and behaviour pattern	VT sustained or VF	Associated with desire for control	+
Follick 1990[32]	277 (17)	59	MI survivors 6–60 days ≥10 VPB/h or ≥5 runs of unsustained VT	Prospective, 12 m follow-up	Depression, anxiety, anger, Type A	VPB on 24 h ECG at baseline and 3, 6, 12 month follow-up	No effects	–
Moss 1991[100]	328		Long QT syndrome	Retrospective	Acute emotional stress	Syncope and ventricular arrhythmia	Commonest precipitant was emotional stress	+
Carney 1993[101]	103		CAD	Cross-sectional	Depression on standardised interview	VT on 24 h ECG	5/21 depressed vs 3/82 non-depressed	+

Abbreviations: CABG = coronary artery bypass graft; CAD = coronary artery disease; CCD = coronary care unit; CHD = coronary heart disease; MI = myocardial infarction; SES = socioeconomic status; VF = ventricular fibrillation; VPB = ventricular premature beats; VT = ventricular tachycardia.

Table 26.6 SES and psychosocial factors: associations with cardiac autonomic function in healthy populations

Study	Total sample (% women)	Age	Study group	Design	Psychosocial factor (A = acute, C = chronic)	Duration, setting of measurement	Cardiac autonomic function		Results	Summary
							Time domain measures	Frequency domain measures		
Rohmert 1973[102]	21		Air traffic controllers	Real life stressor	A: number of planes controlled	50 beats	SDNN	–	HR but not HRV associated with number of planes controlled	+/–
Sekiguchi 1979[103]	46 (0)	22–49	Pilots and air traffic controllers	Real life stressor	A: rest, tracking, air traffic control, flight simulation and actual flying		–	LF, HF	LF at first increased under moderate mental load and then decreased	+
Bronis 1980[104]			Radio broadcasters	Real life stressor	A: live broadcasts	After 3.5 hours of work	SDNN	–	Decreased	+
Mulders 1982[105]			Professional drivers	Real life stressor	C: high versus low absenteeism		SDNN	–	Lower HRV in those with high vs low absenteeism	+
Kamada 1992[106]	19 (0)	21	Healthy students	Laboratory stressor (addition of 2 digit numbers)	C: Type A and Type B	5 min (9 episodes related to tasks)	–	LF, HF	LF/HF 3.9 for Type A vs 2.2 for Type B (P <0.05) resting and during tasks	+
Toivanen 1993[107]	98 (100)	23–60	50 hospital cleaners 48 bank employees	Prospective randomised trial	C: 15 minute relaxation program	2 min, sitting, Valsalva, deep breathing, standing	SDNN	–	3 and 6 month follow-up values were closer to "expected" based on Finnish reference values by age	+
Sloan 1994[108]	35 (13)	36	Volunteers, healthy	Normal daily activities (not specified	C: hostility, sleep/wake	24 h	–	LF, HF	Hostility correlated inversely with HF and directly with LF/ HF among <40 years (N = 19) during daytime only	+
Kawachi 1995[109]	581 (0)	47–86	Volunteers, healthy	Cross-sectional	C: phobic anxiety (Crown–Crisp)	1 min supine,, paced breathing	SDNN, max-min HR	–	SDNN inversely associated with Crown–Crisp score 0–1, 2, 3, ≥4, SDNN 3.54, 3.37, 3.35, 3.11 adjusted for age, heart rate and body mass index, P for trend = 0.03	+

Study	N (%)	Age	Population	Study design	Exposure	Recording		HRV measure	Findings	
McCraty 1995[110]	24 (63)	24–47	Volunteers, healthy	Randomised trial	A: self-induced appreciation or anger	5 min sitting	−	LF, MF, HF	LF increased in anger (0.025–0.072) and appreciation; HF increased in appreciation (0.019–0.031) only	+
DeMeersman 1996[50]	15 (73)	23–48	Volunteer research students	Real life stressor (giving presentation of their own research)	A: anticipated of and presentation with and without audience	30 min before, during 30 min presentation	−	LF, HF	No audience had lower LF (7.6), LF/HF (0.23) and higher HF (32.5) vs audience or anticipation phase	+
Myrtek 1996[111]	50 (100)	23	Students	Normal daily activities (not specified)	Stress of studying	23 h			Lower HRV during university activities	+
Liao 1997[45]	2252 (55)	54	Population based	Cross-sectional	C: SES (education)	2 min supine	SDNN	LF, HF, HF/LF	Low education monotonically, directly associated with LF; less consistent for HF, SDNN	+
Kageyama 1998[48]	223 (0)	30.8	White collar workers	Cross-sectional	C: job stress	2 min supine and standing	−	LF, HF	Job stress not related to HRV	+
Kageyama 1998[112]	223 (0)	30.8	White collar workers	Cross-sectional	C: commuting time, overtime	2 min supine and standing	−	LF, HF	Commuting >90 min or >60 h/month overtime gave a sympathodominant state	+
Sato 1998[113]	16 (100)	20	Students	Laboratory stressor (psychomotor)	C: Type A (N = 8) vs Type B (N = 8)	5 min (×8) recordings	−	LF, HF	LF and LF/HF increased after task in Type A	+
Watkins 1998[114]	93 (47)	25–44	Volunteers, healthy	Cross-sectional	C: anxiety (Spielberger)	5 min normal and paced breathing	−	BRC, RSA	Lower BRC and RSA in high trait anxiety (N = 23) than low (N = 22)	+
Horsten 1999[51]	300 (100)	57.5	Population based	Normal daily activities (not specified)	C: social isolation anger depression	24 h	SDNN	LF, HF, LF/HF	Social isolation and inability to relieve anger by talking to others were associated with low HRV; depression with LF/HF; education not associated	+
Myrtek 1999[49]	86	50	29 blue collar 57 white collar	Normal daily activities (not specified)	C: during home and work	23 h	−		No differences in HRV	+

Abbreviations: HF = high frequency; HRV = heart rate variability; LF = low frequency; MF = mid frequency; SDNN = standard deviation of the normal; SES = socioeconomic status.

Table 26.7 SES and psychosocial factors: associations with cardiac autonomic function in patient populations

Study	Total sample (% women)	Age	Study group	Design	Psychosocial factor (A = acute, C = chronic)	Duration, setting of measurement	Cardiac autonomic function		Results	Summary
							Time domain measures	Frequency domain measures		
Psychiatric patient populations										
Yeragani 1991[115]	49 (42)	33	19 major depression, 30 panic disorder	20 normal controls	C: depression	1 min supine, standing normal and deep breathing	MCR, SDC, MCDC, MCDSDC, PNN50	–	Panic disorder patients had lowest SDC, MCDC, MCDSDC, PNN50	+
Yeragani 1993[116]	21 (67)	20–44	Phobic anxiety	21 normal controls	C: depression (Hamilton), anxiety	5 min supine, standing, standing + deep breathing	SDNN	LF, MF, HF	Panic disorder had lower supine SDNN (3.7 vs 4.9) and lower standing LF (1199 vs 2211) than controls	+
Rechlin 1994[117]	80 (78)	31	16 major depression 16 panic disorder 16 reactive depression 16 amitriptyline-treated	16 normal controls	C: depression (Hamilton), anxiety	5 min supine, standing, paced breathing	CVr, RMSSDr, CVdr, RMSSDdr, MCR	LF, MF, HF	Panic disorder had increased LF (2.8) vs 1.4 control Major depression lower HF (0.6) vs 1.2 controls and RMSSDr	+
Klein 1995[118]	10 (60)	32	Panic disorder	14 normal controls	C: depression	5–10 min	–	LF, HF, Energy Ratio Index	Reduced HF	+
Mezzacappa 1996[119]	175 (0)	15	7 aggressive, 6 anxious	8 normal controls	C: aggression and anxiety (prospective yearly reports since age 10)	1.5 min supine, standing	–	RSA	Aggression less RSA in supine	+
Thayer 1996[120]	34		Anxiety disorder	34 normal controls	C: anxiety	Baseline, relaxation and worry	–	LF, HF	Anxiety associated with lower HF than in controls; lower HF found under conditions of worry	+
Bonnet 1998[121]	12	18–50	Volunteer insomniacs	12 age, sex, weight matched controls	A: sleep	5 min (×100) during stages of sleep	SDNN	LF, HF, HF/TP	Higher LF, lower HF in insomniacs	+
Watkins 1999[52]	56 (70)	50–70	Volunteers with major depression	Cross-sectional	C: depression severity (Beck, Hamilton), anxiety (Spielberger)	5 min normal and paced breathing	–	BRC, RSA	Anxiety, but not depression associated with decreased baroreflex control	+
CAD patient population										
Carney 1988[122]	77		CAD	Normal daily activities (not specified)	C: depression	24 h	SDNN	–	Decreased (non-significantly)	–
Carney 1995[123]	58		N = 19 CAD and depression	N = 19 age, sex, smoking matched controls	C: depression	24 h	SDNN, SDANN, SDNNIDX, PNN50, RMSSD	–	SDNN lower in depressed than controls 74 vs 94	+
Krittayaphong 1997[124]	42 (21)	46–79	CAD	Normal daily activities (not specified)	C: depression (MMPI)	24 h	SDNN	–	Lower SDNN among those with MMPI depression scores above than below the median (114 vs 135) and higher HR	+
Watkins 1999[53]	66 (13)	62	CAD	Cross-sectional	C: depressive symptoms (Beck)	10 min	–	BRC, RSA	Depression associated with decreased baroreflex control	+

Abbreviations: BRC = baroreflex control of heart rate; CVr = coefficient of variation during deep respiration; CVdr = coefficient of variation while resting; HF = high frequency; LF = low frequency; MCDC = mean consecutive difference corrected for heart rate; MCDSDC = standard deviation of the mean consecutive difference; MCR = mean circular resultant; MF = mid frequency; MMPI = Minnesota Multiphasic Personality Interview; PNN50 = percentage of all differences in R-R intervals ≥50 ms; RMSSDr = root mean square of successive differences during deep respiration; RMSSDr = root mean square of successive differences while resting; RSA = respiratory sinus arrhythmia; SDC = standard deviation of R-R intervals corrected for heart rate; SDNN = standard deviation of the normal R-R intervals.

ventricular arrhythmia: QT (4/4), VPB (10/12) and VT/VF (11/12), and cardiac autonomic control healthy populations (17/18) and patient populations (11/12).

Conclusion

Eighty-nine of 96 identified published studies investigating aspects of the psychosocial-arrhythmic risk argument were positive. Causality has not, however, been demonstrated; many of the studies are of poor methodological quality; there are important negative findings and there is likely to be publication bias.

Future research

Given the consistency of the published findings and public health importance of this association, there is an urgent need for better studies. Particular attention is required to:

● *Primary hypotheses* testing the presence and direction of a single *a priori* psychosocial factor-arrhythmic risk association. Existing studies have both made many measurements – risking spurious inferences from multiple comparisons – and neglected certain factors, e.g. SES, social supports and psychosocial work characteristics – that may be causally related to CHD.

● *Populations studied* need to be adequately powered to detect important effects, with attention given to the potential for selection bias. Interlocking studies of different healthy and patient groups is important.

● *Psychosocial factor measurement* should capture real-life acute stressors (for example using diary methods) and chronic psychosocial factors measured as continuous variables (e.g. anxiety and depression).

● *Outcome measurement.* More prospective epidemiological studies of SCD are required. Better markers of arrhythmic risk are required in conjunction with a more systematic investigation of those who are at high arrhythmic risk (e.g. long QT syndrome, patients undergoing electrophsyiological studies).

● *Public health* agencies should develop SCD monitoring datasets analysable by readily available demographic factors such as SES, ethnicity and marital status.

References

1. Escobedo LG, Zack MM. Comparison of sudden and non-sudden coronary deaths in the United States. *Circulation* 1996;**93**:2033–6.

2. Thomas AC, Knapman PA, Krikler DM, Davies MJ. Community study of the causes of "natural" death. *BMJ* 1988;**297**:1453–6.

3. Davies MJ, Thomas A. Thrombosis and acute coronary-artery lesions in sudden cardiac ischemic death. *New Engl J Med* 1984;**310**:1137–40.

4. Kannel WB, Anderson K, McGee DL, Degatano LS, Stampfer MJ. Nonspecific electrocardiographic abnormality as a predictor of coronary heart disease: the Framingham study. *Am Heart J* 1987;**113**:370–6.

5. Meredith IT, Broughton A, Jennings GL, Esler MD. Evidence of a selective increase in cardiac sympathetic activity in patients with sustained ventricular arrhythmias. *New Engl J Med* 1991;**325**:618–24.

6. Barron HV, Lesh MD. Autonomic nervous system and sudden cardiac death [published erratum appears in *J Am Coll Cardiol* 1996;**28**:286]. *J Am Coll Cardiol* 1996;**27**:1053–60.

7. Kaplan GA, Keil JE. Socioeconomic factors and cardiovascular disease: a review of the literature. *Circulation* 1993;**88**:1973–98.

8. Marmot MG, Rose G, Shipley M, Hamilton PJS. Employment grade and coronary heart disease in British civil servants. *J Epidemiol Commun Hlth* 1978;**32**:244–9.

9. Marmot M, Bosma H, Hemingway H, Brunner E, Stansfeld S. Contribution of job control and other risk factors to social variations in coronary heart disease. *Lancet* 1997;**350**:235–40.

10. Hemingway H, Marmot M. Psychosocial factors in the aetiology and prognosis of coronary heart disease: systematic review of prospective cohort studies. *BMJ* 1999;**318**:1460–7.

11. Manuck SB, Marsland AL, Kaplan JR, Williams JK. The pathogenicity of behavior and its neuroendocrine mediation: an example from coronary artery disease. *Psychosom Med* 1995;**57**:275–83.

12. Mittleman MA, Maclure M, Nachnani M, Sherwood JB, Muller JE. Educational attainment, anger and the risk of triggering myocardial infarction onset. The Determinants of Myocardial Infarction Onset Study Investigators. *Arch Intern Med* 1997;**157**:769–75.

13. Skinner JE, Lie JT, Entman ML. Modification of ventricular fibrillation latency following coronary artery occlusion in the conscious pig. *Circulation* 1975;**51**:656–67.

14. Skinner JE, Reed JC. Blockade of frontocortical–brain stem pathway prevents ventricular fibrillation of ischemic heart. *Am J Physiol* 1981;**240**:H156–63.

15. Eisermann K. Long-term heartrate responses to social stress in wild European rabbits: predominant effect of rank position. *Physiol Behav* 1992;**52**:33–6.

16. Candland DK, Bryan DC, Nazar BL, Kopf KJ, Sendor M. Squirrel monkey heart rate during formation of status orders. *J Comp Physiol Psychol* 1970;**70**:417–23.

17. Cherkovich GM, Tatoyan SK. Heart rate (radiotelemetrical registration) in macaques and baboons according to dominant-submissive rank in a group. *Folia Primatol (Basel)* 1973;**20**:265–73.

18. Holst D. Social relations and their health impact in tree shrews. *Acta Physiol Scand Suppl* 1997;**640**:77–82.

19. Kagan A. Predictors of sudden cardiac death among Hawaiian-Japanese men. *Am J Epidemiol* 1989;**130**:268–77.

20. Kawachi I, Colditz GA, Ascherio A *et al.* Prospective study of phobic anxiety and risk of coronary heart disease in men. *Circulation* 1994;**89**:1992–7.

21. Kawachi I, Sparrow D, Vokonas PS, Weiss ST. Symptoms of anxiety and risk of coronary heart disease. *Circulation* 1994;**90**:2225–9.

22. Cebelin MS, Hirsch CS. Human stress cardiomyopathy. Myocardial lesions in victims of homicidal assaults without internal injuries. *Hum Pathol* 1980;**11**:123–32.

23. Talbott E, Kuller LH, Perper J, Murphy PA. Sudden unexpected death in women: biologic and psychosocial origins. *Am J Epidemiol* 1981;**114**:671–82.

24. Leor J, Poole WK, Kloner RA. Sudden cardiac death triggered by an earthquake. *New Engl J Med* 1996;**334**:413–19.

25. Meisel SR, Kutz I, Dayan KI *et al.* Effect of Iraqi missile war on incidence of acute myocardial infarction and sudden death in Israeli civilians. *Lancet* 1991;**338**:660–1.

26. Weisenberg D, Meisel SR, David D. Sudden death among the Israeli civilian population during the Gulf War – incidence and mechanisms. *Isr J Med Sci* 1996;**32**:95–9.

27. Kawachi, I, Colditz GA, Stampfer MJ *et al.* Smoking cessation and time course of decreased risks of coronary heart disease in middle age women. *Arch Intern Med* 1994;**154**:169–75.

28. Rabkin SW, Mathewson FA, Tate RB. Chronobiology of cardiac sudden death in men. *JAMA* 1980;**244**:1357–8.

29. Beard CM, Fuster V, Elveback LR. Daily and seasonal variation in sudden cardiac death, Rochester, Minnesota, 1950–1975. *Mayo Clin Proc* 1982;**57**:704–6.

30. Willich SN, Maclure M, Mittleman M, Arntz HR, Muller JE. Sudden cardiac death. Support for a role of triggering in causation. *Circulation* 1993;**87**:1442–50.

31. Brackett CD, Powell LH. Psychosocial and physiological predictors of sudden cardiac death after healing of acute myocardial infarction. *Am J Cardiol* 1988;**61**:979–83.

32. Follick MJ, Ahern DK, Gorkin L *et al.* Relation of psychosocial and stress reactivity variables to ventricular arrhythmias in the Cardiac Arrhythmia Pilot Study (CAPS). *Am J Cardiol* 1990;**66**:63–7.

33. Toivonen L, Helenius K, Viitasalo M. Electrocardiographic repolarization during stress from awakening on alarm call. *J Am Coll Cardiol* 1997;**30**:774–9.

34. Hemingway H, Shipley M, Macfarlane PW, Marmot M. Impact of socioeconomic status on coronary mortality in people with symptoms, electrocardiographic abnormalities, both or neither. *J Epidemiol Comm Health* 2000;**54**;510–16.

35. Reich P, DeSilva RA, Lown B, Murawski BJ. Acute psychological disturbances preceding life-threatening ventricular arrhythmias. *JAMA* 1981;**246**:233–5.

36. Brodsky MA, Sato DA, Iseri LT, Wolff LJ, Allen BJ. Ventricular tachyarrhythmia associated with psychological stress. The role of the sympathetic nervous system. *JAMA* 1987;**257**:2064–7.

37. Kennedy GJ, Hoffer MA, Cohen D. Significance of depression and cognitive impairment in patients undergoing programmed stimulus of cardiac arrhythmias. *Psychosom Med* 1987;**49**:410–21.

38. Malik M, Camm AJ. Heart rate variability. *Clin Cardiol* 1990;**13**:570–6.

39. Farrell TG, Paul V, Cripps TR *et al.* Baroreflex sensitivity and electrophysiological correlates in patients after acute myocardial infarction. *Circulation* 1991;**83**:945–52.

40. Reaven GM, Lithell H, Landsberg L. Hypertension and associated metabolic abnormalities – the role of insulin resistance and the sympathoadrenal system. *New Engl J Med* 1996;**334**:374–81.

41. Brunner EJ, Marmot MG, Nanchahal K *et al.* Social inequality in coronary risk: central obesity and the metabolic syndrome. Evidence from the Whitehall II study. *Diabetologia* 1997;**40**:1341–9.

42. Gillum RF. The epidemiology of resting heart rate in a national sample of men and women: associations with hypertension, coronary heart disease, blood pressure, and other cardiovascular risk factors. *Am Heart J* 1988;**116**:163–74.

43. Unden AL, Orth-Gomer K, Elofsson S. Cardiovascular effects of social support in the work place: twenty-four-hour ECG monitoring of men and women. *Psychosom Med* 1991;**53**:50–60.

44. Bigger JT, Fleiss JL, Rolnitzky LM, Steinman RC. The ability of several short-term measures of RR variability to predict mortality after myocardial infarction. *Circulation* 1993;**88**:927–34.

45. Liao D, Cai J, Rosamond WD *et al.* Cardiac autonomic function and incident coronary heart disease: a population-based case-cohort study. The ARIC Study. Atherosclerosis Risk in Communities Study. *Am J Epidemiol* 1997;**145**:696–706.

46. Dekker JM, Schouten EG, Klootwijk P, Pool J, Swenne CA, Kromhout D. Heart rate variability from short electrocardiographic recordings predicts mortality from all causes in middle-aged and elderly men: The Zutphen Study. *Am J Epidemiol* 1997;**145**:899–908.

47. Anonymous. Heart rate variability: standards of measurement, physiological interpretation and clinical use. Task Force of the European Society of Cardiology and the North American Society of Pacing and Electrophysiology. *Circulation* 1996;**93**:1043–65.

48. Kageyama T, Nishikido N, Kobayashi T, Kurokawa Y, Kaneko T, Kabuto M. Self-reported sleep quality, job stress, and daytime autonomic activities assessed in terms of short-term heart rate variability among male white-collar workers. *Ind Health* 1998;**36**:263–72.

49. Myrtek M, Fichtler A, Strittmatter M, Brugner G. Stress and strain of blue and white collar workers during work and leisure time: results of psychophysiological and behavioral monitoring. *Appl Ergon* 1999;**30**:341–51.

50. De Meersman R, Reisman S, Daum M, Zorowitz R. Vagal withdrawal as a function of audience. *Am J Physiol* 1996;**270**:H1381–3.

51. Horsten M, Ericson M, Perski A, Wamala SP, Schenck-Gustafsson K, Orth-Gomer K. Psychosocial factors and heart rate variability in healthy women. *Psychosom Med* 1999;**61**:49–57.

52. Watkins LL, Grossman P, Krishnan R, Blumenthal JA. Anxiety reduces baroreflex cardiac control in older adults

with major depression. *Psychosom Med* 1999;**61**:334–40.

53. Watkins LL, Grossman P. Association of depressive symptoms with reduced baroreflex cardiac control in coronary artery disease. *Am Heart J* 1999;**137**:453–7.

54. Lown B, Verrier R, Corbalan R. Psychologic stress and threshold for repetitive ventricular response. *Science* 1973;**182**:834–6.

55. Corbalan R, Verrier R, Lown B. Psychological stress and ventricular arrhythmias during myocardial infarction in the conscious dog. *Am J Cardiol* 1974;**34**:692–6.

56. Johansson G, Jonsson L, Lannek N, Blomgren L, Lindberg P, Poupa O. Severe stress-cardiopathy in pigs. *Am Heart J* 1974;**87**:451–7.

57. Corley KC, Shiel FO, Mauck HP, Clark LS, Barber JH. Myocardial degeneration and cardiac arrest in squirrel monkey: physiological and psychological correlates. *Psychophysiology* 1977;**14**:322–8.

58. Liang B, Verrier RL, Melman J, Lown B. Correlation between circulating catecholamine levels and ventricular vulnerability during psychological stress in conscious dogs. *Proc Soc Exp Biol Med* 1979;**161**:266–9.

59. Natelson BH, Cagin NA. Stress-induced ventricular arrhythmias. *Psychosom Med* 1979;**41**:259–62.

60. Verrier RL, Lown B. Experimental studies of psychophysiological factors in sudden cardiac death. *Acta Med Scand Suppl* 1982;**660**:57–68.

61. Sgoifo A, Stilli D, Aimi B, Parmigiani S, Manghi M, Musso E. Behavioral and electrocardiographic responses to social stress in male rats. *Physiol Behav* 1994;**55**:209–16.

62. Sgoifo A, De Boer SF, Westenbroek C *et al.* Incidence of arrhythmias and heart rate variability in wild-type rats exposed to social stress. *Am J Physiol* 1997;**273**:H1754–60.

63. Sgoifo A, De Boer SF, Buwalda B *et al.* Vulnerability to arrhythmias during social stress in rats with different sympathovagal balance. *Am J Physiol* 1998;**275**:H460–6.

64. Greene WA, Goldstein S, Moss AJ. Psychosocial aspects of sudden death. A preliminary report. *Arch Intern Med* 1972;**129**:725–31.

65. Rahe RH, Bennett L, Romo M, Siltanen P, Arthur RJ. Subjects' recent life changes and coronary heart disease in Finland. *Am J Psychiatry* 1973;**130**:1222–6.

66. Myers A, Dewar HA. Circumstances attending 100 sudden deaths from coronary artery disease with coroner's characteristics. *Br Heart J* 1975;**37**:1133–43.

67. Talbott E, Kuller LH, Detre K, Perper J. Biologic and psychosocial risk factors of sudden death from coronary disease in white women. *Am J Cardiol* 1977;**39**:858–64.

68. Rissanen V, Romo M, Siltanen P. Prehospital sudden death from ischaemic heart disease. A postmortem study. *Br Heart J* 1978;**40**:1025–33.

69. Cottington EM, Matthews KA, Talbott E, Kuller LH. Environmental events preceding sudden death in women. *Psychosom Med* 1980;**42**:567–74.

70. Beard TC, Gray WR, Cooke HM, Baron R. Randomised controlled trial of a no-added-sodium diet for mild hypertension. *Lancet* 1982;454–8.

71. Kirschner RH, Eckner FA, Baron RC. The cardiac pathology of sudden, unexplained nocturnal death in Southeast Asian refugees. *JAMA* 1986;**256**:2700–5.

72. Sexton PT, Jamrozik K, Walsh J. Sudden unexpected cardiac death among Tasmanian men. *Med J Aust* 1993;**159**:467–70.

73. Salonen JT, Alfthan G, Pikkarainen J. Association between cardiovascular death and myocardial infarction and serum selenium in a matched-pair longitudinal study. *Lancet* 1982;**2**:175–9.

74. Hinkle LE, Jr., Thaler HT, Merke DP, Renier-Berg D, Morton NE. The risk factors for arrhythmic death in a sample of men followed for 20. years. *Am J Epidemiol* 1988;**127**:500–15.

75. Bruhn JG, Paredes A, Adsett CA, Wolf S. Psychological predictors of sudden death in myocardial infarction. *J Psychosom Res* 1974;**18**:187–91.

76. Weinblatt E, Ruberman W, Goldberg JD, Frank CW, Shapiro S, Chaudhary B. Relation of education to sudden death after myocardial infarction. *New Engl J Med* 1978;**299**:60–5.

77. Ruberman W, Weinblatt E, Goldberg JD, Chaudhary BS. Education, psychosocial stress and sudden cardiac death. *J Chronic Dis* 1983;**36**:151–60.

78. Ruberman W, Weinblatt E, Goldberg JD, Chaudhary BS. Psychosocial influences on mortality after myocardial infarction. *New Engl J Med* 1984;**311**:552–9.

79. Ahern DK, Gorkin L, Anderson JL *et al.* Biobehavioral variables and mortality or cardiac arrest in the Cardiac Arrhythmia Pilot Study (CAPS). *Am J Cardiol* 1990;**66**:59–62.

80. Thomas SA, Friedmann E, Wimbush F, Schron E. Psychological factors and survival in the Cardiac Arrhythmia Suppression Trial (CAST): a reexamination. *Am J Crit Care* 1997;**6**:116–26.

81. Taggart P, Carruthers M, Somerville W. Electrocardiogram, plasma catecholamines and lipids, and their modification by oxyprenolol when speaking before an audience. *Lancet* 1973;**2**:341–6.

82. Cook TC, Cashman PM. Stress and ectopic beats in ships' pilots. *J Psychosom Res* 1982;**26**:559–69.

83. Rainey JM, Jr., Pohl RB, Bilolikar SG. The QT interval in drug-free depressed patients. *J Clin Psychiatry* 1982;**43**:39–40.

84. Hijzen TH, Slangen JL. The electrocardiogram during emotional and physical stress. *Int J Psychophysiol* 1985;**2**:273–9.

85. Katz C, Martin RD, Landa B, Chadda KD. Relationship of psychologic factors to frequent symptomatic ventricular arrhythmia. *Am J Med* 1985;**78**:589–94.

86. Huang MH, Ebey J, Wolf S. Responses of the QT interval of the electrocardiogram during emotional stress. *Psychosom Med* 1989;**51**:419–27.

87. Lown B, Temte JV, Reich P, Gaughan C, Regestein Q, Hal H. Basis for recurring ventricular fibrillation in the absence of coronary heart disease and its management. *New Engl J Med* 1976;**294**:623–9.

88. Lynch JJ, Thomas SA, Paskewitz DA, Katcher AH, Weir LO. Human contact and cardiac arrhythmia in a coronary care unit. *Psychosom Med* 1977;**39**:188–92.

89. Lown B, DeSilva RA. Roles of psychologic stress and autonomic nervous system changes in provocation of ventricular premature complexes. *Am J Cardiol* 1978;**41**:979–85.

90. Weinblatt E, Ruberman W, Goldberg JD, Frank CW, Shapiro S, Chaudhary BS. Relation of education to sudden death after myocardial infarction. *New Engl J Med* 1978;**299**:60–5.

91. Donlon PT, Meadow A, Amsterdam E. Emotional stress as a factor in ventricular arrhythmias. *Psychosomatics* 1979;**20**:233–40.

92. Orth-Gomer K, Edwards ME, Erhardt L, Sjogren A, Theorell T. Relation between ventricular arrhythmias and psychological profile. *Acta Med Scand* 1980;**207**:31–6.

93. Graboys TB. Celtics fever: playoff-induced ventricular arrhythmia [letter]. *New Engl J Med* 1981;**305**:467–8.

94. Krantz DS, Arabian JM, Davia JE, Parker JS. Type A behavior and coronary artery bypass surgery: intraoperative blood pressure and perioperative complications. *Psychosom Med* 1982;**44**:273–84.

95. Freeman AM, 3d, Fleece L, Folks DG, Cohen-Cole S, Waldo A. Psychiatric symptoms, type A behavior, and arrhythmias following coronary bypass. *Psychosomatics* 1984;**25**:586–9.

96. Jennings JR, Follansbee WP. Type A and ectopy in patients with coronary artery disease and controls. *J Psychosom Res* 1984;**28**:49–54.

97. Tavazzi L, Zotti AM, Rondanelli R. The role of psychologic stress in the genesis of lethal arrhythmias in patients with coronary artery disease. *Eur Heart J* 1986;**7**(Suppl. A): 99–106.

98. Follick MJ, Gorkin L, Capone RJ *et al.* Psychological distress as a predictor of ventricular arrhythmias in a post-myocardial infarction population. *Am Heart J* 1988;**116**:32–6.

99. Hatton DC, Gilden ER, Edwards ME, Cutler J, Kron J, McAnulty JH. Psychophysiological factors in ventricular arrhythmias and sudden cardiac death. *J Psychosom Res* 1989;**33**:621–31.

100. Moss AJ, Schwartz PJ, Crampton RS *et al.* The long QT syndrome. Prospective longitudinal study of 328 families. *Circulation* 1991;**84**:1136–44.

101. Carney RM, Freedland KE, Rich MW, Smith LJ, Jaffe AS. Ventricular tachycardia and psychiatric depression in patients with coronary artery disease. *Am J Med* 1993;**95**:23–8.

102. Rohmert W, Laurig W, Philipp U, Luczak H. Heart rate variability and work-load measurement. *Ergonomics* 1973;**16**: 33–44.

103. Sekiguchi C, Handa Y, Gotoh M, Kurihara Y, Nagasawa Y, Kuroda I. Frequency analysis of heart rate variability under flight conditions. *Aviat Space Environ Med* 1979;**50**:625–34.

104. Bronis M, Vicenik K, Rosik V, Tysler M. Heart rhythm variability during work in radio speakers. *Act Nerv Super (Praha)* 1980;**22**:66–8.

105. Mulders HP, Meijman TF, O'Hanlon JF, Mulder G. Differential psychophysiological reactivity of city bus drivers. *Ergonomics* 1982;**25**:1003–11.

106. Kamada T, Miyake S, Kumashiro M, Monou H, Inoue K. Power spectral analysis of heart rate variability in Type As and Type Bs during mental workload. *Psychosom Med* 1992;**54**:462–70.

107. Toivanen H, Lansimies E, Jokela V, Hanninen O. Impact of regular relaxation training on the cardiac autonomic nervous system of hospital cleaners. *Scand J Work Environ Health* 1993;**19**:319–25.

108. Sloan RP, Shapiro PA, Bigger JT, Bagiella E, Steinman RC, Gorman JM. Cardiac autonomic control and hostility in healthy subjects. *Am J Cardiol* 1994;**74**:298–300.

109. Kawachi I, Colditz GA, Stampfer MJ *et al.* Prospective study of shift work and risk of coronary heart disease in women. *Circulation* 1995;**92**:3178–82.

110. McCraty R, Atkinson M, Tiller WA, Rein G, Watkins AD. The effects of emotions on short-term power spectrum analysis of heart rate variability [published erratum appears in *Am J Cardiol* 1996;**77**:330]. *Am J Cardiol* 1995;**76**:1089–3.

111. Myrtek M, Weber D, Brugner G, Muller W. Occupational stress and strain of female students: results of physiological, behavioral, and psychological monitoring. *Biol Psychol* 1996;**42**:379–1.

112. Kageyama T, Nishikido N, Kobayashi T, Kurokawa Y, Kaneko T, Kabuto M. Long commuting time, extensive overtime, and sympathodominant state assessed in terms of short-term heart rate variability among male white-collar workers in the Tokyo megalopolis. *Ind Health* 1998;**36**:209–7.

113. Sato N, Kamada T, Miyake S, Akatsu J, Kumashiro M, Kume Y. Power spectral analysis of heart rate variability in type A females during a psychomotor task. *J Psychosom Res* 1998;**45**:159–9.

114. Watkins LL, Grossman P, Krishnan R, Sherwood A. Anxiety and vagal control of heart rate. *Psychosom Med* 1998;**60**:498–02.

115. Yeragani VK, Pohl R, Balon R *et al.* Heart rate variability in patients with major depression. *Psychiatry Res* 1991;**37**:35–6.

116. Yeragani VK, Pohl R, Berger R *et al.* Decreased heart rate variability in panic disorder patients: a study of power spectral analysis of heart rate. *Psychiatry Res* 1993;**46**:89–103.

117. Rechlin T, Weis M, Spitzer A, Kaschka WP. Are affective disorders associated with alterations of heart rate variability? *J Affect Disord* 1994;**32**:271–5.

118. Klein E, Cnaani E, Harel T, Braun S, Ben-Haim SA. Altered heart rate variability in panic disorder patients. *Biol Psychiatry* 1995;**37**:18–24.

119. Mezzacappa E, Tremblay RE, Kindlon D *et al.* Relationship of aggression and anxiety to autonomic regulation of heart rate variability in adolescent males. *Ann N Y Acad Sci* 1996;**794**:376–9.

120. Thayer JF, Friedman BH, Borkovec TD. Autonomic characteristics of generalized anxiety disorder and worry. *Biol Psychiatry* 1996;**39**:255–66.

121. Bonnet MH, Arand DL. Heart rate variability in insomniacs and matched normal sleepers. *Psychosom Med* 1998;**60**: 610–15.

122. Carney RM, Rich MW, Freedland KE *et al.* Major depressive disorder predicts cardiac events in patients with coronary artery disease. *Psychosom Med* 1988;**50**:627–33.

123. Carney RM, Saunders RD, Freedland KE, Stein P, Rich MW, Jaffe AS. Association of depression with reduced heart rate variability in coronary artery disease. *Am J Cardiol* 1995;**76**:562–4.

124. Krittayaphong R, Cascio WE, Light KC *et al.* Heart rate variability in patients with coronary artery disease: differences in patients with higher and lower depression scores. *Psychosom Med* 1997;**59**:231–5.

PART III

Clinical studies of risk assessment

27 Risk stratification after myocardial infarction

Yee Guan Yap

Sudden cardiac death (SCD) is defined as instantaneous, unexpected death or death within 1 hour of symptom onset not related to circulatory failure. In the USA, SCD accounted for 200 000 to 400 000 deaths per year.[1,2] There are many causes of SCD,[3] with coronary artery disease being the most common cause of sudden death. About 10% of patients who survive the acute and subacute phases of myocardial infarction (MI) will die during the first year after hospital discharge[4] and death is sudden in most cases. SCD is arguably the most dramatic manifestation of coronary artery disease.

In the last decade, the widespread use of thrombolysis and aspirin has each associated with a reduction in the mortality after MI by approximately 20%.[5] Effective thrombolytic therapy may also prevent the development of an abnormal electrophysiological milieu after myocardial infarction and improve the electrical stability, and hence reduce the risk of fatal arrhythmia and possibly SCD. In addition to thrombolytic therapy, many contemporary treatments, including aspirin, beta-blockers, angiotensin-converting enzyme and lipid-lowering drugs, have also improved the mortality after MI.

Despite these recent developments in the management of myocardial infarction, SCD remains a both a problem for the practising clinician and a public health issue. The prevention of SCD in patients, who survived cardiac arrest or who are believed to be at high risk, remains one of the major challenges facing cardiologists. Risk stratification after MI has therefore attracted much attention among arrhythmologists, in an attempt to identify patients at risk of SCD who may potentially be treated prophylactically with an antiarrhythmic drug or implantable cardiodefibrillator. This is important because most antiarrhythmic agents have the unwelcome adverse effect of pro-arrhythmia and an implantable cardiodefibrillator is expensive. The selection of patients most at risk is therefore crucial to ensure that the prophylactic treatment of SCD is safe and cost-effective. In the last decade, many non-invasive tests have been discovered to be predictive of arrhythmic events (sudden death and life threatening ventricular arrhythmias) with MI being the subject most commonly investigated. Unfortunately, the predictive powers of

some of these tests are limited and the search for a more sensitive and specific non-invasive test continues. The introduction of modern post-MI therapy may have altered the predictive values and clinical relevance of these risk factors, and it is important to discuss risk stratification of post-MI patients in the context of modern therapy. In this chapter, we will review the contemporary tests available in the risk stratification of patients after MI.

Heart rate variability

In a normal heart, the heart rate is not regular but is determined by the balance between vagal and sympathetic activity. Heart rate variability (HRV) is a measure of such spontaneous variability of heart rate and periodic change of the heart rate rhythm. Autonomic activities, such as respiratory sinus arrhythmia and blood pressure regulation, and other factors including thermoregulation, the renin–angiotensin system, and circadian rhythm can all affect the heart rate.[6] The analysis of HRV is an established non-invasive method of assessing autonomic influence on the heart rate at the level of the sinus node.[7] As a general rule, an increased sympathetic or decreased parasympathetic tone is reflected in decreased indices of HRV, whilst decreased sympathetic or increased parasympathetic activity is reflected in increased indices of HRV.[6] When stationary data are analysed, in the frequency domain of HRV, the so-called high-frequency (HF) component of physiologic HRV is almost exclusively mediated by vagal activity, whereas the low frequency (LF) component of HRV is under the influence of both sympathetic and vagal activity.[8] Both HF and LF oscillations interact to modulate target functions and determine their rhythmic properties. In other words, HRV represents a measure of sympathovagal modulation.

In recent years, it has been shown that impaired function of the autonomic nervous system plays an important part in the genesis of ventricular arrhythmias. Therefore, a marker of autonomic control on cardiac electrophysiological properties such as HRV (and baroreflex sensitivity) might provide important information in the risk stratification of patients following MI. HRV can be analysed in the time or frequency domain using 24-h Holter monitoring. Different parameters of time and frequency domain measurements of HRV have been used, most commonly being the standard deviation of RR intervals (SDNN), and their mutual dependency should be considered for better comparability of clinical results.[9–11] A recent publication by the task force of the European Society of Cardiology and the North American Society of Pacing and Electrophysiology has comprehensively discussed the various methods used for measuring HRV and their corresponding normal values.[12]

The earlier landmark study by Kleiger *et al.* showed that decreased HRV was an independent predictor of all-cause mortality after MI, irrespective of demographic background, New York Heart Association functional class, left ventricular ejection fraction (LVEF), and ventricular ectopic activity.[13] For the specific prediction of SCD or ventricular tachyarrhythmias, studies performed in our department demonstrated that HRV, expressed as total number of all RR intervals divided by the height of the histogram of all RR intervals (TI) was a better predictor of sudden deaths and symptomatic ventricular tachycardia than LVEF, whereas both HRV and LVEF performed equally well in predicting all-cause mortality in the postinfarction patients.[14] Among the non-invasive variables including HRV, signal-averaged electrocardiogram (SAECG), ventricular arrhythmias, and LVEF in predicting arrhythmic versus non-arrhythmic mortality, our data showed that arrhythmic death was associated predominantly with depressed HRV and ventricular tachycardic runs, whereas non-arrhythmic death was associated with low ejection fraction, ventricular ectopic beats, and depressed HRV. Thus, reduced HRV implies a lack of an autonomic protection against ventricular arrhythmias and SCD.[15]

For postinfarction risk stratification, the predictive value of HRV is modest, although it appears to be better than other recognised risk factors. Differences in the timing of investigations, method of analysis and specific endpoints makes comparisons of predictive accuracy between studies difficult. For the prediction of arrhythmic events, the sensitivity was 75% with a specificity of 76% for a TI ≤30 U.[13] When analysed using a different HRV parameter, TINN (width of the triangle interpolation of the RR histogram) of <20 ms, HRV had a sensitivity of 92% for the prediction of arrhythmic events (sudden death or life-threatening ventricular arrhythmias), but a specificity of 77% only resulted in a large number of false-positive results and a low positive predictive accuracy of 17%.[16] Among all the HRV measures, time domain HRV provides better prognostic information than the rest, particularly SDNN and TI.[12] A high-risk group may be selected by the dichotomy limits of SDNN <50 ms or TI <15 U. It is recommended that HRV should be measured approximately 1 week after the index infarct.[12]

At present, to improve the predictive value of HRV, it is necessary for HRV to be combined with other risk factors despite its independent risk prediction for mortality and arrhythmic complication.[12] Multivariate analysis showed that the most sensitive combination for the prediction of arrhythmic events was a reduced HRV and a positive SAECG.[16] Such combination had a sensitivity of 58%, a positive predictive accuracy of 33%, and a relative risk of 18 (95% CI, 7–34) and was superior to other combinations, including those incorporating LVEF, exercise ECG, ventricular ectopic beat frequency, and repetitive ventricular forms.

HRV is unaffected by thrombolytic therapy. It continues to retain its independent prognostic significance in postinfarction patients of all ages treated with thrombolysis.[17] On the other hand, beta-blocker increases the RR variance and the normalised power of the high-frequency component (vagal tone) and reduces the low frequency component (sympathetic activity). This may partly explain the beneficial effect of these drugs after myocardial infarction.[18]

The ATRAMI (Autonomic Tone and Reflexes in Acute Myocardial Infarction) study showed that HRV (and baroreflex sensitivity) remained significant predictors of cardiac mortality in patients after myocardial infarction (<28 days) in the thrombolytic era. The full results showed that during 21 months of followed-up, low value of HRV (SDNN <70 ms) and BRS (<3.0 ms/mmHg) carried a significant multivariate risk of cardiac mortality of 3.2 and 2.8 respectively.[19] The association of low SDNN and BRS further increased the risk: the 2-year mortality was 17% when both were below the cut-offs and 2% when both were well preserved (SDNN >105 ms, BRS >6.1 ms/mmHg). Furthermore, the association of low SDNN or BRS with left ventricular ejection fraction (LVEF) below 35% carried a relative risk of 6.7 or 8.7 respectively, compared with LVEF above 35% and less compromised SDNN (≥70 ms) and BRS (≥3 ms). Thus, the ATRAMI results confirm that, after MI, the analysis of autonomic markers has significant independent prognostic value in the thrombolytic era. The combination of low values of autonomic markers and reduced LVEF may help to identify a group of post-MI patients at high risk of cardiac death.

Recently, analysis of the fractal characteristics of short-term RR interval dynamics from the DIAMOND study yields more powerful prognostic information than the traditional measures of HRV for the prediction of arrhythmic death among patients with depressed left ventricular function after an AMI.[20] However, the prognostic value of these new variables of HRV will require further confirmation.

Several studies are currently ongoing to test the effect of prophylactive treatments (pharmacological or non-pharmacological) on survival in post-MI patients stratified using a combination of HRV and othe non-invasive variables. The ALIVE study (AzimiLide postinfarct surVival Evaluation) is a new clinical trial using both reduced LVEF and HRV as predictors to target a post-MI population at high risk of sudden death and examine the potential of azimilide, a novel class III antiarrhythmic, for improving survival in patients with a recent MI (6–21 days).[21] The DINAMIT (Defibrillator In Acute Myocardial Infarction Trial) trial is a multicentre study to evaluate the efficacy of the implantable cardioverter defibrillator (ICD) on all-cause mortality in high-risk patients post-MI patients with reduced LVEF (≤40%) and either impaired HRV (SDNN ≤70 ms) or high resting heart rate. If any of these trials reveals a survival benefit with prophylactic treatment on post-MI patients with depressed HRV, it will be a major step forward in the strategy of risk stratification and clinical practice will need to be changed accordingly.

Baroreflex sensitivity (BRS)

Whilst HRV is a measure of sympathovagal modulation of the autonomic nervous system, BRS assesses the ability of the autonomic nervous system to respond to a stimulus with an increase in acetylcholine release (i.e. vagal reflex activation). BRS can be assessed by studying either the reflex heart rate response to a physiological activation or deactivation of the baroreceptors by a variety of mechanical or pharmacological manipulations, or by analysing the spontaneous fluctuations of the arterial pressure in steady-state condition.[22] The most well-accepted standardised technique involved a bolus injection of phenylephrine as described by Smyth *et al.*[23] and is of proven value in assessing BRS. The slope of the regression line of the beat-to-beat variation in blood pressure (ΔBP) plotted against the beat-to-beat change in the RR interval (ΔRR) following phenylephrine infusion is taken as the BRS.

Earlier studies showed that BRS was more reduced in postinfarction patients with ventricular tachycardia on Holter monitoring or during an exercise stress test compared to those without arrhythmias[24] and in the patients in whom sustained ventricular tachycardia was induced with programmed ventricular stimulation.[25] Indeed, BRS is an independent risk factor for cardiac death, and the risk of dying was 17 times greater for those patients who had a depressed BRS 1 month after a myocardial infarction.[24]

BRS is significantly more reduced in postinfarction patients with three-vessel disease than in those with one-vessel coronary artery disease.[24] In patients with stable coronary disease, the decrease in BRS is correlated with the extent and severity of coronary narrowing.[26] The latest evidence from the ATRAMI study on BRS confirmed that the presence of an open infarct-related artery is associated

with a higher BRS and lower incidence of markedly depressed BRS (<3 ms/mmHg), therefore reducing the risk of post-MI mortality.[27] These data offer new insights into the mechanisms by which coronary artery patency may affect cardiac electrical stability and survival.

BRS is temporarily affected by thrombolytic therapy. The mean BRS at 6 weeks postinfarction was higher in patients treated with thrombolysis compared with non-treated patients, but this difference disappeared at 6 weeks and 3 months subsequently.[28] This finding has been substantiated by the result from a separate ATRAMI report, which showed that there were fewer patients with a markedly depressed BRS in patients who received thrombolytic treatment compared with those who did not.[29]

Farrell *et al.* studied the prognostic significance of BRS on 122 postinfarction patients and reported a sensitivity of 89%, a specificity of 91% and a positive predictive accuracy of 445 for predicting sudden death.[30] As discussed earlier, similar to HRV, the ATRAMI study demonstrated that reduced BRS increases the risk of mortality after AMI, especially if combined with a reduced HRV or LVEF.[19,31]

Late potential

In the genesis of malignant ventricular arrhythmias, the role of re-entry due to slow conduction is important. In regions of experimental infarction, slow conduction is the result of delayed fractionated electrical activity during diastole. These potentials that occur in/or after the end of the QRS complex are known as "ventricular late potentials". They are characterised by multiple low-amplitude spikes, sometimes separated by isoelectric intervals, which can be detected on signal averaged ECG (SAECG).[32] Areas of myocardium from which ventricular late potentials have been detected are thought to be arrhythmogenic electrophysiological substrates for the genesis of re-entry ventricular arrhythmias.

Clinically, among survivors of acute myocardial infarction, the presence of late potential was a significant predictor of spontaneous ventricular arrhythmia or sudden death and induced ventricular tachycardia, independent of both ventricular function and ventricular arrhythmia on Holter monitoring.[33-35] Steinberg and co-workers performed a meta-analysis of all available prospective studies on the use of SAECG after MI. They found that the presence of late potential as assessed with SAECG predicted a six-fold increase in the risk of arrhythmic events independent of left ventricular function, and an eight-fold increase in risk of arrhythmic events independent of Holter results.[33] The total number of patients in the meta-analysis however was small. Recently, in the CAST/SAECG substudy report, late potential predicted serious arrhythmic events in the first year after infarction better than do clinical, ejection fraction and ventricular arrhythmia variables.[36]

The majority of the trials on SAECG were performed in the prethrombolytic era. Thrombolytic therapy had been found to reduce the frequency of SAECG abnormality (filtered QRS duration >120 ms) by 37% and the filtered QRS duration,[37] as well as the predictive value of late potentials on the SAECG.[38] Nevertheless, SAECG remains an independent predictor of arrhythmic events after MI.[39] In a consecutive series of 301 survivors of MI, 68% of who received thrombolytic agents that underwent SAECG examination, 13 patients (4.3%) had an arrhythmic event (SCD and sustained VT) at a median follow-up time of approximately 1 year.[40] A positive SAECG was 64% sensitive (95% CI 36–92%) and 81% specific (95% CI 76–86%) for prediction of arrhythmic events. In another prospective study of 222 patients with AMI in the thrombolytic era, the presence of late potential at discharge was predictive of arrhythmic events (sudden cardiac death, sustained ventricular tachycardia, syncope) during the first year after MI, with a sensitivity of 94% and a specificity of 72%.[41]

Different approaches have been used for the detection of ventricular late potentials: time- and frequency-domain analysis and spectral temporal mapping, which are a combination of time and frequency analyses. Work done in our department showed that time domain analysis is more superior to frequency domain analysis, spectral temporal mapping, and spectral turbulence analysis of the SAECG in predicting arrhythmic events after myocardial infarction,[42–46] although spectral turbulence analysis is more powerful in predicting 1-year mortality. Other investigators have also confirmed the superiority of the time domain analysis.[47] Time-domain SAECG is based on high-gain amplification, bandpass filtering and signal-averaging of a given number of identical beats to eliminate the random noise. The averaged ECG signals of three orthogonal leads are then combined into a vector lead and processed using a digital bidirectional bandpass filter. A SAECG is considered positive if two of the following three parameters are abnormal:

- the duration of the filtered QRS complex;
- the duration of the low amplitude signal (<40 mV) in the terminal QRS;
- the root mean square voltage of the terminal 40 ms of the QRS signal.

It has been suggested that a combined use of time and frequency domain analysis of SAECG should be used to enhance the accuracy of this technique as a screening test for selecting patients for programmed electrical stimulation after MI.[46] Although SAECG had an excellent negative predictive value of late potentials (between 96–99%),

the positive accuracy was low (between 7–27%), which limits its role in risk stratification.[32]

Left ventricular ejection fraction (LVEF)

Earlier studies showed that left ventricular dysfunction, and the presence of frequent or repetitive ventricular premature depolarisations on ambulatory monitoring, were independent risk factors for subsequent mortality amongst survivors of acute myocardial infarction.[48–50] Univariate analysis demonstrated a progressive increase in 1-year mortality following MI as the ejection fraction fell below 40%.[48] Bigger *et al.* showed that after adjusting for other variables, the risk of dying for patients with a LVEF <30% was 3.5 times that for patients with a LVEF ≥30%.[49] There was a high incidence of ventricular arrhythmias and sudden cardiac death in patients with poor left ventricular function following a previous MI.[49] Among variables such as SAECG, complex ventricular ectopic activity, and left ventricular dysfunction, left ventricular dysfunction was the most powerful predictor of subsequent arrhythmic events after MI.[51] It was also one of the most important predictors of prognosis.[52]

Zaret et al. reaffirmed that LVEF remained an important prognostic index in predicting the total and cardiac mortality in patients receiving thrombolytic therapy following a MI from TIMI phase II study,[53] although, when it was compared with the Multicenter Postinfarction Research Group data in the prethrombolytic era,[48] there was a strong difference in survival in the two studies. At any level of ejection fraction, mortality was lower in TIMI II patients than in patients in the prethrombolytic era.

For the prediction cardiac death, a LVEF <35% had a 40% sensitivity, 78% specificity, and 14% positive predictive accuracy.[54] Both ejection fraction and functional class of heart failure were powerful predictors of arrhythmia suppression and cardiac events in patients with ventricular arrhythmia after MI with each providing incremental prediction.[55] The mortality for myocardial infarction survivors with LVEF <40% was 20% over 3.5 years and that half of the deaths were sudden.[56]

We have recently evaluated the value of LVEF in stratifying MI patients in the thrombolytic era in a combined analysis of recently completed survival trials. We pooled the individual placebo patient data from European Myocardial Infarct Amiodarone Trial (EMIAT), Survival With Oral d-Sotalol (SWORD), TRAndolapril Cardiac Evaluation (TRACE) and Danish Investigation of Arrhythmias and Mortality on Dofetilide-Myocardial Infarction (DIAMOND-MI) studies, which recruited patients with LVEF ≤40% after MI. Survival at 2 years was analysed on patients surviving 45 days onwards from MI to allow for different recruitment periods between studies. Short-term survival (from onset of MI to day 44 after MI) was also examined using data from TRACE and DIAMOND MI which recruited patients within 2 weeks of MI. Effect of LVEF was investigated after adjusted for baseline treatment and study effects and other risk factors associated with survival. LVEF significantly predicted 2-year all-cause, arrhythmic and cardiac mortality (Table 27.1). Interestingly, significantly more patients were likely to die of non-arrhythmic than arrhythmic death if LVEF<20%. Thus, LVEF remains a powerful predictor of mortality at 2-year post-MI despite modern treatment. LVEF is not as specific marker for arrhythmic mortality if LVEF<20% compared with LVEF = 31–40%.

Ventricular premature complexes (VPC)

In the prethrombolytic era, the prevalence of ventricular ectopic activity was independently associated with mortality risk after MI.[48,49,57,58] Results from the Multicentre Postinfarction Research Group showed that there was a progressive increase in 1-year cardiac mortality as the frequency of VPC rose above one per hour.[49]

Statters *et al.* reassessed the role of VPC in risk stratification of patient post-myocardial infaction in the thrombolytic era. They examined 680 patients, of whom 379 received early thrombolytic therapy. All patients underwent 24-h Holter monitoring in a drug-free state between 6 and 10 days after AMI. Patients were followed up for 1–8 years. Mean VPC frequency was significantly higher in patients who died of cardiac causes and sudden death, and in those with arrhythmic events during the first year of follow-up. This was also true when patients who did and did not undergo thrombolysis were considered separately. The positive predictive accuracy of VPC frequency in predicting adverse cardiac events was greater in patients who did than in those who did not undergo thrombolysis. At a sensitivity level of 40%, the positive predictive accuracy for cardiac mortality and arrhythmic events for the group with thrombolysis was 19.4% and 25.8%, respectively, compared with 16% and 16% for those without thrombolysis. Thus, VPC frequency appears to be more highly predictive of prognosis after AMI in patients who have undergone thrombolysis than in those who have not, but the optimal dichotomy limit is higher in the former.[59] The GISSI-2 study confirmed that frequent VPBs remained an independent risk factors for SCD after MI in the thrombolytic era. After adjusting for other risk factors, the presence of VPBs >10/h independently predicted total mortality and SCD at 6 months after MI (total mortality: RR = 1.62; 95% CI = 1.16–2.26; SCD: RR = 1.20; 95% CI = 0.80–1.79).[60] Other workers also found that complex premature complexes were the strongest influence on the risk of sudden coronary death.[61]

Nevertheless, the value of VPC as a predictor of SCD remains controversial. Moss *et al.* showed that, whilst complex VPCs were associated with a significantly increased cardiac death rate, they did not discriminate between sudden and non-sudden cardiac death.[62] Data analysis in the placebo patients of the Beta-Blocker Heart Attack Trial showed that a number of patients who had sudden death remained undetected (low sensitivity) when VPCs were used, whereas there were a considerable number of false positive results in the subclass analysis.[63] Furthermore, the CAST studies showed that suppression of VPCs using class Ic antiarrhythmic drugs was associated with increased mortality compared with the placebo.[64,65] Although the pro-arrhythmic effect of sodium channel blockers (class I action) may be partly to blame for the increased mortality risk observed in the treatment group, the CAST studies questioned the hypothesis whether suppression of asymptomatic ventricular ectopy can reduce mortality.[66]

Table 27.1 LVEF and risk of mortality after myocardial infarction

Effect of 10% increase in LVEF on survival	Mortality <45 days Odd ratio (95% CI)	Mortality 45 days – 2 years Hazard ration (95% CI)
All-cause mortality	0.77 (0.56–1.06), p = 0.1	0.58 (0.49–0.68), P <0.001
Arrhythmic mortality	0.72 (0.47–1.09), p = 0.1	0.61 (0.48–0.78), P <0.001
Cardiac mortality	1.01 (0.61–1.68), p = 0.96	0.51 (0.39–0.66), P <0.001

LVEF (%)	No. of patients	Rate (%) per person-year (total events) between 45 days and 2 years		
		All-cause	Arrhythmic	Cardiac
<20	193	23.1	9.4	10.6
21–30	881	17.5	7.7	6.3
31–40	1432	6.8	3.2	2.2

Abbreviations: LVEF = left ventricular ejection fraction.

Non-sustained VT

Although studies performed before the advent of thrombolysis have shown that the presence of non-sustained VT increases the risk of arrhythmic mortality after MI, such as association is less certain in the current thrombolytic era. The large GISSI-2 study reported that the prevalence of non-sustained VT was only 6.8% and its presence is not predictive of SCD at 6 months after MI in the thrombolytic era.[60] Other investigators supported this finding.[67] In this other study where 325 patients were followed-up for 30±22 months, there was a low prevalence (9%) of non-sustained VT shortly after AMI. In a univariate analysis, the presence of non-sustained VT carried a relative risk of 2.6 for the primary study end-point (cardiac death, sustained VT, or resuscitated VF), but was not a significant predictor if only arrhythmic events (SCD, sustained VT, and resuscitated VF) were considered. On multivariate analysis, only HRV, LVEF, and the status of the infarct artery were found to be independent predictors of the primary study end-point.[67]

Coronary perfusion

Successful reperfusion of the infarct-related artery with thrombolysis and/or interventional catheter therapy in patients with AMI reduces the in-hospital as well as out-of-hospital 1-year mortality. Open infarct-related artery results in increased electrical stability of the heart, which in part explains the favourable outcome of these patients. The presence or absence of an open infarct-related artery as assessed by coronary angiography therefore requires a renewed examination.

In a multivariate analysis of 173 post-MI patients, among occluded infarct-related artery, LVEF ≤40%, late potential, ventricular dysarrhythmia, and clinical variables, only the presence or absence of a patent infarct-related artery was an independent predictor of arrhythmic event (SCD, resuscitated VF, sustained VT) during the 12-month follow-up period.[68] Similarly, other workers showed that an occluded infarct-related artery as assessed by coronary angiography was 78% sensitive and 58% specific for the prediction of arrhythmic events (SCD, sustained VT, and unexplained syncope).[69] However, recent investigations into the efficacy of coronary angiography and angioplasty systematically carried out after MI in the thrombolysed patients failed to show any beneficial effects. The result of TIMI II showed that coronary angiography routinely performed after the acute period and the consequent revascularisation when anatomically indicated did not improve the outcome.[70] The result from GISSI-2 trial, which only excluded MI patients contraindicated to thrombolysis or late presentation, supports an individualised conservation approach to coronary angiography.[71]

Traditionally, exercise testing has been used to select post-MI patients at risk of subsequent cardiac events, although its role in risk stratification is still debated. A large meta-analysis with a total of more than 5300 patients, who underwent either a predischarge submaximal or post-discharge maximal exercise test, showed that only inadequate blood pressure response and a low exercise capacity identified a high-risk group.[72] Exercise-induced ST-segment depression only appeared as a significant predictor of death in the subset of patients with inferior–posterior MI. However, most of the studies in this meta-analysis did not include a multivariate analysis. Studies carried out in the thrombolytic era also showed some reservation on the predictive value of exercise testing, when merely interpreted in terms of the presence or absence of ST depression or angina.[73,74] However, when exercise-induced ST depression occurred in patients who also had reduced exercise duration, a significantly increased risk of cardiac death or non-fatal infarction was noted (hazard ratio, 3.4).[74] It is possible that a variable proportion of patients who underwent revascularisations when exertional ST-segment depression or angina was present, may have blunted the prognostic significance of exercise testing. Nevertheless, the strategy of using a positive exercise test or ST-segment depression at rest[74] as an indication for coronary angiography is recommended.

Electrophysiological test

Although an electrophysiological test has been regarded as the golden test for the prediction of ventricular tachyarrhythmias or SCD after MI, such a test has not gained universal popularity as a routine risk stratification tool. This is partly explained by conflicting results previously published on the use of a programmed stimulation test for this purpose. Furthermore, many clinicians are wary of using the provocative invasive test and are apprehensive about its safety. Finally, the proportion of at-risk patients was probably too low, suggesting that stratification on the basis of other risk factors could be used to reduce the proportion of infarct survivors requiring electrophysiological study.

Most studies on programmed stimulation test after MI were performed during the prethrombolytic era. The largest study was that performed by Bourke *et al.*[75] Among 3286 consecutive patients treated for AMI, an electrophysiological test was performed in 1209 survivors (37%) who were free of significant complications at the time of hospital discharge. Sustained monomorphic VT was inducible in only 75 (6.2%) of the patients. Antiarrhythmic therapy was not routinely prescribed regardless of the test results. During the first year of follow-up, significantly more patients (19%) among the infarct survivors with inducible VT experienced spontaneous VT or VF in the absence of new ischaemia than those without inducible VT (2.9%). During the extended follow-up period (median 28 months) of those with inducible ventricular tachycardia, 19 (25%) had a spontaneous electrical event; 37% of these first events were fatal. Thus, it is important to realise that the inducibility of ventricular tachyarrhythmias was low and the mortality among patients with an inducible ventricular tachyarrhythmias was variable. Although the sensitivity and specificity were acceptable, the positive predictive values vary substantially. Furthermore, thrombolysis has substantially reduced the incidence of inducible ventricular tachycardia in infarct survivors.[76] The role of the programmed stimulation test as a predictor of SCD in the general MI population remains unclear.

What is probably clear is that these results suggest that the most cost-effective strategy for predicting arrhythmia will be obtained by restricting electrophysiological testing to infarct survivors who have been preselected on the basis of other risk factors such as low LVEF, etc. Indeed, Pedretti and colleagues demonstrated that the combination of ≥2 variables among LVEF <40%, positive late potential, ≥2 runs of NSVT, and a subsequent positive programmed stimulation test selected a group of post-MI patients at sufficiently high risk with a event rate of 65%.[77] The combined use of non-invasive tests and a programmed stimulation test revealed a sensitivity of 81%, specificity of 97%, positive predictive accuracy of 65%, and negative predictive accuracy of 99%. This strategy is substantiated by the result of Multicenter Unsustained Tachycardia Trial.[78] In this study, high-risk coronary artery disease patients stratified with LVEF ≤40%, non-sustained VT, and an inducible electrophysiological test who received an implantable cardioverter-defibrillator had their risk of cardiac arrest or death from arrhythmia significantly reduced by 73%, compared to patients who did not receive any antiarrhythmics at all. Similarly, the Multicenter Automatic Defibrillator Implantation Trial (MADIT) showed that prophylactic therapy saves lives in high-risk post-MI patients with LVEF ≤35%, NSVT, inducible/non-suppressible ventricular tachycardia at electrophysiological study.[79] Indeed, the FDA has approved the used of ICD in MADIT-defined patients for the prevention of SCD. Thus, the results of this study reiterates the notion that a favourable effect on survival will depend on both the predictive power of the risk parameter itself or a combination of risk parameters as well as the efficacy of the intervention.

Newer variables

The values of newer variables such as QT dispersion, T wave alternans, or heart rate turbulence in the prediction of SCD after MI remains uncertain owing to a lack of large prospective data. In one prospective study, QT dispersion is not predictive of arrhythmic events after MI but this was disputed by others.[80,81]

Conclusion

The identification of patients without a previous spontaneous ventricular tachyarrhythmias or aborted SCD is difficult. Many non-invasive and invasive tests have been introduced to help stratify post-MI patients who are at high risk of sudden cardiac death. These tests remain useful even with contemporary MI treatment. They reflect different risk aspects for sudden cardiac death, including information on coronary anatomy, myocardial perfusion, arrhythmia substrate, myocardial pumping function, and neurohumoral balance. Unfortunately, all these tests have a high negative predictive value but a low positive predictive value when used alone. Although a combination of different tests will improve the predictive value of the test, the positive predictive value is rarely reaching more than 40%. Nevertheless, the results from study such as MUSTT and MADIT have shown that, despite the shortfall of these technologies, it is possible to stratify post-MI patients using a combination of non-invasive and invasive tests, and successfully reduces the risk of SCD with an implantable cardioverter-defibrillator. Data from other ongoing primary prevention studies will provide further insight into the efficacy of certain treatments on high-risk patients stratified using other risk markers. Accordingly, they are likely to change the management of post-MI patients in the primary prevention of arrhythmic or sudden cardiac deaths. Newer risk parameters continue to be introduced and may help further improve the identification of patients at high risk of sudden death.

References

1. Gillum RF. Sudden coronary death in the United States1980-1985. *Circulation* 1989;**79**:756–65.
2. National Center for Health Statistics. Advance report, final mortality statistics. *Monthly Vital Stat Rep 1081*;**33** (Suppl. DHHS):4–5.
3. Myerburg RJ, Castellanos A. Cardiac arrest and sudden cardiac death. In: Braunwald E, ed. *Heart disease, a textbook of cardiovascular disease*, 5th edn. Philadelphia: WB Saunders, pp. 742–79.
4. The Multicentre Postinfarction Research Group. Risk stratification and survival after myocardial infarction. *New Engl J Med* 1983;**309**:331–6.
5. Hennekens CH, O'Donnell CJ, Ridker PM, Marder VJ. Current issues concerning thrombolytic therapy for acute myocardial infarction. *J Am Coll Cardiol* 1995;**25**:18S–22S.

6. Stein PK, Bosner MS, Kleiger RE, Conger BM. Heart rate variability: a measure of cardiac autonomic tone. *Am Heart J* 1994;**127**:1376–81.

7. Schwartz PJ, Randall WC, Anderson EA *et al*. Sudden cardiac death. Nonpharmacologic interventions. *Circulation* 1987;**76**(Suppl. I):I215–19.

8. Malik M, Camm AJ. Components of heart rate variability-what they really mean and what we really measure. *Am J Cardiol* 1993;**72**:821–2.

9. Turner A, Malik M, Camm AJ. Autonomic function following myocardial infarction. *Br J Hosp Med* 1994;**51**:89–96.

10. Malliani A, Lombardi F, Pagani M. Power spectrum analysis of heart rate variability: a tool to explore neural regulatory mechanisms. *B Heart J* 1994;**71**:1–2.

11. Fetsch T, Reinhardt L, Makijarvi M *et al*. Heart rate variability in time domain after acute myocardial infarction. *Clin science* 1996;**91**(Suppl.):136–40.

12. Task Force of the European Society of Cardiology and the North American Society of Pacing and Electrophysiology. Heart rate variability: standard of measurement, physiological interpretation, and clinical use. *Circulation* 1996;**93**:1043–65.

13. Odemuyiwa O, Malik M, Farrell T, Bashir Y, Poloniecki J, Camm AJ. Comparison of the predictive characteristics of heart rate variability index and left ventricular ejection fraction for all-cause mortality, arrhythmic events and sudden death after acute myocardial infarction. *Am J Cardiol* 1991;**68**:434–9.

14. Hartikainen JEK, Malik M, Staunton A, Poloniecki J, Camm AJ. Distinction between arrhythmic and nonarrhythmic death after acute myocardial infarction based on heart rate variability, signal-averaged electrocardiogram, ventricular arrhythmias and left ventricular ejection fraction. *J Am Coll Cardiol* 1996;**28**:296–304.

15. Malik M, Camm AJ. Heart rate variability and clinical cardiology. *B Heart J* 1994;**71**:3–6.

16. Farrel TG, Bashir Y, Cripps T *et al*. Risk stratification for arrhythmic events in postinfarction patients based on heart rate variability, ambulatory electrocardiographic variables and the signal-averaged electrocardiogram. *J Am Coll Cardiol* 1991;**18**:687–97.

17. Zuanetti G, Neilson JMM, Latini R, Santoro E, Maggioni AP, Ewing DJ;on behalf of GISSI-2 investigators. Prognostic significance of heart rate variability in post-myocardial infarction patients in the fibrinolytic era. *Circulation* 1996;**94**:432–6.

18. Sandrone G, Mortara A, Torzillo D, La Rovere MT, Malliani A, Lombardi F. effects of beta blockers (atenolol or metoprolol) on heart rate variability after acute myocardial infarction. *Am J Cardiol* 1994;**74**:340–5.

19. La Rovere MT, Bigger JT, Marcus FI, Mortara A, Schwartz PJ, for the ATRAMI Investigators. Baroreflex sensitivity and heart rate variability in prediction of total cardiac mortality after myocardial infarction. *Lancet* 1998;**351**:478–84.

20. Huikuri HV, Makikallio TH, Peng C-K, Goldberger AL, Hintze U, Moller M, for the DIAMOND Grouo. Fractal correlation properties of the RR interval dynamics and mortality in patients with depressed left ventricular function after an acute myocardial infarction. *Circulation* 2000;**101**:47–53.

21. Camm AJ, Karam R, Pratt CM. The azimilide post-infarct survival evaluation (ALIVE) trial. *Am J Cardial* 1998;**81**:35D-9D.

22. La Rovere MT, Montara A, Schwartz PJ. Baroreflex sensitivity. *J Cardiovas Electrophysiol* 1995;**6**:761–74.

23. Smyth HS, Sleight P, Pickering GW. Reflex regulation of arterial pressure during sleep in man. A quantitative method for assessing baroreflex sensitivity. *Circ Res* 1969;**24**:109–21.

24. La Rovere MT, Specchia G, Mortara A, Schwartz PJ. Baroreflex sensitivity, clinical correlates and cardiovascular mortality among patients with a first myocardial infarction. A prospective study. *Circulation* 1988;**78**:816–24.

25. Farrell TG, Paul V, Cripps TR *et al*. Baroreflex sensitivity and electrophysiological correlates in patients after myocardial infarction. *Circulation* 1991;**83**:945–52.

26. Katsube Y, Saro H, Naka M *et al*. Baroreflex sensitivity in patients with stable coronary artery disease is correlated with the severity of arterial narrowing. *Am J Cardiol* 1996;**78**:1007–10.

27. Mortara A. Specchia G. La Rovere MT *et al*. Patency of infarct-related artery: effect of restoration of anterograde flow on vagal reflexes. ATRAMI (Automatic Tone and Reflexes After Myocardial Infarction) Investigators. *Circulation* 1996;**93**:1114–22.

28. Odemuyiwa O. Farrell T. Staunton A *et al*. Influence of thrombolytic therapy on the evolution of baroreflex sensitivity after myocardial infarction. *Am Heart J* 1993;**125**(2 Pt 1):285–91.

29. La Rovere MT, Mortara A, Bigger JT Jr *et al*. on behalf of the ATRAMI investigators: Effect of thrombolytic therapy on baroreceptors reflexes. *Eur Heart J* 1994;**15**(Abstr.):446.

30. Farrell T, Odemuyiwa O, Bashir Y *et al*. Prognostic value of baroreflex sensitivity testing after acute myocardial infarction. *Br Heart J* 1992;**67**:129–32.

31. La Rovere MT, Bigger JT Jr, Marcus FI *et al*. on behalf of the ATRAMI Investigators. Prognostic value of depressed baroreflex sensitivity. *Circulation* 1995;**9**(Abstr. Suppl. 1):2676.

32. Martinez-Rubio A, Borgrefe M, Fetsch T *et al*. Signal averaging. In: Julian DG, Camm AJ, Fox KM, Hall RJC, Poole-Wilson P eds. *Diseases of the heart*. London: WB Saunders, 1996, pp.228–41.

33. Steinberg JS, Regan A, Sciacca RR *et al*. Predicting arrhythmic events after acute myocardial infarction using the signal-averaged electrocardiogram. *Am J Cardiol* 1992;**69**:13–21.

34. Kuchar DL, Thorburn CW, Sammel NL. Late potentials detected after myocardial infarction: natural history and prognostic significance. *Circulation* 1986;**74**:1280–9.

35. Denniss AR, Richards DA, Cody DV *et al*. Prognostic significance of ventricular tachycardia and fibrillation induced at programmed stimulation and delayed potentials detected on the signal-averaged electrocardiograms of survivors of acute myocardial infarction. *Circulation* 1986;**74**:731–45.

36. El-Sherif N, Denes P, Katz R, Capone R, Mitchell LB, Carlson M, Reynolds-Haertle R. Definition of the best prediction criteria of the time domain signal-averaged electro-

cardiogram for serious arrhythmic events in the postinfarction period. The Cardiac Arrhythmia Suppression Trial/Signal-Averaged Electrocardiogram (CAST/SAECG) Substudy Investigators. *J Am Coll Cardiol* 1995;**25**:908–14.

37. Steinberg JS, Hochman JS, Morgan CD *et al*. Effects of thrombolytic therapy administered 6 to 24 hours after myocardial infarction on the signal-averaged ECG. Results of a multicenter randomized trial. LATE Ancillary Study Investigators. Late Assessment of Thrombolytic Efficacy. *Circulation* 1994;**90**:746–52.

38. Malik M, Kulakowski P, Odemuyiwa O *et al*. Effect of thrombolytic therapy on the predictive value of signal-averaged electrocardiography after acute myocardial infarction. *Am J Cardiol* 1992;**70**:21–5.

39. McClements BM, Adgey AA. Value of signal-averaged electrocardiography, radionuclide ventriculography, Holter monitoring and clinical variables for prediction of arrhythmic events in survivors of acute myocardial infarction in the thrombolytic era. *J Am Coll Cardiol* 1993;**21**:1419–27.

40. McClements BM, Adgey AA. Value of signal-averaged electrocardiography, radionuclide ventriculography, Holter monitoring and clinical variables for prediction of arrhythmic events in survivors of acute myocardial infarction in the thrombolytic era. *J Am Coll Cardiol* 1993;**21**:1419–27.

41. Hermosillo AS, Araya V, Casanova JM. Risk stratification for malignant arrhythmic events in patients with an acute myocardial infarction: role of an open infarct-related artery and the signal-averaged ECG. *Cor Artery Dis* 1995;**6**:973–83.

42. Malik M, Kulakowski P, Poloneicki J *et al*. Frequency versus time domain analysis of signal-averaged electrocardiograms I. Reproducibility of the results. *J Am Coll Cardiol* 1992;**20**:127–34.

43. Kulakowski P, Malik M, Poloniecki J *et al*. Frequency versus time domain analysis of signal-averaged electrocardiogram II. Identification of patients with ventricular tachycardia after myocardial infarction. *J Am Coll Cardiol* 1992;**20**:135–43.

44. Odemuyiwa O, Malik M, Poloniecki J *et al*. Frequency versus time domain analysis of signal-averaged electrocardiogram. III. Stratification of postinfarction patients for arrhythmic events. *J Am Coll Cardiol* 1992;**20**:144–50.

45. Malik M. Kulakowski P. Hnatkova K. Staunton A. Camm AJ. Spectral turbulence analysis versus time-domain analysis of the signal-averaged ECG in survivors of acute myocardial infarction. *J Electrocardiol* 1994;**27**(Suppl.):227–32.

46. Nogami A, Iesaka Y, Akiyama J *et al*. Combined use of time and frequency domain variables in signal-averaged ECG as a predictor of inducible sustained monomorphic ventricular tachycardia in myocardial infarction. *Circulation* 1992;**86**:781–9.

47. Bloomfield DM, Snyder JE, Steinberg JS. A critical appraisal of quantitative spectro-temporal analysis of the signal-averaged ECG: predicting arrhythmic events after myocardial infarction. *PACE* 1996;**19**:768–77.

48. The Multicenter Postinfarction Research Group. Risk stratification and survival after myocardial infarction. *New Engl J Med* 1983;**309**:331–6.

49. Bigger JT, Fleiss JL, Kleiger R, Miller JP, Rolnitzky LM, the Multicenter Post-infarction Research Group. The relationships among ventricular arrhythmias, left ventricular dysfunction, and mortality in the 2 years after myocardial infarction. *Circulation* 1984;**69**:250–8.

50. Mukharji J, Rude RE, Poole WK *et al.*, the MILIS Study Group. Risk factors for sudden death after acute myocardial infarction: two-year follow-up. *Am J Cardiol* 1984;**54**:31–6.

51. Kuchar DL, Thorburn CW, Sammel NL. Prediction of serious arrhythmic events after myocardial infarction: signal-averaged electrocardiogram, Holter monitoring and radionuclide ventriculography. *J Am Coll Cardiol* 1987;**9**:531–8.

52. Bearning J, Hoilund-Carlsen PF, Gadsboll N, Nielsen GG, Marving J. Early risk stratification in acute myocardial infarction by echocardiographic characterisation of left ventricular wall motion profiles (EKKAMI). *Am J Cardiol* 1990;**65**: 567–76.

53. Zaret BL, Wackers FJ, Terrin ML, *et al*. Value of radionuclide rest and exercise left ventricular ejection fraction in assessing survival of patients after thrombolytic therapy for acute myocardial infarction: results of Thrombolysis in Myocardial Infarction (TIMI) phase II study. The TIMI Study Group. *JAMA* 1995;**26**:73–9.

54. Copie X, Hnatkova K, Staunton A, Fei L, Camm AJ, Malik M. Predictive power of increased heart rate versus depressed left ventricular ejection fraction and heart rate variability for risk stratification after myocardial infarction. Results of a two-year follow-up study. *J Am Coll Cardiol* 1996;**27**:270–6.

55. Hallstrom A, Pratt CM, Greene HL *et al*. Relations between heart failure, ejection fraction, arrhythmia suppression and mortality: analysis of the Cardiac Arrhythmia Suppression Trial. *J Am Coll Cardiol* 1995;**25**:1250–7.

56. Stevenson WG, Ridker PM. Should survivors of myocardial infarction with low ejection fraction be routinely referred to arrhythmia specialists. *JAMA* 1996;**276**:481–5.

57. Ruberman W, Weinblatt E, Goldberg JD, Frank CW, Shapiro S. Ventricular premature beats and mortality after myocardial infarction. *New Engl J Med* 1977;**297**:750.

58. The Coronary Drug Project Research Group. Prognostic importance of premature beats following myocardial infarction: experience in the Coronary Drug Project. *JAMA* 1973;**223**:1116.

59. Statters DJ, Malik M, Redwood S, Hnatkova K, Staunton A, Camm AJ. Use of ventricular premature complexes for risk stratification after acute myocardial infarction in the thrombolytic era. *Am J Cardiol* 1996;**77**:133–8.

60. Maggioni AP, Zuanetti G, Franzosi G *et al*. on behalf of GISSI-2 Investigators. Prevalence and prognostic significance of ventricular arrhythmias after acute myocardial infarction in the fibrinolytic era. GISSI-2 results. *Circulation* 1993;**87**:312–22.

61. Ruberman W, Weinblatt E, Goldberg JD, Frank CW, Chaudhary BS, Shapiro S. Ventricular premature complexes and sudden death after myocardial infarction. *Circulation* 1981;**64**:297–305.

62. Moss AJ, Davis HT, DeCamilla J, Bayer LW. Ventricular ectopic beats and their relation to sudden and non-sudden

cardiac death after myocardial infarction. *Circulation* 1979;**60**:998–1003.

63. Kostis JB, Byington R, Friedman LM, Goldstein S, Furberg C, for the BHAT Study Group. Prognostic significance of ventricular ectopic activity in survivors of acute myocardial infarction. *J Am Coll Cardiol* 1987;**10**:231–42.

64. Echt DS, Liebson PR, Mitchell LB *et al.* and the CAST investigators. Mortality and morbidity in patients receiving encanide, flecainide, or placebo; the Cardiac Arrhythmia Suppression Trial. *New Engl J Med* 1991;**324**:781–8.

65. The Cardiac Arrhythmia Suppression Trial II Investigators. Effect of the anti-arrhythmic agent moricizine on survival after myocardial infarction. *New Engl J Med* 1992;**327**:227–33.

66. Lazzara R. From first class to third class: recent upheaval in antiarrhythmic therapy – lesson from clinical trials. *Am J Cardiol* 1996;**78**(4A):28–33.

67. Hohnloser SH, Klingenheben T, Zabel M, Schopperl M, Mauss O. Prevalence, characteristics and prognostic value during long-term follow-up of nonsustained ventricular tachycardia after myocardial infarction in the thrombolytic era. *J Am Coll Cardiol* 1999;**33**:1895–902.

68. Hohnloser SH, Franck P, Klingenheben T, Zabel M, Just H. Open infarct artery, late potentials and other prognostic factors in patients after acute myocardial infarction in the thrombolytic era. A prospective study. *Circulation* 1994;**90**:1747–56.

69. Hermosillo AS, Araya V, Casanova JM. Risk stratification for malignant arrhythmic events in patients with an acute myocardial infarction: role of an open infarct-related artery and the signal-averaged ECG. *Coron Art Dis* 1995;**6**:973–83.

70. The TIMI Group. Comparison of invasive and conservative strategies after treatment with intravenous tissue plasminogen activator in acute myocardial infarction (TIMI) phase II trial. *New Engl J Med* 1989;**320**:618–27.

71. Volpi A, De Vita C, Franzosi MG *et al.* Determinants of mortality in survivors of myocardial infarction after thrombolysis. Result from the GISSI-2 database. *Circulation* 1993;**88**:416–29.

72. Froelicher VF, Perdue S, Pewen W *et al.* Application of meta-analysis using an electronic spread sheet to exercise testing in patients after myocardial infarction. *Am J Med* 1987;**83**:1045–54.

73. Chaitman BR, McMahon RP, Terrin M *et al.* Impact of treatment strategy on predischarge exercise test in the Thrombolysis in Myocardial Infarction (TIMI) II Trial. *Am J Cardiol* 1993;**71**:131–8.

74. Moss AJ, Goldstein RE, Hall WJ *et al.* Detection and significance of myocardial ischemia in stable patients after recovery from an acute coronary event. Multicenter Myocardial Ischemia Research Group. *JAMA* 1993;**269**:2379–85.

75. Bourke JP, Richards DAB, Ross DL, Wallace EM, McGuire MA, Uther JB. Routine programmed electrical stimulation in survivors of acute myocardial infarction for the prediction of spontaneous ventricular tachyarrhythmias during follow-up: results, optimal stimulation protocol and cost-effective screening. *J Am Coll Cardiol* 1991;**18**:780–8.

76. Bourke JP, Young AA, Richards DAB, Uther JB. Reduction of incidence of inducible ventricular tachycardia after myocardial infarction by treatment with streptokinase during infarct evolution. *J Am Coll Cardiol* 1990;**16**:1703–10.

77. Pedrettii R, Etro MD, Laporta A, Braga SS, Caru B. Prediction of late arrhythmic events after acute myocardial infarction from combined use of noninvasive prognostic variables and inducibility of sustained monomorphic ventricular tachycardia. *Am J Cardiol* 1993;**71**:1131–41.

78. Buxton AE, Lee KL, Fisher JD, Josephson ME, Prystowsky EN, Hafley G for the Multicenter Unsustained Tachycardia Trial Investigators. *New Engl J Med* 1999;**341**:1881–90.

79. Moss AJ, Hall WJ, Cannom DS *et al.* and the MADIT Investigators. Improved survival with an implanted defibrillator in patients with coronary disease at high risk for ventricular arrhythmias. *New Engl J Med* 1996;**335**:1933–40.

80. Zabel M, Klingenheben T, Franz MR, Hohnloser SH. Assessment of QT dispersion for prediction of mortality or arrhythmic events after myocardial infarction: results of a prospective, long-term follow-up study. *Circulation* 1998;**97**:2543–50.

81. Yap YG, Yi G, Goa X-H, Aytemir K, Camm AJ, Malik M. Fluctuation of QT dispersion and the optimal timing for its measurement for correlation with arrhythmic events after acute myocardial infarction. *PACE* 1999;**22**(6)(II): A38.

28 Ventricular arrhythmias in chronic heart failure

Steven Lindsay and Jim Nolan

Chronic heart failure is the only major cardiovascular disorder that is increasing in incidence and prevalence in the developed world, and it is a major cause of morbidity and mortality. Even in patients with mild symptoms, the average annual mortality approaches 10%.[1] Heart failure has major socioeconomic impact costing an estimated $20–40 billion a year in the USA[2] and £1 million a day in the United Kingdom.[3] Ventricular arrhythmias are commonly observed in patients with heart failure and many patients with heart failure will die suddenly from presumed ventricular arrhythmias. There is conflicting data relating ventricular arrhythmias to prognosis in heart failure and it has been argued that such arrhythmias are a marker of a dying heart rather than a substrate for the terminal event.[4] In part this conflict may relate to the heterogeneous nature of the populations studied. Dilated cardiomyopathy (DCM) is defined as ventricular dilatation with reduced systolic function. The clinical syndrome of heart failure may or may not be present. Although ventricular dilatation is a common manifestation of many diseases that affect the myocardium, the term "dilated cardiomyopathy" usually excludes ischaemic cardiomyopathy, the commonest aetiology of heart failure in contemporary practice. Whilst there is an extensive list of toxic, metabolic and inflammatory conditions known to cause DCM,[5] in most series of non-ischaemic DCM 40–50% are idiopathic, although this clearly varies depending on how thoroughly the patient is assessed. The age adjusted prevalence of idiopathic DCM in the USA averages 36/100 000[6] with 10 000 deaths annually.[7]

In this review we will discuss ventricular arrhythmias occurring in the setting of heart failure. However, it should be borne in mind that patients with ischaemic cardiomyopathy may differ from those with global ventricular pathology, and arrhythmias may have a different significance in these patients.

Pathophysiology

In the failing heart a variety of extrinsic factors and cellular substrates facilitate the genesis of arrhythmias. These may conspire together to account for the frequency with which ventricular arrhythmias are seen in this condition.

Mechanisms of arrhythmias

After depolarisations and triggered activity

Oscillations in the membrane potentials following the upstroke of the action potential, known as after depolarisations, can induce triggered rhythms.[8] Failing myocardium has a greater propensity to develop after depolarisations. For example, myocardium from failing rabbit hearts develops more delayed after depolarisations and triggered activity than control hearts when exposed to an extracellular solution low in potassium and magnesium and high in norepinephrine.[9] Human myocardium from explanted failing hearts behaves similarly.[9] Action potential prolongation favours the development of early after-depolarisations.[8] In heart failure this may be a consequence of changes in various transmembrane currents (inward rectifier [Iki], transient outward [Ito], and delayed rectifier [Ik]).[10] Other causes of action potential prolongation in heart failure include decreased activity of the ATP dependent Na/K pump[11] and intracellular calcium overload which may cause spontaneous calcium leakage and delayed after depolarisations.[12]

Automaticity

Automaticity arises when a gradually decreasing membrane potential reaches threshold. This is the mechanism of normal cardiac pacemaker activity in the specialised conducting tissues. It also occurs in failing myocardium,[13] although not at a sufficient rate to explain the arrhythmias seen in clinical practice.[9] Changes in the inward rectifying current and the occurrence of a pacemaker current at less negative potentials than normal have been seen in failing ventricular cells.[10]

Re-entry

Re-entry is established as an important mechanism for sustained arrhythmias in patients with myocardial infarction.[14] Not all of these patients had heart failure and other mechanisms may predominate in patients with non-ischaemic cardiomyopathy.[15] Studies in patients undergoing arrhythmia surgery reveal that focal mechanisms may play a role in sustained arrhythmias,[16] although the resolution of these mapping studies does not exclude micro-re-entry as the mechanism for apparently focal arrhythmias.

Slow conduction, short refractory periods, large dispersion of refractory periods, and the presence of unidirectional block favour re-entry. In the failing myocardium a variety of mechanisms may interact to facilitate re-entry. Increased preload, for example, shortens action potential duration and refractory period more than in the normal heart.[17] Intramyocardial fibrosis occurs in heart failure without myocardial infarction[18–20] and provides a substrate for unidirectional block. In perfused papillary muscles from failing rabbit hearts, acute global ischaemia produced more pronounced action potential shortening and a decrease in conduction velocity when compared to control hearts.[21] Thus the patient with ischaemic heart disease and heart failure may be at even greater risk of arrhythmia in the event of acute ischaemia.

Modulating factors

In heart failure important changes in homeostatic mechanisms occur that have the potential to facilitate the onset and maintenance of arrhythmias in interaction with the cellular phenomena noted above.

Autonomic dysfunction

Overactivity of the sympathetic nervous system is a feature of the failing heart manifested by elevated circulating catecholamine levels, reduced myocardial norepinephrine content, and decreased beta receptor density.[22] The changes in beta receptors and neuronal dysfunction are heterogeneous through the myocardium.[23] A correlation between reduced neuronal norepinephrine stores and prolonged refractoriness might explain dispersion of refractoriness that could facilitate re-entry.[24] The prognostic significance of these abnormalities is supported by the dramatic benefits of beta-blockade in recent clinical trials of these drugs in heart failure.[25,26] In addition to sympathetic overactivity there is attenuation of parasympathetic activity. In animal models vagal stimulation protects from ventricular fibrillation (VF).[27,28]

Electrolyte abnormalities

Abnormalities of serum electrolytes are common in heart failure, in part a consequence of diuretic therapy. Hypokalaemia and hyponatraemia predict outcome in heart failure,[29] and hypomagnesaemia often accompanies hypokalaemia and may contribute to arrhythmic risk.[30] Recent data show an increased risk of arrhythmic death from diuretic therapy used in the absence of potassium sparing agents.[31]

Stretch

Acute myocyte stretch can generate arrhythmias via after depolarisations,[32] increase the rate of discharge of Purkinje fibres, and initiate pacemaker activity in other myocardial cells.[33] The failing heart is more susceptible to stretch induced arrhythmias[34] and changes in preload and after-load shorten repolarisation in failing ventricles and increase arrhythmia inducibility.[17]

Prevalence of ventricular arrhythmias in heart failure

Given the above it is no surprise that ventricular arrhythmias are common in patients with heart failure. Their frequency depends on the arrhythmia classification used, the severity of heart failure in the population studied and the method used to look for them. Keogh observed couplets or triplets in 39% and non-sustained ventricular tachycardia (VT) in 41% of 137 patients referred for transplant assessment.[35] Cohn found either frequent couplets or non-sustained VT in 60% of patients in the Ve-HEFT studies.[36] In our own series with 24-h Holter monitoring, we found frequent VPBs (>10/h) in 53% and non-sustained VT in 40% of 417 patients with mild to moderate heart failure, mean EF $42 \pm 17\%$.[37] In the CHF STAT study patients were required to have at least 10 VPB/h prior to entry. Over 80% of these had non-sustained VT on Holter monitoring. In all these studies the populations were heterogeneous with both ischaemic and non-ischaemic aetiologies, although the incidence of ventricular arrhythmias was not influenced by aetiology. In the majority of cases these arrhythmias are unnoticed by the patient.

Sustained ventricular arrhythmias, on the other hand, may present clinically. In a consecutive series of 103 patients with DCM, 11 had a prior history of sustained VT.[38] Mancini reported 10 of 114 patients[39] and Denearez 10 of 51 patients.[40] In these series recurrent sustained ventricular arrhythmias occurred in between 3% and 7% of patients during follow-up periods of around 18 months. In addition there was an incidence of sudden death of up to 8%. It is presumed that the majority of these deaths are due to ventricular arrhythmias, although this assumption has been challenged. The advent of implantable cardiac defibrillators (ICD) with the capacity to store RR intervals or intra-cardiac electrograms has permitted a prospective estimation of the frequency of life-threatening arrhythmias in these high-risk patients. In several studies the incidence of appropriate defibrillator therapy at between two and three years is up to 50%.[41–43] Many of these events would have been deaths had it not been for the defibrillator. This indicates a higher recurrent VT rate than the combination of VT and sudden death reported in the earlier series. However, it must be remembered that most of the patients in the defibrillator studies had a prior history of a clinical arrhythmic event (VT or resuscitated sudden death) and would be expected to be at higher risk for recurrent events.

Correlation of ventricular arrhythmias and ventricular dysfunction

The frequency of ventricular arrhythmias increases with increasing severity of heart failure. Thus 10% of patients with NYHA I heart failure have non-sustained VT on Holter monitoring compared with 70% of NYHA IV patients.[44] We have found similar results in our own series (Fig. 28.1). In the SOLVD database significant relations were found between the frequency of non-sustained VT and left ventricular end-diastolic and end-systolic volumes and left ventricular mass (Fig. 28.2) but not with ejection fraction, wall stress, or wall motion index.[45] This analysis was confined to patients with an ejection fraction <35%. In our own database of heart failure patients with a wide range of ejection fraction, frequency of VPBs was correlated with ejection fraction (Spearman rank correlation coefficient 0.227 P <0.001, UK HEART unpublished observation).

Sudden death in heart failure

Death can be classified as cardiac or non-cardiac and cardiac death further classified as sudden, presumed arrhyth-

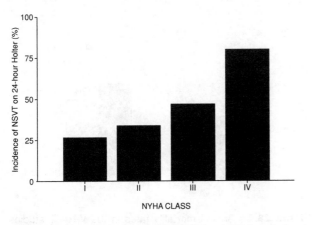

Figure 28.1 Incidence of non-sustained VT in relation to NYHA class in the UK HEART study.[29]

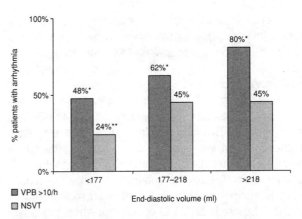

Figure 28.2 Prevalence of ventricular premature beat (VPBs) frequency >10/h and non-sustained VT (NSVT) across tertiles of left ventricular end-diastolic volume. (*P <0.001 versus other two tertiles, ** P = 0.007 versus highest two tertiles.) (Adapted from reference 45.)

mic death, death due to pump failure or progressive heart failure, or death due to myocardial infarction. Sudden death is variably defined as witnessed instantaneous death, death during sleep, death within 1 hour of symptom onset, etc. The incidence of VT and VF as the fatal arrhythmia in patients wearing Holter monitors at the time of death was about 80%.[46,47] Many of these patients had an indication for Holter monitoring and the incidence of fatal ventricular arrhythmias among these patients may be higher than in other groups.

Ultimately all death is sudden, the patient with pump failure may well collapse and die from a fatal arrhythmia, and the substrate for a fatal arrhythmia in a patient with ischaemic cardiomyopathy may be an acute ischaemic event. The latter case may be classified as death from myocardial infarction if the patient presents to medical services before death, or sudden death if found dead in bed the following morning. Pratt demonstrated the difficulties of the classification of sudden death.[48] In 17 patients dying with ICDs and a clinical classification of sudden cardiac death, autopsy found non-arrhythmic causes of sudden cardiac death in seven (myocardial infarction, pulmonary embolism, cerebral infarction, ruptured thoracic and abdominal aortic aneurysms), whilst defibrillator interrogation revealed evidence of discharge in only seven. The situation may be more difficult in a heart failure population. In stable patients with severe heart failure hospitalised for transplant assessment, only 38% of cardiac arrests were due to VT or VF. In the remainder, the rhythm was bradycardia or electromechanical dissociation. No patient with a non-ischaemic cardiomyopathy had a ventricular arrhythmic arrest.[49]

In heart failure the risk of death increases with increasing severity of heart failure. For example, in the V-HeFT studies, mortality among patients with peak oxygen consumption ≤14.5 ml/kg/min was 46% compared to 30% among those with peak oxygen consumption >14.5 ml/kg/min during an average follow-up of 2.3 years.[50] Aetiology did not influence mortality, which was about 36% in patients with coronary disease and 38% in those without. The mortality from DCM in some series reaches 30% at 1 year and 50% at 5 years,[51,52] although in more recent series the 5-year survival is closer to 80%.[53–56] In mild heart failure the commonest cause of cardiac death is sudden death, 50–70% of deaths compared to 10–30% of those in NYHA III or IV[26,44] in whom pump failure is the dominant mechanism (Fig. 28.3). In a review of 15 series of patients with idiopathic DCM, 12% died suddenly (range 8–51%) and sudden death accounted for 28% of all deaths.[5] Again, in the V-HeFT studies there was no evidence that the incidence of sudden death differed between those with and without coronary disease (34.8% compared with 38.5% in V-HeFT II).[50]

Notwithstanding the difficulties of the definition of mechanism of death, many patients with heart failure die suddenly. The Holter studies reveal that fatal VT or VF was often preceded by periods of increasingly frequent ventricular ectopic activity.[46,47] Interest in the prognostic significance of ventricular arrhythmias arises from this presumed relation to the risk of sudden death.

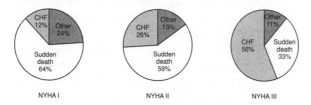

Figure 28.3 Severity of heart failure and mode of death. (Adapted from reference 26.)

Asymptomatic ventricular arrhythmias and prognosis in heart failure

Targeting therapeutic interventions at high-risk groups offers the possibility of maximally effective use of therapies, both pharmaceutical and otherwise, while avoiding unnecessary treatment of lower risk groups. The advent of the ICD mandates the identification of patients at particular risk of arrhythmic sudden death. If asymptomatic ventricular arrhythmias are common in heart failure and more so in severe heart failure and sudden death is due to sustained ventricular arrhythmias in at least some cases, then it is reasonable to ask if the presence of ventricular arrhythmias predict outcome.

All-cause mortality

It is clear that the presence of frequent VPBs or non-sustained VT is associated with an increase in total mortality. Early reviews of the subject in mixed populations found conflicting data[57] with some studies showing a relation between arrhythmias and mortality[58–61] while others did not.[62–64] Analyses from large heart failure populations clearly demonstrate the relation between measures of ventricular arrhythmia and total mortality. In the V-HeFT studies ventricular arrhythmias (couplets or non-sustained VT) were not an independent predictor of all-cause mortality in V-HeFT I but were in V-HeFT II.[36] The presence of non-sustained VT approximately doubled the risk of death (RR 2.06, 95% CI 1.34–3.16, Fig. 28.4).[1] Frequent VPB (>10/h) did not relate to mortality in these studies. In the CHF STAT study, a randomised trial of amiodarone in 666 patients with heart failure and frequent VPBs, non-sustained VT was found in 80% of patients.[65] Although associated with an increased mortality on univariate analysis in a multivariate model, including ejection fraction, NYHA class, diuretic use, type of cardiomyopathy, ventricular dimensions, frequency of VPBs, and use of beta-blockers or amiodarone, only ejection fraction and NYHA class were independent predictors of all-cause mortality.

In another randomised trial of amiodarone in heart failure (GESICA-GEMA), non-sustained VT was an independent predictor of total mortality (RR 1.62 95% CI 1.22–2.16).[66] When aetiology was considered, the presence of non-sustained VT remained a significant predictor total of mortality in patients with non-ischaemic cardiomyopathy and this risk was not significantly different from patients with ischaemic cardiomyopathy. However, there are some problems with this data. Randomisation was stratified so that one-third of patients had non-sustained VT, patients with sustained arrhythmias or with asymptomatic VT of >10 beats in duration were excluded, and 9%

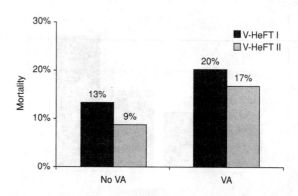

Figure 28.4 Annual mortality rates in the V-HeFT studies for patients with and without ventricular arrhythmias (VA). (Adapted from reference 36.)

of patients had Chagas' disease. This was an independent predictor of the presence of non-sustained VT and could have some influence on the significance of the result, although type of cardiomyopathy was included in the multivariate model. In the PROMISE study, a trial of the inotrope milrinone in over 1000 patients with NYHA grade III or IV heart failure and an ejection fraction <35%, a variety of markers of ventricular arrhythmia on ambulatory monitoring proved to be independent predictors of total mortality.[67]

Sudden death mortality

The early studies generated the same conflicting messages concerning the association between ventricular arrhythmias and mode of death as they did for all-cause mortality, but none of them was large enough to reliably demonstrate any relation between ventricular arrhythmias and cause of death. In the V-HeFT cohorts, the presence of pairs or non-sustained VT were not associated with an increased risk of sudden death.[50] In CHF-STAT ventricular arrhythmias were only univariate predictors of an increased risk of sudden death.[65] In contrast in the GESICA-GEMA study most of the mortality risk associated with non-sustained VT was due to the risk of sudden death (RR 2.77, 95% CI 1.78–4.44) and this was independent of other factors.[66] The PROMISE study confirmed the independent predictive value of ventricular arrhythmias on ambulatory monitoring for risk of sudden death. Frequent VPBs (>30/h) and non-sustained VT (≥3 beats at >100/min) were predictive of sudden death and retained their predictive value in a multivariate model which included age, NYHA class, aetiology, ejection fraction systolic blood pressure, and trial therapy.[67]

These studies generally included patients with more severe heart failure. The mean ejection fraction in V-HeFT was about 30%,[36] in CHF STAT it was nearer 25%,[65] in PROMISE 20%,[67] and in GESICA-GEMA less than 20%.[66] In contrast in our own study (UK HEART) with a mean ejection fraction close to 40% we found non-sustained VT to be an independent predictor of sudden death risk but not all-cause mortality.[29] The other independent predictors of risk of sudden death were left ventricular end-diastolic dimension, cardiothoracic ratio and serum potassium but non-sustained VT had the highest risk ratio at 3.71 (95% CI 1.23–11.22). This is an interesting observation in that it suggests that among patients with milder heart failure ambulatory monitoring may be more useful in identifying patients at greater risk of sudden death than it is in more advanced heart failure. Paradoxically in our study only 33% of deaths were classified as sudden, lower than one might expect. It should also be noted that the majority of our patients had ischaemic cardiomyopathy (76%).

Arrhythmia classification and prognosis

Ventricular arrhythmias on ambulatory monitoring range in severity from isolated and infrequent ventricular ectopics to sustained VT. The modified Lown classification consists of grade I: uniform ventricular ectopics ≤30/h; grade II: >30 VPBs/h; grade III: multiform VPBs; grade IV: couplets, and grade V: R on T ectopics.[68] Non-sustained VT is usually considered to be present when there are three or more ventricular beats in succession with a rate >100/min without haemodynamic instability and <30 s duration (1 min in some cases). Some classify three beats as a triplet and non-sustained VT as more than three beats. It might be suspected that higher grades of arrhythmia are more important, and this is borne out in some of the studies above where non-sustained VT was related to outcome, while frequent VPBs were not. Relatively few studies have considered whether frequency, duration, or rate of non-sustained VT are important.

Doval reported the results of quantitative Holter analysis in 295 patients in GESICA.[66] The number of VPBs or episodes of non-sustained VT did not correlate with mortality. Frequent VPBs (>10/h) or non-sustained VT ≥4 beats were univariate predictors only. Combining the presence of couplets and/or non-sustained VT gave a group with a higher risk ratio (2.2, 95% CI 1.45–3.34 for total mortality and 5.3, 95% CI 2.09–13.4 for sudden death). However, on multivariate analysis only the combined variable was an independent predictor with a risk ratio for sudden death of 10.1 but with 95% CI of 1.91–52.7. In CHF STAT there were no differences in total or sudden death mortality between patients with fast (>120/min) or long (>15 beats/min) non-sustained VT.[65] Teerlink reported the most detailed study of ventricular arrhythmia characteristics and mortality in heart failure.[67] Here frequent VPBs (>30/h), couplets, non-sustained VT, >5 episodes of non-sustained VT, and non-sustained VT >10 beats were all considered alongside clinical predictors of outcome in the PROMISE trial. All ambulatory ECG variables were related to total mortality and sudden death. On multivariate analysis each variable on its own remained independent of clinical variables. The frequency of non-sustained VT was the most powerful Holter variable with a risk ratio of 1.16 (95% CI 1.09–1.24) for sudden death. However, non-sustained VT frequency was not a specific predictor of sudden death as the receiver operator curve shows (Fig. 28.5). A model based on the clinical variables identified 67% of sudden deaths but with a false positive rate of over 80%. The addition of the Holter data did not substantially alter this.

The above studies did not specifically address the issue of aetiology of heart failure, although the inclusion of aetiology in multivariate analysis controls for this to an extent. Reese investigated 122 patients, 51 with ischaemic

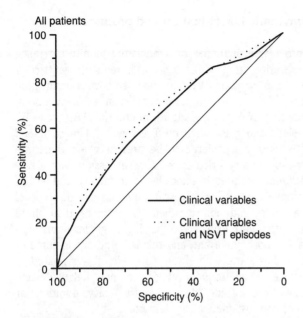

Figure 28.5 Receiver operator curves of sensitivity and specificity of multivariate models including only clinical variables and of clinical variables and NSVT episodes in predicting sudden death in the PROMISE study.[67]

cardiomyopathy and 71 with non-ischaemic heart failure.[69] The presence of non-sustained VT did not predict total mortality in patients with non-ischaemic cardiomyopathy whereas the length of non-sustained VT did. Patients with ≥4 beats of non-sustained VT had a 2–year mortality of 41% compared with 16% for those with <4 beats.

Electrophysiology studies and prognosis in heart failure

Invasive evaluation of ventricular arrhythmias by electrophysiological studies (EPS) can identify patients with life-threatening arrhythmias, such as inducible VT. Turitto reported the outcome of programmed ventricular stimulation in 80 patients with non-sustained VT and idiopathic DCM, 25% with syncope or presyncope, but none with documented sustained ventricular arrhythmia.[70] Inducible VT occurred in 10 patients (13%) and these were all treated with amiodarone. During mean follow-up of 22 months three died suddenly or had a sustained arrhythmia (30%) compared with six of 70 patients without inducible VT (8.5%). There was a trend towards better 2-year arrhythmia-free survival in the group without inducible VT (87% compared with 75%) but this was not significant.

In a prospective and consecutive series of EPS in 103 patients with DCM, 11 patients had prior sustained ven-

tricular arrhythmias of whom eight had inducible VT.[38] Thirty-six had no or infrequent ventricular arrhythmias (VPBs ≤30/h) and none of these had inducible VT. Fifty-six had frequent VPBs of whom 42 had non-sustained VT. Eight of these had inducible ventricular arrhythmias. There were five recurrent events in the spontaneous VT group, four of whom had inducible VT, only one of which had been suppressed by drug therapy. One patient died among those with infrequent VPBs and 14 died among those with frequent VPBs. Three died suddenly, all had inducible VT that was not suppressed by drug therapy. Patients who had sustained VT at follow-up had inducible VT. Serial EPS revealed suppression of induced VT in eight of 16 patients and only one of these died suddenly. In the remaining eight patients VT was always induced and six of these died suddenly and one had recurrent VT.

Even in patients with spontaneous VT up to a third do not have an inducible arrhythmia.[71–74] In a pooled analysis of six studies, including patients without spontaneous VT, 11% of 288 patients had inducible VT.[75] The 2-year risk of sudden death or sustained ventricular arrhythmia was 32% compared with 9% for those without an inducible arrhythmia ($P = 0.004$) but 75% of all deaths occurred in those who were not inducible. Hernandez reported an annual sudden death rate of 17% in patients with ventricular dysfunction due to IHD, non-sustained VT, and a negative EPS. All patients with events had clinical heart failure. This failure of EPS to identify at risk groups is further emphasised by data from Knight *et al.* who described their experience with 14 ICD patients with DCM, unexplained syncope, and a negative EP study.[42] Half of these patients received appropriate shocks for VT during a follow-up of 24 ± 13 months.

Thus while patients whose arrhythmias are suppressed during EPS-guided drug therapy fared better in some studies[38,72,76,77] this was not the case in all[70,71] Rates of suppression vary from 20–70%,[71,72,76–79] and pro-arrhythmic effects are a particular hazard during serial drug testing in patients with impaired ventricular function.[79] There is a paucity of data comparing ambulatory electrocardiographic monitoring with EPS in DCM. In the ESVEM study, data from the intention-to-treat analysis suggested that survival was better in patients with non-ischaemic disease when ambulatory ECG monitoring was used to assess efficacy rather than EPS.[80]

In summary therefore inducible ventricular arrhythmias do identify a group at increased risk of arrhythmic events and sudden death but the majority of these events occur in patients with negative EP studies. In DCM the most potent determinants of both total mortality and sudden death remain the degree of ventricular dysfunction, whether assessed by objective indices or functional class.[81]

Ambulatory ECG monitoring for risk stratification in heart failure

In addition to arrhythmias, ambulatory ECG monitoring can be used to evaluate autonomic dysfunction as assessed by heart rate variability, which may surpass arrhythmia data in identification of at risk patients.[29,82] Research continues on other variables such as 24-hour QT variability. A limitation of heart rate variability analysis is the influence that frequent ventricular ectopics may have on the analysis. Time domain analysis of heart rate variability from 24-h Holter is relatively simple but a proportion of tapes will be unsuitable for analysis because of frequent arrhythmias. In UK HEART we investigated this in 417 patients with no prior history of arrhythmias and not on antiarrhythmic therapy.[37] All of these patients were in sinus rhythm at the time of recruitment. The frequency of arrhythmias and of failure to analyse heart rate variability because of arrhythmias is given in Table 28.1. Atrial arrhythmias whilst more common did not carry an increased risk of mortality while ventricular arrhythmias preventing heart rate variability analysis were independent predictors of all-cause mortality along with NYHA class, cardiothoracic ratio, serum sodium and urea (Fig. 28.6). Thus the ambulatory electrocardiogram is a useful and simple means of identifying patients with heart failure at increased risk of death.

Table 28.1 The prevalence of supraventricular and ventricular arrhythmias and inability to analyse 24-h tapes in the UK HEART study[37]

Rhythm	N (%)
Atrial fibrillation	9 (2.4)
Supraventricular tachycardia	74 (18.2)
VPB >10/h	217 (53.3)
NSVT	161 (39.6)
Unanalysed tape	51 (12.2)
atrial arrhythmias	37 (8.8)
ventricular arrhythmias	14 (3.4)

Abbreviation: NSVT = non-sustained ventricular tachycardia.

Therapeutic interventions in patients with ventricular arrhythmias and heart failure

Antiarrhythmic therapy

Antiarrhythmic therapy has proved disappointing in the management of patients with heart failure. In the CAST study of patients with a history of myocardial infarction class I agents were associated with an increased risk of death in spite of successful suppression of ventricular

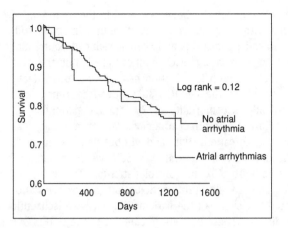

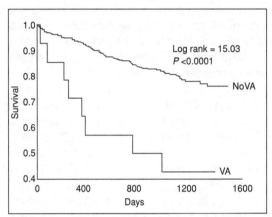

Figure 28.6 Survival curves for patients with tapes suitable and unsuitable for heart rate variability analysis due to frequent atrial arrhythmias or ventricular arrhythmias (VA). Patients with ventricular arrhythmias had significantly reduced survival whereas those with atrial arrhythmias did not.[37]

ectopy.[83] Patients with heart failure were less likely to achieve arrhythmia suppression in the first place (58% compared with 75%) and had a higher mortality than those who did achieve suppression and therefore were randomised to therapy.[84] The incidence of drug toxicity during the open label phase was higher in patients with heart failure. Among those randomised to therapy the adverse effects of treatment were greater in those with more frequent VPCs, higher heart rates, or taking diuretics.[85] Similar experiences were reported in the Stroke Prevention Atrial Fibrillation trials.[86] Here patients with non-valvar atrial fibrillation receiving antiarrhythmic drug therapy had a 4.7-fold increase in risk of cardiac death and a 3.7-fold increase in risk of arrhythmic death if they had a history of heart failure compared to those without. In patients with DCM similar adverse effects of class I agents in patients with asymptomatic arrhythmias have been described.[4,79] The limitations of EPS-guided drug therapy have been discussed above.

Amiodarone has also been evaluated in the treatment of patients with arrhythmias and heart failure. In small studies of mixed populations amiodarone reduced ventricular ectopy on ambulatory ECG monitoring,[87,88] but this was not associated with a reduction in total or sudden death mortality.[87,89] In the GESICA study low-dose amiodarone reduced all-cause mortality by 28% in 516 patients with heart failure.[90] The effect of amiodarone on mortality was comparable in patients with and without non-sustained VT at baseline (2-year survival was 59% with amiodarone, compared with 45% in control patients). The effect of amiodarone in different aetiological groups was not reported but over half the patients did not have ischaemic heart disease. These data are in contrast to the CHF STAT study.[89] Here 2-year survival was 69% with amiodarone and 71% in control patients, half the deaths were sudden, and there were no differences in the incidence of sudden death or sustained VT between treatment groups. Amiodarone suppressed non-sustained VT from 77% to 33%, but there was no difference in outcome between those with suppression of non-sustained VT and those without. There was a trend towards improved survival in those with non-ischaemic heart failure. The differences in the two studies are difficult to explain. Patients in CHF STAT had less severe heart failure (43% NYHA III or IV compared with 79%) and this, together with the differences in aetiology, may be relevant. A meta-analysis of five trials of amiodarone therapy in 1452 patients with heart failure showed a 17% (95% CI 1%-30%) reduction in all-cause mortality with treatment.[91] The risk of sudden death was reduced by 23% (95% CI −1–41%). This relative risk reduction was not different between patients with and without frequent VPBs or non-sustained VT or with more severe heart failure. The group at highest risk of arrhythmic/sudden death, and therefore with the highest absolute risk reduction, was that with NYHA grade III/IV heart failure.

Heart failure treatment

The most effective strategy for the prevention of arrhythmias in heart failure may well be optimisation of heart failure treatment. ACE inhibitors prolong ventricular refractoriness and repolarisation in patients with ischaemic heart failure and VT[92] and reduce the incidence of ventricular arrhythmias.[93–95] ACE inhibitors also favourably influence baroreflex sensitivity,[96,97] heart rate variability,[98,99] and QT dispersion,[100] all of which may contribute to their antiarrhythmic effect. That said, among mortality trials, only V-HeFT showed a reduction in sudden death.[101] Non-potassium sparing diuretics are associated with an increased incidence of sudden death,[31] whilst spironolactone has been shown to improve heart rate variability[102] and reduce the incidence of ventricular arrhythmias on ambulatory ECG monitoring.[103] In the RALES study, a randomised trial of spironolactone in severe heart failure, there was a significant reduction in total and sudden death mortality but no reduction in hospital admission for VT or VF.[104]

Beta-blockade dramatically reduces total mortality and sudden death in patients with heart failure.[25,26] It has been argued that these benefits reflect the anti-ischaemic properties of beta-blockade as IHD was the dominant aetiology in these trials.[105] In CIBIS-II the incidence of VT and VF was also significantly reduced and, in the earlier CIBIS study, the frequency of VT on ambulatory ECG monitoring was reduced by beta-blockade.[106,107]

Implantable cardiac defibrillators

The ICD now has a clear role in the management of patients with haemodynamically significant VT or VF.[108] There are also data for patients with ischaemic heart disease, impaired ventricular function, and asymptomatic non-sustained VT who had an inducible tachycardia that could not be suppressed by procainamide.[109] This showed a 1-year survival of 96% in the defibrillator group compared with 76% in those given empirical drug therapy (usually amiodarone).

In small series of patients with a history of cardiac arrest or recurrent refractory VT or VF and mixed aetiologies of heart failure, the incidence of sudden death is reduced,[110,111] as it was in patients with DCM.[73] Some 20% of the patients in AVID did not have ischaemic heart disease, but a separate analysis was not performed for DCM patients. A potential limitation to the use of ICDs in patients with advanced heart failure is that total mortality may not differ from patients managed with antiarrhythmic therapy or heart failure therapy alone, in spite of a reduction in sudden death because of the high rate of pump failure deaths.[112] Knight has reported the benefits of "empirical" ICD therapy in patients with DCM, unexplained syncope and a negative EPS.[42] There are no meaningful data on the use of the ICD in patients with asymptomatic ventricular arrhythmias in the setting of DCM. The limitations of EPS in this group would argue against such an approach until data from prospective randomised trials, such as the German cardiomyopathy trial, are available.[113]

Conclusions

Ventricular arrhythmias are a common manifestation of the failing heart and are often asymptomatic. They are independent markers of an increased risk of death, particularly sudden death, and this relation is independent of the aetiology of heart failure. However, as sudden death is more prevalent in patients with milder heart failure, ventricular arrhythmias may be more useful as a prognostic marker in this group. In more advanced heart failure they add little to conventional clinical markers of prognosis. In patients with sustained ventricular arrhythmias, the ICD reduces the risk of sudden death. In heart failure patients without ischaemic heart disease, current data do not support the prophylactic use of the ICD and empirical amiodarone may be a better choice.

References

1. Carson P, Johnson G, Fletcher R, Cohn J. Mild systolic dysfunction in heart failure (left ventricular ejection fraction >35%): baseline characteristics, prognosis and response to therapy in the Vasodilator in Heart Failure Trials (V-HeFT). *J Am Coll Cardiol* 1996;**27**:642–9.

2. Massie BM, Shah NB. Evolving trends in the epidemiological factors of heart failure: rationale for preventive strategies and comprehensive disease management. *Am Heart J* 1997;**133**:703–12.

3. McMurray J, Hart W, Rhodes G. An evaluation of the economic cost of heart failure to the National Health Service in the United Kingdom. *Br J Med Econ* 1993;**6**:99–110.

4. Packer M. Lack of relation between ventricular arrhythmias and sudden death in patients with chronic heart failure. *Circulation* 1992;**85**:I50–6.

5. Dec GW, Fuster V. Idiopathic dilated cardiomyopathy. *New Engl J Med* 1994;**331**:1564–75.

6. Codd MB, Sugrue DD, Gersh BJ, Melton LJ. Epidemiology of idiopathic dilated and hypertrophic cardiomyopathy. A population-based study in Olmsted County, Minnesota, 1975–1984. *Circulation* 1989;**80**:564–72.

7. Gillum RF. Idiopathic cardiomyopathy in the United States, 1970-1982. *Am Heart J* 1986;**111**:752–5.

8. Fozzard HA. After-depolarizations and triggered activity. *Basic Res Cardiol* 1992;**87**(Suppl. 2):105–13.

9. Vermeulen JT, McGuire MA, Opthof T *et al.* Triggered activity and automaticity in ventricular trabeculae of failing human and rabbit hearts. *Cardiovasc Res* 1994;**28**:1547–54.

10. Beuckelmann DJ, Nabauer M, Erdmann E. Alterations of K^+ currents in isolated human ventricular myocytes from patients with terminal heart failure. *Circ Res* 1993;**73**:379–85.

11. Houser SR, Freeman AR, Jaeger JM *et al.* Resting potential changes associated with Na-K pump in failing heart muscle. *Am J Physiol* 1981;**240**:H168–76

12. Lakatta EG. Functional implications of spontaneous sarcoplasmic reticulum Ca^{2+} release in the heart. *Cardiovasc Res* 1992;**26**:193–214.

13. Gilmour RFJ, Heger JJ, Prystowsky EN, Zipes DP. Cellular electrophysiologic abnormalities of diseased human ventricular myocardium. *Am J Cardiol* 1983;**51**:137–44.

14. de Bakker JM, van Capelle FJ, Janse MJ *et al.* Reentry as a cause of ventricular tachycardia in patients with chronic ischemic heart disease: electrophysiologic and anatomic correlation. *Circulation* 1988;**77**:589–606.

15. Pogwizd SM. Nonreentrant mechanisms underlying spontaneous ventricular arrhythmias in a model of nonischemic heart failure in rabbits. *Circulation* 1995;**92**:1034–48.

16. Pogwizd SM, Hoyt RH, Saffitz JE *et al.* Reentrant and focal mechanisms underlying ventricular tachycardia in the human heart. *Circulation* 1992;**86**:1872–87.

17. Pye MP, Cobbe SM. Arrhythmogenesis in experimental models of heart failure: the role of increased load. *Cardiovasc Res* 1996;**32**:248–57.

18. Weber KT, Pick R, Silver MA *et al.* Fibrillar collagen and remodeling of dilated canine left ventricle. *Circulation* 1990;**82**:1387–401.

19. Brilla CG, Maisch B, Zhou G, Weber KT. Hormonal regulation of cardiac fibroblast function. *Eur Heart J* 1995;**16**(Suppl. C):45–50.

20. Unverferth DV, Baker PB, Pearce LI, Lautman J, Roberts, WC. Regional myocyte hypertrophy and increased interstitial myocardial fibrosis in hypertrophic cardiomyopathy. *Am J Cardiol* 1987;**59**:932–6.

21. Vermeulen JT, Tan HL, Rademaker H *et al.* Electrophysiologic and extracellular ionic changes during acute ischemia in failing and normal rabbit myocardium. *J Mol Cell Cardiol* 1996;**28**:123–31.

22. Bristow MR, Ginsburg R, Minobe W *et al.* Decreased catecholamine sensitivity and beta-adrenergic-receptor density in failing human hearts. *New Engl J Med* 1982;**307**:205–11.

23. Pierpont GL, Francis GS, DeMaster EG *et al.* Heterogeneous myocardial catecholamine concentrations in patients with congestive heart failure. *Am J Cardiol* 1987;**60**:316–21.

24. Calkins H, Allman K, Bolling S *et al.* Correlation between scintigraphic evidence of regional sympathetic neuronal dysfunction and ventricular refractoriness in the human heart. *Circulation* 1993;**88**:172–9.

25. CIBIS-II Investigators. The Cardiac Insufficiency Bisoprolol Study II (CIBIS-II): a randomised trial. *Lancet* 1999;**353**:9–13.

26. Merit-HF Study Group. Effect of metoprolol CR/XL in chronic heart failure: Metoprolol CR/XL Randomised Intervention Trial in Congestive Heart Failure (MERIT-HF). *Lancet* 1999;**353**:2001–7.

27. Kolman BS, Verrier RL, Lown B. Effect of vagus nerve stimulation upon excitability of the canine ventricle. Role of sympathetic–parasympathetic interactions. *Am J Cardiol* 1976;**37**:1041–5.

28. Zipes DP, Levy MN, Cobb LA *et al.* Sudden cardiac death. Neural–cardiac interactions. *Circulation* 1987;**76**:I202–7.

29. Nolan J, Batin PD, Andrews R *et al.* Prospective study of heart rate variability and mortality in chronic heart failure; results of the United Kingdom Heart Failure Evaluation and Assessment of Risk Trial (UK-HEART). *Circulation* 1998;**98**:1510–16.

30. Douban S, Brodsky MA, Whang DD, Whang R. Significance

of magnesium in congestive heart failure. *Am Heart J* 1996;**132**:664–71.

31. Cooper HA, Dries DL, Davis CE, Shen YL, Domanski MJ. Diuretics and risk of arrhythmic death in patients with left ventricular dysfunction. *Circulation* 1999;**100**:1311–15.

32. Franz MR, Cima R, Wang D, Profitt D, Kurz R. Electrophysiological effects of myocardial stretch and mechanical determinants of stretch-activated arrhythmias. *Circulation* 1992;**86**:968–78.

33. Vermeulen JT. Mechanisms of arrhythmias in heart failure. *J Cardiovasc Electrophysiol* 1998;**9**:208–21.

34. Wang Z, Taylor LK, Denney WD, Hansen DE. Initiation of ventricular extrasystoles by myocardial stretch in chronically dilated and failing canine left ventricle. *Circulation* 1994;**90**:2022–31.

35. Keogh AM, Baron DW, Hickie JB. Prognostic guides in patients with idiopathic or ischemic dilated cardiomyopathy assessed for cardiac transplantation. *Am J Cardiol* 1990;**65**:903–8.

36. Cohn JN, Johnson GR, Shabetai R *et al.* Ejection fraction, peak exercise oxygen consumption, cardiothoracic ratio, ventricular arrhythmias, and plasma norepinephrine as determinants of prognosis in heart failure. The V-HeFT VA Cooperative Studies Group. *Circulation* 1993;**87**:VI5–16.

37. Lindsay SJ, Brooksby P, Batin PD *et al.* Ambulatory electrocardiography provides independent prognostic information in patients with congestive heart failure in whom heart rate variability cannot be measured. *Eur Heart J* 1998;**19**:429(Abstr.)

38. Brembilla-Perrot B, Donetti J, de la Chaise AT, Sadoul N, Aliot E, Juilliere Y. Diagnostic value of ventricular stimulation in patients with idiopathic dilated cardiomyopathy. *Am Heart J* 1991;**121**:1124–31.

39. Mancini DM, Wong KL, Simson MB. Prognostic value of an abnormal signal-averaged electrocardiogram in patients with nonischemic congestive cardiomyopathy. *Circulation* 1993;**87**:1083–92.

40. Denereaz D, Zimmermann M, Adamec R. Significance of ventricular late potentials in non-ischaemic dilated cardiomyopathy. *Eur Heart J* 1992;**13**:895–901.

41. Grimm W, Marchlinski FE. Shock occurrence and survival in 49 patients with idiopathic dilated cardiomyopathy and an implantable cardioverter-defibrillator. *Eur Heart J* 1995;**16**:218–22.

42. Knight BP, Goyal R, Pelosi F *et al.* Outcome of patients with nonischemic dilated cardiomyopathy and unexplained syncope treated with an implantable defibrillator. *J Am Coll Cardiol* 1999;**33**:1964–70.

43. Lessmeier TJ, Lehmann MH, Steinman RT *et al.* Outcome with implantable cardioverter-defibrillator therapy for survivors of ventricular fibrillation secondary to idiopathic dilated cardiomyopathy or coronary artery disease without myocardial infarction. *Am J Cardiol* 1993;**72**:911–15.

44. Kjekshus J. Arrhythmias and mortality in congestive heart failure. *Am J Cardiol* 1990;**65**:42I–8I.

45. Koilpillai C, Quinones MA, Greenberg B *et al.* Relation of ventricular size and function to heart failure status and ventricular dysrhythmia in patients with severe left ventricular dysfunction. *Am J Cardiol* 1996;**77**:606–11.

46. Nikolic G, Bishop RL, Singh JB. Sudden death recorded during Holter monitoring. *Circulation* 1982;**66**:218–25.

47. Bayes de Luna A, Coumel P, Leclercq JF. Ambulatory sudden cardiac death: mechanisms of production of fatal arrhythmia on the basis of data from 157 cases. *Am Heart J* 1989;**117**:151–9.

48. Pratt CM, Greenway PS, Schoenfeld MH, Hibben ML, Reiffel, JA. Exploration of the precision of classifying sudden cardiac death. Implications for the interpretation of clinical trials. *Circulation* 1996;**93**:519–24.

49. Luu M, Stevenson WG, Stevenson LW, Baron K, Walden J. Diverse mechanisms of unexpected cardiac arrest in advanced heart failure. *Circulation* 1989;**80**:1675–80.

50. Goldman S, Johnson G, Cohn JN, Cintron G, Smith R, Francis G. Mechanism of death in heart failure. The Vasodilator-Heart Failure Trials. *Circulation* 1993;**87**:VI24–31

51. Fuster V, Gersh BJ, Giuliani ER *et al.* The natural history of idiopathic dilated cardiomyopathy. *Am J Cardiol* 1981;**47**:525–31.

52. Diaz RA, Obasohan A, Oakley CM. Prediction of outcome in dilated cardiomyopathy. *Br Heart J* 1987;**58**:393–9.

53. Komajda M, Jais JP, Reeves F *et al.* Factors predicting mortality in idiopathic dilated cardiomyopathy. *Eur Heart J* 1990;**11**:824–31.

54. Sugrue DD, Rodeheffer RJ, Codd MB, Ballard DJ, Fuster V, Gersh BJ. The clinical course of idiopathic dilated cardiomyopathy. A population-based study. *Ann Inter Med* 1992;**117**:117–23.

55. Di Lenarda A, Secoli G, Perkan A *et al.* Changing mortality in dilated cardiomyopathy. The Heart Muscle Disease Study Group. *Br Heart J* 1994;**72**:S46–51.

56. Ikram H, Williamson HG, Won M, Crozier IG, Wells EJ. The course of idiopathic dilated cardiomyopathy in New Zealand. *Br Heart J* 1987;**57**:521–7.

57. Francis GS. Development of arrhythmias in the patient with congestive heart failure: pathophysiology, prevalence and prognosis. *Am J Cardiol* 1986;**57**:3B–7B.

58. Meinertz T, Hofmann T, Kasper W *et al.* Significance of ventricular arrhythmias in idiopathic dilated cardiomyopathy. *Am J Cardiol* 1984;**53**:902–7.

59. Holmes J, Kubo SH, Cody RJ, Kligfield P. Arrhythmias in ischemic and nonischemic dilated cardiomyopathy: prediction of mortality by ambulatory electrocardiography. *Am J Cardiol* 1985;**55**:146–51.

60. Chakko CS, Gheorghiade M. Ventricular arrhythmias in severe heart failure: incidence, significance, and effectiveness of antiarrhythmic therapy. *Am Heart J* 1985;**109**:497–504.

61. Unverferth DV, Magorien RD, Moeschberger ML, Baker PB, Fetters JK, Leier CV. Factors influencing the 1-year mortality of dilated cardiomyopathy. *Am J Cardiol* 1984;**54**:147–52.

62. Huang SK, Messer JV, Denes P. Significance of ventricular tachycardia in idiopathic dilated cardiomyopathy: observations in 35 patients. *Am J Cardiol* 1983;**51**:507–12.

63. Wilson JR, Schwartz JS, Sutton MS *et al.* Prognosis in severe heart failure: relation to hemodynamic measurements and ventricular ectopic activity. *J Am Coll Cardiol* 1983;**2**:403–10.

64. von Olshausen K, Schafer A, Mehmel HC, Schwarz F, Senges J, Kubler W. Ventricular arrhythmias in idiopathic dilated cardiomyopathy. *Br Heart J* 1984;**51**:195–201.

65. Singh SN, Fisher SG, Carson PE, Fletcher RD. Prevalence and significance of nonsustained ventricular tachycardia in patients with premature ventricular contractions and heart failure treated with vasodilator therapy. *J Am Coll Cardiol* 1998;**32**:942–7.

66. Doval HC, Nul DR, Grancelli HO *et al.* Nonsustained ventricular tachycardia in severe heart failure. Independent marker of increased mortality due to sudden death. GESICA-GEMA Investigators. *Circulation* 1996;**94**:198–203.

67. Teerlink JR, Jalaluddin M, Anderson S *et al.* Ambulatory ventricular arrhythmias in patients with heart failure do not specifically predict an increased risk of sudden death. *Circulation* 2000;**101**:40–6.

68. Lown B, Wolf M. Approaches to sudden death from coronary heart disease. *Circulation* 1971;**44**:130–42.

69. Reese DB, Silverman ME, Gold MR, Gottlieb SS. Prognostic importance of the length of ventricular tachycardia in patients with nonischemic congestive heart failure. *Am Heart J* 1995;**130**:489–93.

70. Turitto G, Ahuja RK, Caref EB, el-Sherif N. Risk stratification for arrhythmic events in patients with nonischemic dilated cardiomyopathy and nonsustained ventricular tachycardia: role of programmed ventricular stimulation and the signal-averaged electrocardiogram. *J Am Coll Cardiol* 1994;**24**:1523–8.

71. Milner PG, DiMarco JP, Lerman BB. Electrophysiological evaluation of sustained ventricular tachyarrhythmias in idiopathic dilated cardiomyopathy. *Pacing Clin Electrophysiol* 1988; **11**:562–8.

72. Liem LB, Swerdlow CD. Value of electropharmacologic testing in idiopathic dilated cardiomyopathy and sustained ventricular tachyarrhythmias. *Am J Cardiol* 1988;**62**:611–16.

73. Fazio G, Veltri EP, Tomaselli G, Lewis R, Griffith LS, Guarnieri T. Long-term follow-up of patients with nonischemic dilated cardiomyopathy and ventricular tachyarrhythmias treated with implantable cardioverter defibrillators. *Pacing Clin Electrophysiol* 1991;**14**:1905–10.

74. Naccarelli GV, Prystowsky EN, Jackman WM, Heger JJ, Rahilly GT, Zipes DP. Role of electrophysiologic testing in managing patients who have ventricular tachycardia unrelated to coronary artery disease. *Am J Cardiol* 1982;**50**:165–71.

75. Wilber DJ. Evaluation and treatment of nonsustained ventricular tachycardia. *Curr Opin Cardiol* 1996;**11**:23–31.

76. Rae AP, Spielman SR, Kutalek SP, Kay HR, Horowitz LN. Electrophysiologic assessment of antiarrhythmic drug efficacy for ventricular tachyarrhythmias associated with dilated cardiomyopathy. *Am J Cardiol* 1987;**59**:291–5.

77. Poll DS, Marchlinski FE, Buxton AE, Josephson ME. Usefulness of programmed stimulation in idiopathic dilated cardiomyopathy. *Am J Cardiol* 1986;**58**:992–7.

78. Poll DS, Marchlinski FE, Buxton AE *et al.* Sustained ventricular tachycardia in patients with idiopathic dilated cardiomyopathy: electrophysiologic testing and lack of response to antiarrhythmic drug therapy. *Circulation* 1984;**70**:451–6.

79. Pratt CM, Eaton T, Francis M *et al.* The inverse relationship between baseline left ventricular ejection fraction and outcome of antiarrhythmic therapy: a dangerous imbalance in the risk-benefit ratio. *Am Heart J* 1989;**118**:433–40.

80. Anderson KP, Hartz VL, Hahn EA, Moon TE. Design and analysis of the ESVEM Trial. *Prog Cardiovasc Dis* 1996;**38**:489–502.

81. Tamburro P, Wilber D. Sudden death in idiopathic dilated cardiomyopathy. *Am Heart J* 1992;**124**:1035–45.

82. Ponikowski P, Anker SD, Chua TP *et al.* Depressed heart rate variability as an independent predictor of death in chronic congestive heart failure secondary to ischemic or idiopathic dilated cardiomyopathy. *Am J Cardiol* 1997;**79**: 1645–50.

83. The Cardiac Arrhythmia Suppression Trial (CAST) Investigators. Preliminary report: effect of encainide and flecainide on mortality in a randomized trial of arrhythmia suppression after myocardial infarction. *New Engl J Med* 1989;**321**:406–12.

84. Hallstrom A, Pratt CM, Greene HL *et al.* Relations between heart failure, ejection fraction, arrhythmia suppression and mortality: analysis of the Cardiac Arrhythmia Suppression Trial. *J Am Coll Cardiol* 1995;**25**:1250–7.

85. Anderson JL, Platia EV, Hallstrom A *et al.* Interaction of baseline characteristics with the hazard of encainide, flecainide, and moricizine therapy in patients with myocardial infarction. A possible explanation for increased mortality in the Cardiac Arrhythmia Suppression Trial (CAST). *Circulation* 1994;**90**:2843–52.

86. Flaker GC, Blackshear JL, McBride R, Kronmal RA, Halperin JL, Hart RG. Antiarrhythmic drug therapy and cardiac mortality in atrial fibrillation. The Stroke Prevention in Atrial Fibrillation Investigators. *J Am Coll Cardiol* 1992;**20**:527–32.

87. Neri R, Mestroni L, Salvi A, Pandullo C, Camerini F. Ventricular arrhythmias in dilated cardiomyopathy: efficacy of amiodarone. *Am Heart J* 1987;**113**:707–15.

88. Nicklas JM, McKenna WJ, Stewart RA *et al.* Prospective, double-blind, placebo-controlled trial of low-dose amiodarone in patients with severe heart failure and asymptomatic frequent ventricular ectopy. *Am Heart J* 1991;**122**:1016–21.

89. Singh SN, Fletcher RD, Fisher SG *et al.* Amiodarone in patients with congestive heart failure and asymptomatic ventricular arrhythmia. Survival Trial of Antiarrhythmic Therapy in Congestive Heart Failure. *New Engl J Med* 1995;**333**:77–82.

90. Doval HC, Nul DR, Grancelli HO, Perrone SV, Bortman GR, Curiel R. Randomised trial of low-dose amiodarone in severe congestive heart failure. Grupo de Estudio de la Sobrevida en la Insuficiencia Cardiaca en Argentina (GESICA). *Lancet* 1994;**344**:493–8.

91. Amiodarone Trials Meta-Analysis Investigators. Effect of prophylactic amiodarone on mortality after acute myocardial infarction and in congestive heart failure: meta-analysis of individual data from 6500 patients in randomised trials. *Lancet* 1997;**350**:1417–24.

92. Bashir Y, Sneddon JF, O'Nunain S *et al.* Comparative electrophysiological effects of captopril or hydralazine combined with nitrate in patients with left ventricular dysfunction and inducible ventricular tachycardia. *Br Heart J* 1992;**67**:355–60.

93. Cleland JG, Dargie HJ, Hodsman GP *et al.* Captopril in heart failure. A double blind controlled trial. *Br Heart J* 1984;**52**:530–5.

94. Webster MW, Fitzpatrick MA, Nicholls MG, Ikram H, Wells, JE. Effect of enalapril on ventricular arrhythmias in congestive heart failure. *Am J Cardiol* 1985;**56**:566–9.

95. Fletcher RD, Cintron GB, Johnson G, Orndorff J, Carson, Cohn JN. Enalapril decreases prevalence of ventricular tachycardia in patients with chronic congestive heart failure. The V-HeFT II VA Cooperative Studies Group. *Circulation* 1993;**87**:VI49–55

96. Marakas SA, Kyriakidis MK, Vourlioti AN, Petropoulakis PN, Toutouzas PK. Acute effect of captopril administration on baroreflex sensitivity in patients with acute myocardial infarction. *Eur Heart J* 1995;**16**:914–21.

97. Bonaduce D, Petretta M, Morgano G *et al.* Effects of converting enzyme inhibition on baroreflex sensitivity in patients with myocardial infarction. *J Am Coll Cardiol* 1992;**20**:587–93.

98. Kamen PW, Krum H, Tonkin AM. Low-dose but not high-dose captopril increases parasympathetic activity in patients with heart failure. *J Cardiovasc Pharmacol* 1997;**30**:7–11.

99. Binkley PF, Haas GJ, Starling RC *et al.* Sustained augmentation of parasympathetic tone with angiotensin-converting enzyme inhibition in patients with congestive heart failure. *J Am Coll Cardiol* 1993;**21**:655–61.

100. Barr CS, Naas AA, Fenwick M, Struthers AD. Enalapril reduces QTc dispersion in mild congestive heart failure secondary to coronary artery disease. *Am J Cardiol* 1997;**79**:328–33.

101. Cohn JN, Johnson G, Ziesche S *et al.* A comparison of enalapril with hydralazine–isosorbide dinitrate in the treatment of chronic congestive heart failure. *New Engl J Med* 1991;**325**:303–10.

102. MacFadyen RJ, Barr CS, Struthers AD. Aldosterone blockade reduces vascular collagen turnover, improves heart rate variability and reduces early morning rise in heart rate in heart failure patients. *Cardiovasc Res* 1997;**35**:30–4.

103. Barr CS, Lang CC, Hanson J, Arnott M, Kennedy N, Struthers AD. Effects of adding spironolactone to an angiotensin-converting enzyme inhibitor in chronic congestive heart failure secondary to coronary artery disease. *Am J Cardiol* 1995;**76**:1259–65.

104. Pitt B, Zannad F, Remme WJ *et al.* The effect of spironolactone on morbidity and mortality in patients with severe heart failure. Randomized Aldactone Evaluation Study Investigators. *New Engl J Med* 1999;**341**:709–17.

105. Poole-Wilson PA. The Cardiac Insufficiency Bisoprolol Study II. *Lancet* 1999;**353**:1360–1.

106. Copie X, Pousset F, Lechat P, Jaillon P, Guize L, Le Heuzey JY. Effects of beta-blockade with bisoprolol on heart rate variability in advanced heart failure: analysis of scatterplots of RR intervals at selected heart rates. *Am Heart J* 1996;**132**:369–75.

107. Pousset F, Copie X, Lechat P *et al.* Effects of bisoprolol on heart rate variability in heart failure. *Am J Cardiol* 1996;**77**:612–17.

108. The Antiarrhythmics versus Implantable Defibrillators (AVID) Investigators. A comparison of antiarrhythmic-drug therapy with implantable defibrillators in patients resuscitated from near-fatal ventricular arrhythmias. *N Engl J Med* 1997;**337**:1576–83.

109. Moss AJ, Hall WJ, Cannom DS *et al.* Improved survival with an implanted defibrillator in patients with coronary disease at high risk for ventricular arrhythmia. Multicenter Automatic Defibrillator Implantation Trial Investigators. *New Engl J Med* 1996;**335**:1933–40.

110. Tchou PJ, Kadri N, Anderson J, Caceres JA, Jazayeri M, Akhtar M. Automatic implantable cardioverter defibrillators and survival of patients with left ventricular dysfunction and malignant ventricular arrhythmias. *Ann Intern Med* 1988;**109**:529–34.

111. Fogoros RN, Elson JJ, Bonnet CA, Fiedler SB, Burkholder, JA. Efficacy of the automatic implantable cardioverter–defibrillator in prolonging survival in patients with severe underlying cardiac disease. *J Am Coll Cardiol* 1990;**16**:381–6.

112. Sweeney MO, Ruskin JN, Garan H *et al.* Influence of the implantable cardioverter/defibrillator on sudden death and total mortality in patients evaluated for cardiac transplantation. *Circulation* 1995;**92**:3273–81.

113. The Cardiomyopathy Trial Investigators. Cardiomyopathy trial. *Pacing Clin Electrophysiol* 1993;**16**:576–81.

29 Ventricular arrhythmias in hypertrophic cardiomyopathy

Gang Yi and William J McKenna

Clinical characteristics of hypertrophic cardiomyopathy

Hypertrophic cardiomyopathy is defined clinically as an idiopathic heart muscle condition characterised by a hypertrophied and non-dilated left and/or right ventricle in the absence of a cardiac or systemic cause.[1] Scientifically, the condition is now recognised to be a disease of the sarcomere and is caused by mutations in genes encoding cardiac sarcomeric proteins.[2,3] Hypertrophic cardiomyopathy is a relatively common disease with a prevalence estimated of at least 0.2%.[4] It is characterised by a predisposition to fatal cardiac arrhythmia, and is an important cause of sudden death in individuals aged less than 35 years. All forms of clinical presentation may be observed from almost asymptomatic hypertrophy to severe familial forms with multiple cases of sudden death. The main problem for clinicians is to assess the risk of arrhythmic complications, especially in adolescents and young adults.

Arrhythmias in hypertrophic cardiomyopathy

Supraventricular and ventricular arrhythmias, particularly non-sustained ventricular tachycardia and supraventricular arrhythmias (i.e. paroxysmal or persistent atrial fibrillation) are common findings in patients with hypertrophic cardiomyopathy. Non-sustained ventricular tachycardia occurs in 25% of adults.[5,6] The incidence detected during 48-hour ambulatory ECG monitoring is age-related, up to 32% in patients aged 46–60 (Fig. 29.1). Sustained ventricular tachycardia is uncommon and is sometimes associated with apical aneurysms, which may develop as a consequence of mid-ventricular obstruction.[7] Premature sudden unexpected death has been regarded as a critical feature of the natural history.[8,9] Annual mortality varies from 1% to 6% depending on the characteristics of the cohort studied.[9–13] Data from referral centres suggest an overall annual mortality of 2%, with maximum of 4–6% during childhood and adolescence,[9,10] whereas studies from non-referral populations suggest a mortality of approximately

1% per annum.[11–13] Sudden death occurs even in those who have previously been symptom free.[9] Most patients (about 60%) experience sudden death during or just after mild to moderate physical exertion, including competitive sports.[14] While the arrhythmogenic substrate in patients with hypertrophic cardiomyopathy is incompletely understood, it is suggested that several mechanisms may be involved in sudden death: ventricular arrhythmias, supraventricular arrhythmias leading to cardiac collapse, abnormal vascular response leading to hypotension, bradycardias, and ischaemia.

Identification of high risk for arrhythmic events

Clinical risk factors

It has been recognised that young age at diagnosis (<16 years), a family history of multiple premature sudden

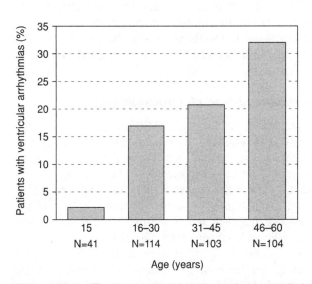

Figure 29.1 The frequency of non-sustained ventricular tachycardia at different ages in a consecutively referred population at St George's Hospital, London (unpublished data).

death from hypertrophic cardiomyopathy and recurrent syncope episodes are risk factors for sudden death. In children and adolescents with hypertrophic cardiomyopathy, recurrent unexplained syncope is an ominous symptom, particularly when it occurs in individuals with a family history of premature sudden death.[9] Although severe hypertrophy (≥30 mm) is an adverse prognostic feature, such patients are uncommon (≤10%) and most patients who die suddenly do not have severe left ventricular hypertrophy.[14] Other obvious disease features such as left ventricular outflow tract obstruction and severe symptoms of functional limitation are also not sensitive markers to identify the high-risk patients.[14] Recently, genotype phenotype studies have suggested that particular mutations may influence clinical outcomes. Some sarcomeric protein mutations are associated with a high incidence of sudden death, for example the beta-myosin heavy chain Arg403Gln and cardiac troponin T mutations.[15] However, this "genetic stratification" based on DNA diagnosis has not yet become available in clinical practice and must be considered preliminary until confirmed with larger numbers of genotyped patients.

Electrocardiographic markers of the risk for sudden death

Standard 12-lead ECG, Holter monitoring ECG, signal-averaged ECG, and exercise ECG are commonly used non-invasive techniques in clinical practice to detect cardiac electrical instability. Several ECG findings are generally recognised as markers of cardiac electrical instability, including abnormal ECG morphology (bundle branch block, ST-T abnormalities), complex ventricular arrhythmias, abnormalities in depolarisation or ventricular repolarisation, and alterations in the autonomic nervous system, which may lead to life-threatening arrhythmias.

Standard 12-lead electrocardiogram

Abnormalities of conventional ECG parameters may be the initial manifestation of hypertrophic cardiomyopathy, appearing even before left ventricular hypertrophy is detectable by echocardiography,[16,17] but the ECG abnormalities are highly variable and often non-specific in hypertrophic cardiomyopathy.[18] Although it is clinically used as a diagnostic tool, standard 12-lead ECG is of limited utility in identifying arrhythmic risk.

In patients with hypertrophic cardiomyopathy, it has been shown that both QTc interval and QT dispersion are increased,[19–21] and that QT dispersion was significantly greater in patients with than without ventricular arrhythmias on Holter or sudden cardiac death.[20] The value of these early studies[19,20] is, however, limited by their retrospective nature and small size (N <30). In a relatively larger population (N = 83), the association between QT dispersion measurements and the recognised risk factors for sudden death was examined, but this study did not demonstrate any significant association between them.[21] In a recent study, 254 initial ECGs of hypertrophic cardiomyopathy patients were retrospectively analysed.[22] No differences in QT dispersion were found between survivors and either sudden death or disease related mortality. Although some studies have shown that QT dispersion is of prognostic value in patients after myocardial infarction,[23] initial studies do not suggest a usefulness of QT dispersion measurements in prospective identification of patients with hypertrophic cardiomyopathy at risk of sudden death.

Signal-averaged electrocardiogram

The signal-averaged ECG plays a limited role in determining risk of sudden death in patients with hypertrophic cardiomyopathy.[24–26] An early study[24] showed that an abnormal signal-averaged ECG was common (20%) in hypertrophic cardiomyopathy and signal-averaged ECG had a sensitivity of 50%, a specificity of 93%, and a positive predictive accuracy of 77% in detecting patients with electrical instability (defined as a history of cardiac arrest or the presence of non-sustained ventricular tachycardia on Holter, or both). It seemed that the signal-averaged ECG might be a useful adjunct to the non-invasive assessment of patients with hypertrophic cardiomyopathy. However, this study was conducted in only 64 patients with hypertrophic cardiomyopathy, 26 of whom (41%) were receiving amiodarone therapy, which was later shown to induce late potentials.[27,28] Kulakowski *et al.*[25] found that conventional analysis of ventricular late potentials was not helpful in identifying hypertrophic cardiomyopathy patients with ventricular tachyarrhythmias or sudden cardiac death. This later study consisted of a larger population of well-categorised patients with hypertrophic cardiomyopathy (N = 121) and excluded patients who were receiving amiodarone therapy. The low incidence (6–8%) of late potentials and the lack of association between late potentials and catastrophic events in hypertrophic cardiomyopathy shown by the late study[25] did not support the hypothesis that late potentials analysis could be useful in risk stratification of patients with hypertrophic cardiomyopathy, at least using conventional time domain analysis. Wavelet decomposition analysis, a recently proposed alternative method of analysing the signal-averaged ECG, did not improve the predictive ability of the signal-averaged ECG for sudden death or ventricular fibrillation in patients with hypertrophic cardiomyopathy.[26]

Exercise electrocardiogram

Routine analysis of exercise ECG for ST segment changes, exercise-induced arrhythmias, and exercise capacity, does not help with risk stratification, while assessment of the blood pressure response during upright exercise plays an important role in risk stratifying patients with hypertrophic cardiomyopathy, particularly for the young. To investigate the incidence of abnormal exercise blood pressure response in hypertrophic cardiomyopathy and the potential role of haemodynamic instability as a determinant of sudden death, 129 consecutive patients with hypertrophic cardiomyopathy underwent maximal symptom-limited treadmill exercise testing with continuous cuff blood pressure recording.[29] Exercise-induced hypotension occurred in a third of patients with hypertrophic cardiomyopathy. Its importance is underlined by the fact that a significant proportion of sudden cardiac deaths occur during or shortly after exercise.[14] The observation of an abnormal blood pressure response during exercise in 4 of 6 patients who had experienced failed sudden cardiac death led a prospective study to assess the prognostic significance in young patients with hypertrophic cardiomyopathy.[30] Maximum symptom-limited treadmill exercise testing with continuous blood pressure monitoring was performed in 161 consecutive patients aged 8–40 years old (mean 27 ± 9). A normal exercise blood pressure response was shown to identify low-risk young patients with hypertrophic cardiomyopathy, whilst significantly more patients with abnormal blood pressure response died suddenly during follow-up (Fig. 29.2). The data indicate that the high negative predictive accuracy (97%) in the study population allows reassurance of young patients with a normal blood pressure response.[30] An abnormal blood pressure response identifies the high-risk cohort; the low positive predictive accuracy (15%), however, indicates the need for additional risk stratification. These data have recently been confirmed in a large Italian study.[31]

Holter monitoring electrocardiogram

The role of non-sustained ventricular tachycardia as a marker of the high-risk patient continues to cause controversy. The finding of episodes of non-sustained ventricular tachycardia on Holter monitoring ECG was considered to be the most useful marker of the high risk for sudden death in adult patients with hypertrophic cardiomyopathy.[32] In the early 1980s, simultaneous observation from two independent centres was reported that adults with non-sustained ventricular tachycardia have 7–8-fold increased mortality from sudden cardiac death. Of 169 consecutive unoperated patients from the National Institute of Health, Bethesda, Maryland and the Hammersmith Hospital, London, 13 died suddenly during three years, nine of whom had non-sustained ventricular tachycardia. In both studies, this arrhythmia was significantly more common in these who died suddenly.[5,6] The pooled data of theses two studies are summarised in Fig. 29.3. The finding of non-sustained ventricular tachycardia on Holter monitoring has a sensitivity of 69%, a specificity of 80% and a positive predictive accuracy of 22% for the prediction of sudden cardiac death.[32] Although this does not prove a causal relation, it does establish that ventricular tachycardia is a marker in adults who are at particular risk of sudden cardiac death. Spirito, however, has pro-

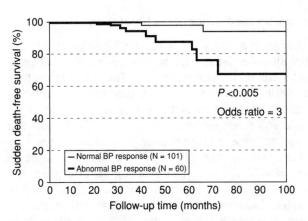

Figure 29.2. Kaplan–Meier survivor curves for sudden cardiac death in patients with hypertrophic cardiomyopathy. The bold line indicates the patients with an abnormal blood pressure (BP) response and the fine line indicates the patients with a normal blood pressure response during exercise testing. (Adapted from reference 30.)

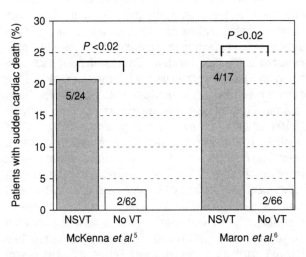

Figure 29.3 Pooled data from two studies showing the association between non-sustained ventricular tachycardia (NSVT) on Holter monitoring ECG and the occurrence of sudden cardiac death in adult patients with hypertrophic cardiomyopathy (modified from references 5 and 6). No VT, no ventricular tachycardia on Holter.

posed that significant risk is only conferred if episodes are fast or repetitive.[33] He studied a highly selected cohort of 151 asymptomatic or mildly symptomatic patients with hypertrophic cardiomyopathy and reported that non-sustained ventricular tachycardia on Holter monitoring had a benign prognosis in asymptomatic patients with a relative risk for sudden death of 2.4. This study was limited by the fact that few patients died suddenly during relatively short follow-up (mean 4.8 years). In addition, analysis of the characteristics of non-sustained ventricular tachycardia episodes by Monserrat *et al.*[34] has failed to confirm Spirito's logical suggestion that episodes are only significant if they are fast or repetitive.

Nevertheless, patients with non-sustained ventricular tachycardia are heterogeneous and do not all have the same risk. Cecchi *et al.*[35] treated patients with either adverse arrhythmia characteristics or additional risk factors and documented few sudden deaths in the patients with non-sustained ventricular tachycardia who were not treated. This is consistent with the St. George's Hospital experience of a marked increase in risk when additional risk factors are present.[36] Overall in adults the finding of non-sustained ventricular tachycardia confers a relative risk of approximately 2.5. Particular subsets however such as the young (<30 years), those with other risk factors, and perhaps those with repetitive or rapid episodes are at greater risk, which is sufficient to warrant prophylactic treatment.

Assessment of autonomic function

Heart rate variability analysis. Impaired autonomic function plays an important role in arrhythmogenesis. Autonomic dysfunction is a powerful predictor of arrhythmic events and sudden death after myocardial infarction. In hypertrophic cardiomyopathy some preliminary findings indicate that hypertrophic cardiomyopathy patients have impaired autonomic function. Studies of heart rate variability in patients with hypertrophic cardiomyopathy have been inconclusive.[37–39] Counihan *et al.*[38] performed heart rate variability analysis (non-spectral and spectral analysis) in 104 patients with hypertrophic cardiomyopathy in sinus rhythm, 10 of whom experienced catastrophic events (ventricular fibrillation or sudden cardiac death) during follow-up. Indices of heart rate variability in patients with subsequent serious arrhythmias were similar to those in patients who survived without events. Similarly, no significant difference in heart rate variability was found between 14 sudden death victims and 10 age- and gender-matched low-risk patients in the study of Fei *et al.*[39] Analysis of heart rate variability has so far not been found to be a reliable prognostic marker in hypertrophic cardiomyopathy.

Tilt test. Head-up tilt testing has been shown to be a valuable diagnostic tool for the evaluation of unexplained syncope in patients with structurally normal hearts. Conflicting results were reported regarding whether this may also be so in patients with hypertrophic cardiomyopathy. Gilligan *et al.*[40] performed the head-up tilt testing in 17 hypertrophic cardiomyopathy patients with a history of syncope, 19 without syncope, and 9 normal subjects. They used unconventional criteria for a positive tilt test, defining it as the occurrence of a progressive fall in systolic blood pressure to <90 mmHg associated with impairment of consciousness with or without bradycardia. Reflex hypotension with or without bradycardia, associated with syncope or presyncope, during head-up tilt was induced in 41% of syncopal patients compared with 11% of non-syncopal patients and 22% of control subjects ($P = 0.05$). They interpreted their data to indicate that patients with hypertrophic cardiomyopathy and a history of syncope frequently display hypotension during head-up tilt, suggesting that head-up tilt may yield information about the mechanisms of syncope. Others have not confirmed their findings. Sneddon *et al.*[41] studied 46 patients with hypertrophic cardiomyopathy and applied more strict criteria for a positive tilt test, which was defined as loss of consciousness or a progressive and sustained decrease in systolic blood pressure <60 mmHg. A tilt test was found positive in 15, 17 and 30% of patients with unexplained syncope, explained syncope, and no syncope, respectively. The rate of positive tilts is low in patients with syncope and the high-false positive rate severely compromises the specificity of the test. There is so far no proven role of the head-up tilt test in risk stratification of patients with hypertrophic cardiomyopathy.

Electrophysiological studies

Programmed electrical stimulation

The role of programmed electrical stimulation in the identification of high-risk patients with hypertrophic cardiomyopathy has been controversial.[42–45] The largest series from a single centre reported that programmed ventricular stimulation using up to three premature stimuli in the right and/or left ventricle produced sustained ventricular arrhythmia (i.e. lasting for more than 30 seconds or associated with hypotension) in 43% of patients selected on the basis of a history of previous cardiac arrest, syncope, palpitation, or non-sustained ventricular tachycardia on Holter. Inducible sustained ventricular arrhythmia was associated with a reduced survival.[44,45] Studies from other centres failed to confirm these findings.[43,46] Kuck *et al.*[43] performed a prospective study in 54 patients with hypertrophic cardiomyopathy who underwent electrophysiological studies. Ventricular arrhythmias could be induced in 18 patients (five sustained ventricular tachycardia, three primary ventricular fibrillation). Induction of these arrhythmias was independent of the presence or absence of spontaneous sustained ventricular arrhythmias. Sustained ventricular tachycardia or ventricular fibrillation was inducible not only in patients with documented cardiac arrest or syncope but also in asymptomatic patients. The induction of these arrhythmias is not specific in patients with hypertrophic cardiomyopathy. Similar results and conclusion were obtained from our centre based on data of programmed electrical stimulation from 52 consecutive patients with hypertrophic cardiomyopathy.[46] The use of programmed electrical stimulation adds little if anything to simple non-invasive tests, such as Holter monitoring or exercise testing in the clinical assessment of arrhythmic risk in hypertrophic cardiomyopathy (Table 29.1).

Table 29.1 Predictive power of clinical tests for risk stratification in hypertrophic cardiomyopathy

	Sensitivity (%)	Specificity (%)	PPA (%)	NPA (%)
NSVT[5,6]	69	80	22	97
ABPR[30]	75	66	15	97
PES[46]	33	78	17	90

Abbreviations: ABPR = abnormal blood pressure response during upright exercise testing; NPA = negative predictive accuracy; NSVT = non-sustained ventricular tachycardia; PES = programmed electrical stimulation; PPA = positive predictive accuracy.

Electrocardiogram fractionation

Electrocardiogram fractionation is an electrophysiological research technique designed to analyse the homogeneity of intraventricular conduction. It has been hypothesised that myofibrillar and myocytes disarray create a spectrum of conduction velocities and refractory periods within the myocardium that acts as a substrate for re-entrant tachycardia.[47] Saumarez *et al.* have shown that patients with a history of ventricular fibrillation have marked prolongation ("fractionation") of the paced electrocardiogram at relatively long extrastimulus coupling intervals, whereas patients with no risk factors exhibit very little changes in electrogram morphology. The patients with non-sustained ventricular tachycardia on Holter monitoring or a family history of sudden cardiac death spanned the range from ventricular fibrillation survivors to controls.[46,47] These data require confirmation in prospective studies. In its present form it remains a research tool that is dependent on a prolonged invasive procedure and complex data analysis. Nevertheless, this technique does provide the theoretical basis for non-invasive studies of inhomogeneity of ven-

tricular depolarisation and repolarisation to aid risk factor stratification in hypertrophic cardiomyopathy.

Risk stratification and patient management

Despite relatively low prevalence of hypertrophic cardiomyopathy (1:500), it retains a high profile because it is a common cause of unexpected sudden death in young persons, especially in those engaged in athletic competition.[8,9] Clinical risk stratification in patients with hypertrophic cardiomyopathy is based on the premise that if sudden death can be prevented, the natural history of the disease for most patients is relatively benign. It is also apparent that not all patients within the disease spectrum are at equal risk of premature death, and indeed in some individuals the disease seems to convey little or no added risk.[5,6,48] Risk stratification should be done on an individualised basis.

There are many prognostic factors of sudden death, a reflection of the multifactorial character of sudden death in hypertrophic cardiomyopathy. Five major risk factors have been recognised to be associated with increased risk of sudden cardiac death:

- a family history of premature sudden cardiac death due to hypertrophic cardiomyopathy;[8,9]
- a history of recurrent syncope;[9,45]
- non-sustained ventricular tachycardia on Holter monitoring in adults;[5,6,34]
- an abnormal blood pressure response during upright exercise testing;[29–31]
- severe left ventricular hypertrophy (≥30 mm).[49]

In addition to these recognised risk factors, other markers for sudden death are considered to be young age at diagnosis, myocardial ischaemia (particularly in the young), and clinical or inducible sustained monomorphic ventricular tachycardia.[50]

Conclusive data on the relative value of different risk factors for sudden death are emerging.[36] It is our practice to consider patients with two or more conventional risk factors for prophylactic therapy. In our institution, the presence of two or more risk factors is associated with a 3–4% annual mortality, which is sufficient in the young to initiate prophylactic treatment with low dose amiodarone and/or an implantable cardioverter defibrillator. Both are likely to reduce mortality, although the efficacy of treatment remains to be proven and neither treatment will be universally successful. There is no established management protocol in cases with a single risk factor. Very short runs of non-sustained ventricular tachycardia do not warrant treatment in the absence of any other high-risk factors or identifiable potential triggers for sudden death. Management of patients with a single risk factor is done on an individualised basis. Patients with a single risk factor, i.e. one three-beat episode of non-sustained ventricular tachycardia, a single unexplained syncope episode, or an abnormal blood pressure response on exercise may not require treatment, whilst the same risk factor if recurrent or severe may in some patients be sufficient to warrant treatment.

Conclusions

Ventricular arrhythmias are common in hypertrophic cardiomyopathy, and are associated with sudden death. Identification of patients with hypertrophic cardiomyopathy who are at high risk of sudden death remains the major challenge in clinical management. Non-invasive risk stratification is currently possible although the algorithms need to be refined in relation to age. Based on the non-invasive markers, high-risk patients can be identified and effectively treated.

References

1. WHO report. Report of the 1995 World Health Organisation/International Society and Federation of Cardiology Task Force on the Definition and Classification of Cardiomyopathies. *Circulation* 1996;**93**:841–2.
2. Spirito P, Seidman CE, McKenna WJ, Maron BJ. The management of hypertrophic cardiomyopathy. *New Engl J Med* 1997;**336**:775–85.
3. Marian AJ, Roberts R. Molecular genetics of hypertrophic cardiomyopathy. *Ann Rev Med* 1995;**46**:213–22.
4. Maron BJ, Gardin JM, Flack JM *et al*. Prevalence of hypertrophic cardiomyopathy in a population of young adults. Echocardiographic analysis of 4111 subjects in the CARDIA study (Coronary Artery Risk Development in (Young) Adults). *Circulation* 1995;**92**:785–9.
5. McKenna WJ, England D, Doi JL, Deanfield JE, Oakley C, Goodwin JF. Arrhythmia in hypertrophic cardiomyopathy. I. Influence on prognosis. *Br Heart J* 1981;**46**:168–72.
6. Maron BJ, Savage DD, Wolfson JF, Epstein SE. Prognostic significance of 24-hour ambulatory monitoring in patients with hypertrophic cardiomyopathy: A prospective study. *Am J Cardiol* 1981;**48**:252–7.
7. Alfonso F, Frenneaux MP, McKenna WJ. Clinical sustained uniform ventricular tachycardia in hypertrophic cardiomyopathy: association with left ventricular apical aneurysm. *Br Heart J* 1989;**61**:178–81.
8. Maron BJ, Lipson LC, Roberts WC, Savage DD, Epstein SE. "Malignant" hypertrophic cardiomyopathy: identification of a subgroup of families with unusually frequent premature death. *Am J Cardiol* 1978;**41**:1133–40.
9. McKenna WJ, Deanfield JE, Faruqui A, England D, Oakley C, Goodwin J. Prognosis in hypertrophic cardiomyopathy: Role of age and clinical, electrocardiographic and haemodynamic features. *Am J Cardiol* 1981;**47**:532-8.
10. Frank S, Braunwald E. Idiopathic hypertrophic subaortic stenosis. Clinical analysis of 126 patients with emphasis on the natural history. *Circulation* 1968;**37**:759–88.
11. Spirito P, Chiarella F, Carratino L, Berisso MZ, Bellotti P, Vecchio C. Clinical course and prognosis of hypertrophic cardiomyopathy in an outpatient population. *New Engl J Med* 1989;**320**:749–55.
12. Cecchi F, Olivotto I, Montereggi A, Santoro G, Dolara A, Maron BJ. Hypertrophic cardiomyopathy in Tuscany: clinical course and outcome in an unselected regional population. *J Am Coll Cardiol* 1995;**26**:1529–36.
13. Cannan CR, Reeder GS, Bailey KR, Melton LJ 3rd, Gersh BJ. Natural history of hypertrophic cardiomyopathy. A population-based study, 1976 through 1990. *Circulation* 1995;**92**:2488–95.
14. Maron BJ, Roberts WC, Epstein SE. Sudden death in hypertrophic cardiomyopathy: Profile of 78 patients. *Circulation* 1982;**65**:1388–94.
15. Watkins H, McKenna WJ, Thierfelder L *et al*. Mutations in the genes for cardiac troponin T and alpha-tropomyosin in hypertrophic cardiomyopathy. *New Engl J Med* 1995;**332**:1058–64.
16. Panza JA, Maron BJ. Relation of electrocardiographic abnormalities to evolving left ventricular hypertrophy in hypertrophic cardiomyopathy in childhood. *Am J Cardiol* 1989;**63**:1258–65.
17. Ryan MP, Cleland JG, French JA *et al*. The standard electrocardiogram as a screening test for hypertrophic cardiomyopathy. *Am J Cardiol* 1995;**76**:689–94.
18. Maron BJ, Wolfson JK, Ciro E, Spirito P. Relation of electrocardiographic abnormalities and patterns of left ventricular hypertrophy identified by 2-dimensional echocardiography in patients with hypertrophic cardiomyopathy. *Am J Cardiol* 1983;**51**:189–94.
19. Dritsas A, Gilligan D, Sbarouni E, Nihoyannopoulos P, Oakley CM. QT-interval abnormalities in hypertrophic cardiomyopathy. *Clin Cardiol* 1992;**15**:739–42.
20. Buja G, Miorelli M, Turrini P, Melacini P, Nava A. Comparison of QT dispersion in hypertrophic cardiomyopathy between patients with and without ventricular arrhythmias and sudden death. *Am J Cardiol* 1993;**72**:973–6.
21. Gang Yi, Elliott PM, McKenna WJ *et al*. QT dispersion and risk factors for sudden death in patients with hypertrophic cardiomyopathy. *Am J Cardiol* 1998;**82**:1514–19.
22. Maron BJ, Leyhe MJ, Gohman TE, Casey SA, Crow RS, Hodges M. QT dispersion is not a predictor of sudden cardiac death in hypertrophic cardiomyopathy as assessed in an unselected patient population. *J Am Coll Cardiol* 1999;**33**:129A(abstr.).
23. Perkiömäki JS, Koistinen J, Yli-Mäyry S, Huikuri HV. Dispersion of QT interval in patients with and without susceptibility to ventricular tachyarrhythmias after previous myocardial infarction. *J Am Coll Cardiol* 1995;**26**:174–9.
24. Cripps TR, Counihan PJ, Frenneaux MP, Ward DE, Camm AJ, McKenna WJ. Signal-averaged electrocardiography in hypertrophic cardiomyopathy. *J Am Coll Cardiol* 1990;**15**:956–61.
25. Kulakowski P, Counihan PJ, Camm AJ, McKenna WJ. The value of time and frequency domain, and spectral temporal

mapping analysis of the signal-averaged electrocardiogram in identification of patients with hypertrophic cardiomyopathy at increased risk of sudden death. *Eur Heart J* 1993;**14**:941–50.

26. Englund A, Hnatkova K, Kulakowski P, Elliott PM, McKenna WJ, Malik M. Wavelet decomposition analysis of the signal averaged electrocardiogram used for risk stratification of patients with hypertrophic cardiomyopathy. *Eur Heart J* 1998;**19**:1383–90.

27. Borbola J, Denes P. Oral amiodarone loading therapy. I. The effect on serial signal-averaged electrocardiographic recordings and the QTc in patients with ventricular tachyarrhythmias. *Am Heart J* 1988;**115**:1202–8.

28. Goedel ML, Hofmann M, Schmidt G *et al.* Amiodarone-efficacy and late potentials during long-term therapy. *Int J Pharmacol Ther Toxicol* 1990;**28**:449–54.

29. Frenneaux P, Counihan PJ, Caforio ALP, Chikamori T, McKenna WJ. Abnormal blood pressure response during exercise in hypertrophic cardiomyopathy. *Circulation* 1990;**82**:1995–2002.

30. Sadoul N, Prasad K, Elliott P, Bannerjee S, Frenneaux M, McKenna WJ. Prospective prognostic assessment of blood pressure response during exercise in patients with hypertrophic cardiomyopathy. *Circulation* 1997;**96**:2987–91.

31. Olivotto I, Maron BJ, Montereggi A, Mazzuoli F, Dolara A, Cecchi F. Prognostic value of systemic blood pressure response during exercise in a community-based patient population with hypertrophic cardiomyopathy. *J Am Coll Cardiol* 1999;**33**:2044–51.

32. McKenna WJ, Camm AJ. Sudden death in hypertrophic cardiomyopathy: Assessment of patients at high risk. *Circulation* 1989;**80**:1489–92.

33. Spirito P, Rapezzi C, Autore C *et al.* Prognosis of asymptomatic patients with hypertrophic cardiomyopathy and non-sustained ventricular tachycardia. *Circulation* 1994;**90**:2743–7.

34. Monserrat L, Elliott PM, Penas-Lado M, Castro-Beiras A, McKenna WJ. Prognostic value of non-sustained ventricular tachycardia in adult patients with hypertrophic cardiomyopathy. *Eur Heart J* 1999;**20**:17(abstr.).

35. Cecchi F, Olivotto I, Montereggi A, Squillatini G, Dolara A, Maron BJ. Prognostic value of non-sustained ventricular tachycardia and the potential role of amiodarone treatment in hypertrophic cardiomyopathy: assessment in an unselected non-referral based patient population. *Heart* 1998;**79**:331–6.

36. Elliott PM, Poloniecki J, Sharma S, Dickie S, McKenna WJ. Non-invasive risk stratification in hypertrophic cardiomyopathy. *Heart* 1998;**79**:3 (abstr.).

37. Ajiki K, Murakawa Y, Yanagisawa-miwa A *et al.* Autonomic nervous system activity in idiopathic dilated cardiomyopathy and in hypertrophic cardiomyopathy. *Am J Cardiol* 1993;**71**:1316–20.

38. Counihan PJ, Fei L, Bashir Y, Farrel TG, Haywood GA, McKenna WJ. Assessment of heart rate variability in hypertrophic cardiomyopathy: association with clinical and prognostic features. *Circulation* 1993;**88**:1682–90.

39. Fei L, Slade AK, Prasad K, Malik M, McKenna WJ, Camm AJ. Is there increased sympathetic activity in patients with hypertrophic cardiomyopathy? *J Am Coll Cardiol* 1995;**26**:472–80.

40. Gilligan DM, Nihoyannopoulos P, Chan WL, Oakley CM. Investigation of a haemodynamic basis for syncope in hypertrophic cardiomyopathy. Use of a head-up tilt test. *Circulation* 1992;**85**:2140–8.

41. Sneddon JF, Slade A, Seo H, Camm AJ, McKenna WJ. Assessment of the diagnosis value of head-up tilt testing in the evaluation of syncope in hypertrophic cardiomyopathy. *Am J Cardiol* 1994;**73**:601–4.

42. Geibel A, Brugada P, Zehender M, Stevenson W, Waldecker B, Wellens HJ. Value of programmed electrical stimulation using a standardised ventricular stimulation protocol in hypertrophic cardiomyopathy. *Am J Cardiol* 1987;**60**:738–9.

43. Kuck KH, Kunze KP, Schluter M, Neinaber CA, Costard A. Programmed electrical stimulation in hypertrophic cardiomyopathy: Results in patients with and without cardiac arrest or syncope. *Eur Heart J* 1988;**9**:177–85.

44. Fananapazir L, Tracy C, Leon M. Electrophysiological abnormalities in patients with hypertrophic cardiomyopathy: A consecutive analysis of 155 patients. *Circulation* 1989;**80**:1259–68.

45. Fananapazir L, Chang AC, Epstein SE, McAreavey D. Prognostic determinants in hypertrophic cardiomyopathy. Prospective evaluation of a therapeutic strategy based on clinical, Holter, haemodynamic, and electrophysiological findings. *Circulation* 1992;**86**:730–40.

46. Saumarez R, Slade AKB, Grace AA, Sadoul N, Camm AJ, McKenna WJ. The significance of paced electrogram fractionation in hypertrophic cardiomyopathy: a prospective study. *Circulation* 1995;**91**:2762–8.

47. Saumarez R, Camm AJ, Panagos A *et al.* Ventricular fibrillation in hypertrophic cardiomyopathy is associated with increased fraction of paced right ventricular electrograms. *Circulation* 1992;**86**:467–74.

48. Watkins H, Rosenzweig A, Hwang DS *et al.* Characteristics and prognostic implications of myosin missense mutations in familial hypertrophic cardiomyopathy. *New Engl J Med* 1992;**326**:1108–14.

49. Spirito P, Maron BJ. Relation between extent of left ventricular hypertrophy and occurrence of sudden cardiac death in hypertrophic cardiomyopathy. *J Am Coll Cardiol* 1990;**15**:1521–6.

50. Kuck KH. Arrhythmias in hypertrophic cardiomyopathy. *PACE* 1997;**20**:2706–13.

30 Ventricular arrhythmias in apparently healthy athletes

Francesco Furlanello, Fredrick Fernando, Amedeo Galassi and Annalisa Bertoldi

The definition of a normal heart at times is difficult especially when severe arrhythmias are life-threatening occurring in apparently healthy and asymptomatic subjects with no previously identified underlying cardiac disease. In this instance athletes are usually considered the best expression of a healthy subject.[1-5] In addition, athletes as opposed to normal healthy subjects usually undergo regular medical visits; this is seen particularly in Italy where Italian legislation requires annual visits to determine their eligibility to participate in competitive sport activities and where the sports physician can be liable for an athlete's health in case of dramatic events.[6,7]

Every kind of arrhythmia has been observed in the athletic population. including life-threatening ones, arrhythmic syncope, cardiac arrest, and sudden death, and it is not unusual to discover arrhythmias during a routine sports medical visit; this then usually poses major problems in the decision on an athlete's eligibility.[8,9] Sudden exercise-related death in athletes is still rare (<1% in the adult), but, when it does occur, it is a devastating event with a tremendous impact on the media, that can, at times, lead to forensic consequences for the sports physician and sometimes trigger off new legislations and medical recommendations.[6,9] Even the presence of important arrhythmic events, such as syncope and cardiac arrest during sports activity, or the cessation of a sports career owing to arrhythmias always seem an impossibility because athletes are, by definition, healthy subjects.

For this reason we believe that the analysis of a population of athletes with severe ventricular arrhythmias, previously considered eligible to compete on the basis of certification, can represent a valid study model transposable to the population of arrhythmic subjects with apparently normal hearts.[5,10-12]

However, athletes should also be differentiated with regards to age, since there are different age-related pathologies, such as increased incidence of coronary heart disease over 35 years. For this reason it is important to give a rigorous definition of what an athlete is.

To avoid confusion about the meaning of the word "athlete", we adhered to an accepted definition of a competitive athlete as reported at the 26th Bethesda Conference (1994):

Anyone who participates in an organised team or individual sport that requires regular competition against others as a central component, places a high premium on excellence and achievement, and requires some form of systematic training.[9]

To this definition we have added some further selection criteria unique to Italy:[5]

- The athlete must have a valid sports certificate, requested annually by Italian law, which declares whether he or she is eligible to participate in a specific sport activity.
- The athlete must be younger than 35 years of age at the time of the cardiovascular evaluation

In this study there is also data regarding a subgroup of elite athletes (world, Olympic, and national champions) with complex ventricular arrhythmias that endangered their sports career.[4,5,11,13] The aim of this contribution is to provide useful information for risk stratification of ventricular arrhythmias in apparently normal hearts on the basis of our 25 years' experience

Presentation of referring athletic population

Since 1974 we have continuously evaluated competitive athletes, performing different types of sports, referred to us for significant arrhythmias. The inclusion criteria for these athletes was very rigorous: only athletes who were under 35 years of age, considered until then to be eligible to take part in competitive sports activities, were included.

All these athletes underwent an individualised risk assessment by arrhythmological study protocol including non-invasive and invasive diagnostic techniques (Box 30.1).[5,11-18]

At the last update, January 1999, the study population consisted of 1952 competitive athletes (1637 males and 315 females) with an average age of 21 years, who had been followed up for 3 months to over 10 years (Table 30.1).

In this group 161 elite athletes were included (134 males, 27 females) with an average age of 25 years, with minimum-maximum follow-up of 3 months to just over 9

Box 30.1   Risk assessment in competitive athletes with ventricular arrhythmias

- Family and personal history
- Clinical visit
- Routine blood tests (including thyroid function tests)
- Resting and stress test ECG
  - T wave alternans*
- Holter recording, also during intense physical activity
  - heart rate variability*
  - QT dynamics*
- 2 Doppler colour flow echocardiography
  - stress echo, pharmacological and during exercise
  - transoesophageal echocardiography
- Magnetic resonance imagining (MRI)
- Nuclear cardiology
  - myocardial perfusion imaging
  - radionuclide angiography
  - MIBG scintigraphy
- Signal averaged ECG time and frequency domain analysis
- Uphead tilt-test
- Specific blood test (e.g. for myocarditis)
- Search for illicit substances (e.g. amphetamines, anabolic steroids, corticosteroids, cocaine, etc)
- Pharmacological testing
  - ajmaline, procainamide, flecainide administration
  - isoproterenol infusion
- Genetic testing
- Transoesophageal electrophysiological study
- Endocavitary electrophysiological study
- Cardiac catheterisation and angiography, endomyocardial biopsy

*Investigational in athletes

years; all had previously been competing at international level, including world, Olympic, European and national championships (Table 30.1).

Major cardiac events

Cardiac arrest

Among the 1952 competitive arrhythmic athletes, 52 had cardiac arrest, fatal in 21, resuscitated with successful CPR in 31 (Table 30.2).

Resuscitated cardiac arrest occurred during physical or athletic activity in all but two at rest, one had a Wolff–Parkinson–White (WPW) syndrome and experienced cardiac arrest at night (Table 30.2), another with dilated cardiomyopathy had a cardiac arrest during an emotional episode.

Ventricular tachycardia (VT) and ventricular fibrillation (VF)

VT and VF were the leading arrhythmic causes of cardiac arrest in 28/31 (90.4%) resuscitated athletes (Fig. 30.1).

VT/VF was documented in 21/28 athletes, but seven with WPW had a pre-excited atrial fibrillation followed by VF and cardiac arrest. VT was due to a torsade de pointes

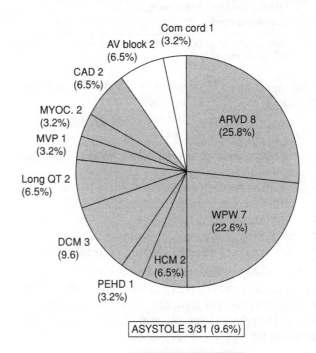

Figure 30.1 Cardiac abnormalities and arrhythmic causes of cardiac arrest in 31 athletes with average age 26 years. Abbreviations: ARVD = Arrhythmogenic right ventricular dysplasia; CAD = Coronary artery disease; Com cord = Commotio cordis; DCM = Dilated cardiomyopathy; HCM = Hypertrophic cardiomyopathy; Long QT = long QT syndrome; MVP = Mitral valve prolapse; MYOC = Myocarditis; PEHD = Primary electrical heart disease

Table 30.1   Young competitive athletes with arrhythmias studied from 1974 to 1999

	No. athletes	Male	Female	Average age (years)	Follow-up (months)	Sudden death (%)	Cardiac arrest (%)
Total athletes	1952	1637	315	21.4	3–123	21 (1.1)	31 (1.6)
Elite athletes	161	134	27	25.1	3–109	3 (1.9)	4 (2.5)

Table 30.2   Fatal and resuscitated cardiac death in 52 young competitive athletes

Disease	Sudden death		Cardiac arrest	
	Total athletes	% of total SD	Total athletes	% of total CA
ARVD	5	23.8	8	25.8
WPW	2	9.5	7	22.5
Dilated cardiomyopathy	2	9.5	3	9.5
Hypertrophic cardiomyopathy			2	6.5
Mitral valve prolapse	2	9.5	1	3.2
Myocarditis	5	23.8	2	6.5
Coronary artery disease	4	19	2	6.5
Unknown cardiomyopathy	1	0.6		
Long QT			2	6.5
AV block			2	6.5
Primary electrical heart disease			1	3.2
Commotio cordis			1	3.2

Abbreviations: ARVD = arrhythmogenic right ventricular dysplasia; AV = atrioventricular; WPW = Wolff–Parkinson–White syndrome

in congenital long QT syndrome in one and acquired long QT (from myocarditis) in the other.

A structural cardiac abnormality was diagnosed in 18 athletes previously considered healthy:

- arrhythmogenic right ventricular dysplasia (ARVD) in eight (25.8%);
- hypertrophic cardiomyopathy (HCM) in two (6.5%);
- dilative cardiomyopathy (DCM) in three (9.6%);
- myocarditis in two (3.2%);
- mitral valve prolapse (MVP) in one (3.2%);
- coronary artery disease (CAD) in two (6,5%).

One athlete, a basketball player, with previously complex ventricular ectopic beats (VEBs), had cardiac arrest while playing; she had inducible VF and was considered a bearer of a "primary electrical heart disorder"; an ICD was implanted for high risk of recurrences.

Asystole

Asystole was a cause of cardiac arrest in only 3/31 athletes (9.6%): from a paroxysmal AV block in two with Lev–Lenegre concealed disease and from asystolic commotio cordis in one[5,19] (thoracic impact in a rugby player with an opponent during competition).

Follow-up

The follow-up was a minimum 3 months and maximum 15 and a half years. Of the 31 athletes resuscitated after the episode of cardiac arrest, 27 are still alive:

- six had successful RF catheter ablation of the accessory pathway;
- seven required an ICD implantation;
- two had a pacemaker implantation;
- 11 are under intense antiarrhythmic drug treatment.

Four athletes suffered sudden death during the follow-up period, because of the evolution of the underlying heart disease in two (one athlete with ARVD and another with DCM), whilst the other two athletes died during exercise (which had been banned by the physician) – one with a DCM and another with MVP.

Five athletes with CA have to be considered elite athletes since they were previously competing at international level: one had asystolic commotio cordis, one had an ARVD, one had DCM, one had HCM, whilst the fifth had WPW – cardiac arrest was due in this athlete to rapid pre-excited atrial fibrillation, which degenerated into VF at night.[12]

Sudden death

Among the 1952 competitive arrhythmic athletes, 21 suffered sudden death (1.1%) (Table 30.2 and Fig. 30.2).

In 19 of 21 athletes with SCD, an underlying structural heart disease was documented:

- ARVD in five (23%);
- myocarditis in five (23%);
- CAD in four (19%);
- DCM in two (9.5%) in one post-myocarditis;
- complex MVP in two (9.5%);
- cardiomyopathy of unknown origin in one (autopsy results were not available);
- WPW in two (9.5%).

These last two athletes had WPW and were at high risk; this has been previously documented, but both refused any treatment and suffered sudden death at rest (one at night).

Timing of sudden death

Seven athletes (33%) had sudden death as a first event: four had myocarditis (one at night) and three had CAD

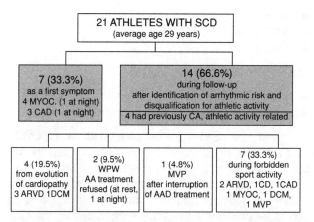

Figure 30.2 Timing of sudden death in 21 competitive young athletes. (AA = antiarrhythmic; AAD = antiarrhythmic drugs; ARVD = arrhythmogenic right ventricular dysplasia; CA = cardiac death; DCM = dilated cardiomyopathy; MVP = mitral valve prolapse; MYOC = myocarditis; SCD = sudden cardiac death; WPW = Wolff–Parkinson–White syndrome.)

(one at night). Fourteen (66.6%) had sudden death during the follow-up period after identification of the arrhythmic risk, and consequently considered non-eligible to take part in competitive sports (Fig. 30.1). Four of these had a previous exercise-related CA.

Only four (19.5%) died from evolution of the identified cardiac disease (three ARVD, one DCM). The other 10 died during the follow-up period, disregarding medical recommendations for treatment (two WPW, one MVP) and for interruption of athletic activity. In fact seven had sudden death during banned sporting activities (two ARVD, one unknown cardiomyopathy, one CAD, one myocarditis, one DCM, and one MVP).

Three athletes who suffered sudden death were previously elite level ones: two identified as high risk had sudden death during the follow-up period whilst exercising, even though they had been told not to, but one was a rugby player who died suddenly at night, and this was a first symptom with documented CAD at pathological examination.

Risk stratification for severe cardiac events in apparently healthy competitive athletes with ventricular arrhythmic manifestations

Ventricular ectopic beats (VEBs)

VEBs are quite common in athletes and are frequently benign. In a previous study in elite athletes with arrhythmias, the prevalence of VEBs was 63.7% of all types of identified rhythm disturbances.[4]

In a 5-year Holter study conducted on the soccer players of the Italian National Team, the prevalence of VEBs was 54.1% (complex in 14.6%): none of these athletes had an identified underlying cardiac disease[20] and they are all asymptomatic after 10 years' follow-up. Another 5-year follow-up study conducted on endurance athletes with VEB but without evidence of cardiovascular abnormalities showed a good prognosis.[21] The presence of asymptomatic VEBs in otherwise healthy athletes does not seem to increase the risk of SCD.[8] However, the detection in competitive athletes of numerous or complex forms of VEBs or exercise-induced ectopy and/or with arrhythmic symptoms may induce a careful investigation for a structural heart disease or other arrhythmogenic causes (i.e. use of illicit drugs,[22] metabolic disorders, thyroid dysfunction, etc.).

Particular attention should be paid to the spatial cardiac origin of ventricular ectopy, since right bundle branch block (RBBB) morphology may be a sign of ARVD, or left BBB (LBBB) morphology may suggest HCM, DCM, complex MVP, or myocarditis.

Repolarisation abnormalities in 12-lead ECG may be a sign of some underlying arrhythmogenic heart disease:

- T wave inversion in V1–V3 may be present in ARVD.[15,17,23,24]
- RBBB and ST elevation in the right precordial leads has been described in the Brugada syndrome.[25,26]
- QT prolongation is diagnostic for long QT syndrome.
- QT dispersion does not seem to increase in elite athletes with normal "athletic heart".[27]

Family and personal history, clinical visit, Holter monitoring (also with intense physical activity), stress test ECG, 2D colour flow echocardiography signal averaged ECG (Box 30.1), are the fundamental non-invasive diagnostic techniques,[4,5,6,8,10,27,31] MRI, nuclear cardiology, cardiac catheterisation, and angiography may reveal some undetected subclinical silent cardiac abnormalities such as early stages of ARVD, DCM, HCM myocarditis, and congenital and atherosclerotic CAD.[32–37]

An electrophysiological endocavitary study may induce sustained VT/VF also in asymptomatic athletes with silent arrhythmogenic cardiopathy at high risk of, for example, Brugada syndrome[25] or ARVD.[13,15,23]

Life-threatening ventricular arrhythmias in competitive athletes

There is sufficient evidence to say that even elite athletes, previously considered eligible to participate in strenuous physical activity, may have life-threatening arrhythmias, which could be the cause of severe cardiac events, such as arrhythmic syncope, cardiac arrest, and sudden death; in the majority of the cases studies, these were exercise-related.[3,10,11,12,38-43] These arrhythmias are usually represented by sustained fast VT mono- or polymorphic, torsade de pointes[1] with or without long QT syndrome (short coupled variant of torsade de pointes), or pre-excited atrial fibrillation in WPW that degenerates in VF (Box 30.2).[44,45]

Ventricular fibrillation can be the first or last manifestation of life-threatening arrhythmia as results from our analysis in athletes (younger than 35 years of age) with cardiac arrest where VF is the cause in 90% of the cases vs 10% asystolic arrest cases. (Fig. 30.1). VF in the competitive athlete occurs with structural heart disease or primary electrical disorder present.[16,17,41,42] In our 31 competitive athletes younger than 35 years of age with exercise-induced cardiac arrest, an underlying cardiac disease was present. These were:

- ARVD in one
- HCM in two
- DCM in three

Box 30.2 Life-threatening ventricular arrhythmias in competitive athletes able to induce CA and SD

- Monopolymorphic, torsade de pointes, VF
  - in structural heart disease also in early phases
    - ARVD, DCM, HCM, CAD, myocarditis etc.
  - from primary electrical disorders
    - torsade de pointes in congenital long QT syndrome
    - idiopathic VT/VF (in apparently intact heart)
    - short coupled variant of torsade de pointes with normal QT
    - Brugada syndrome
  - Commotio cordis from to VF

Abbreviations: ARVD = arrhythmogenic right ventricular dysplasia; CAD = coronary artery disease; DCM = dilated cardiomyopathy; HCM = hypertrophic cardiomyopathy; VF = ventricular fibrillation; VT = ventricular tachycardia; WPW = Wolff–Parkinson–White syndrome.

Notes: **Brugada syndrome**: right bundle branch block complete or incomplete, ST elevation in right precordial leads, clinical and/or inducible VT/VF, high risk of recurrences and SD.
Commotio cordis: CA or SD from non-penetrating chest wall trauma during athletic activity in young athletes (prevalently male) in the absence of structural injury to the thoracic wall and myocardium. The mechanism is an FV induced by the impact during critical vulnerable period (like R on T phenomenon) of repolarization.[19] Some cases with asystole were documented.[5]
Life-threatening arrhythmias in athletes: usually exercise-sport activity related. Sometimes (e.g. WPW, CAD, Brugada syndrome) may occur at rest.

- myocarditis in two
- MVP in one
- CAD in two.

Primary electrical disorders included:

- WPW in seven
- long QT in two (one congenital, one acquired).

Only in a young ex-basketball player with complex VEBs with a cardiac arrest from VF during physical activity was the final diagnosis "primary electrical heart disease".

A recognised underlying heart disease responsible for arrhythmic sudden death was observed in 21 athletes except for two with a preceding electrophysiological diagnosis of high-risk WPW.

The cardiac diseases

The main underlying cardiac diseases in young competitive athletes who experience sudden death are HCM in North America (11%)[46] and ARVD in Northern Italy.[47,48] The later data are confirmed by the fact that in our analysis ARVD was the underlying pathology in 25% of our 31 athletes resuscitated from cardiac arrest and 23% in the 21 athletes who had sudden death. Even myocarditis is a frequent cause of sudden death in athletes[49,50] and had a prevalence of 23% (5/21) in our group of sudden death athletes.

CAD is the major cause of sudden death in athletes older than 35 years[51-57] but can also occur as a first symptom in younger athletes.[11,40,58,59] In our population an atherosclerotic CAD was present in 2/31 (6.4%) of the athletes who were resuscitated from cardiac arrest and in 4/21 (19%) of the athletes who had sudden death.

Of the totally silent arrhythmogenic pathologies and those with a high risk of sudden death in athletes, both CAD and myocarditis were present in all of our seven competitive athletes younger than 35 years of age and who had a sudden death as first event (Fig. 30.2).

Evaluation of competitive athletes with life-threatening arrhythmias

Evaluation may include the basal non-invasive investigations[5,6,16,60] (Box 30.I), nuclear cardiology imaging, cardiac MRI (particularly useful in the diagnosis of ARVD), cardiac catheterisation and coronarography to rule out atherosclerotic or congenital coronary disease, and myocardial biopsy in selected cases of suspected myocarditis (not useful for the active forms), ARVD, or DCM.[61]

An endocavitary electrophysiological study can confirm the diagnosis, establish the site of origin and mechanism of VT, when inducible, and provides information for the implantation of an ICD, which is considered more effective than an antiarrhythmics in those young patients with a high risk of recurrence of cardiac arrest. An ICD was implanted in seven of our athletes resuscitated from a cardiac arrest and in two elite athletes with ARVD at risk of VT and cardiac arrest.

It is important to identify subjects with warning prodromal symptoms such as syncope, which is usually the most important symptom.[17,62,63]

Recently genetic testing has been performed on a restricted number of hereditary cardiac pathologies causing sudden death,[64] such as long QT syndrome in its various forms,[65,66] ARVD,[67] HCM, and particularly the Brugada syndrome,[25,64] an arrhythmic pathology not yet described in athletes.

In HCM recent results of molecular genetic studies indicate the probable existence of different subgroups of families with different prognosis, at low or high risk respectively.[68] Also some arrhythmic pathologies exist in the young athlete previously described as idiopathic and at the present time as "primary electrical disorder". They are characterised by ventricular tachyarrhythmias in a structurally normal heart where the electrical instability is caused by a genetic defect concerning ion channels; the best known is the Brugada syndrome where a frequent finding is the mutation of the sodium channel genes.[25,64] The Brugada syndrome is an hereditary disorder characterised by ST elevation in V1–V3, associated with complete or incomplete RBBB and with clinical and/or inducible VT/VF. There are even asymptomatic latent forms in which the ECG pattern can be reproduced by testing with drugs such as procainamide, ajmaline, and flecainide (drugs that have an electrophysiological effect on the sodium channels). This is an arrhythmic pathology in an apparently healthy subject with a high risk of sudden death and a good indication for the implantation of an ICD.

Sports activity and life-threatening arrhythmias in athletes

There is sufficient evidence to suggest that exercise can have a trigger effect in the induction of life-threatening arrhythmias leading to cardiac arrest and sudden death in those athletes with silent underlying arrhythmogenic pathologies. The importance of exercise as a cause of sudden death has been extensively described in subjects with ARVD,[13,15,23,47] HCM,[3] and myocarditis.

From our experience cardiac arrest nearly always occurred during exercise, competion or practice, except in two cases in which it occurred at rest during the night (subject with WPW at risk) and another, with DCM, at rest during a stressful occasion. In particular, each of seven athletes, in the subgroup banned from taking part of any type of sport because of the high risk (i.e. two had had cardiac arrest on field), succumbed to sudden death during forbidden competition or practice (Fig. 30.1)

Both the Italian[6,7] guidelines and North American[9] ones preclude banning competitive sport activity in athletes who have had a cardiac arrest from ventricular arrhythmias, unless the arrhythmyic cause is not completely resolved. In fact in six athletes in our study with cardiac arrest from pre-excited atrial fibrillation in WPW syndrome, athletic activity was allowed after successful RF catheter ablation of the accessory pathway.

Finally, the population of ex-athletes identified at high risk for arrhythmogenic pathologies need to be strictly prevented from sporting activity, the decision based on periodical clinical surveillance, life-styles, interventional and pharmacological therapies, with particular regards for what concerns the use of RF catheter ablation, when possible, and ICD implantation in cases of high risk of VT, cardiac arrest, and sudden death.

Conclusions

Young competitive athletes, especially top level ones, are considered by the public to be the epitomy of health with a normal heart. It is, however, not a rare finding to record, during a routine visit or observe in some athletes during their sporting career, ventricular arrhythmias that are usually benign but in some cases can be life-threatening and can lead to cardiac arrest or sudden death.

Usually in these subjects an underlying arrhythmogenic cardiac pathology or some primary electrical disorders (such as WPW and long QT syndrome) are present, until then silent and ignored. There are also some cases in which no underlying cardiac disease can be found, even after pathological examination; maybe in these cases there are hereditary genetic defects, such as in the Brugada syndrome (which has not yet been described in competitive athletes). Genetic testing will certainly have a future, especially in the detection of initial and subclinical forms, especially if hereditary.

Athletes with significant ventricular arrhythmias have to undergo a careful comprehensive medical examination with invasive and if necessary non-invasive diagnostic techniques in order to:

- make a detailed diagnostic and prognostic individuation of the suspected arrhythmias;
- search for any underlying structural heart disease or primary arrhythmic disorders recognised as a cause of life-threatening arrhythmias;
- exclude any infectious, metabolic, electrolytic, toxic, or use of banned drugs;

- classify the recognised arrhythmias concerning sport eligibility;
- take the final decisions for sport eligibility or non-eligibility;
- implement a prolonged clinical surveillance and pharmacological and/or interventional treatment (RFCA, ICD implantation), particularly in athletes at risk of recurrences of tachyventricular arrhythmias, cardiac arrest, or sudden death.

References

1. Jordaens L, Tavernier R, Kazmierczak J, Dimmer C. Ventricular arrhythmias in apparently health subjects. *PACE* 1997;20:2692–8.
2. Maron BJ, Thompson PD, Puffer JC et al. Cardiovascular preparticipation screening of competitive athletes. *Circulation* 1996;**94**:850–6.
3. Maron BJ. Scope of the problem of sudden death in athletes: definitions, epidemiology and socioeconomic implications. In: Bayes de Luna A, Furlanello F, Maron BJ, Zipes DP eds. *Arrhythmias and sudden death in athletes.* Dordrecht: Kluwer Academic Publishers, 2000, Ch. 1, pp. 1–10.
4. Bertoldi A, Furlanello F, Fernando F et al. Cardio-arrhythmologic evaluation of symptoms and arrhythmic manifestations in 110 top level consecutive professional athletes. *New Trends Arrhyth* 1993;**9**:199–209.
5. Furlanello F, Bertoldi A, Fernando F, Biffi A. Competitive athletes with arrhythmias. Classification, evaluation and treatment. In: Bayes de Luna A, Furlanello F, Maron BJ, Zipes DP eds. *Arrhythmias and sudden death in athletes.* Dordrecht: Kluwer Accademic Publishers, 2000, Ch. 7, pp. 89–105.
6. Comitato Organizzativo Cardiologico per l'idoneità allo Sport (COCIS). Protocolli cardiologici per il giudizio di idoneità allo sport agonistico 1995. *G Ital Cardiol* 1996;**26**:949–83.
7. Biffi A, Furlanello F, Caselli G, Bertoldi A, Fernando F. Italian guidelines for competitive athletes with arrhythmias. In: Bayes de Luna A, Furlanello F, Maron BJ, Zipes DP eds. *Arrhythmias and sudden death in athletes.* Dordrecht: Kluwer Academic Publishers, 2000, Ch. 10, pp. 153–60.
8. Al Sheikh T, Zipes D. Guidelines for competitive athletes with arrhythmias. In: Bayes de Luna A, Furlanello F, Maron BJ, Zipes DP eds. *Arrhythmias and sudden death in athletes.* Dordrecht: Kluwer Academic Publishers, 2000, Ch. 9, pp. 119–51.
9. Maron B.J, Mitchell J. 26th Bethesda Conference. Recommendations for determining eligibility for competition in athletes with cardiovascular abnormalities. *J Am Coll Cardiol* 1994;**24**:848–99.
10. Furlanello F, Bettini R, Cozzi F. et al. Ventricular arrhythmias and sudden death in athletes. Clinical aspects of life-threatening arrhythmias. *Ann NY Acad Sci* 1984;**427**:253–79.
11. Fur Ianello F, Bertoldi A, Bettini R, Dallago M, Vergara G. l. Life threatening tachyarrhythmias in athletes. *PACE* 1992;**15**:1403–12.
12. Furlanello F, Bertoldi A, Galassi A et al. Management of severe cardiac arrhythmic events in elite athletes. *PACE,* 1999;**22**:A165.
13. Furlanello F, Bertoldi A, Bettini R, Durante G.B, Vergara G. The disease in competitive athletes. In: Nava A, Rossi L, Thiene G eds. eds. *Arrhythmogenic right ventricular cardiomyopathy/dysplasia.* Amsterdam: Elsevier Science BV, 1997, pp. 477–87.
14. Furlanello F, Bertoldi A, Dallago M et al. Atrial fibrillation in elite athletes. *J Cardiovasc Electrophysiol* 1998;**9**: 563–8(Suppl.).
15. Furlanello F, Bertoldi A, Dallago M et al. Cardiac arrest and sudden death in competitive athletes with arrhythmogenic right ventricular dysplasia. *PACE* 1998;**21**:331–5.
16. Furlanello F, Bertoldi A. Le aritmie nello sportivo: gestione clinica. *Cardiologia* 1998;**43**(Suppl.2):263–71.
17. Bertoldi A, Furlanello F, Fernando F et al. Young competitive athletes resuscitated from cardiac arrest on field: What have we learned and what can be done? *New Trends Arrhyth* 1996;1–4:20–30.
18. Furlanello F, Bertoldi A, Fernando F. Current criteria for evaluation of athletes with arrhythmias. In: Pelliccia A, Caselli G, Bellotti P, eds. *Advances in sports cardiology.* Milano: Springer-Verlag Italia, 1997, pp. 67–72.
19. Link M, Maron B, Estes M. Commotio cordis. In: Estes NAM, Salem DN, Wang PJ, eds. *Sudden cardiac death in the athlete.* Armonk, NY: Futura Publishing Co. Inc., 1998, pp. 515–28.
20. Furlanello F, Bettini R, Resina A et al. Mondiali di calcio 1990: 5 anni di sorveglianza aritmologica in calciatori della Nazionale Italiana. In: D'Alessandro LC ed. *Heart surgery.* Roma: CESI, 1989, pp. 631–4.
21. Palatini P, Scanavacca G, Bongiovi S et al. Prognostic significance of ventricular extrasystoles in healthy professional athletes: results of a 5-year follow-up. *Cardiology* 1993;**82**:286.
22. Kloner R. Illicit drug use in the athlete as a contributor to cardiac events. In: Estes NAM, Salem DN, Wang PJ, eds. *Sudden cardiac death in the athlete.* Armonk, NY: Futura Publishing Co. Inc., 1998, pp. 441–51.
23. Nava A, Rossi L, Thiene G eds. *Arrhythmogenic right ventricular cardiomyopathy/dysplasia.* Amsterdam: Elsevier Science BV, 1997.
24. Leclercq JF, Coumel P. Changes in surface ECG and signal-averaged ECG with time right ventricular dysplasia. Evidence for an evolving disease. *G Ital Cardiol* 1998; **28**(Suppl. 1):488–92.
25. Brugada J, Brugada P, Brugada R. The syndrome of right bundle branch block, ST segment elevation in V1 to V3 and sudden death. The Brugada syndrome. *Europace* 1999;**1**:156–66.
26. Corrado D, Basso C, Buja G, Nava A, Thiene G. Right bundle branch block, right precordial ST segment elevation and sudden death in the young. *G Ital Cardiol* 1998;(Suppl. 1):566–8.
27. Biffi A, Verdile L, Pelliccia A et al. QT dispersion in elite

athletes with and without ventricular arrhythmias. *G Ital Cardiol* 1999;**29**(Suppl. 5).

28. Biffi A, Verdile L, Caselli G. *et al.* Ventricular arrhythmias in athletes: markers of subclinical heart disease. *G Ital Cardiol* 1998;**28**(Suppl. 1): 519–21.

29. Zeppilli P, Santini C. L'ecocardiogramma nell'atleta. In: Zeppilli P, ed. *Cardiologia dello sport*. Roma: CESI, 1995, pp. 197–242.

30. Bettini R, Bonato P, Furlanello F. Prevalence of late potentials in normal and arrhythmic athletes. In: Santini M, ed. *International symposium on progress in clinical pacing*. Armonk, NY: Futura Media Service, 1994, p. 707.

31. Folino F, Dal Corso L, Oselladore Luca, Nava A. Signal-averaged electrocardiogram. In: Nava A, Rossi L, Thiene G, eds. *Arrhythmogenic right ventricular cardiomyopathy/dysplasia*. Amsterdam: Elsevier Science BV, 1997, pp. 210–23.

32. Wichter T, Lentschig M.G, Reimer P, Borggrefe M, Breithard G. Magnetic resonance imaging. In: Nava A, Rossi L, Thiene G, eds. *Arrhythmogenic right ventricular cardiomyopathy/dysplasia*. Amsterdam: Elsevier Science BV, 1997, pp. 269–84.

33. Penco M, Di Cesare E, Aurigemma G. *et al.* l. Arrhythmogenic right ventricular dysplasia: which diagnostic role for magnetic resonance imaging? *G Ital Cardiol* 1998;**28**(Suppl.1):475–81.

34. Corrodi JG, Udelson EJ. Noninvasive imaging techniques to assess cardiac disease in the athlete. In: Estes NAM, Salem DN, Wang PJ, eds. *Sudden cardiac death in the athlete*. Armonk, NY: Futura Publishing Co. Inc., 1998, pp. 159–87.

35. Le Guludec D, Slama M, Faraggi M *et al.* Radionuclide angiography. In: Nava A, Rossi L, Thiene G, eds. *Arrhythmogenic right ventricular cardiomyopathy/dysplasia*. Amsterdam: Elsevier Science BV, 1997, pp. 285–97.

36. Bettini R, Camerani M, Severi S, Furlanello F. MIBG scintigraphy in sportsmen. In: Nava A, Rossi L, Thiene G, eds. *Arrhythmogenic right ventricular cardiomyopathy/dysplasia*. Amsterdam: Elsevier Science BV, 1997, pp. 463–76.

37. Witchter T, Hindricks G, Lerch H *et al.* Regional myocardial sympathetic dysinnervation in arrhythmogenic right ventricular cardiomyopathy. An analysis using ^{123}I-meta-iodobenzylguanidine scintigraphy. *Circulation* 1994;**89**:667–83.

38. Maron BJ, Shirani J, Poliac L.C. *et al.* Sudden death in young competitive athletes: Clinical, demographic and pathological profiles. *JAMA* 1996;**276**:199–204.

39. Maron BJ. Hypertrophic cardiomyopathy as a cause of sudden death in the young competitive athlete. Clinical, demographic and pathological profiles, *JAMA* 1996;**16**:301–17.

40. Corrado D, Basso C, Thiene G. Pathologic findings in victims of sports-related sudden cardiac death. *New Trends Arrhyth* 1995;**11**:30–2.

41. Furlanello F, Bertoldi A, Dallago M *et al.* Aborted sudden death in competitive athletes. *Progr Clini Pacing* 1994;**51**: 733–41.

42. Furlanello F, Bertoldi A, Fernando F, Dallago M, Inama G, Vergara G. Estudio cardioaritmologico de jovenes atletas resucitados de una muerte subita en el campo de juego. *Ed Lat Electrocard* 1996;**2**:25–37.

43. Furlanello F, Bettini R, Bertoldi A *et al.* Competitive sports and cardiac arrhythmias. In: Luderitz B, Saksena S eds. *Interventional electrophysiology*. Mount Kisco, NY: Futura Publishing, 1991, pp. 41–7.

44. Vergara G, Furlanello F, Disertori M *et al.* Induction of supraventricular tachyarrhythmia at rest and during exercise with transesophageal atrial pacing in the electrophysiological evaluation of asymptomatic athletes with WPW syndrome. *Eur Heart J* 1988;**9**:1119–26.

45. Furlanello F, Bertoldi A, Vergara G *et al.* Cardiac preexcitation: what one should do in the selection and in the follow-up of an athlete. *Int J Sports Cardiol* 1992;**1**:11–16.

46. Maron BJ. Cardiovascular causes and pathology of sudden death in athletes: American experience. In: Bayes de Luna A, Furlanello F, Maron BJ, Zipes DP eds. *Arrhythmias and sudden death in athletes*. Dordrecht: Kluwer Academic Publishers, 2000, Ch. 4, pp. 31–48.

47. Thiene G, Basso C, Corrado D. Pathology of sudden death in young athletes: European experience. In: Bayes de Luna A, Furlanello F, Maron BJ, Zipes DP eds. *Arrhythmias and sudden death in athletes*. Dordrecht: Kluwer Academic Publishers, 2000, Ch. 5, pp. 49–69.

48. Thiene G, Basso C, Corrado D. Is prevention of sudden death in young athletes feasible? *Cardiologia* 1999;**44**: 497–505.

49. Portugal D, Smith J. Myocarditis and the athlete. In: Estes NAM, Salem DN, Wang PJ eds. *Sudden cardiac death in athlete*. Armonk, NY: Futura Publishing Company, 1998, pp. 349–71.

50. Valente M, Basso C, Calabrese F, Thiene G. Viral myocarditis and sudden death. *G Ital Cardiol* 1999;**29**(Suppl.5): 54–8.

51. Cantwell JD. The athlete's heart syndrome. *Int J Cardiol* 1987;**17**:1.

52. Opie LH. Sudden death and sport. *Lancet* 1975;**1**:263.

53. Maron BJ, Epstein SE, Roberts WC. Causes of sudden death in competitive athletes. *J Am Coll Cardiol* 1986;**7**:204.

54. Waller BF, Roberts WC. Sudden death while running in conditioned runners aged 40 years or over. *Am J Cardiol* 1980;**45**:1292.

55. Hawley DA, Slentz K, Clarke MA *et al.* Athletic fatalities. *Am J Forensic Med Pathol* 1990;**11**:124.

56. Virmani IR, Rabinowitz M, McAllister HA. Nontraumatic death in joggers: a series of 30 patients at autopsy. *Am J Med* 1982;**72**:874.

57. Northcote RJ, Evans ADB, Ballantyne D. Sudden death in squash players. *Lancet* 1984;**1**:148.

58. Corrado D, Thiene G, Nava A, Rossi L, Pennelli N. Sudden cardiac death in young competitive athletes: clinicopathologic correlation in 22 cases. *Am J Med* 1990;**89**:588.

59. Furlanello F, Bertoldi A, Dallago M *et al.* Evaluacion cardioarritmologica del atleta. In: Bayes De Luna A, Furlanello F, Maron BJ, Serra Grima JR eds. *Cardiologia deportiva*. Barcelona: Doyma Libros, 1994, pp. 172–81.

60. Myerburg RJ, Mitrani R, Interian A, Castellanos A. Identification of risk of cardiac arrest and sudden cardiac death in athletes. In: Estes NAM, Salem D, Wang P eds. *Sudden cardiac death in the athlete*. Armonk, NY: Futura Publishing Company, 1998, pp. 25–55.

61. Angelini A, Basso C, Turrini P, Thiene G. Clinical and

pathological relevance of endomyocardial biopsy. In: Nava A, Rossi L, Thiene G. *Arrhythmogenic right ventricular cardiomyopathy/dysplasia*. Amsterdam: Elsevier Science BV, 1997, pp. 257–68.

62. Olshansky B. Evaluation of syncope in the athlete. *G Ital Cardiol* 1999;**29**(Suppl.5):344–51.

63. Corrado D, Basso C, Thiene G. Sudden arrhythmic death in young people: warning symptoms and pathologic substrates. *G Ital Cardiol* 1999;**29**(Suppl.5):52–4.

64. Priori S, Cerrone M. Molecular bases of juvenile sudden cardiac death. *G Ital Cardiol* 1999;**29**(Suppl.5):430–3.

65. Schwartz PJ. Gene therapy for long QT syndrome: fact or fiction? In: Raviele A ed. *Cardiac arrhythmias 1999*, Vol. I. Milano: Springer-Verlag Italia, 2000, pp. 306–10.

66. Priori SG, Crotti L. Brugada and long QT syndrome are two different disease: true or false? In: Raviele A ed. *Cardiac arrhythmias 1999*, Vol. I. Milano: Springer-Verlag Italia, 2000, pp. 291–8.

67. Nava A, Bauce B, Villanova C *et al*. Arrhythmogenic right ventricular cardiomyopathy: a report of 162 familial cases. *G Ital Cardiol* 1998;**28**(Suppl. 1):492–6.

68. Basso C, Corrado D, Thiene G. Hypertrophic cardiomyopathy and sudden death in the young. *G Ital Cardiol* 1999;**29**(Suppl.5):46–8.

31 Paroxysmal atrial fibrillation

Johan EP Waktare

The patient population that suffers from paroxysmal atrial fibrillation (AF) is substantially different from that which suffers from persistent or permanent forms of the disorder; they are younger and likely to be free of structural heart disease. This difference arises for two reasons. Patients with paroxysmal AF may have distinct mechanisms for AF that do not require the more diffuse atrial myopathy and/or disturbance of atrial electrophysiology that predispose to sustained forms of the arrhythmia. Secondly, paroxysmal AF can represent the initial presentation of AF, which progresses over time to persistent and finally permanent AF. Thus the issues pertaining to risk assessment in this population also differ significantly.

This chapter will describe the population at risk of paroxysmal AF, based upon clinical characteristics, and describe current methods of risk assessment. It will also discuss the clinical application of these tests and the prognostic importance of paroxysmal AF itself.

Mechanisms, and their implication for risk assessment

There are two competing mechanisms of paroxysmal AF currently at the fore. The first is the concept of multiple wavelet re-entry within the atria, which was originally proposed by Moe four decades ago.[1,2] This holds that AF is sustained by multiple re-entrant wavefronts of depolarisation. These rotate around native barriers to conduction (caval orifices and atrioventricular valves), but are also dependent on creating areas of functional block and slow conduction by depolarising the atria close to their effective refractory period. Slowing of atrial conduction and atrial enlargement will be manifest on the surface ECG, and the signal averaged derivative thereof, as increased P wave duration.

More recently the concept of focally mediated AF has been introduced.[3–12] Haissaguerre *et al.* have demonstrated that atrial triggers, in the form of either repeatedly firing ectopic foci or atrial tachycardias, are important in a substantial proportion of patients with paroxysmal AF.[5] Their conclusions are now supported by several other authors, with short- to medium-term cure of paroxysmal AF by ablation of such foci.[6–12] The initial reports from Haisaguerre and others focused on patients with very frequent atrial premature beats (typically >700/day),[5] but more recent experience suggests that this frequency criterion may not be needed. Some preliminary studies have investigated the identification of this patient population,[13] but as yet no widespread experience exists.

A third but less well defined mechanism for paroxysmal AF is triggering by fluctuations in autonomic tone, usually enhanced vagal activity, in some patient subgroups.[14–16] Patients with autonomically mediated paroxysmal AF are encountered in clinical practice, but systematic data regarding them is sparse. They are described as young, frequently male, suffering AF episodes postprandially, in the evenings and at night, and having a low propensity to progress to sustained AF.[15,17] Conventional time and frequency domain analysis of beat interval files have been used to study this phenomenon.[18–21]

The progression of AF from paroxysmal episodes to non-self-terminating episodes of persistent AF to permanent AF is well recognised.[22] However, whether this represents an inevitable decline in atrial function or is due to the inadequacy of current treatment is unknown. The concept that "atrial fibrillation begets atrial fibrillation"[23] is reaching prominence in current strategies of managing AF: allowing the arrhythmia to perpetuate causes remodelling of the atria, such that the atria sustain the arrhythmia better while effective disease-suppressing therapy may cause "reverse remodelling" over time. It is likely that progression to sustained forms of AF is most likely in those with the highest arrhythmia burden and most disturbed atrial electrophysiology.

Finally, the mechanism of harm from AF arises predominantly from thromboembolism, but the precise risk poorly established in those with the paroxysmal AF,[24–27] in contrast to the overwhelming data in those with sustained AF.[28–30] Tachycardiomyopathy may also occur in those who suffer prolonged episodes of AF if the AF results in high ventricular rates.[31–35]

Terminology used

In keeping with other chapters herewith, *paroxysmal AF* is taken to mean AF that exhibits a predominant pattern of self-terminating episodes of AF lasting minutes, hours, or occasionally days.[36,37] *Persistent AF* (non-self-terminating but responding to medical intervention to restore sinus rhythm) and *permanent AF* (attempts to maintain sinus rhythm ineffective or abandoned) will be collectively be described as *sustained AF*. Unfortunately, this terminology is not universally recognised, and in the published literature some authors term AF that requires DC cardioversion or intravenous pharmacological agents to restore sinus rhythm as paroxysmal AF. Often no clear definition is actually given in the published work. In view of the significant differences in the population effected, the frequency of coexistent cardiovascular disease and the mechanism of the arrhythmia, every effort has been made to clarify how closely each given study population adheres to our preferred terminology.

Patient population at risk of paroxysmal AF

Epidemiology

The prevalence of AF is estimated to be of the order of 1% of the general population but shows a significant age relationship. Feinberg *et al.*[38] calculated that there were 2.2 million persons in the USA with some form of atrial fibrillation (= 0.9% population). The prevalence rises with age such that 10% of those aged between 64 and 89 years old have AF.[38,39] The proportion of AF subjects who have the paroxysmal form of the disorder is suggested to be as high as 90% amongst those with "lone AF".[40] However those with structural heart disease and older patients, who constitute most AF sufferers are more likely to experience a sustained form of the arrhythmia. Determining the frequency of paroxysmal AF is difficult, owing to the substantial numbers of patients who have asymptomatic arrhythmias. Short runs of paroxysmal AF are not infrequently seen on ambulatory recordings performed for other purposes, and, amongst patients who suffer from symptomatic paroxysmal AF, as few as one in 12 episodes are noticed.[41] Overall, it is likely that one-third of all AF treated is paroxysmal, and this is supported by data from anticoagulation trials in AF.[42] However, this figure must be regarded as an estimate because of the inherent inability of point screening to determine accurately the prevalence of paroxysmal arrhythmias, the inherent ascertainment bias of studies performed for other purposes, and the high prevalence of clinically undetected AF.

Whether the very striking age dependence of overall AF incidence holds true for paroxysmal AF is less certain. It seems likely that paroxysmal AF is proportionately commoner amongst younger subjects, as the paroxysmal form of the disorder is the initial presentation of a disease that progresses over months and years from paroxysmal to persistent and finally to permanent AF (although by no means all subjects exhibit this pattern, Fig. 31.1). Also, younger

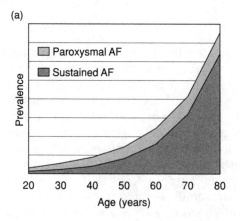

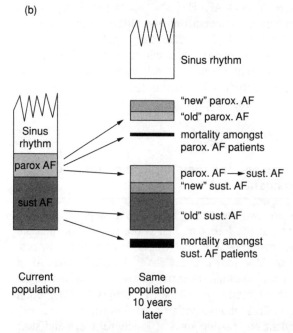

Figure 31.1 The age dependence of the prevalence of paroxysmal AF, and its relationship to the prevalence of sustained AF. (a) Both paroxysmal and sustained AF increase in prevalence with age. However the rate of rise in sustained AF is much greater, resulting in a drop in the proportion with paroxysmal AF. (b) The rise in the proportion with sustained AF arises from both progression of paroxysmal AF to sustained AF and *de novo* cases of sustained AF. Note that, owing to the lack of precise data and poor differentiation of paroxysmal from sustained AF, data have been taken from multiple sources and no precise numbers are given.

subjects are more likely to have structurally normal hearts, which is much more frequently associated with the paroxysmal form of the disorder: 80% of patients with sustained AF have associated structural heart disease, but this is true of only 50% of patients with paroxysmal AF (Fig. 31.2).[43]

Hypertension

Hypertension has a consistent association with AF throughout multiple studies.[44–46] The mechanism of this is as yet unproven. It may be that the same primary vascular abnormality that leads to essential hypertension also causes an atrial myopathy. More likely is that the increased left atrial pressure, which results from ventricular hypertrophy and consequent reduced diastolic compliance, increases the probability of paroxysmal atrial fibrillation through structural remodelling.

Sick sinus syndrome and pacemaker patients

Sick sinus syndrome has a close interrelationship with paroxysmal AF, with AF often representing the "tachycardia" component of the "tachy-brady" syndrome. Even if

there is no evidence of AF at presentation, a substantial proportion of patients with sick sinus syndrome go on to suffer from AF following pacemaker implantation.[47,48] Centurion *et al.*[49] found that patients with sick sinus syndrome without paroxysmal AF had abnormal atrial electrograms restricted to the high and mid-right atrium, whilst those who also experienced AF had evidence of wider disease. The histological appearance of both conditions is characterised by loss of atrial myocytes, fibrosis, and variable amyloid protein deposition, whether restricted to the sinus node region in sick sinus syndrome or more diffusely in AF patients. Thus the two conditions probably represent ends of the same spectrum, although additional factors are involved in paroxysmal AF for some patients. A lower rate of progression to sustained AF, if patients receive atrially rather than ventricularly based pacing for sick sinus syndrome,[47,48] suggests that the disease progression can be affected by whether the pacing therapy maintains optimal electrophysiological and haemodynamic physiology.

Whether paroxysmal AF is related to AV nodal block is much less clear-cut. Few data are available, but a prospective trial currently underway such as the UK-Pace study will at least clarify the role of pacing modality on the risk of developing AF.

Post-myocardial infarction

Atrial fibrillation occurs during the acute postinfarction phase in about 10% of patients,[50] but the observed incidence varies widely between studies.[51–53] Most of these studies do not discriminate paroxysmal AF from sustained AF, and there is sometimes difficulty in determining whether the AF is new or pre-existing. Studies in the mid-1970s suggested that supraventricular arrhythmia of some description complicated as many as 44% of myocardial infarctions,[52] and this group was found to have a greatly increased mortality (33 versus 9% in controls). Goldberg *et al.*[53] found that the incidence of new atrial fibrillation rose from 1975 to 1986 in successive time-grouped cohorts. Eldar *et al.*[50] specifically investigated whether this proportion has fallen in the post-thrombolytic era using data from a number of Coronary Care Units in Israel collected in the early 1980s (5803 patients) and the 1990s (2866 patients). Overall the proportion had fallen slightly (from 9.9 to 8.9%), but the occurrence of paroxysmal AF had become more closely associated with other adverse risk factors such as advanced age and congestive heart failure. While paroxysmal AF was associated with a worse outcome and higher death rates, a logistic model revealed that the relationship was less strong and no longer statistically significant after correction for appropriate clinical features of increased risk (prior MI, diabetes, etc.) with

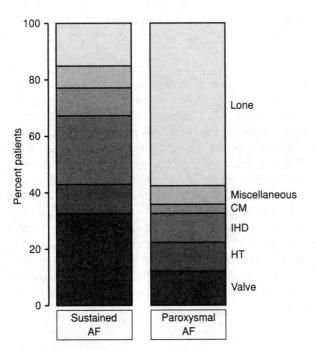

Figure 31.2 The frequency of lone AF and of underlying cardiac diseases in patients with sustained and paroxysmal AF. Abbreviations: CM = cardiomyopathy; IHD = ischaemic heart disease; HT = hypertension; valve = valvular heart disease. (Modified from reference 40, with permission.)

an odds ratio of 1.32 (95% CI 0.92–1.87). Stroke risk was higher in those with paroxysmal AF even after adjustment for other predictors (corrected OR 4.6, 95% CI 1.9–10.8).

In summary therefore paroxysmal AF postinfarction appears to predominantly be a marker of increased risk.[50,51,53] The adverse haemodynamic effects of the arrhythmia may have a marginal direct effect on mortality, but there appears to be a particular risk of stroke related to paroxysmal AF in this population.

Postoperative (especially cardiac surgery)

Both paroxysmal and persistent AF occur during the postoperative phase, with the highest incidence being in cardiac surgery owing to direct physical insult to the atria and the greater haemodynamic sequelae of these types of operation. AF occurs in about one-third of patients undergoing coronary artery surgery.[54] As with myocardial infarction, paroxysmal AF during the postoperative phase appears to be a non-specific marker of increased risk of complications rather than a mechanism. In contrast, persistent AF can cause major management difficulties and is independently associated with a longer hospital stay.[54,55]

Cardiomyopathy, valvular and congenital heart disease

The cardiomyopathies, and valvular and congenital heart disease are associated with atrial fibrillation through mechanisms of pressure overload, atrial scarring, and possibly primary atrial muscle involvement. As with the other predisposing conditions and associations, data regarding the precise relationship to paroxysmal rather than other forms of AF are imprecise. However, it is very clear that paroxysmal AF has a particularly important prognostic importance in these conditions.[56]

Arrhythmia risk stratification tests for paroxysmal AF

In the context of paroxysmal AF, risk stratification techniques may be employed towards three goals. The first is deciding who will get paroxysmal AF, both within the general population and also with defined high-risk groups: patients with known cardiac disease. Amongst patients who suffer from paroxysmal AF, it is desirable to be able to decide who is likely to suffer from an increased arrhythmia burden. This may be in the form of increasing frequency of paroxysms or progression to persistent AF. Finally, although paroxysmal AF is an unpleasant and often difficult to treat disorder, it is not usually associated with

severe morbidity or mortality. There are, however, a few patients at risk of adverse outcomes, and it is important to be able to identify them.

12-lead ECG

The reduced atrial conduction velocity found in AF patients,[57,58] which will be reflected in surface recordings, and the wide availability of the 12-lead ECG makes it attractive as a modality for patient identification.

Suggested parameters are maximum P wave duration and P wave dispersion. P wave duration reflects intra-atrial and interatrial conduction time, and hence reflects the ability of the atria to sustain AF. The electrophysiological basis of P wave dispersion is less well defined but it is likely that it reflects delay in depolarising of areas of the atria remote from the sinus node.

Snoeck et al.[59] made surface ECG P wave measurements at pacemaker implantation to predict atrial fibrillation in VVI paced patients. Their population consisted of 126 patients with symptomatic atrioventricular block and 56 with sick sinus syndrome. They found that P wave duration in V1 correlated with the incidence of atrial fibrillation during follow-up (5 years). Mean V1 P wave duration was 114.6 ms in patients developing atrial fibrillation and 91.9 ms in those who did not. As would be expected, the incidence of AF was higher in sick sinus syndrome than in AV block, with, for example, an incidence of 33% and 8% respectively for a P wave duration in lead V1 of more than 110 ms.

In a recent study, Dilaveris et al.[60] compared ECG parameters of 60 patients presenting with AF of up to 2 days duration with 40 age- and sex-matched controls. Although these were termed paroxysmal AF sufferers, 30% underwent electrical cardioversion to restore sinus rhythm and active pharmacological agents were given to most of the others. In this population, the maximum P wave duration was 123 ± 16 ms in AF patients and 101 ± 10 ms in controls. The authors quote a sensitivity of 88%, a specificity of 75% and a positive predictive accuracy of 84% for this test, but the latter two figures are of uncertain meaning because of the randomly chosen control population of an arbitrary size. P wave duration measured from a single lead does not appear to be sufficient to allow discrimination between paroxysmal AF patients and controls, however.[61]

P wave signal averaged ECG (P-SAECG)

P wave signal averaging has been used in a number of studies to identify prospectively patients at risk of paroxysmal AF, or at risk of progression from paroxysmal to persistent AF. Early studies proved negative,[62] probably because R wave triggering was used. In this methodology, the beat-to-beat variation in PR interval prevents the accurate averaging of the P wave. Utilisation of the P wave itself for triggering is clearly optimal, but the lower signal-to-noise ratio of the P wave compared to the R wave presents technical challenges (see Chapter 15).

P-SAECGs from 42 patients with paroxysmal AF were compared to 50 controls by Fukunami *et al.*.[61] The P-SAECG was based upon modified X, Y, and Z leads, which were combined to give a spatial magnitude after filtering (40–300 Hz pass-band), analogue-to-digital conversion, and signal averaging. The root mean square voltage of the final 10, 20, and 30 ms of the averaged P wave was found to be lower, and the duration of the averaged P wave longer in paroxysmal AF patients than controls (Fig. 31.3). In contrast, the duration of the conventional P wave and the left atrial diameter did not differ greatly, irrespective of coexistent structural heart disease.

Since the incidence of paroxysmal AF in the general population is low, and the immediate morbidity is low, unselected screening is not appropriate. The best studied area is the field of postoperative atrial fibrillation. Amongst 45 patients undergoing coronary artery bypass surgery, Klein *et al.*[63] found that a P-wave duration on a P wave signal-averaged ECG was longer, at 163 ± 19 ms, than that of those who did not develop AF, at 144 ± 16 ms ($P < 0.0005$). A cut-off duration of 155 ms yielded a sensitivity of 69%, specificity of 79%, and a positive predictive accuracy of 65%. The same authors found that left atrial enlargement by standard ECG criteria was also of predictive value. However, using the conventional ECG yielded inferior discriminatory power and is unlikely to be independent of the P-SAECG, although this was not formally assessed. In an earlier study, Steinberg *et al.*[64] found broadly similar results in 130 patients undergoing

cardiac surgery. The discriminatory power was slightly less (sensitivity 77%, specificity 55%, PPA 37%), perhaps reflecting their more mixed population, which included 16% undergoing valve surgery. There are significant differences in the technology employed between the studies, reflected by the shorter P wave duration (AF = 152 ± 18 ms, no AF = 139 ± 17 ms), and this may also have influenced the results. A prior history of AF is a strong predictor of postoperative AF,[65] and the frequency of the complication rises with age.[65-67] Finally, AF occurs more frequently following valve surgery.[67] Thus, the combination of clinical features and PW-SAECG provides good risk assessment for this troublesome postoperative complication. With emerging strategies for AF prevention, such as pharmacotherapy[68] and preventative pacing,[69] a targeted approach is now possible.

Ambulatory monitoring and heart rate variability

Ambulatory monitoring has been widely used to study the mechanisms of paroxysmal AF, and shows promise for the clinical evaluation of patients, but its precise role in risk stratification is not yet established.

Ambulatory recordings have been used to study the autonomic hypothesis of paroxysmal AF, but with inconsistent findings. In an unselected population of patients with paroxysmal AF, Hnatkova *et al.*[18] found no evidence from heart rate changes before AF onset to suggest increasing vagal tone, either in their overall population or in individuals with frequent AF episodes. Kok *et al.*[70] also found bradycardia dependent onset to be rare.

Frequency domain analysis of a beat interval series provides a useful non-invasive methodology for examining autonomic tone, and fluctuations thereof, in human studies. However, when applied to the sinus rhythm preceding

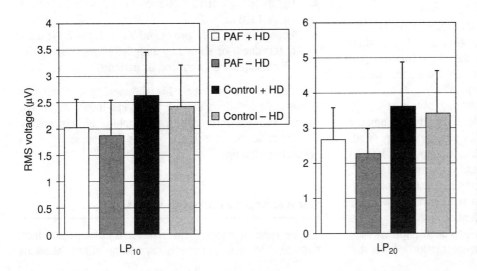

Figure 31.3 The root mean square (RMS) voltage during the last 10 ms and last 20 ms of the signal averaged P wave (LP_{10} and LP_{20} respectively, mean±SD) from paroxysmal AF patients and controls with or without concomitant structural heart disease (HD).[61]

AF onset, analysis may be unreliable because of the increasingly frequent atrial premature beats prior to AF onset. Although interpolation techniques allow the preservation of a contiguous time series, the effect of this interpolation on the results of the mathematical calculations used to derive the frequency spectrum is unpredictable. Thus either significant interpolation must be accepted, or only episodes with infrequent ectopics can be used. A few studies have attempted to use the technique none-the-less. Hnatkova *et al.*[71] and Herweg *et al.*[72] both found a shift towards vagal dominance before paroxysmal AF onset. Hnatkova *et al.*[71] examined pooled data from patients with clinical paroxysmal AF, and selected the subset of patients with few ectopics; there was a modest shift towards vagal predominance prior to AF onset. A broadly similar approach was taken by Herweg *et al.*,[72] who also divided the episodes according to time of onset. They described a much more marked shift to vagal dominance in episodes occurring at night. In contrast, however, Capucci *et al.*[21] found no evidence of increasing vagal tone prior to the onset of AF in 15 subjects who had a clinical history of vagal AF and in whom AF onset was recorded during sleep.

Sopher *et al.*[73] examined 296 AF episodes from 42 Holter recordings and found episodes lasting more than 30 seconds were slightly more frequent at night (165 versus 131) but of shorter duration (median 1.15 min versus 1.5 min) at night. As would be expected, the preceding ventricular rate was slower at night (62 bpm versus 76 bpm). Yamashita *et al.* plotted the diurnal variation in AF frequency[74] and found this fitted well to a sinusoidal function, with the nadir for onset frequency occurring at approximately 11 am. These authors concluded that AF episodes were of longer duration if they began in the early evening rather than at night. However, since mean AF duration rather than median was quoted, there may have been bias from long episodes, compounded by the fitting and finishing of recordings of Holters occurring during the working day.

Thus, although there are undoubtedly patients who tend to suffer from AF episodes beginning at times when vagal dominance is expected, the data regarding the precise autonomic shifts that occur are conflicting and modes of onset are not consistent in individuals.

Ambulatory recording has monitoring uses in preventing complications of paroxysmal AF. First, it is commonly used to assess arrhythmia burden as only a minority of AF episodes are symptomatic[41] and drug therapy may lead to conversion of symptomatic into asymptomatic AF episodes.[75,76] Although thromboembolic risk from paroxysmal AF is probably less than from sustained AF, whether episodes are noticed by the patient is irrelevant to the risk. If, therefore, the patient is felt to be at high risk (see criteria in next section), then documentation of arrhythmia suppression by ambulatory monitoring is necessary before considering withdrawal of thromboembolic prophylaxis. Also atrial fibrillation can cause a tachycardia induced cardiomyopathy ("tachycardiomyopathy") if the ventricular rate is poorly controlled over prolonged periods.[31–35] While this complication probably occurs most commonly in sustained forms of AF, there are data to show left ventricular impairment can occur in paroxysmal AF.[77] What is currently undetermined is the rate and amount of paroxysmal AF that will induce a tachycardiomyopathy. The risk is probably minimal if ventricular rates are below 120 bpm during episodes and episodes constitute the minority of the cardiac rhythm. In sustained forms of AF more aggressive rate control is needed (see Chapters 32 and 33), but, in all cases, ambulatory recordings will provide a fuller rate profile than sedentary ventricular rate assessment.

Echocardiography and invasive evaluation

Although this text focuses on non-invasive ECG techniques, it is important to remember that the majority of the morbidity and mortality arising from atrial fibrillation is as a result of thromboembolic complications. Thus echocardiography must form a vital part of the evaluation of patients with paroxysmal AF. Controversy exists regarding whether paroxysmal AF confers a significant thromboembolic risk.[24–27] Since it is suggested that AF of less than 24 hours duration may safely be cardioverted without antecedent anticoagulation, by logical extension, paroxysmal AF with episodes lasting for similar or shorter periods probably conveys negligible risk. While some recommend anticoagulation for all patients with paroxysmal AF who meet conventional AF anticoagulation criteria, the author restricts anticoagulation to selected subgroups:

- prior thromboembolism;
- significant left atrial dilatation or severe left ventricular dysfuction;
- known or possible prolonged AF paroxysms (clinical determined, or shown by ambulatory monitoring that AF episodes are unnoticed by patient)

Paroxysmal AF is rarely life threatening in itself, but important exceptions are the Wolff–Parkinson–White syndrome and patients with hypertrophic cardiomyopathy. Risk stratification for these groups is discussed in the respective chapters.

Clinical application of the tests

At the time of writing, the risk stratification tools most applicable to patients with paroxysmal atrial fibrillation are ambulatory recording and P wave SAECG. The 12-lead ECG provides baseline electrocardiographic data, and because of its low cost and wide availability, should always be included. It will document coexistent cardiac conditions, such as prior myocardial infarction or Wolff–Parkinson–White syndrome. Finally, biatrial pacing for patients with a P wave duration of greater than 120 ms is a suggested treatment modality for a subset of patients.[78,79]

Ambulatory recordings

Ambulatory recording provides diverse information, and what is taken from it by individual clinicians depends partially on their interest and therapeutic focus. All will be interested in arrhythmia burden, the frequency of symptomatic versus asymptomatic episodes, and ventricular rate during AF paroxysms. The heart rate trend graph (tachogram) provides a useful summary of much of the information of interest (Fig. 31.4). When patients are being assessed for therapy, the mode of AF onset can provide useful information. Onset at times of slow atrial rates or associated with heart rate deceleration suggests that atrial pacing may provide benefit, while tachycardic onset would favour antiarrhythmic therapy and perhaps specifically agents with beta-blocking actions. The value of such guided therapy has not been systematically prospectively validated, and it important to capture the onset of more than one AF episode, as patients do not exhibit consistent modes of onset.[18]

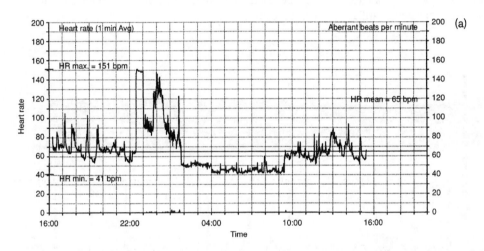

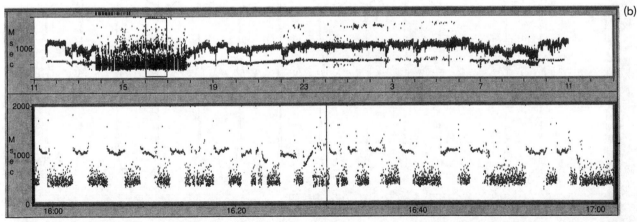

Figure 31.4 Tachograms from patients with paroxysmal AF. (a) Patient who experienced a single episode of AF during the recording. Note that at the onset of the episode the tachycardia has a relatively constant rate of 150 bpm, and the electrogram was consistent with atrial flutter. This patient was completely asymptomatic from the tachycardia; his clinical complaint was syncope. This proved to be due to prolonged sinus arrest after AF terminated. The tachogram in (b) Analysis package of another company. Note that the vertical axis denotes RR interval duration rather than ventricular rate. The lower frame demonstrates a "zoom" of 1 hour. The patient had complained of a prolonged episode of AF, but the tachogram demonstrates that there were in fact numerous onsets and terminations.

With increasing interest in the radiofrequency ablation of paroxysmal AF triggers, ambulatory monitoring is likely to become a useful tool in assessment of patients. At our institution, digital Holters (6632 Altair-DISC Recorder, SpaceLabs Burdick Inc, East Syracuse, NY, USA) are being used to assess patients with paroxysmal AF. The very high resolution signal (0.15 µV at ≥500 Hz sampling) allows identification of atrial ectopic morphology and demonstration that it is the beats of the same morphology that are seen prior to the majority of AF episodes and are seen remote from AF onset (Fig. 31.5).

P wave SAECG

As has been described earlier, PW-SAECG has been extensively evaluated for identification of patients at risk of paroxysmal AF. Because of the low prevalence of paroxysmal AF, PW-SAECG has optimal use for patient stratification in high-risk situations such as following cardiac

surgery. In this setting, several interventions have either been shown to be beneficial in preventing paroxysmal AF or are currently under evaluation. These include continuing beta-blocker therapy in the perioperative period,[80–82] use of amiodarone,[68] and atrial pacing therapies.[69]

Conclusion

The risk stratification of paroxysmal AF has great clinical value but stage of development of the various methodologies is currently very varied. The simple 12-lead ECG and analogue ambulatory recording provide much useful information, but systematic data on how the data should be used are currently lacking. The P-SAECG has, in contrast, been subject to much fuller technical evaluation. What is currently lacking are prospective data on how these data can be used to helpfully intervene to alter the patients clinical course.

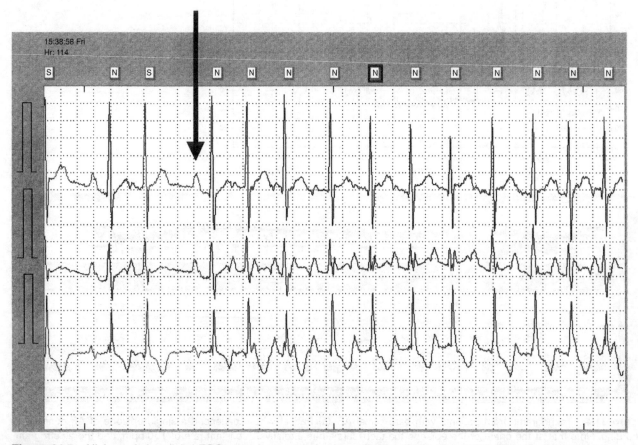

Figure 31.5 High-resolution digital ECG example, recorded using a Burdick 6632 Altair-DISC Recorder. The resolution, signal-to-noise quality, and frequency response of the system allows the identification of distinct P-waves for several seconds into the onset of this episode of paroxysmal AF. Later in the same episode typical fibrillation waves are apparent. The last sinus beat is marked with an arrow. The morphology of the atrial tachycardia at the onset of AF is identical to the morphology of bigeminal beats before AF onset.

References

1. Moe GK, Abildskov JA. Atrial fibrillation as a self-sustaining arrhythmia independent of focal discharge. *Am Heart J* 1959;**58**:59–70.
2. Moe GK. On the multiple wavelet hypothesis of atrial fibrillation. *Arch Int Pharmacodyn Ther* 1962;**140**:183–8.
3. Haissaguerre M, Marcus FI, Fischer B, Clementy J. Radiofrequency catheter ablation in unusual mechanisms of atrial fibrillation: report of three cases. *J Cardiovasc Electrophysiol* 1994;**5**:743–51.
4. Jais P, Haissaguerre M, Shah DC *et al*. A focal source of atrial fibrillation treated by discrete radiofrequency ablation. *Circulation* 1997;**95**:572–6.
5. Haissaguerre M, Jais P, Shah DC *et al*. Spontaneous initiation of atrial fibrillation by ectopic beats originating in the pulmonary veins. *New Engl J Med* 1998;**339**:959–66.
6. Hwang C, Karagueuzian HS, Chen PS. Idiopathic paroxysmal atrial fibrillation induced by a focal discharge mechanism in the left superior pulmonary vein: possible roles of the ligament of Marshall. *J Cardiovasc Electrophysiol* 1999;**10**:636–48.
7. Tsai CF, Chen SA, Tai CT *et al*. Bezold–Jarisch-like reflex during radiofrequency ablation of the pulmonary vein tissues in patients with paroxysmal focal atrial fibrillation. *J Cardiovasc Electrophysiol* 1999;**10**:27–35.
8. Chen SA, Tai CT, Yu WC *et al*. Right atrial focal atrial fibrillation: electrophysiologic characteristics and radiofrequency catheter ablation. *J Cardiovasc Electrophysiol* 1999;**10**:328–35.
9. Chen SA, Hsieh MH, Tai CT *et al*. Initiation of atrial fibrillation by ectopic beats originating from the pulmonary veins: electrophysiological characteristics, pharmacological responses, and effects of radiofrequency ablation. *Circulation* 1999;**100**:1879–86.
10. Chen S-A, Tai C-T, Wu W-C, Chen Y-J, Chang M-S. Radiofrequency catheter of right atrial focal atrial fibrillation: characterizing the successful ablation site electrogram. *Pacing Clin Electrophysiol* 1998;**21**:984.
11. Arentz T, Ott P, Stockinger J, Blum T, von Rosenthal J, Kalusche D. Radiofrequency catheter of focal atrial fibrillation. *Pacing Clin Electrophysiol* 1998;**21**:963.
12. Chen PS, Wu TJ, Ikeda T *et al*. Focal source hypothesis of atrial fibrillation. *J Electrocardiol* 1998;**31**:32–4.
13. Hill MRS, Hammill S, Mehra R. Morphological analysis of atrial premature beats associated with the spontaneous onset of atrial fibrillation. *Pacing Clin Electrophysiol* 1997;**20**:1066.
14. Coumel P, Attuel P, Lavall,e JP, Flammang D, Leclercq JF, Slama R. Syndrome d'arrythmie auriculaire d'origine vagale. *Arch Mal Coeur* 1978;**71**:645–56.
15. Coumel P. Neural aspects of paroxysmal atrial fibrillation. In: Falk RH, Podrid PJ eds. *Atrial fibrillation: mechanisms and management*. New York: Raven Press Ltd, 1992, pp. 109–25.
16. Coumel P. Paroxysmal atrial fibrillation: a disorder of autonomic tone? *Eur Heart J* 1994;**15**:9–16.
17. Coumel P, Friocourt P, Mugica J, Attuel P, Leclercq JF. Long-term prevention of vagal atrial arrhythmias by atrial pacing at 90/minute: experience with 6 cases. *Pacing Clin Electrophysiol* 1983;**6**:552–60.
18. Hnatkova K, Waktare JE, Murgatroyd FD *et al*. Analysis of the cardiac rhythm preceding episodes of paroxysmal atrial fibrillation. *Am Heart J* 1998;**135**:1010–19.
19. Sopher SM, Waktare JEP, Hnatkova K *et al*. Influence of time of onset on paroxysmal atrial fibrillation duration. *Arch Mal Coeur Vaiss* 1998;**91**(Suppl. 3):283.
20. Hnatkova K, Gallagher MM, Murgatroyd FD *et al*. Onset and termination of paroxysmal atrial fibrillation – time domain analysis. *Arch Mal Coeur Vaiss* 1998;**91**(Suppl. 3):115–18.
21. Capucci A, Coccagna G, Santarelli A, Bauleo S, Boriani G. Prevalence of the sympathetic influence before atrial fibrillation onset in the so-called "vagal paroxysmal atrial fibrillation" patients. *J Am Coll Cardiol* 1998;**31**:A184.
22. Godtfredsen J. Atrial fibrillation: course and prognosis – a follow-up study of 1212 cases. In: Kulbertus HE, Olsson SB, Schlepper M eds. *Atrial fibrillation*. Mölndal, Sweden: AB Hassle, 1982, pp. 134–45.
23. Wijffels MCEF, Kirchhof CJHJ, Dorland R, Allessie MA. Atrial fibrillation begets atrial fibrillation: A study in awake chronically instrumented goats. *Circulation* 1995;**92**:1954–68.
24. Petersen P. Thromboembolic complications in atrial fibrillation. *Stroke* 1990;**21**:4–13.
25. Thyagarajan VS. Antithrombotic therapy in paroxysmal atrial fibrillation. *Chest* 1994;**105**:971–2.
26. Stoddard MF. Risk of thromboembolism in new onset or transient atrial fibrillation. *Prog Cardiovasc Dis* 1996;**39**:69–80.
27. Lip GYH, Lowe GDO, Rumley A, Dunn FG. Fibrinogen and fibrin D-dimer levels in paroxysmal atrial fibrillation: Evidence for intermediate elevated levels of intravascular thrombogenesis. *Am Heart J* 1996;**131**:724–30.
28. Wolf PA, Abbot RD, Kannel WB. Atrial fibrillation a major contributor to stroke in the elderly. *Arch Intern Med* 1987;**147**:1561–4.
29. Wolf PA, Dawber TR, Thomas HE, Kannel WB. Epidemiologic assessment of chronic atrial fibrillation and risk of stroke: the Framingham study. *Neurology* 1978;**28**:973–7.
30. Chesebro JH, Fuster V, Halperin JL. Atrial fibrillation – risk marker for stroke. *New Engl J Med* 1990;**323**:1556–8.
31. Rodriguez LM, Smeets JL, Xie B *et al*. Improvement in left ventricular function by ablation of atrioventricular nodal conduction in selected patients with lone atrial fibrillation. *Am J Cardiol* 1993;**72**:1137–41.
32. Grogan M, Smith HC, Gersh BJ, Wood DL. Left ventricular dysfunction due to atrial fibrillation in patients initially believed to have idiopathic dilated cardiomyopathy. *Am J Cardiol* 1992;**69**:1570–3.
33. Haiat R, Halphen C, Stoltz JP, Leroy G, Soussana C. Auricular fibrillation: a cause of reversible myocardiopathy. *Ann Cardiol Angeiol*. 1987;**36**:417–19.
34. Peters KG, Kienzle MG. Severe cardiomyopathy due to chronic rapidly conducted atrial fibrillation: complete recovery after restoration of sinus rhythm. *Am J Med* 1988;**85**:242–4.

35. Van Den Berg MP, van Veldhuisen DJ, Crijns HJ, Lie KI. Reversion of tachycardiomyopathy after beta-blocker. *Lancet* 1993;**341**:1667.

36. Gallagher MG, Camm AJ. Classification of atrial fibrillation. *Pacing Clin Electrophysiol* 1997;**20**:1603–5.

37. Waktare JEP, Camm AJ. Atrial fibrillation. In: Jackson G ed. *Difficult cardiology III*. London: Martin Dunitz, 1997.

38. Feinberg WM, Blackshear JL, Laupacis A, Kronmal R, Hart RG. Prevalence, age distribution, and gender of patients with atrial fibrillation. Analysis and implications. *Arch Intern Med* 1995;**155**:469–73.

39. Wolf PA, Benjamin EJ, Belanger AJ, Kannel WB, Levy D, D'Agostino RB. Secular trends in the prevalence of atrial fibrillation: The Framingham Study. *Am Heart J* 1996;**131**:790–5.

40. Murgatroyd FD, Camm AJ. Atrial arrhythmias. *Lancet* 1993;**341**:1317–22.

41. Page RL, Wilkinson WE, Clair WK, McCarthy EA, Pritchett EL. Asymptomatic arrhythmias in patients with symptomatic paroxysmal atrial fibrillation and paroxysmal supraventricular tachycardia. *Circulation* 1994;**89**:224–7.

42. Flaker GC, Fletcher KA, Rothbart RM, Halperin JL, Hart RG. Clinical and echocardiographic features of intermittent atrial fibrillation that predict recurrent atrial fibrillation. Stroke Prevention in Atrial Fibrillation (SPAF) Investigators. *Am J Cardiol* 1995;**76**:355–8.

43. Murgatroyd FD, Curzen NP, Aldergather J, Ward DE, Camm AJ. Clinical features and drug therapy in patients with paroxysmal atrial fibrillation: results of the CRAFT multi-center database. *J Am Coll Cardiol* 1993;**21**:380A.

44. Takahashi N, Seki A, Imataka K, Fujii J. Clinical features of paroxysmal atrial fibrillation. An observation of 94 patients. *Jap Heart J* 1981;**22**:143–9.

45. Benjamin EJ, Levy D, Vaziri SM, D'Agostino RB, Belanger AJ, Wolf PA. Independent risk factors for atrial fibrillation in a population-based cohort. The Framingham Heart Study. *JAMA* 1994;**271**:840–4.

46. Krahn AD, Manfreda J, Tate RB, Mathewson FAL, Cuddy TED. The natural history of atrial fibrillation: incidence, risk factors, and prognosis in the Manitoba follow-up study. *Am J Med* 1995;**98**:476–84.

47. Andersen HR, Neilsen JC, Thomsen PEB *et al.* Long term follow-up of patients from a randomised trial of atrial versus ventricular pacing for sick sinus syndrome. *Lancet* 1997;**350**:1210–16.

48. Andersen HR, Thuesen L, Bagger JP, Vesterlund T, Bloch Thomsen PE. Atrial versus ventricular pacing in sick sinus syndrome. A prospective randomized trial in 225 consecutive patients. *Eur Heart J* 1993;**14**:252.

49. Centurion OA, Fukatani M, Konoe A *et al.* Different distribution of abnormal endocardial electrograms within the right atrium in patients with sick sinus syndrome. *Br Heart J* 1992;**68**:596–600.

50. Eldar M, Canetti M, Rotstein Z *et al.* Significance of paroxysmal atrial fibrillation complicating acute myocardial infarction in the thrombolytic era. SPRINT and Thrombolytic Survey Groups. *Circulation* 1998;**97**:965–70.

51. Cristal N, Peterburg I, Szwarcberg J. Atrial fibrillation developing in the acute phase of myocardial infarction. Prognostic implications. *Chest* 1976;**70**:8–11.

52. Cristal N, Szwarcberg J, Gueron M. Supraventricular arrhythmias in acute myocardial infarction. Prognostic importance of clinical setting; mechanism of production. *Ann Intern Med* 1975;**82**:35–9.

53. Goldberg RJ, Seeley D, Becker RC *et al.* Impact of atrial fibrillation on the in-hospital and long-term survival of patients with acute myocardial infarction: a community-wide perspective. *Am Heart J* 1990;**119**:996–1001.

54. Aranki SF, Shaw DP, Adams DH *et al.* Predictors of atrial fibrillation after coronary artery surgery. Current trends and impact on hospital resources. *Circulation* 1996;**94**:390–7.

55. Mathew JP, Parks R, Savino JS *et al.* Atrial fibrillation following coronary artery bypass graft surgery: predictors, outcomes, and resource utilization. MultiCenter Study of Perioperative Ischemia Research Group. *JAMA* 1996;**276**:300–6.

56. Spirito P, Seidman CE, McKenna WJ, Maron BJ. The management of hypertrophic cardiomyopathy. *New Engl J Med* 1997;**336**:775–85.

57. Tanigawa M, Fukatani M, Konoe A, Isomoto S, Kadena M, Hashiba K. Prolonged and fractionated right atrial electrograms during sinus rhythm in patients with paroxysmal atrial fibrillation and sick sinus node syndrome. *J Am Coll Cardiol* 1991;**17**:403–8.

58. Centurion OA, Isomoto S, Fukatani M *et al.* Relationship between atrial conduction defects and fractionated atrial endocardial electrograms in patients with sick sinus syndrome. *Pacing Clin Electrophysiol* 1993;**16**:2022–33.

59. Snoeck J, Decoster H, Vrints C *et al.* Predictive value of the P wave at implantation for atrial fibrillation after VVI pacemaker implantation. *Pacing Clin Electrophysiol* 1992;**15**:2077–83.

60. Dilaveris PE, Gialafos EJ, Sideris SK *et al.* Simple electrocardiographic markers for the prediction of paroxysmal idiopathic atrial fibrillation. *Am Heart J* 1998;**135**:733–8.

61. Fukunami M, Yamada T, Ohmori M *et al.* Detection of patients at risk for paroxysmal atrial fibrillation during sinus rhythm by P wave-triggered signal-averaged electrocardiogram. *Circulation* 1991;**83**:162–9.

62. Engel TR, Vallone N, Windle J. Signal-averaged electrocardiograms in patients with atrial fibrillation or flutter. *Am Heart J* 1988;**115**:592–7.

63. Klein M, Evans SJ, Blumberg S, Cataldo L, Bodenheimer MM. Use of P-wave-triggered, P-wave signal-averaged electrocardiogram to predict atrial fibrillation after coronary artery bypass surgery. *Am Heart J* 1995;**129**:895–901.

64. Steinberg JS, Zelenkofske DO, Wong S, Gelernt M, Sciacca R, Menchavez E. Value of the P-wave signal-averaged ECG for predicting atrial fibrillation after cardiac surgery. *Circulation* 1993;**88**:2618–22.

65. Hashimoto K, Ilstrup DM, Schaff HV. Influence of clinical and hemodynamic variables on risk of supraventricular tachycardia after coronary artery bypass. *J Thorac Cardiovasc Surg* 1991;**101**:56–65.

66. Leitch JW, Thomson D, Baird DK, Harris PJ. The importance of age as a predictor of atrial fibrillation and flutter

after coronary artery bypass grafting. *J Thorac Cardiovasc Surg* 1990;**100**:338–42.

67. Creswell LL, Schuessler RB, Rosenbloom M, Cox JL. Hazards of postoperative atrial arrhythmias. *Ann Thorac Surg* 1993;**56**:539–49.

68. Daoud EG, Strickberger SA, Man KC *et al.* Preoperative amiodarone as prophylaxis against atrial fibrillation after heart surgery. *New Engl J Med* 1997;**337**:1785–91.

69. Orr WP, Tsui SSL, Stafford PJ, Pillai R, Bashir Y. Synchronised bi-atrial pacing prevents atrial fibrillation after coronary artery bypass surgery. *Heart* 1999;**81**(Suppl. 1):31.

70. Kok LC, Rohleder A, Haines EE. Bradycardia-dependent onset of paroxysmal atrial fibrillation is uncommon. *Circulation* 1998;**98**:SS87.

71. Hnatkova K, Waktare JEP, Murgatroyd FD, Baiyan X, Camm AJ, Malik M. Fluctuations in autonomic tone before atrial fibrillation onset: assessment by fast Fourier transformation. *Pacing Clin Electrophysiol* 1997;**20**:1515.

72. Herweg B, Dalal P, Nagy B, Schweitzer P. Power spectral analysis of heart period variability of preceding sinus rhythm before initiation of paroxysmal atrial fibrillation. *Am J Cardiol* 1998;**82**:869–74.

73. Sopher SM, Hnatkova K, Waktare JE, Murgatroyd FD, Camm AJ, Malik M. Circadian variation in atrial fibrillation in patients with frequent paroxysms. *Pacing Clin Electrophysiol* 1998;**21**:2445–9.

74. Yamashita T, Murakawa Y, Sezaki K *et al.* Circadian variation of paroxysmal atrial fibrillation. *Circulation* 1997;**96**:1537–41.

75. Wolk R, Kulakowski P, Karczmarewicz S *et al.* The incidence of asymptomatic paroxysmal atrial fibrillation in patients treated with propranolol or propafenone. *Int J Cardiol* 1996;**54**:207–11.

76. Murgatroyd FD, Gibson SM, Baiyan X *et al.* Double-blind placebo-controlled trial of digoxin in symptomatic paroxysmal atrial fibrillation. *Circulation* 1999;**99**:2765–70.

77. Brignole M, Gianfranchi L, Menozzi C *et al.* Assessment of atrioventricular junction ablation and DDDR mode-switching pacemaker versus pharmacological treatment in patients with severely symptomatic paroxysmal atrial fibrillation: a randomized controlled study. *Circulation* 1997;**96**:2617–24.

78. Daubert C, Mabo P, Berder V, Le Breton H, Leclercq C, Gras D. Permanent dual atrium pacing in major interatrial conduction blocks: a four years experience. *Pacing Clin Electrophysiol* 1993;**16**:885.

79. Daubert C, Mabo P, Berder V, Gras D, Leclercq C. Atrial tachyarrhythmias associated with high degree interatrial conduction block: prevention by permanent atrial resynchronization. *Eur J Cardiac Pacing Electrophysiol* 1994;**4**:35–44.

80. White HD, Antman EM, Glynn MA *et al.* Efficacy and safety of timolol for prevention of supraventricular tachyarrhythmias after coronary artery bypass surgery. *Circulation* 1984;**70**:479–84.

81. Daudon P, Corcos T, Gandjbakhch I, Levasseur JP, Cabrol A, Cabrol C. Prevention of atrial fibrillation or flutter by acebutolol after coronary bypass grafting. *Am J Cardiol* 1986;**58**:933–6.

82. Stephenson LW, MacVaugh H, Tomasello DN, Josephson ME. Propranolol for prevention of postoperative cardiac arrhythmias: a randomized study. *Ann Thorac Surg* 1980;**29**:113–16.

32 Persistent atrial fibrillation

Joseph T Dell'Orfano and Gerald V Naccarelli

Atrial fibrillation is the most common arrhythmia likely to be encountered in primary care practice. It presents in a variety of forms. Traditionally, it has been divided into acute and chronic forms. The chronic forms may be further divided into chronic paroxysmal, chronic persistent, and permanent atrial fibrillation.[1] Paroxysmal atrial fibrillation is defined by recurrent episodes of atrial fibrillation which resolve spontaneously (see Chapter 31), whereas persistent atrial fibrillation requires cardioversion (either direct current or pharmacological) for reversion to sinus rhythm.[1] Permanent atrial fibrillation is either refractory to attempts at cardioversion or cardioversion is not attempted. In this chapter, we will focus on chronic persistent forms of atrial fibrillation.

Pathophysiology of persistent atrial fibrillation

Although we do not fully understand the mechanisms responsible for the onset and maintenance of atrial fibrillation, research efforts have increased our knowledge base. Recently, a gene locus for familial atrial fibrillation has been identified, suggesting that certain types of atrial fibrillation may have a genetic basis.[2] It is generally held that the electrophysiological mechanism for atrial fibrillation is multiple wavelets of re-entry. Several recent investigations, including high-density epicardial mapping studies in humans undergoing surgery for Wolff–Parkinson–White syndrome, have provided compelling evidence in support of this hypothesis.[3-7] In order to support multiple re-entrant wavelets, there appears to be a critical mass of excitable tissue necessary to allow the re-entrant wavelets to propagate. If refractory tissue is encountered, then the wavelet will extinguish and the arrhythmia will not be sustained (see Fig. 32.1). This occurs under two conditions: increased conduction velocity of the atrial tissue (which allows the re-entrant circuit them to "catch up" to refractory tissue left behind by previous wavelets and extinguish) and increased refractory period of the atrial tissue (which prevents recovery of the atrial tissue before another wavelet is encountered). Thus, factors that decrease conduction velocity and decrease refractoriness

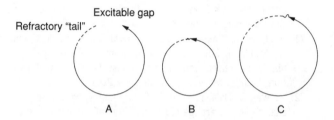

Figure 32.1 The effects of wavelength on maintenance of re-entry. In diagram A, re-entry is maintained because there is a gap of excitable tissue between the leading edge of the re-entrant wave and the refractory tail. However, if conduction velocity increases, the wavelength decreases and the excitable gap is closed, extinguishing the circuit (B). Alternatively, the refractory tail may lengthen (C), again closing the excitable gap and extinguishing the re-entrant wave.

of the atrial tissue will promote persistent atrial fibrillation. Conduction velocity may be decreased by electrolyte abnormalities, ischaemia, fibrosis, or inflammation. Increased sympathetic and increased vagal tone both decrease the atrial refractory period, as does thyrotoxicosis. Additionally, factors that increase the atrial size, thus allowing wavelets with larger wavelengths to exist, will promote persistent atrial fibrillation. These processes include valvular heart disease, ischaemic heart disease, and dilated cardiomyopathy.

In addition to these mechanisms, it appears that atrial fibrillation itself promotes persistent atrial fibrillation. This process is known as electrical remodelling and was first demonstrated by Wijffels in a goat model of sustained atrial fibrillation. These investigators proved that the longer atrial fibrillation is maintained, the easier it is to induce it in the future. Furthermore, after frequent inductions of atrial fibrillation, the arrhythmia tends to convert into a persistent form.[8] With maintenance of atrial fibrillation, the atrial tissue shows fibrosis with loss of myofibrils and the atrial refractory period decreases. Thus, atria become remodelled owing to chronic atrial fibrillation and favour the maintenance of atrial fibrillation. To quote Dr Allessie, "Atrial fibrillation begets atrial fibrillation."

Electrical remodelling has recently been examined.[9,10] Several investigators have shown that calcium channel blockade may minimise electrical remodeling. In a study by Tieleman and colleagues, electrical remodelling of the atrium during rapid atrial pacing was attenuated (P <0.001) by verapamil.[11] This study noted a minimal induction of atrial fibrillation by verapamil (34%) versus control (39%), $P = 0.03$. This suggests that electrical remodelling may be at least partially triggered by high calcium influx during rapid atrial pacing rates. Yu and colleagues demonstrated in 60 patients that the effective refractory period of the atrium at the appendage decreases with atrial pacing (cycle lengths of 400, 350, 300 and 250 ms for 10 minutes) and with paroxysmal atrial fibrillation. This finding is consistent with Wijffels' initial observations. This effect was attenuated by verapamil, but not by class I and III antiarrhythmic agents (including procainamide, propafenone, sotalol, amiodarone, and the beta-blocker propranolol).[10] In a human study by Daoud and co-workers, verapamil attenuated shortening of atrial refractory periods after atrial fibrillation; procainamide was ineffective in preventing this remodelling. Further studies by Wijffels showed that electrical remodelling was not mediated by changes in autonomic tone, ischaemia, stretch, or atrial natriuretic factor.[12] In this study, verapamil also shortened the time course of postatrial fibrillation. Finally, Tieleman demonstrated that sinus rhythm may be maintained for longer periods of time in patients pretreated with calcium channel blocking agents.[13] Although still speculative at this time, there is data to suggest that calcium channel blockade may be helpful in the prevention, or at least the attenuation of, atrial remodelling.

There is some data suggesting that electrical remodelling is associated with the progression from paroxysmal to persistent atrial fibrillation.[14] Furthermore, changes in the atrial refractory period associated with remodelling were reversed after successful RF ablation of a focal trigger of atrial fibrillation.[14]

Clinical consequences of persistent atrial fibrillation

Persistent atrial fibrillation has two major effects on the heart. First, the atrioventricular node is subjected to a much higher frequency of stimulation. This translates into a faster than usual ventricular heart rate. The ventricular response to atrial fibrillation depends upon the conduction properties of the AV node and the presence or absence of an accessory pathway. Ventricular rates may be as high as 300–400 bpm in patients with the Wolff–Parkinson–White (WPW) syndrome. In patients without WPW, the ventricular response may be as high as

180–200 bpm. In some patients this may cause haemodynamic instability and sudden cardiac death. In other patients, the tachycardia may be haemodynamically tolerated. Patients with chronic tachycardia from atrial fibrillation are at risk to develop tachycardia-induced cardiomyopathy.

The second effect of a chaotic atrial rhythm is loss of atrial transport. This may have significant haemodynamic effects, especially in patients who already have a cardiomyopathy. This is believed to be one of the reasons why patients develop decreased exercise tolerance even with rate controlled atrial fibrillation. The loss of atrial contraction also allows blood to become stagnant, especially in the atrial appendage, thus favouring thrombus formation. The ejection of atrial thrombus into the systemic circulation is the cause for stroke in these patients.

Because atrial fibrillation is so heterogeneous, patients may experience a variety of symptoms ranging from palpitations to syncope. Other patients may remain asymptomatic.[15] Additionally, patients with persistent atrial fibrillation may experience different symptoms than those with paroxysmal forms.[16] Thus it is often difficult to estimate the onset, duration, or severity of atrial fibrillation by history alone. Furthermore, treatment strategies will vary, depending upon the patient's symptoms and clinical syndrome. Major goals of therapy include prevention of stroke, prevention of cardiomyopathy, reduction of symptoms, and overall improvement of mortality. To this end, management may include heart rate control, rhythm control, anticoagulation, or a combination of these strategies.

Treatment of persistent atrial fibrillation

Ventricular rate control

When a patient presents with haemodynamically stable atrial fibrillation, one of the first goals of therapy should be control of the ventricular rate. This can be accomplished with calcium channel blockers such as diltiazem or verapamil, or beta-blockers such as metoprolol, esmolol, or digoxin. Intravenous calcium channel blockers and beta-blockers have the advantage of rapid onset of action. Digoxin on the other hand has an onset of action between 4–6 h (see Table 32.1). When the heart rate is controlled, oral medications may be used (see Table 32.2). Again, calcium channel blockers, beta-blockers, or digoxin may be used, often in combination.

Digoxin is perhaps the oldest form of therapy for persistent atrial fibrillation. Its effects are primarily mediated through the autonomic nervous system.[17] At therapeutic doses, vagal tone is enhanced by actions on the central and peripheral parasympathetic nervous system. Digoxin is

Table 32.1 Intravenous agents used for ventricular rate control

Drug	Loading dose	Onset	Maintenance dose	Major side effects
Digoxin	0.25 mg iv q2 hours, up to 1.5 mg	2 hours	0.125–0.25 mg qd	Digitalis toxicity, heart block, bradycardia
Diltiazem	0.25 mg/kg iv over 2 minutes	2–7 minutes	5–15 mg/h infusion	Hypotension, heart block, heart failure
Verapamil	0.075–0.15 mg/kg iv over 2 minutes	3–5 minutes	n/a	Hypotension, heart block, heart failure
Esmolol	0.5 mg/kg iv over 1 minute	5 minutes	0.05–0.2 mg/kg/min	Hypotension, heart block, bradycardia, asthma, heart failure
Metoprolol	2.5–5 mg iv bolus over 2 minutes, up to 3 doses	5 minutes	n/a	Hypotension, heart block, bradycardia, asthma, heart failure
Propranolol	0.15 mg/kg iv	5 minutes	n/a	Hypotension, heart block, bradycardia, asthma, heart failure

Table 32.2 Oral agents used for ventricular rate control

Drug	Loading dose	Onset	Maintenance dose	Major side effects
Digoxin	0.25 mg po q2 hours, up to 1.5 mg	2 hours	0.125–0.25 mg qd	Digitalis toxicity, heart block, bradycardia
Diltiazem	n/a	2–4 hours	120–360 mg daily in divided doses; slow release available	Hypotension, heart block, heart failure
Verapamil	n/a	1–2 hours	120–360 mg daily in divided doses; slow release available	Hypotension, heart block, heart failure
Metoprolol	n/a	4–6 hours	25–100 mg bid	Hypotension, heart block, bradycardia, asthma, heart failure
Propranolol	n/a	60–90 minutes	80–240 mg daily in divided doses	Hypotension, heart block, bradycardia, asthma, heart failure
Sotalol	n/a	4–6 hours	80–160 mg bid	Pro-arrhythmia, heart block, bradycardia, asthma, heart failure
Amiodarone	800 mg daily for 1 week 600 mg daily for 1 week 400 mg daily for 4–6 weeks	1–3 weeks	200 mg daily	Pulmonary toxicity, skin discoloration, hypothyroidism, pro-arrhythmia

therefore not as effective in ventricular rate control when catecholamines are increased. In a review of 139 episodes of paroxysmal atrial fibrillation on Holter monitor, digoxin failed to control the ventricular rate.[18] However, some improvement in heart rate response to atrial fibrillation has been documented. Digoxin was recently shown to reduce the frequency and severity of atrial fibrillation recurrences, presumably because of its effect on heart rate response.[19] Furthermore, in the Digitalis and Acute Atrial Fibrillation (DAAF) trial, digoxin slowed heart rate statistically ($P = 0.001$) within 2 hours of administration. This rate control was maintained throughout the observation.[20]

In summary, ventricular rate can be controlled with a variety of medications, including beta-blockers, calcium channel blockers, or digoxin. In patients with drug-resistant tachycardia from persistent atrial fibrillation, radiofrequency ablation of the atrioventricular junction with implantation of a pacemaker may be performed (see below).

Maintenance of sinus rhythm

By definition, patients with persistent atrial fibrillation will require cardioversion if restoration of sinus rhythm is desired. In contrast, patients with paroxysmal atrial fibrillation will revert to sinus rhythm without intervention (see Chapter 31). Additionally, up to 50% of patients presenting acutely with atrial fibrillation will convert to sinus rhythm spontaneously.[15,21] In the remaining patients, either direct current or pharmacologic cardioversion may be used. Pharmacologic alternatives include ibutilide, procainamide, quinidine, or intravenous amiodarone (see Table 32.3).

Type IA medications: procainamide and quinidine

Intravenous procainamide appears to result in conversion in 43–58% of patients.[22,23] Its main side effects include hypotension and QRS and/or QT prolongation. Procainamide is given as an i.v. infusion of up to 1 g over 1 hour and should be discontinued if the arrhythmia is terminated or if the patient develops side effects, including widening of the QRS or QT intervals. Oral quinidine may be used for the acute termination of atrial fibrillation. Its effectiveness has not been well studied.

Class 1C medications: flecainide and propafenone

Intravenous flecainide has been studied for acute conversion of atrial fibrillation. The conversion rate after a 2 mg/kg, 30-min infusion given with digoxin was 57% within 1 hour, versus 14% for the placebo arm.[24,25] Side effects include hypotension and rare bradyarrhythmias. QRS widening may also occur. Initial studies of oral fle-

cainide have demonstrated its efficacy and safety in the chronic treatment of atrial tachycardia and atrial fibrillation.[26] Oral flecainide (<400 mg within 3 hours) has a conversion rate of 68% at 3 hours and 91% at 8 hours.[27] In a placebo-controlled trial comparing oral flecainide, propafenone, and placebo in 181 patients with recent onset atrial fibrillation, the 3-h conversion rate was 59, 51, and 18% for flecainide, propafenone, and placebo respectively (P <0.001). At 8 hours, 78% of patients given flecainide and 72% of the patients with propafenone had converted, versus 39% for placebo.[28] Intravenous propafenone restored sinus rhythm in 71% of patients.[29] Oral propafenone (600 mg) has been shown to be superior to placebo in a randomised study of 240 patients (76% versus 37% at 8 hours).[30] Oral propafenone (600 mg as a single dose or divided every 4 hours) was as effective as oral flecainide; both are more effective than placebo.[28]

In all of these trials, observation periods were short. It is possible that spontaneous conversion rates equal pharmacological conversion rates over a period of 24 hours or more.

Class III medications: amiodarone, sotalol and ibutilide

Patients treated with intravenous amiodarone do not have a higher conversion rate than placebo.[31] In 100 patients with recent onset atrial fibrillation, there was a 68% conversion rate amongst patients treated with i.v. amiodarone versus a 60% conversion rate amongst the placebo group (P = 0.5).[32] Side effects include hypotension and bradyarrhythmias. In a study of intravenous flecainide versus intravenous amiodarone, flecainide resulted in faster cardioversion (59% versus 34% within 2 hours). However, after 8 hours, there was no statistical difference between

Table 32.3 Antiarrhythmic strategies for acute cardioversion and chronic maintenance of sinus rhythm

Type	Medication	Dose	Acute conversion rate (%)	Time to cardioversion	Chronic efficacy (%)
IA	Procainamide	10–15 mg/kg iv at 25 mg/min	20	1 hour	50
	Quinidine	324–648 mg po q8	38–86	3–6 hours	47–60
IC	Propafenone	600 mg po as a single dose or q4	51–76	3–8 hours	50–60
	Flecainide	400 mg po	68–91	3–8 hours	40–74
III	Amiodarone	150 mg iv over 10 minutes then 30–60 mg/h	43–68	8–24 hours	55–65
	Sotalol	160–320 mg po daily	20–52	3–8 hours	50–60
	Ibutilide	0.01 mg/kg iv over 10 minutes may repeat once after 30 minutes	33–45	1 hour	n/a
Other	DC cardioversion	100–360 joules	67–94	Immediate	n/a

patients receiving flecainide, amiodarone, or placebo, with an overall conversion rate of 56–68%.[24] In a study of 129 patients with chronic persistent atrial fibrillation treated with oral amiodarone, 18% were found to be in sinus rhythm after a 4-week loading period of 600 mg/day. In patients who continued to be in atrial fibrillation, the ventricular rate decreased from 100 ± 25 to 87 ± 27 bpm. No patient in this study discontinued the medication because of side effects.[33] In 30 patients with chronic rheumatic atrial fibrillation after mitral valve surgery, 77% were successfully cardioverted back to sinus rhythm, 40% with oral amiodarone alone and an additional 37% with DC cardioversion after taking oral amiodarone for 4 weeks.[34]

Sotalol appears to be ineffective for terminating atrial fibrillation. This is probably because it tends to prolong atrial refractoriness more at a slow rate as opposed to during tachycardia. This phenomenon is known as reverse use dependence. In a comparison of sotalol with quinidine and digoxin, 52% of patients taking sotalol and 86% of those taking quinidine converted to sinus rhythm, although 39% of patients in the sotalol group required DC cardioversion and 14% of the patients receiving quinidine underwent DC cardioversion.[35]

Ibutilide is a new class III agent with a very short half-life. It is currently indicated for the acute termination of atrial fibrillation and flutter. Ibutilide prolongs repolarisation by enhancing the slow inward depolarising Na^+ current in the plateau phase of repolarisation. Ibutilide has little to no effect on the conduction velocity of the atrial tissue.[36] Conversion rates are between 33 and 45% within the first 70 minutes. Ibutilide is administered as 0.01 mg/kg i.v. over 10 minutes: 70% of all conversions occurred within 20 minutes of infusion. If the first dose doesn't work, a second may be administered. Side effects include significant QT prolongation with *torsade de pointes* in 1.7% of patients. A 4-h observation period is recommended in patients who have received ibutilide.

In the past, digoxin has been recommended for termination and prevention of atrial fibrillation. However, in a trial by Falk and colleagues, 50% of 18 patients who received digoxin reverted to sinus rhythm in a mean of 5.1 hours; however, in the placebo group 8 of 18 (44%) reverted to sinus rhythm in a mean of 3.3 hours.[37] In the third Propafenone in Atrial Fibrillation Italian Trial (PAFIT3), patients with recent-onset (1–72 h) atrial fibrillation were randomised to receive a 10-min i.v. infusion of either propafenone 2 mg/kg, digoxin 0.007 mg/kg, or placebo. After 1 hour, 49% of patients treated with propafenone converted versus 32% in the digoxin group and 14% in the placebo group.[38] Recent data from the Digitalis and Acute Atrial Fibrillation (DAAF)[20] trial showed that intravenous digoxin reverted 51% of patients to sinus rhythm within 16 hours versus 46% in the placebo group. This difference was not statistically differ-

ent. Thus, digoxin has not been shown effective in either terminating atrial fibrillation or maintaining sinus rhythm.

DC cardioversion

External electrical cardioversion remains the safest, most effective means of terminating atrial fibrillation. It is certainly the method of choice for haemodynamically unstable atrial fibrillation. During elective cardioversion, a short-acting benzodiazepine or a short-acting barbiturate may be used for conscious sedation during the procedure. The risks of cardioversion include the risks of conscious sedation and pro-arrhythmia. However, if the shock is synchronised to the QRS complex, ventricular arrhythmias are rare. The efficacy of external DC shocks is 67–94%.

Electrical and pharmacological cardioversion both carry a risk of embolic events including stroke. However, the risk is very small in patients who have been in atrial fibrillation for less than 48 hours. In a study of 357 patients who underwent cardioversion (95.2% success rate), three patients suffered thromboembolic events (0.8%).[39]

It has recently been suggested that transoesophageal echocardiography (TEE) may be used to exclude the presence of thrombus in the atria of patients being considered for cardioversion. A pilot study examining 126 patients with chronic persistent atrial fibrillation were randomised to receive either conventional therapy, including three weeks of warfarin therapy prior to DC cardioversion followed by 4 weeks of warfarin, versus transoesophageal-guided cardioversion followed by 4 weeks of warfarin therapy. The investigators found that 13% of patients randomised to the TEE arm had atrial thrombus. Of the remaining 45 patients who underwent immediate DC cardioversion, 84% had a successful cardioversion and none experienced an embolic event.[40] Furthermore, with a decision-analytic model to examine the cost-effectiveness of TEE-guided cardioversion, it was found that TEE-guided therapy may actually be a more cost-effective alternative to conventional therapy.[41]

In those patients who fail DC cardioversion, pretreatment with antiarrhythmic medications is often helpful. In a study of 49 patients who had failed DC cardioversion and were subsequently loaded with oral amiodarone, 18% converted during the loading period and 59% had successful repeat cardioversions. After 12 months, 52% of patients maintained sinus rhythm on 200 mg/day of amiodarone.[42] More recently, ibutilide has been shown effective in facilitating DC cardioversion.[43]

Maintenance therapy

Once sinus rhythm has been re-established, maintenance therapy must be considered. The decision to initiate maintenance therapy should be based upon the number of recurrences the patient has experienced and how symptomatic the patient is. Patients with rare recurrences of atrial fibrillation may be followed without antiarrhythmic medications. Patients with frequent symptomatic recurrences should be considered candidates for antiarrhythmic therapy. This decision should be made only after careful consideration of the potential risks and benefits of therapy. The only proven benefit of antiarrhythmic therapy is a reduction in the number of recurrences of symptomatic atrial fibrillation. A theoretical (but unproven) benefit of antiarrhythmic therapy may include a reduction in thromboembolic risk. There is currently no data to prove that antiarrhythmic therapy improves survival in patients with chronic persistent atrial fibrillation. In fact, the potential risk of antiarrhythmic therapy is pro-arrhythmia.[44,45] For example, patients with a history of CHF who are treated with antiarrhythmic medications have a relative risk of cardiac death equal to 3.3 according to the SPAF investigators.[44] Additionally, many antiarrhythmic medications require inpatient monitoring during the initial loading phase. Finally, patients on antiarrhythmic therapy may experience side effects, which are poorly tolerated. Thus, the risks and benefits of antiarrhythmic therapy must be carefully weighed prior to starting therapy.

Although we have several different antiarrhythmic agents available, they are only partially efficacious (see Table 32.3). In a small study of sotalol versus placebo for maintenance of sinus rhythm, about 50% of patients reverted to atrial fibrillation within the first 6 months after cardioversion.[46] In a retrospective study of 110 patients refractory to class I agents given low dose amiodarone for maintenance of sinus rhythm, 25% had recurrence of atrial fibrillation or atrial flutter. The actuarial probability of remaining in sinus rhythm was 87, 70, and 55% after 1, 3, and 5 years, respectively; 82% of the patients with recurrences were patients with paroxysmal atrial flutter. However, 15% of patients experienced adverse effects that necessitated withdrawal of amiodarone, including skin discoloration (4.5%) and pulmonary fibrosis (3.6%).[47]

Flecainide was compared to quinidine in a randomised placebo-control, crossover study of 19 patients without structural heart disease and with paroxysmal atrial fibrillation. Both medications prolonged the time to recurrence by 40% (flecainide) and 47% (quinidine).[48] In another study of 239 patients with chronic paroxysmal atrial fibrillation or flutter, flecainide and quinidine were shown to have similar efficacy in controlling symptomatic attacks. Patients reported that they were symptom-free for up to 74% of the time that they were being treated. However, patients receiving quinidine were more likely to discontinue their medication because of adverse effects, most commonly diarrhoea. There were no life-threatening side effects noted in either group.[49]

A randomised, placebo-control study of propafenone was carried out in 100 patients with paroxysmal SVT or atrial fibrillation/flutter which showed that patients treated with 300 mg bid of propafenone were 6.8 times more likely to maintain sinus rhythm than those patients treated with placebo.[50] In a study of 102 patients with chronic persistent atrial fibrillation who had undergone successful cardioversion and were maintained on either oral propafenone (150 mg tid) versus placebo, 67% of patients on propafenone maintained sinus rhythm versus 35% of those receiving placebo ($P < 0.01$). Furthermore, the time to recurrence was significantly longer in the propafenone group.[51]

In a study comparing propafenone versus sotalol for control of paroxysmal atrial fibrillation, both showed about a 75% efficacy at 3 months.[52] However, in a meta-analysis comparing sotalol with quinidine, the 6-month efficacy was 50% with sotalol versus 53% with quinidine.[53]

Recent data suggests that amiodarone is the most effective agent for maintaining sinus rhythm. Kochiadakis and colleagues demonstrated 60% recurrence rates in patients treated with sotalol versus only 29% in patients on amiodarone ($P = 0.008$).[54] Initial findings of the Canadian Trial of Atrial Fibrillation (CTAF) shows that patients treated with amiodarone had a lower recurrence rate (35%) versus sotalol or propafenone (63%).[55] In a retrospective analysis of 124 patients who had received amiodarone over a 10-year period, 73, 65, and 62% had significant improvement of their atrial arrhythmias at 1, 2, and 3 years, respectively. The cumulative incidence of amiodarone-related adverse effects was 5.8 per 100 patient-years. 9,7% of patients had symptoms requiring drug withdrawal.[56]

Until more data are available, the decision to maintain sinus rhythm in patients with chronic atrial fibrillation must be made on an individualised basis with a clear understanding of the symptoms being treated.

Stroke prevention in persistent atrial fibrillation

Patients with atrial fibrillation have a stroke rate of 1.8–5.5% per year[57–64] and the overall mortality rate is 5–8%.[60,61] Patients with lone atrial fibrillation appear to have a stroke rate of about 1.6% (ages 60–69 years), 2.1% in ages 70–79 and 3.0% in patients older than 80 years.[65] There appears to be no difference in stroke rate in chronic persistent versus paroxysmal atrial fibrillation.[65] Recent trials have identified several risk factors for thromboembolism during atrial fibrillation. In an analysis of data pooled from five major randomised clinical trials, it appears that increasing age, previous stroke or TIA, history of hypertension, and history of diabetes are all independent risk factors for stroke from atrial fibrillation.[65] In an analysis of the Stroke Prevention in Atrial Fibrillation

Study (SPAF), congestive heart failure was also identified as a significant risk factor, as were left ventricular dysfunction and left atrial enlargement on 2-D echocardiography.[66,67]

There have been five major randomised trials examining the issue of stroke prevention in atrial fibrillation, all of which confirm the usefulness of chronic anticoagulation with warfarin in reducing the risk of stroke in atrial fibrillation. Although the SPAF trial showed a modest benefit to adult dose aspirin, the SPAF III trial, which randomised 1044 patients with chronic atrial fibrillation and at least one risk factor for thromboembolic events to low-intensity, fixed dose warfarin plus aspirin versus adjusted dose warfarin (INR 2.0–3.0), showed an ischaemic stroke and systemic embolism rate of 7.9% per year in the combination group versus 1.9% in the adjusted dose group (P <0.0001).[68] This clearly shows the benefits of warfarin over aspirin and suggests that aspirin is inadequate therapy for stroke prevention in atrial fibrillation.

Despite the overwhelming data in support of chronic warfarin use in patients suffering from chronic persistent, permanent, and paroxysmal atrial fibrillation, it is widely underused. The Cardiovascular Health Study, a population-based longitudinal study of risk factors for coronary disease and stroke in 5201 men and women aged 65 and over found that, despite a relatively high prevalence of atrial fibrillation in the elderly (as high as 9.1% in men and women with coexisting clinical cardiovascular disease), 62% of patients in which warfarin was indicated received nether warfarin nor aspirin.[69] In a retrospective analysis of 95 patients discharged from the hospital with a diagnosis of atrial fibrillation, 48% of those in whom warfarin was indicated were receiving neither warfarin nor aspirin.[70]

Non-pharmacological therapy for persistent atrial fibrillation

Several non-pharmacological treatments exist for atrial fibrillation. They are generally divided into procedures to control heart rate and procedures to maintain sinus rhythm. The most common procedure used to control heart rate during atrial fibrillation is *catheter ablation of the atrioventricular junction with permanent pacemaker implantation*.[71–73] This method provides absolute control of the heart rate during atrial fibrillation. However, it also renders the patient pacemaker-dependent. Since the atria continue to fibrillate, anticoagulation is also maintained. It is sometimes possible to modify the AV node and avoid the need for a pacemaker.[74] Nevertheless, patients who undergo this procedure generally report improved exercise tolerance and quality of life.[75,76] Additionally, some investigators have reported an improvement in ventricular function.[77,78]

Currently, there are several procedures being investigated for the maintenance of sinus rhythm in patients with atrial fibrillation. The *Cox–Maze procedure* represents the first major advance in the surgical treatment of atrial fibrillation. During this open-heart procedure, the right and left atria are compartmentalised with surgical suture lines. The lines are placed in such a way as to allow a sinus impulse to activate both atria. However, the suture lines also prevent the maintenance of multiple re-entrant wavelets. Overall, the procedure has been over 90% successful in maintaining sinus rhythm.[79] Furthermore, atrial transport appears to be preserved as well.[79]

Because of the success of the Cox–Maze procedure, several investigators have been devising methods of reproducing this procedure using catheter techniques. Results have been disappointing because of long procedure times, unacceptable complication rates, and relatively low chronic efficacy.[80] However, newer approaches, including *ablation of focal triggers of atrial fibrillation*, show more promise.[81]

Another approach to non-pharmacological therapy is the *implantable atrial defibrillator*. This implanted device is a patient activated system for terminating atrial fibrillation. It does not prevent recurrent atrial fibrillation. Initial trials have been promising for selected patients.[82,83]

Atrial fibrillation is a topic of intense research. New therapies, pharmacological and non-pharmacological, are currently under development.

A rational approach to the management of persistent atrial fibrillation

Given this wealth of data, it is possible to develop rational, literature-based guidelines for the treatment of persistent atrial fibrillation. It is important to note that despite our current understandings of atrial fibrillation, there is surprisingly little data to support many of our current practices in the treatment of atrial fibrillation. For example, although we believe that maintenance of sinus rhythm is a worthwhile goal of our therapy, it has never been demonstrated that this will increase survival in patients suffering from atrial fibrillation, nor has it been shown that this will reduce the risk of thromboembolism and stroke. There are three ongoing trials designed to assess whether maintenance of sinus rhythm does indeed result in long-term benefit to the patient. These trials are AFFIRM (Atrial Fibrillation Follow-Up: Investigation of Rhythm Management), PIAF (Progress In Atrial Fibrillation) and RACE (Rate Control versus Electrical Cardioversion for Atrial Fibrillation).

AFFIRM is by far the largest of these trials and plans to randomise 5300 patients at high risk for stroke and randomise them to receive either rate control with anticoagulation or rhythm control and anticoagulation. Patients will be followed for an average of 3.5 years. The primary end-point is total mortality with secondary end-points including stroke, cost of therapy and quality of life.[45]

PIAF and RACE are smaller trials currently underway in Europe.[1,84] Preliminary results of the PIAF trial demonstrate that, although amiodarone-treated patients had a higher conversion rate and maintained sinus rhythm, there were no differences in symptoms between patients on antiarrhythmic therapy and rate control therapy.

However, patients in sinus rhythm did experience an improvement in exercise tolerance compared to those in atrial fibrillation. When the final results of these trials become available, they should provide valuable insight into these current problems in the management of patients with chronic atrial fibrillation.

Until more data are available, therapy of atrial fibrillation should be tailored to the individual patient (see Fig. 32.2). The patient's stroke risk must be evaluated and compared to the risk of bleeding from chronic warfarin therapy. In addition, the patient's symptoms must be con-

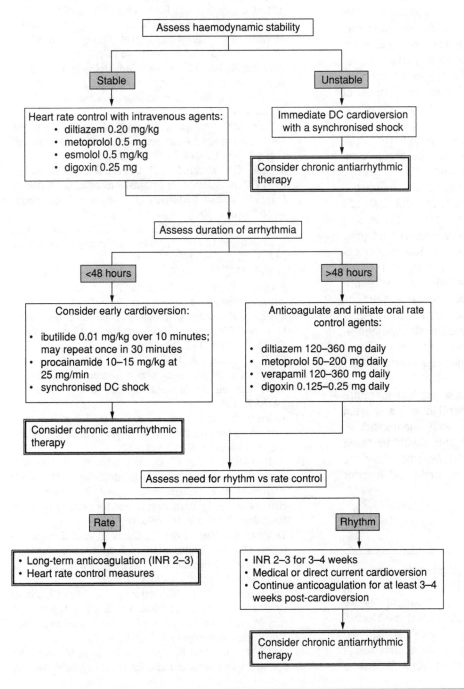

Figure 32.2 An algorithm for the treatment of atrial fibrillation.

sidered. A patient who has disabling palpitations during episodes of paroxysmal atrial fibrillation is a candidate for aggressive rhythm control, whereas a patient who is symptom-free during atrial fibrillation may be a candidate for simply heart rate control with anticoagulation.

In patients presenting with acute atrial fibrillation, i.e. the first episode of atrial fibrillation lasting for less than 48 hours, primary cardioversion without prior anticoagulation is safe. These patients may undergo DC cardioversion or chemical cardioversion using ibutilide. There is some evidence to suggest that cardioversion is prothrombotic because it causes atrial stunning.[85-87] Therefore, warfarin should be used for 3–6 weeks following a successful cardioversion, maintaining the INR at 2.0–2.5. Following successful cardioversion, patients should be monitored closely for symptoms of recurrent atrial fibrillation. An evaluation for structural heart disease, including echocardiography as well as an evaluation for causes of secondary atrial fibrillation, such as thyroid disorders, should be pursued as well.

Patients experiencing the first occurrence of atrial fibrillation in whom the onset either cannot be documented (e.g. in asymptomatic patients) or the onset is greater than 48 hours prior to presentation, require at least 3 weeks of anticoagulation with warfarin (INR 2.0–2.5) prior to cardioversion. As discussed above, it may be safe and cost-effective to perform cardioversion without prior anticoagulation if TEE is performed and fails to demonstrate intracardiac thrombus.

A second recurrence of atrial fibrillation in the absence of a treatable underlying disorder probably warrants attempts at rhythm control with antiarrhythmic medications as well as long-term anticoagulation with warfarin. A chronotropic agent such as a beta-blocker or a calcium channel blocker may be necessary for rate control during recurrences.

Patients with chronic forms of atrial fibrillation require long-term warfarin for stroke prevention and may need medications for heart rate control as well. The decision to pursue rhythm control in these patients should be based upon the patients symptoms and lifestyle, since there are currently no data to suggest that one strategy is superior to the other.

Conclusion

Atrial fibrillation is a common arrhythmia associated with significant morbidity and mortality. Its presentation, symptoms, and sequelae vary from patient to patient. As we continue to define and understand the underlying electrophysiological mechanisms responsible for this arrhythmia, our methods of treatment can become more effective. A rational approach to the treatment of atrial fibrillation requires a clear definition of the problem in each patient so that the treatment may be individualised to provide the most effective, safe therapy available. Ongoing trials such as AFFIRM will undoubtedly help us in the management of these difficult but common patients.

References

1. Gallagher MM, Camm AJ. Long-term management of atrial fibrillation. *Clinical Cardiology* 1997;**20**:381–90.
2. Brugada R, Tapscott T, Czernuszewicz GZ *et al.* Identification of a genetic locus for familial atrial fibrillation. *New Engl J Med* 1997;**336**:905–11.
3. Murgatroyd FD, Camm AJ. Current concepts in atrial fibrillation. *Br J Hosp Med* 1993;**49**:546–57.
4. Hoekstra BP, Diks CG, Allessie MA, DeGoede J. Nonlinear analysis of epicardial atrial electrograms of electrically induced atrial fibrillation in man. *J Cardiovasc Electrophysiol* 1995;**6**:419–40.
5. Allessie MA, Konings KTS, Kirchhof CJHJ, Wijffels M. Electrophysiologic mechanisms of perpetuation of atrial fibrillation. *Am J Cardiol* 1996;**77**:10A–23A.
6. Konings KTS, Kirchhof CJHJ, Smeets JRLM, Wellens HJJ, Penn OC, Allessie MA. High-density mapping of electrically induced atrial fibrillation in humans. *Circulation* 1994;**89**:1665–80.
7. Ferguson TB, Schuessler RB, Hand DE, Boineau JP, Cox JL. Lessons learned from computerized mapping of the atrium. *J Electrocardiol* 1993;**26**:210–19.
8. Wijffels MC, Kirchhof CJ, Dorland R, Allessie MA. Atrial fibrillation begets atrial fibrillation. A study in awake chronically instrumented goats. *Circulation* 1995;**92**:1954–68.
9. Goette A, Honeycutt C, Langberg JJ. Electrical remodeling in atrial fibrillation. Time course and mechanisms. *Circulation* 1996;**94**:2968–74.
10. Yu W-C, Chen S-A, Lee S-H *et al.* Tachycardia-induced change of atrial refractory period in humans: rate dependency and effects of antiarrhythmic drugs. *Circulation* 1998;**97**:2331–7.
11. Tieleman RG, De Langen C, Van Gelder IC *et al.* Verapamil reduces tachycardia-induced electrical remodeling of the atria. *Circulation* 1997;**95**:1945–53.
12. Wijffels MC, Kirchhof CJ, Dorland R, Power J, Allessie MA. Electrical remodeling due to atrial fibrillation in chronically instrumented conscious goats: roles of neurohumoral changes, ischemia, atrial stretch, and high rate of electrical activation. *Circulation* 1997;**96**:3710–20.
13. Tieleman RG, Van Gelder IC, Crijns HJ *et al.* Early recurrences of atrial fibrillation after electrical cardioversion: a result of fibrillation-induced electrical remodeling of the atria? *J Am Coll Cardiol* 1998;**31**:167–73.
14. Hobbs WJ, Van Gelder IC, Fitzpatrick AP, Crijns HJ, Garratt CJ. The role of atrial electrical remodeling in the progression of focal atrial ectopy to persistent atrial fibrillation. *J Cardiovasc Electrophysiol* 1999;**10**:866–70.
15. Dell'Orfano JT, Patel H, Wolbrette DL, Luck JC, Naccarelli GV. Acute treatment of atrial fibrillation: spontaneous con-

version rates and cost of care. *Am J Cardiol* 1999;**83**:788–90, A10.

16. Levy S, Maarek M, Coumel P, Guize L, Lekieffre J, Medvedowsky JL, Sebaoun A. Characterization of different subsets of atrial fibrillation in general practice in France: the ALFA study. The College of French Cardiologists. *Circulation* 1999;**99**:3028–35.

17. Watanabe AM. Digitalis and the autonomic nervous system. *J Am Coll Cardiol* 1985;**5**:35A–42A.

18. Rawles JM, Metcalfe MJ, Jennings K. Time of occurrence, duration and ventricular rate of paroxysmal atrial fibrillation: the effect of digoxin. *Br Heart J* 1990;**63**:225–7.

19. Murgatroyd FD, Gibson SM, Baiyan X et al. Double-blind placebo-controlled trial of digoxin in symptomatic paroxysmal atrial fibrillation. *Circulation* 1999;**99**:2765–70.

20. The Digitalis in Acute Atrial Fibrillation (DAAF) Trial Group Investigators. Intravenous digoxin in acute atrial fibrillation. Results of a randomized, placebo-controlled multicentre trial in 239 patients. The Digitalis in Acute Atrial Fibrillation (DAAF) Trial Group. *Eur Heart J* 1997;**18**:649–54.

21. Danias PG, Caulfield TA, Weigner MJ, Silverman DI, Manning WJ. Likelihood of spontaneous conversion of atrial fibrillation to sinus rhythm. *J Am Coll Cardiol* 1998;**31**:588–92.

22. Fenster PE, Comess KA, Marsh R, Katzenberg C, Hager WD. Conversion of atrial fibrillation to sinus rhythm by acute intravenous procainamide infusion. *Am Heart J* 1983;**106**:501–4.

23. Halpern SW, Ellrodt G, Singh BN, Mandel WJ. Efficacy of intravenous procainamide infusion in converting atrial fibrillation to sinus rhythm: relation to left atrial size. *Br Heart J* 1980;**44**:589–95.

24. Donovan KD, Power BM, Hockings BE, Dobb GJ, Lee KY. Intravenous flecainide versus amiodarone for recent-onset atrial fibrillation. *Am J Cardiol* 1995;**75**:693–7.

25. Donovan KD, Dobb GJ, Coombs LJ et al. Reversion of recent-onset atrial fibrillation to sinus rhythm by intravenous flecainide. *Am J Cardiol* 1991;**67**:137–41.

26. Berns E, Rinkenberger RL, Jeang MK, Dougherty AH, Jenkins M, Naccarelli GV. Efficacy and safety of flecainide acetate for atrial tachycardia or fibrillation. *Am J Cardiol* 1987;**59**:1337–41.

27. Capucci A, Lenzi T, Boriani G et al. Effectiveness of loading oral flecainide for converting recent-onset atrial fibrillation to sinus rhythm in patients without organic heart disease or with only systemic hypertension. *Am J Cardiol* 1992;**70**:69–72.

28. Capucci A, Boriani G, Botto GL et al. Conversion of recent-onset atrial fibrillation by a single oral loading dose of propafenone or flecainide. *Am J Cardiol* 1994;**74**:503–5.

29. Bianconi L, Boccadamo R, Pappalardo A, Gentili C, Pistolese M. Effectiveness of intravenous propafenone for conversion of atrial fibrillation and flutter of recent onset. *Am J Cardiol* 1989;**64**:335–8.

30. Boriani G, Biffi M, Capucci A et al. Oral propafenone to convert recent-onset atrial fibrillation in patients with and without underlying heart disease. A randomized, controlled trial. *Ann Intern Med* 1997;**126**:621–5.

31. Horner SM. A comparison of cardioversion of atrial fibrillation using oral amiodarone, intravenous amiodarone and DC cardioversion. *Acta Cardiolog* 1992;**47**:473–80.

32. Galve E, Rius T, Ballester R et al. Intravenous amiodarone in treatment of recent-onset atrial fibrillation: results of a randomized, controlled study. *J Am Coll Cardiol* 1996;**27**:1079–82.

33. Tieleman RG, Gosselink ATM, Crijns HJGM et al. Efficacy, safety and determinants of conversion of atrial fibrillation and flutter with oral amiodarone. *Am J Cardiol* 1997;**79**:53–7.

34. Skoularigis J, Rothlisberger C, Skudicky D, Essop MR, Wisenbaugh T, Sareli P. Effectiveness of amiodarone and electrical cardioversion for chronic rheumatic atrial fibrillation after mitral valve surgery. *Am J Cardiol* 1993;**72**:423–7.

35. Halinen MO, Huttunen M, Paakkinen S, Tarssanen L. Comparison of sotalol with digoxin–quinidine for conversion of acute atrial fibrillation to sinus rhythm (the Sotalol–Digoxin–Quinidine Trial). *Am J Cardiol* 1995;**76**:495–8.

36. Naccarelli GV, Lee KS, Gibson JK, VanderLugt J. Electrophysiology and pharmacology of ibutilide. *Am J Cardiol* 1996;**78**:12–16.

37. Falk RH, Knowlton AA, Bernard SA, Gotlieb NE, Battinelli NJ. Digoxin for converting recent-onset atrial fibrillation to sinus rhythm. A randomized, double-blinded trial. *Ann Intern Med* 1987;**106**:503–6.

38. Bianconi L, Mennuni M. Comparison between propafenone and digoxin administered intravenously to patients with acute atrial fibrillation. PAFIT-3 Investigators. The Propafenone in Atrial Fibrillation Italian Trial. *Am J Cardiol* 1998;**82**:584–8.

39. Weigner MJ, Caulfield TA, Danias PG, Silverman DI, Manning WJ. Risk for clinical thromboembolism associated with conversion to sinus rhythm in patients with atrial fibrillation lasting less than 48 hours. *Ann Intern Med* 1997;**126**:615–20.

40. Klein AL, Grimm RA, Black IW et al. Cardioversion guided by transesophageal echocardiography: the ACUTE pilot study. *Ann Intern Med* 1997;**126**:200–9.

41. Seto TB, Taira DA, Tsevat J, Manning WJ. Cost-effectiveness of transesophageal echocardiographic-guided cardioversion. *J Am Coll Cardiol* 1997;**29**:122–30.

42. Opolski G, Stanislawska J, Gorecki A, Swiecicka G, Torbicki A, Kraska T. Amiodarone in restoration and maintenance of sinus rhythm in patients with chronic atrial fibrillation after unsuccessful direct-current cardioversion. *Clin Cardiol* 1997;**20**:337–40.

43. Oral H, Souza JJ, Michaud GF et al. Facilitating transthoracic cardioversion of atrial fibrillation with ibutilide pretreatment. *New Engl J Med* 1999;**340**:1849–54.

44. Flaker GC, Blackshear JL, McBride R, Kronmal RA, Halperin JL, Hart RG. Antiarrhythmic drug therapy and cardiac mortality in atrial fibrillation. The Stroke Prevention in Atrial Fibrillation Investigators. *J Am Coll Cardiol* 1992;**20**:527–32.

45. The Planning and Steering Committees of the AFFIRM Study for the NHLBI AFFIRM Investigators. Atrial fibrilla-

tion follow-up investigation of rhythm management – the AFFIRM study design. *Am J Cardiol* 1997;**79**:1198–202.

46. Singh S, Saini RK, DiMarco J, Kluger J, Gold R, Chen YW. Efficacy and safety of sotalol in digitalized patients with chronic atrial fibrillation. The Sotalol Study Group. *Am J Cardiol* 1991;**68**:1227–30.

47. Chun SH, Sager PT, Stevenson WG, Nademanee K, Middlekauff HR, Singh BN. Long-term efficacy of amiodarone for the maintenance of normal sinus rhythm in patients with refractory atrial fibrillation or flutter. *Am J Cardiol* 1995;**76**:47–50.

48. Lau CP, Leung WH, Wong CK. A randomized double-blind crossover study comparing the efficacy and tolerability of flecainide and quinidine in the control of patients with symptomatic paroxysmal atrial fibrillation. *Am Heart J* 1992;**124**:645–50.

49. Naccarelli GV, Dorian P, Hohnloser SH, Coumel P. Prospective comparison of flecainide versus quinidine for the treatment of paroxysmal atrial fibrillation/flutter. The Flecainide Multicenter Atrial Fibrillation Study Group. *Am J Cardiol* 1996;**77**:53A–59A.

50. UK Propafenone PSVT Study Group. A randomized, placebo-controlled trial of propafenone in the prophylaxis of paroxysmal supraventricular tachycardia and paroxysmal atrial fibrillation. *Circulation* 1995;**92**:2550–7.

51. Stroobandt R, Stiels B, Hoebrechts R. Propafenone for conversion and prophylaxis of atrial fibrillation. *Am J Cardiol* 1997;**79**:418–23.

52. Lee SH, Chen SA, Tai CT *et al.* Comparisons of oral propafenone and sotalol as an initial treatment in patients with symptomatic paroxysmal atrial fibrillation. *Am J Cardiol* 1997;**79**:905–8.

53. Southworth MR, Zarembski D, Viana M, Bauman J. Comparison of sotalol versus quinidine for maintenance of normal sinus rhythm in patients with chronic atrial fibrillation. *Am J Cardiol* 1999;**83**:1629–32.

54. Kochiadakis GE, Igoumenidis NE, Marketou ME, Solomou MC, Kanoupakis EM, Vardas PE. Low-dose amiodarone versus sotalol for suppression of recurrent symptomatic atrial fibrillation. *Am J Cardiol* 1998;**81**:995–8.

55. Roy D, Talajic M, Thibault B *et al.* Pilot study and protocol of the Canadian Trial of Atrial Fibrillation (CTAF). *Am J Cardiol* 1997;**80**:464–8.

56. Lee KL, Tai Y-T. Long-term low-dose amiodarone therapy in the management of ventricular and supraventricular tachyarrhythmias: efficacy and safety. *Clin Cardiol* 1997;**20**:372–7.

57. Wolf PA, Abbott RD, Kannel WB. Atrial fibrillation as an independent risk factor for stroke: the Framingham Study. *Stroke* 1991;**22**:983–8.

58. Albers GW, Atwood JE, Hirsh J, Sherman DG, Hughes RA, Connolly SJ. Stroke prevention in nonvalvular atrial fibrillation. *Ann Intern Med* 1991;**115**:727–36.

59. The Boston Area Anticoagulation Trial for Atrial Fibrillation Investigators. The effect of low-dose warfarin on the risk of stroke in patients with non-rheumatic atrial fibrillation. *New Engl J Med* 1990;**323**:1505–11.

60. Ezekowitz MD, Bridgers SL, James KE *et al.* Warfarin in the prevention of stroke associated with nonrheumatic atrial

fibrillation. Veterans Affairs Stroke Prevention in Nonrheumatic Atrial Fibrillation Investigators. *New Engl J Med* 1992;**327**:1406–12.

61. European Atrial Fibrillation Trial Study Group. Secondary prevention in non-rheumatic atrial fibrillation after transient ischaemic attack or minor stroke. EAFT (European Atrial Fibrillation Trial) Study Group. *Lancet* 1993;**342**:1255–62.

62. Peterson P, Boysen G, Godtfredsen J, Andersen ED, Andersen B. Placebo-controlled, randomised trial of warfarin and aspirin for prevention of thromboembolic complications in atrial fibrillation: the Copenhagen AFASAK study. *Lancet* 1989;**1**:175–8.

63. Connolly SJ, Laupacis A, Gent M. Canadian Atrial Fibrillation Anticoagulation (CAFA) Study. *J Am Coll Cardiol* 1991;**18**:349–55.

64. Stroke Prevention in Atrial Fibrillation Investigators. Stroke Prevention in Atrial Fibrillation Study: final results. *Circulation* 1991;**84**:527–39.

65. Atrial Fibrillation Investigators. Risk factors for stroke and efficacy of antithrombotic therapy in atrial fibrillation. Analysis of pooled data from five randomized controlled trials. *Arch Intern Med* 1994;**154**:1449–57.

66. Stroke Prevention in Atrial Fibrillation Investigators. Predictors of thromboembolism in atrial fibrillation: I. Clinical features of patients at risk. The Stroke Prevention in Atrial Fibrillation Investigators. *Ann Intern Med* 1992;**116**:1–5.

67. Stroke Prevention in Atrial Fibrillation Investigators. Predictors of thromboembolism in atrial fibrillation: II. Echocardiographic features of patients at risk. The Stroke Prevention in Atrial Fibrillation Investigators. *Ann Intern Med* 1992;**116**:6–12.

68. Stroke Prevention in Atrial Fibrillation III Investigators. Adjusted-dose warfarin versus low-intensity, fixed-dose warfarin plus aspirin for high-risk patients with atrial fibrillation: Stroke Prevention in Atrial Fibrillation III randomised clinical trial. *Lancet* 1996;**348**:633–8.

69. Furberg CD, Psaty BM, Manolio TA, Gardin JM, Smith VE, Rautaharju PM. Prevalence of atrial fibrillation in elderly subjects (the Cardiovascular Health Study). *Am J Cardiol* 1994;**74**:236–41.

70. Bath PM, Prasad A, Brown MM, MacGregor GA. Survey of use of anticoagulation in patients with atrial fibrillation. *BMJ* 1993;**307**:1045.

71. Carbucicchio C, Tondo C, Fassini G *et al.* Modulation of the atrioventricular node conduction to achieve rate control in patients with atrial fibrillation: long-term results. *Pacing Clin Electrophysiol* 1999;**22**:442–52.

72. Marshall HJ, Harris ZI, Griffith MJ, Holder RL, Gammage MD. Prospective randomized study of ablation and pacing versus medical therapy for paroxysmal atrial fibrillation: effects of pacing mode and mode-switch algorithm. *Circulation* 1999;**99**:1587–92.

73. Mera F, DeLurgio DB, Patterson RE, Merlino JD, Wade ME, Leon AR. A comparison of ventricular function during high right ventricular septal and apical pacing after His-bundle ablation for refractory atrial fibrillation. *Pacing Clin Electrophysiol* 1999;**22**:1234–9.

74. Feld GK. Radiofrequency catheter ablation versus modification of the AV node for control of rapid ventricular response in atrial fibrillation. *J Cardiovasc Electrophysiol* 1995;**6**:217–28.

75. Kay GN, Bubien RS, Epstein AE, Plumb VJ. Effect of catheter ablation of the atrioventricular junction on quality of life and exercise tolerance in paroxysmal atrial fibrillation. *Am J Cardiol* 1988;**62**:741–4.

76. Twidale N, Sutton K, Bartlett L *et al*. Effects on cardiac performance of atrioventricular node catheter ablation using radiofrequency current for drug-refractory atrial arrhythmias. *Pacing Clin Electrophysiol* 1993;**16**:1275–84.

77. Rodriguez LM, Smeets JL, Xie B *et al*. Improvement in left ventricular function by ablation of atrioventricular nodal conduction in selected patients with lone atrial fibrillation. *Am J Cardiol* 1993;**72**:1137–41.

78. Heinz G, Siostrzonek P, Kreiner G, Gossinger H. Improvement in left ventricular systolic function after successful radiofrequency His bundle ablation for drug refractory, chronic atrial fibrillation and recurrent atrial flutter. *Am J Cardiol* 1992;**69**:489–92.

79. Cox JL, Schuessler RB, Lappas DG, Boineau JP. An 8½ year clinical experience with surgery for atrial fibrillation. *Ann Surg* 1996;**224**:267–75.

80. Haissaguerre M, Jais P, Shah DC *et al*. Right and left atrial radiofrequency catheter therapy of paroxysmal atrial fibrillation. *J Cardiovasc Electrophysiol* 1996;**7**:1132–44.

81. Haissaguerre M, Jais P, Shah DC *et al*. Spontaneous initiation of atrial fibrillation by ectopic beats originating in the pulmonary veins. *New Engl J Med* 1998;**339**:659–66.

82. Sra J, Jazayeri MR, Dhala A, Blanck Z, Deshpande S, Akhtar M. Implantable atrial defibrillator for atrial fibrillation. *Wisconsin Med J* 1998;**97**:37–6.

83. Wellens HJ, Lau CP, Luderitz B *et al*. Atrioverter: an implantable device for the treatment of atrial fibrillation. *Circulation* 1998;**98**:1651–6.

84. Hohnloser SH, Kuck KH. Atrial fibrillation-maintaining sinus rhythm versus ventricular rate control: the PIAF trial. Pharmacological Intervention in Atrial Fibrillation. *J Cardiovasc Electrophysiol* 1998;**9**:S121–6.

85. Omran H, Jung W, Rabahieh R *et al*. Left atrial chamber and appendage function after internal atrial defibrillation: a prospective and serial transesophageal echocardiographic study. *J Am Coll Cardiol* 1997;**29**:131–8.

86. Fatkin D, Kuchar DL, Thorburn CW, Feneley MP. Transesophageal echocardiography before and during direct current cardioversion of atrial fibrillation: evidence for "atrial stunning" as a mechanism of thromboembolic complications. *J Am Coll Cardiol* 1994;**23**:307–16.

87. Manning WJ, Silverman DI, Katz SE *et al*. Impaired left atrial mechanical function after cardioversion: relation to the duration of atrial fibrillation. *J Am Coll Cardiol* 1994;**23**:1535–40.

33 Permanent atrial fibrillation

Isabelle C Van Gelder and Harry JGM Crijns

Permanent atrial fibrillation is a form of chronic atrial fibrillation. Patients with permanent atrial fibrillation have resisted previous electrical cardioversion from either shock failure or therapy-resistant recurrences. However, most patients with permanent atrial fibrillation have not even undergone cardioversion because persistence of sinus rhythm was not expected, or cardioversion was refused. Atrial fibrillation is not a benign disease. This holds especially for permanent atrial fibrillation because the very factors predicting shock resistance also point to excess morbidity: older age, longer arrhythmia history, and worse functional class.[1] In addition, the same factors that predict cardioversion failure also predict thromboembolic complications (Fig. 33.1) and hence cerebrovascular and cardiovascular morbidity and death.[2]

Atrial fibrillation may negatively affect quality of life. In addition, all patients with longer lasting atrial fibrillation develop left ventricular dysfunction even those without underlying heart disease. This is indicated as tachycardiomyopathy. Conversely, many patients with atrial fibrillation have pre-existent heart failure. Especially patients with severe heart failure resist (serial) cardioversions. It recently appeared that the serial cardioversion strategy does not reduce the incidence of heart failure in patients with persistent atrial fibrillation.[3]

Therapy for permanent atrial fibrillation focuses on:

- adequate rate control to reduce complaints and prevent or reverse ventricular dysfunction, and
- prevention of thromboembolic complications using warfarin or aspirin.

The present chapter will deal with this type of atrial fibrillation, i.e. permanent atrial fibrillation that is defined as atrial fibrillation in which restoration of sinus rhythm has failed or is considered not feasible anymore.[4]

Heart failure frequently causes atrial fibrillation

In the Framingham study, of all men developing atrial fibrillation during 38 years of follow-up, 20.6% had congestive heart failure at inclusion versus only 3.2% of those without atrial fibrillation. These figures were 26.0% and 2.9% in women, respectively[5] In patients referred for treatment of heart failure, the 2–3 year incidence of atrial fibrillation is 5–10%.[6–8] During almost 2 years' follow-up, Pozzoli *et al.* found that 28 out of 344 heart failure patients (NYHA class II–III) developed atrial fibrillation. We found similar results.[8] Pedersen *et al.*[7] observed a 2.4-year incidence of 5.3% in patients with left ventricular dysfunction after acute myocardial infarction. Interestingly, the angiotensin converting enzyme inhibitor trandolapril reduced this figure to 2.8%. At present it is not certain whether the *onset* of atrial fibrillation has a negative impact on prognosis. Available data suggest that atrial fibrillation does not independently affect prognosis in patients with severe heart failure (class III–IV), whereas it may be a preterminal event in those with mild failure.[8]

The prevalence of atrial fibrillation in heart failure populations has become evident from the large heart failure trials (Table 33.1).

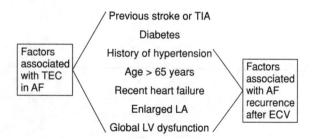

Figure 33.1 Clinical characteristics associated with thromboembolism overlap strongly with those predicting cardioversion failure. If present, these characteristics correspond to an annual stroke risk up to 5–7%, as well as failure to maintain sinus rhythm in 90% of cases at 4 years after cardioversion. ECV: electrical cardioversion; LA and LV: left atrium and left ventricle; TEC: thromboembolic complications; TIA: transient ischaemic attack.

Table 33.1 Prevalence of atrial fibrillation in randomised clinical trials in patients referred for management of heart failure. Prevalence increases as functional class worsens

Trials	NYHA class	Prevalence (%)
SOLVD-prevention[13]	I	4
SOLVD-treatment[13]	II–III	10
Prime II[8]	III–IV	21
Consensus I[26]	IV	50

Atrial fibrillation complicated by heart failure

Data on the incidence of heart failure during permanent atrial fibrillation are sparse. In the Reykjavik study,[9] 25 subjects with chronic atrial fibrillation (found in a population of 9062, prevalence 0.28%) were followed for 14 years. Prevalence of congestive heart failure was 12% compared to 0% in a matched control group of 50 subjects in sinus rhythm. At the end of follow-up, 36% of permanent atrial fibrillation individuals had developed heart failure versus only 2.1% of controls. In a prospective cohort study 3983 pilots during and after World War II were included in 1948.[10] Mean age at inclusion was 31 ± 6 years. Over 44 years of follow-up 299 men (7.5%) developed atrial fibrillation. During a median follow-up of 4.5 years after onset of atrial fibrillation, the arrhythmia independently increased the risk for heart failure. Thirty-five men with atrial fibrillation developed heart failure (12%) versus 258 men in the total population (6.5%, during the total follow-up of 44 years, RR 2.98).[10] In patients with persistent atrial fibrillation undergoing serial electrical cardioversion 45 of 342 patients (13%) developed (progression of) heart failure or died from heart failure (22 patients, 6%) during 3.4 ± 1.6 years.[3] At the end of follow-up 33 of these 45 patients (73%) with a heart failure complication failed the serial cardioversion strategy and were in permanent atrial fibrillation. In contrast, 184 of the 297 patients (62%) without a heart failure complication had relapsed into permanent atrial fibrillation ($P = 0.03$).

The latter suggests that intensive arrhythmia treatment does not prevent heart failure in patients with persistent atrial fibrillation. In addition, atrial fibrillation patients with heart failure tend to resist cardioversions. In these patients the arrhythmia usually is accepted and treatment focuses on heart failure. Nevertheless the issue is still unsettled as to whether a serial cardioversion strategy aiming at maintenance of sinus rhythm is more effective in preventing heart failure compared to simple rate control. Results from randomised studies like AFFIRM[11] are awaited to elucidate this issue. In addition, from future studies it may appear that beta-blockade is beneficial, in particular in atrial fibrillation (rather than sinus rhythm) patients with heart failure, since these drugs not only blunt neurohumoral activation but at the same time control heart rate.

Mortality in permanent atrial fibrillation

Several cohort and retrospective studies have shown that the relative risk of death in subjects with (predominantly permanent?) atrial fibrillation is roughly twice that found in subjects in sinus rhythm.[5,9,10] In the above mentioned Manitoba cohort study,[10] cardiovascular mortality was significantly higher in the pilots who developed atrial fibrillation (N = 92, 31% versus N = 662, 17%, RR 1.41), whereas non-cardiovascular mortality was comparable between the groups (N = 44, 15% versus N = 941, 24%, RR 1.1). In the Framingham Heart Study 5209 residents of Framingham were enrolled. During a follow-up of 40 years, 296 men and 325 women developed atrial fibrillation. Atrial fibrillation was associated with a 1.5- (men) to 1.9 (women)-fold mortality risk after adjustment for pre-existing cardiovascular conditions with which atrial fibrillation was related.[5] It is believed that the reduced survival relates to progression of the underlying cardiovascular disease and stroke rather than the arrhythmia itself. Nevertheless, even after adjustment for arrhythmia-related underlying cardiovascular disorders, the Framingham data suggest that atrial fibrillation adversely affects prognosis.

The prognostic impact of permanent atrial fibrillation in patients with heart failure is uncertain.[8,12,13] Stevenson *et al.* suggested that atrial fibrillation does not affect survival in heart failure patients,[12] whereas a significant impact was seen in a previous paper from the same group.[14] This discrepancy was considered to be caused by a change in drugs from vasodilators and class I drugs to angiotensin converting enzyme inhibitors and amiodarone.[12] Similarly we did not find an impact on survival in a retrospective analysis of PRIME-II data.[8] By contrast, Dries *et al.* showed a significant impact of atrial fibrillation on survival in their retrospective analysis of the SOLVD. In SOLVD patients with asymptomatic (N = 4228) and symptomatic (N = 2569) left ventricular dysfunction were randomised to either placebo or enalapril. At inclusion 419 (6%) were in atrial fibrillation. Compared to those in sinus rhythm, in these patients the rate of non-ischaemic cardiomyopathy was higher (24 versus 7%), and the rate of underlying coronary artery disease lower (44 versus 81%). During an average of 33 months, patients with atrial fibrillation had a higher all-cause mortality (34 versus 23%) and death attributed to pump failure (16.7 versus 9.4%). No differences, however, were observed in arrhythmic death (7 versus 6%).[13] Taken together the data suggest that in heart failure populations with a preserved left ventricular function, atrial fibrillation may have an independent impact on mortality whereas it lacks such influence in advanced heart failure.

Importance of recognising tachycardia-related cardiomyopathy

It is important to distinguish patients with (predominantly) tachycardiomyopathy from those with heart failure complicated by atrial fibrillation. The former group may show substantial improvement of left ventricular function and exercise tolerance (and hence quality of life) after control of the rate and regularisation of the rhythm. Recognition of these patients is challenging (Box 33.1). The chicken and egg problem is especially difficult to resolve in the patients with presumed tachycardiomyopathy (top column). Recruitable contractility (dobutamine stress echocardiography) has been suggested for identifying atrial fibrillation patients with reversible left ventricular dysfunction after successful cardioversion. Whether the onset of atrial fibrillation is a preterminal event propbably depends on the functional class.

Paelinck *et al.* suggested that low-dose dobutamine echo-

cardiography may be helpful in this respect.[15] Of 13 patients with atrial fibrillation and heart failure, eight demonstrated a marked increase of the left ventricular ejection fraction during low dose dobutamine (from 33 to 56%). In these eight patients left ventricular ejection fraction normalised (62%) during follow-up after restoration of sinus rhythm. In the other five patients stress echocardiography did not reveal recruitable wall motion. In these patients ejection fraction was unchanged during follow-up (27 and 29%).[15] This study suggests that stress echocardiography may differentiate between tachycardia-induced cardiomyopathy and left ventricular dysfunction complicated by atrial fibrillation. Such a diagnostic test may be of importance for treatment. In tachycardiomyopathy patients, much effort should be directed to restoration and maintenance of sinus rhythm to prevent further disease. If chronic sinus rhythm cannot be achieved, His bundle ablation and pacemaker implantation should be considered.

Thromboembolic complications during permanent atrial fibrillation

Atrial fibrillation is the most common cardiac cause of systemic emboli, usually cerebrovascular. In the presence of atrial fibrillation, the risk of stroke shows an approximately 5-fold increase unrelated to age. On the other hand, the risk of stroke increases also with age, whether or not atrial fibrillation is present. The proportion of atrial fibrillation-related stroke to total stroke increases significantly with age from 6.7% for ages 50–59 years to 36.2% for ages 80–89 years.[16] The risk for stroke in lone atrial fibrillation is still uncertain.

The cardiac embolus often results in occlusion of a major cerebral artery. The ensuing infarct is often large and may be fatal. Apart from symptomatic strokes, atrial fibrillation has been associated with an increased risk of silent strokes. Risk factors for stroke in atrial fibrillation include rheumatic heart disease, age >65 years, hypertension, previous stroke or transient ischaemic attack, diabetes, recent heart failure, and echocardiographic atrial or ventricular enlargement (Box 33.1).[2]

Quality of life

Atrial fibrillation may severely affect quality of life: palpitations, chest pain, dyspnoea, and fatigue. Presyncope or even drop attacks in particular at arrhythmia onset or termination may occur in patients with paroxysmal atrial fibrillation. The autonomic nervous system is an important mediator for quality of life in these patients. Especially impaired baroreflex function with low vagal activity pre-

---

Box 33.1

Tachycardiomyopathy

- Difficult to recognise
    - AF onset usually unclear
    - patients present with HF
    - recruitable contractility
- HF easy-to-treat
- Prognosis: good
- Prevention: stop AF
- Management: RC or regularisation of rhythm
    - cardioversion
    - neg chronotropic drugs
    - His ablation and PM

AF complicating HF

- Easy to recognise
    - AF onset clear
    - AF onset after HF onset
    - no recruitable contractility
- AF difficult-to-treat
- Preterminal event?
- Prevention: maximal HF treatment
- Management:
    - HF treatment
    - RC: usually digitalis

Abbreviations: AF = atrial fibrillation; HF = heart failure; PM = implantable artificial pacemaker; RC = rate control.

dicts dizziness and hence impaired quality of life.[17] Many clinicians share the impression that, after transition from paroxysmal to permanent atrial fibrillation, severity of symptoms decreases. So far, only limited data on quality of life during permanent atrial fibrillation are available. Preliminary data show that especially low scores were found for physical and emotional role limitations. This indicates that these patients not only feel unable to perform everyday activities but in addition dislike to be active. Of even more importance is that patients with permanent atrial fibrillation show similar low scores for physical and mental role limitations to disabled rheumatoid arthritis patients (unpublished data).

Treatment: control of the ventricular response

Therapy should aim to reduce complaints by adequate control of the ventricular rate and prevention or reversion of symptoms of left ventricular dysfunction. There is no accepted definition for adequate rate control at rest or exercise. The optimal heart rate may vary from one patient to the other. In general, patients with permanent atrial fibrillation practise only lower intensities of exercise. Special attention must therefore be paid to adequate pharmacological ventricular rate control during the lower stages of exercise. Therapy effectiveness may be assessed reliably by 24-h Holter monitoring. In general, a heart rate below 90 bpm at rest and below 110 bpm during light to moderate exercise is usually accepted. Peak exercise heart rate should remain below or at the normal peak value for the patient corrected for age and sex.

Rate control can be achieved by negative chronotropic drugs like digoxin, non-dihydropyridine calcium channel blockers, and beta-blockers. If patients are asymptomatic, have a normal ventricular function, and a normal ventricular response, also during (the lower stages of) exercise, negative chronotropic treatment is not needed. Digoxin monotherapy usually does not prevent rapid ventricular rates during exercise and addition of a calcium antagonist or a beta-blocker may improve rate control.[18–20] Only recently, a systematic comparison of standardised drug regimens on 24-h ventricular response control has been reported. Twelve patients with permanent atrial fibrillation were randomly treated for 2 weeks with (a) 0.25 mg digoxin, (b) 240 mg diltiazem CD, (c) 50 mg atenolol, (d) 0.25 mg digoxin + 240 mg diltiazem CD, and (e) 0.25 mg digoxin + 50 mg atenolol. After 2 weeks of treatment the ventricular rate response during daytime and during exercise was significantly lower during treatment in group (e) as compared to either digoxin, or diltiazem, or atenolol alone.[20] Thus, preferably during permanent atrial fibrillation, treatment should contain a combination of digitalis and a beta-blocker. Whether a combination of a calcium channel blocker and a beta-blocker is even more beneficial remains to be established.

Digoxin is accepted as primary rate control treatment in atrial fibrillation complicated by heart failure, but this advice lacks a solid scientific basis. In view of the positive studies on beta-blockers in heart failure it seems worthwhile to evaluate their rate-controlling effects in this setting.

Class IA antiarrhythmic drugs like disopyramide and quinidine may enhance the atrioventricular nodal conduction during atrial fibrillation leading to high ventricular rates because of their anticholinergic (parasympaticolytic) effect. The same holds for class IC antiarrhythmic drugs.[21] Therefore no class I antiarrhythmic drugs should be instituted during permanent atrial fibrillation. Although class III drugs, like amiodarone and sotalol, may decrease the ventricular rate during atrial fibrillation,[22] these drugs have no significant advantage above the conventional negative chronotropic drugs. Above all, these drugs may induce severe adverse effects like ventricular pro-arrhythmia (sotalol) or thyroid dysfunction or pulmonary toxicity (amiodarone).

In some patients rate-control drugs are ineffective or not tolerated. These patients are ideal candidates for pacemaker implantation and subsequent catheter ablation of the His bundle. Such therapy may dramatically improve systolic function and quality of life. Whether atrioventricular node ablation with implantation of a pacemaker deserves a more prominent role in permanent atrial fibrillation remains to be determined. The beneficial effects of atrioventricular node modification seems to be only temporary and minor as compared to complete atrioventricular node ablation.[23]

Prevention of thromboembolic complications

Warfarin as well as aspirin may prevent ischaemic stroke in patients with atrial fibrillation. Warfarin, however, is substantially more effective than aspirin but bleeding complications and lack of control of the INR level importantly decrease its applicability. It was shown that both advanced age and more intense anticoagulation increased the risk of major haemorrhage in patients treated with warfarin.[24] The SPAF III study[25] randomised patients with atrial fibrillation and at least one risk factor for thromboembolic complications to either a combination of low-intensity fixed-dose warfarin (INR 1.2–1.5) and aspirin (325 mg/day) or adjusted-dose warfarin (INR 2.0–3.0). This study was stopped prematurely because of a higher incidence of thromboembolic complications in those who received the combination therapy. These results encourage to use of warfarin aiming at an INR between 2.0 and 3.0. Patients without risk factors may be left untreated or may be given aspirin.

References

1. Van Gelder IC, Crijns HJGM, Tieleman RG *et al.* Value and limitation of electrical cardioversion in patients with chronic atrial fibrillation – importance of arrhythmia risk factors and oral anticoagulation. *Arch Intern Med* 1996;**156**:2585–92.

2. Risk factors for stroke and efficacy of antithrombotic therapy in atrial fibrillation. Analysis of pooled data from five randomized controlled trials. *Arch Intern Med* 1994;**154**:1449–57.

3. Tuinenburg AE, Van Gelder IC, Van Den Berg MB, Brügemann J, Crijns HJGM. Lack of prevention of heart failure by serial electrical cardioversion therapy in patients with persistent atrial fibrillation. *Heart* 1999;**82**:486–93.

4. Gallagher MM, Camm AJ. Classification of atrial fibrillation. *Pacing Clin Electrophysiol* 1997;**20**:1603–5.

5. Benjamin EJ, Levy D, Vaziri SM, D'Agostino RB, Belanger AJ, Wolf PA. Independent risk factors for atrial fibrillation in a population-based cohort. The Framingham study. *JAMA* 1994;**271**:840–4.

6. Pozzoli M, Cioffi G, Traversi E, Pinna GD, Cobelli F, Tavazzi L. Predictors of primary atrial fibrillation and concomitant clinical and hemodynamic changes in patients with chronic heart failure: a prospective study in 344 patients with baseline sinus rhythm. *J Am Coll Cardiol* 1998;**32**:197–204.

7. Pedersen OD, Bagger H, Kober L, Torp-Pedersen C. Trandolapril reduces the incidence of atrial fibrillation after acute myocardial infarction in patients with left ventricular dysfunction. *Circulation* 1999;**100**:376–80.

8. Crijns HJGM, Tjeerdsma G, De Kam PJ *et al.* Prognostic value of presence and development of atrial fibrillation in patients with advanced chronic heart failure. *Eur Heart J* 2000;**21**:1238–45.

9. Önundarson PT, Thorgeirsson G, Jonmundsson E, Sigfusson N, Hardarson Th. Chronic atrial fibrillation – epidemiological features and 14 years follow-up: a case control study. *Eur Heart J* 1987;**8**:521–7.

10. Krahn AD, Manfreda J, Tate RB, Mathewson FAL, Cuddy TE. The natural history of atrial fibrillation: incidence, risk factors, and prognosis in the Manitoba follow-up study. *Am J Med* 1995;**98**:476–84.

11. The planning and Steering Committees of the AFFIRM Study for the NHLBI AFFIRM Investigators. Atrial fibrillation follow-up investigation of rhythm management – the AFFIRM study design. *Am J Cardiol* 1997;**97**:1198–202.

12. Stevenson WG, Stevenson LW, Middlekauff HR *et al.* Improving survival for patients with atrial fibrillation and advanced heart failure. *J Am Coll Cardiol* 1996;**28**:1458–63.

13. Dries DL, Exner DV, Gersh BJ, Domanski MJ, Waclawiw MA, Stevenson LW. Atrial fibrillation is associated with an increased risk for mortality and heart failure progression in patients with asymptomatic and symptomatic left ventricular systolic dysfunction: a retrospective analysis of the SOLVD trials. Studies of Left Ventricular Dysfunction. *J Am Coll Cardiol* 1998;**32**:695–703.

14. Middlekauf HR, Stevenson WG, Stevenson LW. Prognostic significance of atrial fibrillation in advanced heart failure. A study of 390 patients. *Circulation* 1991;**84**:40–8.

15. Paelinck B, Vermeersch P, Stockman D, Convens C, Vaerenberg M. Usefulness of low-dose dobutamine stress echocardiography in predicting recovery of poor left ventricular function in atrial fibrillation dilated cardiomyopathy. *Am J Cardiol* 1999;**83**:1668–715.

16. Wolf PA, Abbott RD, Kannel WB. Atrial fibrillation: a major contributor to stroke in the elderly. *Arch Intern Med* 1987;**147**:1561–4.

17. Van den Berg MP, HassinkRJ, Tuinenburg AE *et al.* Quality of life in patients with paroxysmal atrial fibrillation and its predictors. Importance of the autonomic nervous system. *Eur Heart J* 2000; (in press).

18. David D, Segni ED, Klein HO *et al.* Inefficacy of digitalis in the control of heart rate in patients with chronic atrial fibrillation: beneficial effect of an added beta adrenergic blocking agent. *Am J Cardiol* 1979;**44**:1378–82.

19. Lundstrom T, Rydén L. Ventricular rate control and exercise performance in chronic atrial fibrillation: effects of diltiazem and verapamil. *J Am Coll Cardiol* 1990;**16**:86–90.

20. Farshi R, Kistner D, Sarma JSM, Longmate JA, Singh BN. Ventricular rate control in chronic atrial fibrillation during daily activity and programmed exercise: a crossover open-label study of five drug regimens. *J Am Coll Cardiol* 1999;**33**:304–10.

21. Feld GK, Chen PS, Nicod P *et al.* Possible atrial pro-arrhythmic effects of class IC antiarrhythmic drugs. *Am J Cardiol* 1990;**66**:378–83.

22. Juul-Möller S, Edvardsson N, Rehnquist-Ahlberg N. Sotalol versus quinidine for the maintenance of sinus rhythm after direct current conversion of atrial fibrillation. *Circulation* 1990;**82**:1932–9.

23. Lee SH, Chen SA, Tai CT *et al.* Comparisons of quality of life and cardiac performance after complete atrioventricular junction ablation and atrioventricular junction modification in patients with medically refractory atrial fibrillation. *J Am Coll Cardiol* 1998;**31**:637–44.

24. Stroke Prevention in Atrial Fibrillation Investigators. Warfarin versus aspirin for prevention of thromboembolism in atrial fibrillation: Stroke Prevention in Atrial Fibrillation II study. *Lancet* 1994;**343**:687–91.

25. The Stroke Prevention in Atrial Fibrillation Investigators. Adjusted-dose warfarin versus low intensity, fixed dose warfarin plus aspirin for high-risk patients with atrial fibrillation: stroke prevention of atrial fibrillation III randomised clinical trial. *Lancet* 1996;**348**:633–8.

26. The CONSENSUS trial study group. Effects of enalapril on mortality in severe congestive heart failure. Results of the Cooperative North Scandinavian Enalapril Survival Study (CONSENSUS). *New Engl J Med* 1987;**316**:1429–35.

34 Arrhythmias associated with the long QT syndrome

Peter J Schwartz

The identification of subgroups of patients at particularly high risk for life-threatening arrhythmias remains an important but elusive task for most cardiac disorders, and the long QT syndrome (LQTS) is no exception. Generalities leave room for exceptions and, when diseases are being dealt with that are characterised by a high degree of lethality, the failure to identify these exceptions usually results in the sudden death of the unfortunate patient. This grim picture should not lead to a nihilistic approach, which could be easily exploited by someone who might feel entitled to recommend an Implantable Cardioverter Defibrillator (ICD) for every patient affected by LQTS. The widely different prognosis among individual patients warrants a major effort in the direction of risk stratification. We should not be deterred by the objective difficulties and unavoidable failures because the reward will be a better quality and duration of life for the vast majority of patients and their families.

With this in mind, the outline of this brief chapter will be the following:

- a brief overview about LQTS and its genetic basis;
- risk factors unrelated to genotype;
- risk factors related to genotype;
- therapeutic implications.

It will be seen that, at variance with the impressive and scientifically rigorous progress in the molecular biology of LQTS, therapeutic choices based on risk stratification are still gross and reflect an unsatisfactory level of discrimination between low- and high-risk patients. Having said that, it is fair to say that the overall efficacy of the available therapies is very good. In referral centres, such as ours, with long-term experience and a large population of LQTS patients followed personally on a regular basis, the current mortality rate is below 3% over 10 years from the first syncope. This represents a dramatic improvement compared to the mortality rates of 50–60% observed 15 years ago among untreated patients.[1] There is certainly room for improvement and specific subgroups at particularly high risk may now be identified and treated more aggressively in order to further reduce mortality, while preserving as much as possible the quality of life of these patients, who, for the vast majority, are children or teenagers.

LQTS and its genetic basis

The congenital long QT syndrome is characterised by prolongation of the QT interval on the surface ECG and by propensity for syncope or cardiac arrest primarily under stressful conditions.[2,3] Among symptomatic and untreated patients the risk of sudden death is very high, exceeding 20% in the first year from the initial syncope.[1]

Until 1995 LQTS was dealt with as a single disease. It was only with the identification of some of the genes responsible for the disease, and with the realisation that they all encode different ion channels,[4] that a novel concept began to emerge. Namely, that under the umbrella of LQTS several diseases – all due to abnormalities involving specific ion currents – might exist and be characterised by a similar phenotype despite a different genotype. So far, six loci have been related to LQTS and five genes have been identified. Two of them, *minK* and *Mirp1*, responsible respectively for LQT5 and LQT6, are rare. The most common forms, responsible respectively for LQT1, LQT2, and LQT3 depend on mutations on *KvLQT1* (encoding the I_{Ks} current), on *HERG* (encoding the I_{Kr} current), and on *SCN5A* (encoding the Na^+ current). The data available for genotype–phenotype correlation studies on adequate numbers are limited to LQT1, LQT2, and LQT3. Therefore a new terminology has now to be used in order not to miss these differences that are important for a molecular understanding of the underlying defects and mechanisms, and for a more specific and effective clinical management. All this refers to Romano–Ward patients, with normal hearing. Patients with the Jervell and Lange-Nielsen (J–LN) variant, associated with congenital deafness, have two mutations, identical (homozygotes) or different (compound heterozygotes). Importantly, these mutations have so far always involved the genes *KvLQT1* or *KCNE1*, which, when co-assembled, form the I_{Ks} current. On this basis, we have previously hypothesised[5] that the "triggers" for cardiac events were likely to be similar for LQT1 and for J–LN patients.

The consequences of the mutations involved in the main LQTS subtypes are important for the understanding of the mechanisms involved in the onset of the life-threatening arrhythmias of LQTS and, hopefully, for the design of novel preventive strategies. The mutations on the K^+ channels lead to losses in repolarising current (loss of function), whereas most of the mutations on the Na^+ channel lead to increases in late Na^+ inward current (gain of function). The consequence in both cases is a prolongation of action potential duration, which manifests clinically in the prolongation of the QT interval. Based on this information, in 1995 we had already begun to explore the possibility for gene-specific therapies in LQTS.[6]

The perception that the prevalence of LQTS might be much higher than anticipated has grown over the years. The original hypothesis that some patients might have been affected by LQTS despite a seemingly normal QT interval[7] was initially supported by data from the International Registry.[8,9] Final confirmation came with the molecular evidences that among a few LQTS families there were gene carriers with a normal QT[10] and that apparently "sporadic" cases were actually hereditary, because their families included several gene carriers with a normal QT interval as a consequence of low penetrance (Fig. 34.1).[11] This results in a potentially large number of gene carriers with a normal QT interval and low probability of symptoms, unless exposed to drugs containing I_{Kr} blockers.[12]

Risk factors unrelated to genotype

Prior to the identification of some of the LQTS genes, life was simpler and physicians could deal with all the affected patients as a whole, as if they had been affected by one single disease. This approach remains important in clinical management because the reality is that most cardiologists have to make their first decisions when still do not know the genotype of the patient, and sometimes do not even know if the suspected patient is a gene carrier or a non-gene carrier with a borderline QT interval.

Also, for a long time physicians have been starting their risk stratification process from a simple, binary, question: "Has my patient already suffered a cardiac event (syncope, cardiac arrest) or is he/she still asymptomatic?" The answer to this basic question was opening two broad areas, with different approaches. Therapy was always initiated in symptomatic patients, whereas with asymptomatic patients the decision was more complex and often involved personal views or, sadly, medicolegal considerations. In my own case, considering what I then thought to be best for these young patients, I tended to be rather conservative and recommended initiation of therapy under six specific conditions.[13] This has now changed.

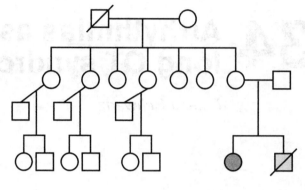

Clinical diagnosis

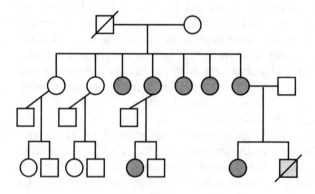

Molecular diagnosis
Penetrance 14% (25%)

Figure 34.1 Clinical (*upper panel*) and molecular diagnosis (*lower panel*) in the same LQTS family. It is evident that six members with normal QT and no symptoms (i.e. non-affected at clinical examination) are gene carriers of the disease. These apparently healthy subjects are at risk if exposed to drugs containing I_{Kr} blockers.

Indeed, this binary approach has been superseded by the recent realisation of the actual risk of sudden death during the first episode. Based on the 160 families regularly followed at our centre in Pavia, and on the almost 600 family members (we have excluded the generations that included the grandparents for the difficulty of correct ascertainment of negative clinical histories), some rather unexpected and disquieting information is now available to us. Excluding events in the first year of life, we have observed an incidence of 10% of cardiac arrests/sudden deaths at first episode among these families; when the first year of life is included, this figure reaches 14%. At this point it becomes unacceptable to leave the patients diagnosed as affected by LQTS without therapy based on the reasoning, which I have accepted for quite some time, that the vast majority of asymptomatic patients will either remain asymptomatic or will develop a non-lethal first cardiac event; this will allow the institution of effective therapy, thus avoiding the need of an unnecessary life-long treatment in many young individuals. It follows that, when anyone recognised as affected by LQTS is being treated, one can now look at various possible risk factors, integrating them appropriately with the knowledge of prior cardiac events if necessary.

QT duration

One would logically expect that the longer the QT, the greater the risk. To some extent this is true, as patients with very long QT intervals (QTc >600 ms) almost never remain asymptomatic. Similarly, patients with QTc in excess of 500 ms tend to be more symptomatic than those with a lower value of QTc. All this makes sense but does not help too much because patients with QTc values of 460–480 can easily have syncope or cardiac arrest. Practically, one can use QT duration to determine only the degree of urgency in making decisions because – probability-wise – it is just less likely that a 15-year-old boy, discovered to have a QTc of 450 ms, will develop a major cardiac event in the next 2 weeks compared to, say, his cousin with a QTc of 580 ms.

The duration of the QT interval, exceeding or not the upper limits of normal, has acquired significance for the gene carriers without QT prolongation. It is also of importance in the first week of life as a major risk factor for sudden death in the first few months of life when – in absence of an ECG – it is often labelled as sudden infant death syndrome[14] and may actually represent undiagnosed cases of LQTS due to *de novo* mutations.[15]

T wave alternans

Since its first recognition as an integral part of the most typical ECG aspects of LQTS,[16] macroscopic T wave alternans (Fig. 34.2) has been regarded as an important marker of electrical instability and of risk of impending ventricular fibrillation. It is important to remember that T wave alternans is an episodic phenomenon, which may easily escape detection if it occurs while the ECG is not recorded; accordingly, no inference for risk should be made when it is not observed. On the other hand, its occurrence has all the importance of any positive finding in biology. Patients observed to have T wave alternans are expected to become symptomatic at any time, if they are not already. The observation of T wave alternans in patients already under treatment is cause for concern; however, it should not be equated to inadequacy or failure of therapy (these definitions should be reserved for recurrence of syncope and for occurrence of cardiac arrest or sudden death, respectively).

T wave notches

Notches on the T wave (Fig. 34.3) have progressively acquired importance for their diagnostic value,[17] particularly when the prolongation of the QT interval is modest. Relevant here is the fact that, among patients, they are more frequently observed in those with cardiac events.[17]

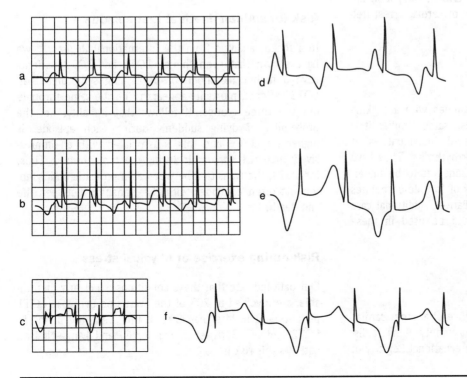

Figure 34.2 Examples of T wave alternans in LQTS patients. (a) and (b), 9-year-old girl: alternation of T wave occurred during an unintentionally induced episode of fear. (c), 3-year-old boy (modified from ref. 16). (d) and (e), 14-year-old girl 1 minute (d) and 3 minutes (e) after induced fright (modified from Fraser GR *et al.* *Q J Med* 1964;**33**:361–85). (f), 7-year-old girl: T wave alternans occurred during exercise (modified from Jervell A. *Adv Intern Med* 1971;**17**:425–38).

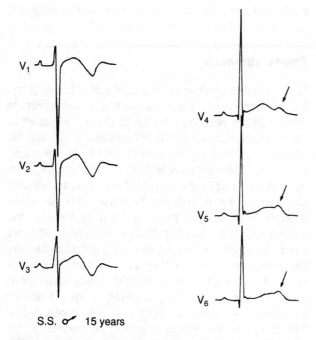

S.S. ♂ 15 years

Figure 34.3 Example of different T wave morphologies across the precordial leads in the same LQTS patient. In leads V2–V4, the T wave is distinctly biphasic, while in V5 and V6 a clear notch is visible, as indicated by the arrow, which produces a TU complex. (From ref. 17.)

Echocardiographic abnormalities

The peculiar abnormalities in the motion of the posterior ventricular wall, which we have described, carry a significantly greater probability of syncope or cardiac arrest (relative risk 2.75).[18,19]

Sudden death in the family

Unquestionably, there are LQTS families with a striking rate of sudden deaths. Within these same families it is reasonable to consider any affected individual as at unusually high risk for malignant arrhythmias. They have the same mutation, which, for reasons yet to be understood, results in a higher probability of torsade de pointes to deteriorate into ventricular fibrillation. Additional care for a fully protective therapy should be used in these families.

Resuscitated cardiac arrest

A cardiac arrest predicts the recurrence of another cardiac arrest, a phenomenon observed in a variety of heart diseases. A recent analysis from the International Registry of

LQTS, which we established with Arthur Moss in 1979, indicates that the patients who have already suffered a cardiac arrest are those at higher risk of recurrence (13% at 5 years), even when they are treated with beta-blockers.[20] This analysis is limited by having also included patients who were off therapy for months or years; 30% of those who died were in this condition. It follows that these data actually overestimate the failure of beta-blockers. The main implication is that when a patient has already suffered a cardiac arrest, beta-blockers do not provide a sufficient degree of safety, and a mortality risk close to 10% in a population with an average age between 10 and 15 years is unacceptable. On this basis, for this subgroup of patients at truly high risk, we now recommend an ICD, in addition to antiadrenergic therapy.

Risk factors related to genotype

If the patient has been genotyped, and if the genotype happens to be one of the three most frequently encountered, namely LQT1, LQT2, or LQT3, then a number of novel information and attending options for management have become available. Of special relevance is the fact that we have recently demonstrated that conditions ("triggers") associated with a major cardiac event are largely genotype-specific.[21] The fact that our most current data are based on almost 800 symptomatic patients of known genotype lends an unusual level of credibility to the related findings.

Risk for sudden death at first episode

In a recent analysis from the International Registry,[22] we have shown that even though LQT1 and LQT2 patients have a higher likelihood of developing symptoms than LQT3 patients, mortality appears to be the same throughout the three groups. It follows that lethality, i.e. the probability of dying suddenly during each episode, is higher for LQT3, and this is associated with an impressively high risk for death during the first episode. Thus, for LQT3, the transition between asymptomatic and symptomatic often coincides with the transition between life and death.

Risk during exercise or physical stress

Our data indicate that these conditions, so clearly identifiable, are involved in 70% of the events occurring in LQT1 patients and in less than 20% of the events occurring in LQT2 and LQT3 patients. For Jervell and Lange-Nielsen patients this risk is 50%.

Risk during emotional stress, including arousal

This risk is approximately 25% for LQT1 patients and close to 50% for J–LN patients. It accounts for 50% and for 30% of the triggering events for LQT2 and LQT3, respectively.

Risk at rest or sleep, without known arousal

LQT1 and J–LN are very seldom at risk in this condition, about 5%. This is in striking contrast with LQT2 and LQT3 patients, who, under these conditions, have approximately 35% and 50% of their episodes, respectively.

Risk during acoustic stimuli

An initial report based only on LQT1 and on LQT2 patients,[23] is now confirmed in our much larger population which also encloses LQT3 patients. Our own data indicate that, whereas acoustic stimuli, including noises producing arousals from sleep, account for 25% of the cardiac events among LQT2, this figure decreases to 8% among LQT3 and is practically – and very curiously – absent among LQT1 patients.

Age as a risk factor

The data from our large cooperative study also provide information relating genotype and a differential risk according to age. The J–LN patients are those who first start to become symptomatic, so that by age 6 almost 80% of those destined to be symptomatic have had their first episode. In our series, based on over 100 J–LN patients, only 4% became symptomatic over age 15. LQT1 patients become symptomatic relatively early, and males earlier than females – a phenomenon already observed in the non-genotyped LQTS population.[24] By age 25, 90% of the symptomatic patients have had their first event. LQT2 and LQT3 patients behave similarly and have a later onset of the symptoms; by age 20, about 35% of the symptomatic patients were still asymptomatic.

Risk of drug-induced torsade de pointes

On this specific point there are almost no data available. The first two patients, described because drug-induced long QT syndrome was found to have mutations on LQTS genes, had them on *KvlQt1*[25] and on *HERG*.[26] Clearly, there is room only for speculation. I would like to offer here one such, perhaps tenable, speculation. It is based on the fact that most agents producing drug-induced torsade de pointes are I_{Kr} blockers. LQT2 patients with "dominant negative" mutations and with major reductions in I_{Kr} current are clearly more dependent on other repolarising currents for the completion of their repolarisation. Administration of an I_{Kr} blocker could, perhaps, do only limited damage, because there was only a limited amount of I_{Kr} still available for block. In contrast, patients whose QT prolongation is secondary to mutations affecting I_{Ks} or delaying inactivation of I_{Na} would be highly dependent on I_{Kr}, and therefore extremely sensitive to even relatively small blocking doses of a compound producing a partial block of I_{Kr}. In theory, one could even propose the opposite; namely, that patients with an already compromised I_{Kr} current cannot tolerate any further reduction. This would actually make LQT2 the group at highest risk for drug-induced torsade de pointes. Time will tell.

Implications for management and therapy

For non-genotyped individuals, the most important recent information is represented by the evidence for an unexpectedly high incidence of sudden death at first episode (14%) and by the relatively high recurrence rate after cardiac arrest, often despite beta-blocker therapy. The two direct consequences for appropriate management are the need to initiate therapy, with beta-blockers, in every patient diagnosed as affected by the LQTS, and to implant an ICD, for safety reasons, in any patient who, independently of being on or off therapy, has had a cardiac arrest.

For genotyped patients, the situation is more complex and less well defined, because of the need to increase data and follow-up. At this time, most of the new considerations should reflect commonsense applied to the growing data on genotype–phenotype correlation.

LQT1 patients should avoid situations involving strenuous exercise, competitive sports, and physical stress in general. They appear to be particularly responsive to beta-blockers and should be treated with full-dose beta-blockade. To a large extent, this applies to the J–LN patients as well, given the implications of having mutations affecting the same current.

LQT2 should avoid, as much as possible within the constraints of modern life, the use of alarm clocks,[23,27] and to receive phone calls while they are asleep.

The only potential note of concern comes from the observation that most LQT3 patients have a tendency toward marked QT prolongation at long cardiac cycles,[2] as it happens during bradycardia or sleeping periods. This observation is in agreement with the increased risk that LQT3 patients have when they are at rest or asleep,[5,21] and raises the disturbing possibility that, not only may they not benefit from beta-blockers, but they may actually be at higher risk during beta-blocker treatment because of the long cardiac cycles. This has led our group to treat these patients with left cardiac sympathetic denervation because this procedure, besides being quite effective in all LQTS patients,[28] exerts its powerful antiadrenergic and antifibrillatory effect without reducing heart rate.[29] If beta-blockers are used in association with a pacemaker, then the potentially adverse effects of the reduction in heart rate are avoided. It is also fair to remember that, for those LQT3 patients with mutations causing a delayed inward Na+ current, drugs such as mexiletine may be very useful in shortening the QT interval.[2,6]

Initiating therapy in an adult genotyped asymptomatic patient may still be an issue. Above the age of 20, the probability of becoming symptomatic is minimal, if the patient has the Jervell and Lange-Nielsen syndrome, and is very modest if the patient is a male with LQT1. This is not true with the other genotypes.

Finally, there is the new complication represented by gene carriers with a normal QT interval. Should they be treated or be left alone? Cardiac events, mostly syncopal episodes, are known to occur in some of these individuals. We do not have as yet sufficient data to make sound decisions. Our current choice, after performance of repeated ECGs and Holter recordings to exclude even transient repolarisation abnormalities such to suggest arrhythmic risk, is not to initiate therapy in gene carriers with a consistently normal QT interval. We are actively pursuing a much needed epidemiological survey to generate adequate prospective data.

It seems fair to conclude that it is becoming possible to look at the arrhythmic risk for LQTS patients in a different way. The novel information provided by the genotype–phenotype studies provides new insights for a better tailored approach to therapy for the individual patient affected by the long QT syndrome.

References

1. Schwartz PJ. Idiopathic long QT syndrome: Progress and questions. *Am Heart J* 1985;**109**:399–411.
2. Schwartz PJ, Priori SG, Napolitano C. The long QT syndrome. In: Zipes DP, Jalife J eds. *Cardiac electrophysiology. From cell to bedside.* 3rd edn. Philadelphia: WB Saunders Co., 2000, pp. 597–615.
3. Priori SG, Barhanin J, Hauer RNW *et al.* Genetic and molecular basis of cardiac arrhythmias: impact on clinical management. Part I and II. *Circulation* 1999;**99**:518–28; Part III. *Circulation* 1999;**99**:674–81; and *Eur Heart J* 1999;**20**:174–95.
4. Abbott GW, Sesti F, Splawski I *et al.* MiRP1 forms I_{Kr} potassium channels with *HERG* and is associated with cardiac arrhythmia. *Cell* 1999;**97**:175–87.
5. Schwartz PJ, Moss AJ, Priori SG *et al.* Gene-specific influence on the triggers for cardiac arrest in the long QT syndrome. *Circulation* 1997;**96**(Abstr. Suppl.):212.
6. Schwartz PJ, Priori SG, Locati EH *et al.* Long QT syndrome patients with mutations on the *SCN5A* and *HERG* genes have differential responses to Na+ channel blockade and to increases in heart rate. Implications for gene-specific therapy. *Circulation* 1995;**92**:3381–6.
7. Schwartz PJ. The long QT syndrome. In: Kulbertus HE, Wellens HJJ eds. *Sudden death.* The Hague: M Nijhoff, 1980, pp. 358–78.
8. Moss AJ, Schwartz PJ, Crampton RS *et al.* The long QT syndrome: prospective longitudinal study of 328 families. *Circulation* 1991;**84**:1136–44.
9. Schwartz PJ, Moss AJ, Locati E *et al.* The long QT syndrome international prospective registry. *J Am Coll Cardiol* 1989;**13**(Suppl. A):20A.
10. Vincent GM, Timothy KW, Leppert M, Keating M. The spectrum of symptoms and QT intervals in carriers of the gene for the long QT syndrome. *N Engl J Med* 1992;**327**:846–52.
11. Priori SG, Napolitano C, Schwartz PJ. Low penetrance in the long QT syndrome. Clinical impact. *Circulation* 1999;**99**:529–33.
12. Napolitano C, Schwartz PJ, Brown AM *et al.* Evidence for a cardiac ion channel mutation underlying drug-induced QT prolongation and life threatening arrhythmias. *J Cardiovasc Electrophysiol* 2000;**11**:691–6.
13. Schwartz PJ, Locati EH, Napolitano C, Priori SG. The long QT syndrome. In: Zipes DP, Jalife J eds. *Cardiac electrophysiology. From cell to bedside.* 2nd edn. Philadelphia: WB Saunders Co., 1995, pp. 788–811.
14. Schwartz PJ, Stramba-Badiale M, Segantini A *et al.* Prolongation of the QT interval and the sudden infant death syndrome. *N Engl J Med* 1998;**338**:1709–14.
15. Schwartz PJ, Priori SG, Dumaine R *et al.* A molecular link between the sudden infant death syndrome and the long QT syndrome. *N Engl J Med* 2000;**343**:262–7.
16. Schwartz PJ, Malliani A. Electrical alternation of the T-wave: clinical and experimental evidence of its relationship with the sympathetic nervous system and with the long Q-T syndrome. *Am Heart J* 1975;**89**:45–50.
17. Malfatto G, Beria G, Sala S, Bonazzi O, Schwartz PJ. Quantitative analysis of T wave abnormalities and their prognostic implications in the idiopathic long QT syndrome. *J Am Coll Cardiol* 1994;**23**:296–301.
18. Nador F, Beria G, De Ferrari GM *et al.* Unsuspected echocardiographic abnormality in the long QT syndrome: diagnostic, prognostic, and pathogenetic implications. *Circulation* 1991;**84**:1530–42.
19. De Ferrari GM, Nador F, Beria G, Sala S, Lotto A, Schwartz PJ. Effect of calcium channel block on the wall motion abnormality of the idiopathic long QT syndrome. *Circulation* 1994;**89**:2126–32.
20. Moss AJ, Zareba W, Hall WJ *et al.* Effectiveness and limitations of beta-blocker therapy in congenital long QT syndrome. *Circulation* 2000;**101**:616–23.
21. Schwartz PJ, Priori SG, Spazzolini C *et al.* Genotype–phenotype correlation in the long QT syndrome. Gene-specific

triggers for life-threatening arrhythmias. *Circulation* (In press).

22. Zareba W, Moss AJ, Schwartz PJ *et al.* for the International Long-QT Syndrome Registry Research Group. Influence of the genotype on the clinical course of the long QT syndrome. *N Engl J Med* 1998;**339**:960–5.

23. Wilde AA, Jongbloed RJ, Doevendans PA *et al.* Auditory stimuli as a trigger for arrhythmic events differentiate *HERG*-related (LQTS2) patients from *KVLQT1*-related patients (LQTS1). *J Am Coll Cardiol* 1999;**33**:327–32.

24. Locati EH, Zareba W, Moss AJ *et al.* Age- and sex-related differences in clinical manifestations in patients with congenital long QT syndrome. Findings from the International LQTS Registry. *Circulation* 1998;**97**:2237–44.

25. Napolitano C, Priori SG, Schwartz PJ *et al.* Identification of a long QT syndrome molecular defect in drug-induced tor-sades de pointes. *Circulation* 1997;**96**(Abstr. Suppl.):I–211.

26. Schulze-Bahr E, Haverkamp W, Hordt M, Wedekind H, Borggrefe M, Funke H. Do mutations in cardiac ion channel genes predispose to drug-induced (acquired) long QT syndrome? *Circulation* 1997;**96**(Abstr. Suppl.):I–211.

27. Wellens HJJ, Vermeulen A, Durrer D. Ventricular fibrillation occurring on arousal from sleep by auditory stimuli. *Circulation* 1972;**46**:661–5.

28. Schwartz PJ, Locati EH, Moss AJ, Crampton RS, Trazzi R, Ruberti U. Left cardiac sympathetic denervation in the therapy of congenital long QT syndrome: a worldwide report. *Circulation* 1991;**84**:503–11.

29. Schwartz PJ. The rationale and the role of left stellectomy for the prevention of malignant arrhythmias. *Ann NY Acad Sci* 1984;**427**:199–221.

35 Arrhythmia associated with other cardiac diseases

Patrick Lam and Paul Schweitzer

Many cardiac conditions are associated with arrhythmia risk but clinically less well defined. Most of them are secondary to haemodynamic changes of the underlying conditions. The arrhythmia risk is usually related to the severity of the underlying disease. In this chapter we will be discussing valvular heart diseases, pericardial diseases, endocarditis, congenital heart diseases, arrhythmogenic right ventricular dysplasia, and sarcoidosis.

Arrhythmia risk of mitral valve disease

Mitral valve prolapse (MVP) is an important cause of mitral regurgitation and is a common disease.[1,2] It was reported as the leading cause of mitral regurgitation requiring surgery. Both diseases have been associated with a spectrum of arrhythmia and even sudden death.[3-4] Virtually all types of arrhythmia have been reported in MVP.[5-6] Paroxysmal supraventricular tachycardia is the most common sustained tachyarrhythmia in patients with MVP and may be related to the left atrioventricular bypass tract.[7] P wave-triggered signal average ECG may be a useful technique in detecting patients with idiopathic mitral valve prolapse at risk of paroxysmal supraventricular arrhythmia.[8] The most common ventricular arrhythmias are ventricular premature beats.[5]

The relationship between MVP and malignant ventricular arrhythmia and sudden death is not clear. The risk appears low.[9] Although mitral valve prolapse is a generally benign disorder, there is certainly a small subgroup of patients who may be at risk for sudden death and complications. Delayed after-depolarisation-induced triggered activity may be the mechanism of ventricular tachycardia in some patients with mitral valve prolapse. The trigger is provided by ventricular premature beats.[10] The arrhythmia also appeared to be sensitive to catecholamines and exercise.[11,12] Kligfield *et al.* identified the following as potential risks for sudden death in MVP:

- the presence of significant mitral regurgitation
- complex ventricular arrhythmia
- prolongation of QT interval, and
- a history of syncope and palpitation[7] (Box 35.1).

Even in the absence of QT prolongation, QT dispersion is greater in patients with mitral valve prolapse and ventricular arrhythmia than in controls.[13] It may be a useful marker in patients with mitral valve prolapse of cardiovascular morbidity and mortality from complex ventricular arrhythmia.[14] Mitral valve prolapse is also frequently detected in patients with idiopathic ventricular tachycardia.[15] The value of signal averaged electrocardiogram in patients with mitral valve prolapse is unclear.[16]

MVP has been called MVP syndrome for the variety of non-specific complaints associated with it.[17] It is not uncommon to discover arrhythmia on routine ECG.[2] A decision has to be made if further investigations are necessary: 24-h Holter monitoring is the most common tool to document arrhythmia and to evaluate correlation with symptoms. Exercise test is indicated when symptoms are precipitated by exercise or when ischaemia heart disease is suspected in patients with chest pain. The role of electrophysiology testing is not well understood in MVP.[18] EPS is certainly indicated in patients with aborted sudden death and complex ventricular arrhythmia.

Mitral regurgitation burdens the left ventricle with excessive volume and leads to a series of compensatory changes.[19] The left ventricle gradually enlarges and systolic functions progressively declines. The risk of malignant ventricular arrhythmia increases as the LV systolic functions decreases.[20] Complex atrial and ventricular arrhythmia are common in patients with non-ischaemic mitral regurgitation irrespective of aetiology; the arrhythmia are more strongly associated with haemodynamic important mitral regurgitation than with MVP alone.[21] Ultralow-frequency heart rate variability, as measured by the 5-min mean RR interval, correlates with right and left ventricular performance and predicts development of atrial fibrillation, mortality, and the progression to valve surgery in patients with chronic severe mitral regurgitation.[21] The risk of atrial fibrillation also increases as the left atrial enlarges and LV systolic function decreases.[22]

Mitral stenosis is classically associated with atrial fibrillation. Atrial fibrillation usually develops in the presence of pre-existent ECG evidence of left atrial enlargement and is related to the size and the extent of fibrosis of the left atrial myocardium, the duration of atriomegaly, and the age of the patient.[23] When ventricular arrhythmia occurs in mitral stenosis patients, the possibility of associated heart disease causing the arrhythmia like LV dysfunction should be excluded.

Arrhythmia risk of aortic valve disease

Atrial fibrillation or atrial flutter occurs in fewer than 10% of patients with severe aortic stenosis. When such arrhythmia is observed in patients with aortic stenosis, the possibility of associated mitral valve disease should be considered.[24] Conduction defects, however, are common in elderly patients with aortic stenosis.[25] It is commonly associated with mitral annular calcification and calcification of the intraventricular conduction system.

Although aortic stenosis is classically associated with sudden death, the risk is very low in asymptomatic patient.[26] Of 229 asymptomatic patients with critical aortic stenosis, only 5 (2%) died suddenly.[27] However, ambulatory electrocardiogram frequently showed complex ventricular arrhythmia, particularly in patients with myocardial dysfunction.[28] To risk-stratify these patients, symptoms like angina, syncope, and heart failure are important. Once aortic stenosis patients become symptomatic with angina or syncope, the average survival is 2–3 years, whereas with congestive failure the average survival is 1.5 years.[29,30] In an analysis of the elderly patients with severe aortic stenosis and symptoms of heart failure who declined surgery, 50% had died by 18 months of follow-up; the ejection fraction correlated inversely with survival.[31] Von Olshausen *et al.*[32] examined Holter findings in seven patients with severe aortic stenosis and sudden death. Six of the deaths were due to ventricular tachyarrhythmia (monomorphic or polymorphic ventricular tachycardia or torsade de pointes); only one death was associated with bradyarrhythmia. Increased ectopic activity with complex forms (couplets and non-sustained ventricular tachycardia) and a significant acceleration in heart rate was observed in the last hours before tachyarrhythmic sudden death. However, all these patients had moderate to severe heart failure and impaired left ventricular systolic dysfunction; the arrhythmia could be more related

to left ventricular dysfunction than to the outflow obstruction.[32] Several studies also support that left ventricular hypertrophy may provide the substrate for malignant arrhythmia and sudden death, independently of aetiology.[33–35] Although the prevalence of late potential in patients with aortic stenosis is higher than control,[36] the prognostic valve of late potential in aortic stenosis by signal average ECG is unclear.

Aortic regurgitation is classically not associated with arrhythmia, sudden death, or syncope. The left ventricle generally undergoes gradual enlargement while the patients remain asymptomatic. Symptoms usually occur only after considerable cardiomegaly and myocardial dysfunction. Severe arrhythmias are frequently a sign of impaired left ventricular function.[37] Recently Freed *et al.*[38] reported that reduced ultralow-frequency heart rate variability is strongly related to the progression to valve surgery in asymptomatic and minimally symptomatic patients with chronic aortic regurgitation.

Although aortic valve replacement usually results in clinical improvement, sudden death still remains a common cause of late death, accounting for 20% of the postoperative death.[39,40] The patients who are at the highest risk of late postoperative sudden death are those characterised by:

- lack of improvement of impairment of systolic function, or
- left ventricular function deteriorates after valve replacement.[41]

Heart rate variability, a reflex of autonomic dysfunction, tends to normalise within a year after aortic valve replacement.[42] This finding may reflect the vulnerability to ventricular arrhythmia and reflects the remodelling of the left ventricle after aortic valve replacement.

Arrhythmia risk in pericardial disease

Pericardial disease is classically associated with atrial arrhythmia, particularly atrial fibrillation.[43] However, the incidence is very low. When atrial fibrillation or significant arrhythmia occurs in patients with patients with pericarditis, concomitant heart disease should be excluded.[44] Even in constrictive pericarditis, atrial fibrillation is reported in less than half of the patients.[45] Cardiac tamponade is usually not associated with arrhythmia but electrocardiagraphic abnormality or even electromechanical dissociation.

Arrhythmia risk in infective endocarditis

Infective endocarditis is generally not associated with arrhythmia. However, conduction abnormality can develop and is usually associated with perivalvular invasive infection. Although the sensitivity of new-onset conduction or persistent electrocardiographic conduction abnormalities is reported as only 28%, the specificity is as high as 85–90%.[46] It is more likely to develop in aortic valve infection than mitral valve infection.[47] Evidence of first-degree heart block usually suggests an abscess near the non-coronary sinus of Valsalva, and evidence of complete heart block usually suggests an abscess in the membranous septum.[48]

Arrhythmia risk in congenital heart disease

Arrhythmia in congenital heart disease can be divided into two categories. The first category is congenital heart abnormality associated with supraventricular abnormality; the second abnormality is congenital heart abnormality associated with malignant ventricular abnormality. The arrhythmia may be further divided into:

- primary association with the congenital abnormality that may or may not be corrected after reparative surgery, or
- arrhythmia that develop after the reparative surgery.

The supraventricular arrhythmia are associated with congenital abnormality-included atrial septal defect, Ebstein's anomaly, and sequelae of intra-atrial corrective surgery.

Atrial fibrillation and atrial flutter are well-known sequelae of atrial septal defect.[49–51] Atrial arrhythmia often persists at late follow-up in patients who have undergone surgical repair after childhood.[49,52,53] The risk of atrial flutter or atrial fibrillation in adults with atrial septal defects is related to the age at the time of surgical repair and the pulmonary arterial pressure.[54]

Ebstein's anomaly is associated with multiple electrophysiological abnormalities including accessory pathway, atrial fibrillation, atrial flutter and supraventricular tachycardia.

The intra-atrial baffle operations like the Mustard and Senning operation are classically associated with postoperative atrial arrhythmia. Because the arterial switch operations do not involve intra-atrial reconstruction, the risk of atrial tissue damage and subsequent atrial arrhythmia is less.

An increased risk of sudden cardiac death from arrhythmia has been found predominantly in four congenital conditions (Box 35.2):

- tetralogy of Fallot
- transposition of the great arteries
- aortic stenosis, and
- pulmonary vascular obstruction.

Box 35.2 Congenital conditions associated with sudden death

- Tetralogy of Fallot
- Transposition of the great arteries
- Aortic stenosis
- Pulmonary vascular obstruction

Adapted from Zipes D, Hein J[40] p. 2340.

Sudden cardiac death has also been described as a late complication after surgical repair of complex congenital cardiac lesions, such as tetralogy of Fallot and transposition of the great arteries, and in patients with primary or secondary pulmonary hypertension.[40] In tetralogy of Fallot, QRS prolongation relates to right ventricular size and predicts patients at risk for sudden cardiac death [55]

Arrhythmia risk in arrhythmogenic right ventricular dysplasia

Arrhythmogenic right ventricular dysplasia is a particular form of arrhythmogenic right ventricular cardiomyopathy associated with sudden death in young individuals and adults. The macroscopic pattern consists of dilatation of the so-called "triangle of dysplasia": right ventricular inflow, apex, and the right ventricular outflow. It occurs as a familial disorder in about 30% of cases in an autosomal dominant inheritance. The genetic defect has recently been localised to chromosomes 1 and 14 q23-q24.[56,57] During the sinus rhythm, intraventricular conduction may be sufficiently slow to produce a terminal notch on the QRS complex, which Fontaine called the epsilon wave. The ventricular tachycardia has a left bundle branch block contour, with the frontal plane axis reflecting the site of origin in the "triangle of dysplasia".

The ventricular arrhythmia in arrhythmogenic right ventricular dysplasia can be precipitated by strenuous exercise. An increase in the vasosympathetic balance with an increased sympathetic tone causes an increased heart rate and shortening of the coupling intervals of the first cycles before the tachycardia.[58] Exercise testing is usually used to determine the arrhythmic risk of ventricular arrhythmia. In the absence of bundle branch block, the extent of abnormality of signal-average ECG variables is in proportion to right ventricular cavity enlargement and thus is indicative of the severity of right ventricular dysfunction.[59]

Arrhythmia risk in sarcoidosis

Sudden death is one of the most common manifestations of cardiac sarcoidosis.[60] The risk of sudden death appears to be greatest in patients with extensive myocardial involvement.[61] Myocardial imaging with thallium-201 is usually helpful in assessment of sarcoid infiltration of the myocardium.[62] Sustained ventricular tachycardia is usually easily induced by programmed ventricular stimulation in high-risk patients.[63] Implantation of an automated implantable antitachycardia device should be considered in high-risk patients.[62,63]

References

1. Levy D, Savage DD. Prevalence and clinical features of mitral valve prolapse. *Am Heart J* 1987;**113**:1281.

2. Savage DD, Garrism RJ, Devereaux RB *et al*. Mitral valve prolapse in general population. 1. Epidemiological features: The Framingham Study. *Am Heart J* 1983;**106**:571–6.

3. Kligfield P, Hochreiter C, Niles N *et al*. Relation of sudden death in pure mitral regurgitation with and without mitral valve prolapse, to repetitive ventricular arrhythmias and right and left ventricular ejection fraction. *Am J Cardiol* 1987;**60**:397.

4. Pocock W A, Bosman CK, Chesler E *et al*. Sudden death in primary mitral valve prolapse. *Am Heart J* 1984;**107**:378.

5. Levy S. Arrhythmia in the mitral valve prolapse syndrome: clinical significance and management. *PACE* 1992;**15**:1080–7.

6. Kligfield P, Levy D, Devoroux RB *et al*. Arrhythmia and sudden death in mitral valve prolapse. *Am Heart J* 1987;**113**:1298–307.

7. Kligfield, P, Devereux, RB. Arrhythmia in mitral valve prolapse. In: Podrid PR, Kowey PR, eds. *Cardiac arrhythmia: mechanisms, diagnosis and management.* Baltimore: Williams and Wilkins Co., 1995, p. 1253.

8. Banasiala W, Pagal I, Ponikewski P *et al*. P wave signal average electrocardiogram in patients with idiopathic mitral valve prolapse syndrome and supraventricular arrhythmia. *Int J Cardiol* 1995;**50**:175–80.

9. Freed LA, Levy D, Levine R *et al*. Prevalence and clinical outcome of mitral valve prolapse. *New Engl J Med* 1999;**341**:1–7.

10. Wilde A, Duren D, Hauer R. Mitral valve prolapse and ventricular arrhythmia: observations. Observations in a patient with a 20 year history. *J Cardiol Electrophysiol* 1997;**8**:307–16.

11. Kochiadakins G, Parthenakis F, Zuridakis E. Is there increased sympathetic activity in patients with mitral valve prolapse? *PACE* 1996;**19**:1872–6.

12. Davies AO, Mares A, Pool JL, Taylor AA. Mitral valve prolapse with symptoms of beta-adrenergic hypersensitivity. Beta$_2$-adrenergic receptor supercoupling with desensitization on isoproterenol exposure. *Am J Med* 1987;**82**:193.

13. Tileman R, Crigins H, Wiesfeld A *et al*. Increased dispersions of refractories in the absence of QT prolongation in patients with mitral valve prolapse and ventricular arrhythmia. *Br Heart J* 1995;**73**:37–40.

14. Kuulan K, Komsuoglu B, Tuncer C. Significance of QT dispersion on ventricular arrhythmia in mitral valve prolapse. *Int J Cardiol* 1996;**54**:251–7.

15. Vecchia L, Ometto R, Centofemite P *et al*. Arrhythmia profile: ventricular function, and histomorphometric findings in patients with idiopathic ventricular tachycardia and mitral valve prolapse: clinical and prognostic evaluation. *Clin Cardiol* 1998;**21**:731–5.

16. Nomuva M, Nalaaya Y, Kishi F *et al*. Signal average electrocardiogram after exercise in patients with mitral valve prolapse. *J Med* 1997;**28**:62–74.

17. Boudoulas H, Kolibash AJ Jr, Baker P *et al*. Mitral valve prolapse and the mitral valve prolapse syndrome: A diagnostic classification and pathogenesis of symptoms. *Am Heart J* 1989;**118**:796.

18. Morady F, Shan E, Bhandari A *et al*. Programmed ventricular stimulation in mitral valve prolapse: analysis of 36 patients. *Am J Cardiol* 1984;**53**:135–8.

19. Braunwald, E. Vascular heart disease. In: Braunwald E. *Heart disease: a textbook of cardiovascular medicine.* Philadelphia: WB Saunders Co., 1997, p. 1020.

20. Kligfield P, Hochreiter L, Kramer H *et al*. Complex arrhythmia in mitral regurgitation with and without mitral valve prolapse: contrast to arrhythmia in mitral valve prolapse with mitral regurgitation. *Am J Cardiol* 1985;**55**:1545–9.

21. Stein K, Boren J, Hochreiter C *et al*. Prognostic valve and physiological correlates of heart rate variability in chronic severe mitral regurgitation. *Circulation* 1993;**88**:127–35.

22. Vaziri SM, Lawson MG, Benjamin E *et al*. Echocardiographic predictors of non rheumatic atrial fibrillation. The Framingham Heart Study. *Circulation* 1991;**89**:724–30.

23. Probst P, Goldschlager N, Selzer A. Left atrial size and atrial fibrillation in mitral stenosis: factors influencing their relationship. *Circulation* 1973;**48**:1281.

24. Braunwald, E. Valvular Heart Disease. In: Braunwald E. *Heart disease: a textbook of cardiovascular medicine.* Philadelphia: WB Saunders Co., 1997, p. 1042.

25. Nair CK, Aoronow WS, Stokke K *et al*. Cardiac conduction defects in patients older than 60 years with aortic stenosis with and without mitral annular calcification. *Am J Cardiol* 1984;**53**:169–72.

26. Braunwald E. Valvular heart disease. In: Braunwald E. *Heart disease: a textbook of cardiovascular medicine.* Philadelphia: WB Saunders Co., 1997, p. 1045.

27. Pellikka PA, Nishimura RA, Bailey KR, Tajik AJ. The natural history of adults with asymptomatic hemodynamically significant aortic stenosis. *J Am Coll Cardiol* 1990;**15**:1012.

28. Klein RC. Ventricular arrhythmias in aortic valve disease: analysis of 102 patients. *Am J Cardiol* 1984;**53**:1079.

29. Ross J Jr, Braunwald E. The influence of corrective operations on the natural history of aortic stenosis. *Circulation* 1968;**37**(Suppl. V):61.

30. Frank S, Johnson A, Ross J Jr. Natural history of valvular aortic stenosis. *Br Heart J* 1973;**35**:41.

31. Aronow WS, Ahn C, Kronson I, Nanna M. Prognosis of congestive heart failure in patients aged > 62 years with unoperated severe valvular aortic stenosis. *Am J Cardiol* 1993;**72**:846.

32. Von Olshausen K, Witt T, Pop T *et al.* Sudden cardiac death while wearing Holter monitor. *Am J Cardiol* 1991;**67**:381–6.

33. Ghali, JK, Kadakia S, Cooper RS *et al.* Impact of left ventricular hypertrophy on ventricular arrhythmia in absence of coronary artery disease. *J Am Coll Cardiol* 1991;**17**:1277–82.

34. Messerli FH, Ventura HO, Elizardi DJ *et al.* Hypertension and sudden death: Increased ectopic activity in left ventricular hypertrophy. *Am J Med* 1984;**77**:18–22.

35. Levy D, Keaven MA, Savage DD *et al.* Risk of ventricular arrhythmias in left ventricular hypertrophy. The Framingham Heart Study. *Am J Cardiol* 1987;**60**:560–5.

36. Sorgato A, Faggiano P, Simmoncelli U *et al.* Prevalence of late potentials in adult aortic stenosis. *Int J Cardiol* 1996;**53**:55–9.

37. Von Olshausen K, Schwarz F, Apfelbach J *et al.* Determinants of the incidence and severity of ventricular arrhythmias in aortic valve disease. *Am J Cardiol* 1983;**51**:1103–9.

38. Freed L, Stein K, Borer J *et al.* Relation of ultra-low frequency heart rate variability to the clinical course of chronic aortic regurgitation. *Am J Cardiol* 1997;**79**:1482–7.

39. Lund O. Pre-operative risk evaluation and stratification of long term survival after valve replacement for aortic stenosis: reason for earlier operative intervention. *Circulation* 1990;**82**:124–39.

40. Zipes D, Hein J. Sudden cardiac death. *Circulation* 1998;**98**:2334–51.

41. Sorgato A, Faggiano P, Aurigemma G *et al.* Ventricular arrhythmia in adult aortic stenosis: prevalence, mechanism, and clinical relevance. *Chest* 1998;**113**:482–91.

42. Vukasovic J, Florenzano F, Adriazola P *et al.* Heart rate variability in severe aortic stenosis. *J Heart Valve Dis* 1999;**8**:143–8.

43. Falk RH. Atrial fibrillation. In: Podrid PJ, eds. *Cardiac arrhythmia: mechanism, diagnosis, and management.* Baltimore: Williams and Wilkins, 1995, p. 805.

44. Spodick DH. Significant arrhythmias during pericarditis are due to concomitant heart disease. *J Am Coll Cardiol* 1998;**32**:551–2.

45. Lorell B. Pericardial diseases. In: Braunwald E. *Heart disease: a textbook of cardiovascular medicine.* Philadelphia: WB Saunders Co., 1997, p. 1500.

46. Karchmer AW. Infective endocarditis. In: Braunwald E. *Heart disease: a textbook of cardiovascular medicine.* Philadelphia: WB Saunders Co., 1997, p. 1094.

47. DiNubile MJ, Calderwood SB, Steinhaus DM *et al.* Cardiac conduction abnormalities complicating native valve active infective endocarditis. *Am J Cardiol* 1986;**58**:1213–17.

48. Roberts NK, Somerville J. Pathological significance of electrocardiographic changes in aortic valve endocarditis. *Br Heart J* 1969;**31**:395–6.

49. Murphy JG, Gersh BJ, McGoon MD *et al.* Long-term outcome after surgical repair of isolated atrial septal defect: follow-up at 27 to 32 years. *New Engl J Med* 1990;**323**:1645–50.

50. Craig RJ, Selzer A. Natural history and prognosis of atrial septal defect. *Circulation* 1968;**37**:805–15.

51. Campbell M. Natural history of atrial septal defect. *Br Heart J* 1970;**32**:820–6.

52. Horvath KA, Burke RP, Collins JJ Jr, Cohn LH. Surgical treatment of adult atrial septal defect: early and long-term results. *J Am Coll Cardiol* 1992;**20**:1156–9.

53. Konstantinides S, Geibel A, Olschewski M *et al.* A comparison of surgical and medical therapy for atrial septal defect in adults. *New Engl J Med* 1995;**333**:469–73.

54. Gatzoulis MA, Freeman MA, Siu SC, Webb GD, Harris L. Atrial arrhythmia after surgical closure of atrial septal defects in adults. *New Engl J Med* 1999;**340**:839–46.

55. Gatzoulis MA, Till JA, Somerville J, Redington AN. Mechanoelectrical interaction in tetralogy of Fallot: QRS prolongation relates to right ventricular size and predicts malignant ventricular arrhythmias and sudden death. *Circulation* 1995;**92**:231–7.

56. Carrado D, Basso C, Schiavon M *et al.* Screening for hypertrophic cardiomyopathy in young athletes. *New Engl J Med* 1998;**339**:364–9.

57. Carrado D, Basso C, Thiene G *et al.* Spectrum of clinicopathologic manifestatons of arrhythmogenic right ventricular cardiomyopathy/dysplasia: a multicenter study. *J Am Coll Cardiol* 1997;**30**:1512–20.

58. Leclercq J, Potenza S, Maison-Blanche P *et al.* Determinants of spontaneous occurrence of sustained monomorphic ventricular tachycardia in right ventricular dysplasia. *J Am Coll Cardiol* 1996;**28**:720–4.

59. Mentha D, Goldman M, David O *et al.* Value of quantitative measurement of signal-averaged electrocardiographic variables in arrhythmogenic right ventricular dysplasia: correlation with echocardiographic right ventricular cavity dimensions. *Am J Coll Cardiol* 1996;**28**:713–19.

60. Shamma R, Movahed A. Sarcoidosis of the heart. *Clin Cardiol* 1993;**16**:462.

61. Wynne J, Braunwald E. The cardiomyopathies and myocarditis. In: Braunwald E. *Heart disease: a textbook of cardiovascular medicine.* Philadelphia: WB Saunders Co., 1997, p. 1431.

62. Yamamoto N, Gotoh K, Yagi Y *et al.* Thallium–201 myocardial SPECT findings at rest in sarcoidosis. *Ann Nucl Med* 1993;**7**:97.

63. Winters S, Cohen M, Greenberg S *et al.* Sustained ventricular tachycardia associated with sarcoidosis: assessment of the underlying cardiac anatomy and the prospective utility of programmed ventricular stimulation, drug therapy and an implantable antitachycardia device. *J Am Coll Cardiol* 1991;**18**:937–43.

36 Arrhythmias associated with non-cardiac disease

Josef Kautzner

Ventricular arrhythmias are believed to be major cause of sudden death in a broad spectrum of cardiac diseases. However, much less is known about their prognostic importance in various non-cardiogenic diseases. From a pathophysiological point of view, the following groups of conditions associated with ventricular arrhythmias can be recognised:

● systemic diseases with frequent cardiac involvement;
● major heredofamilial neuromyopathic disorders in which heart disease is an inherent part;
● endocrine and nutritional disorders;
● metabolic disturbances;
● acute cerebral disorders accompanied by cardiovascular abnormalities.

In addition, various drugs used to treat non-cardiac diseases may also cause ventricular arrhythmias. Despite the fact that many of these associations are rare, making a correct diagnosis is often essential for further prognosis of affected individuals. This may be quite difficult because of the systemic nature of these conditions and many patients being initially under the care of other specialists, who are not necessarily familiar with the disorder. Supraventricular arrhythmias associated with the above diseases include predominantly atrial fibrillation or various types macro-re-entrant tachycardias. In some conditions, serious brady-arrhythmias may become a clinical problem and even lead to sudden death. Thus, this chapter is intended to discuss the most important non-cardiac diseases or drugs potentially leading to arrhythmias, with a particular emphasis on prognostically important ones.

Systemic diseases with frequent cardiac involvement

Sarcoidosis

This is a multisystemic granulomatous disease of unknown cause, and may affect the heart in approximately 20–50% cases. However, cardiac involvement only gives rise to clinical manifestations in about 5% of patients.[1] The reason for this is that sarcoid myocardial involvement is mostly limited to a small portion of the heart. Although sarcoidosis has a low mortality rate, the prognosis is significantly worse when the heart is involved. Clinical presentation includes various kinds of brady- or tachy-arrhythmias, and/or congestive heart failure. The most common manifestation of myocardial involvement is sudden death, which may even be an initial manifestation of the disease.[2] It occurs more frequently as a result of ventricular tachyarrhythmia rather than that of complete heart block. Sarcoid granulomas may either become foci for abnormal automaticity or a substrate for intramyocardial re-entry. Diagnosis requires clinical suspicion and may be supported by ECG, echocardiography, thallium imaging, gallium-67 scanning, or myocardial biopsy. About 60% of cases appear to have elevated angiotensin-converting enzyme levels. The incidence of ECG abnormalities among sarcoidosis patients is more frequent compared with control subjects, reaching up to 50%.[3,4] These include repolarisation changes, conduction abnormalities, and arrhythmias. Data from a limited series of patients have shown that antiarrhythmic drugs are associated with a high rate of arrhythmia recurrences or sudden death. Therefore, implantation of an ICD should be considered as primary therapy.[5,6]

Amyloidosis

This is a term describing a heterogeneous group of disorders that result from extracellular deposition of amyloid fibrils. These are composed of low molecular weight protein subunits derived from a variety of normal and abnormal serum proteins.[7] The heart is commonly infiltrated by amyloid in primary amyloidoses (AL amyloidosis), and in certain familial or age-related amyloidoses. On the contrary, it is rarely involved in secondary amyloidosis (AA amyloidosis). Clinical manifestation of the disease reflects the site of intracardiac deposition. For instance, interstitial deposition reduces ventricular compliance and leads to symptomatic congestive heart failure. Amyloid fibrils deposited in intramyocardial vessels may give rise to ischaemic syndromes. Amyloid depositions are also frequently associated with fibrosis of specialised cardiac conduction tissue. As a result, both brady- and tachyarrhythmias have been reported in association with the disease. However, there are conflicting reports regarding the incidence of ventricular arrhythmias among patients with AL amyloidosis.[8] In some studies, complex ventricular arrhythmias were detected in up to 50% cases, suggesting a possible relationship to sudden death.[9] More recently, analysis of a large series of 133 patients with AL amyloidosis revealed cardiac death in 68% of cases, 22 of whom died suddenly.[10] Whilst the presence of late potentials on signal-averaged ECG was found to predict independently sudden death in this series, high-grade ventricular ectopy or the presence of non-sustained ventricular tachycardia on the Holter recording failed to do so. However, as 53% of patients died suddenly during a 1-year follow-up without having positive late potentials, a certain proportion of these deaths may have occurred from bradyarrhythmias. This notion seems to be supported by previous findings from the same institution that the HV interval prolongation was an independent predictor of sudden death even in the absence of overt conduction abnormalities on the surface ECG.[11]

Another important issue is that ventricular arrhythmias may be the first clinical manifestation of the disease (Fig. 36.1). Therefore, primary amyloidosis should be considered in all cases of malignant arrhythmias that occur in the setting of no documented heart disease (as assessed by routine diagnostic work-up). Endomyocardial biopsy is then the best technique to establish correct diagnosis.[12]

Major heredofamilial neuromyopathic disorders

Duchenne muscular dystrophy

This is a sex-linked recessive disorder passed from mother to one-half of her sons as an overt disease and to one-half of her daughters as a carrier state. It is the most frequent of progressive muscular dystrophies with the average incidence in general population being 1 in 3000–5000 male births. The disease is caused by a defective X chromosome-linked gene that codes the high molecular-weight protein, called dystrophin.[13] This protein product, normally localised in sarcolemmal membrane of skeletal muscle, is absent in affected individuals. Clinical manifestations usually begin in early childhood and comprise reduced muscular strength, often masked by seemingly good muscle development. Patients are likely to succumb to pulmonary infections in the second decade; however, some die of cardiac causes. Cardiac involvement is characterised by a

unique predilection for specific regions of the heart – the posterobasal and lateral left ventricular walls. These regions are the initial and most extensive sites of myocardial fibrosis. The resulting loss of electromotive force appear to explain characteristic ECG pattern of tall right precordial R waves with increased R/S amplitude ratios and deep Q waves in leads I, aVL, and $V_{5,6}$.[14] Despite the high incidence of cardiac involvement, many patients remain asymptomatic. Cardiac symptoms may be present in about a quarter of patients under the age of 18 with overt cardiac involvement and in about half thereafter.[15] The incidence of ventricular arrhythmias varies in different series from 30 to 48%,[16] and appears to increase with the clinical severity of skeletal muscle involvement.[16,17] Complex ventricular arrhythmias have been found to occur more frequently in patients who subsequently die of sudden death.[16,17] These patients also had left ventricular dysfunction more frequently.[18,19] Importantly, late potentials were found to be a fair predictor of ventricular arrhythmias in this condition.[19] However, as the major determinant of prognosis is respiratory failure, it is uncertain whether prophylaxis of ventricular arrhythmias can improve survival of affected individuals.

X-linked Becker muscular dystrophy

This differs from Duchenne dystrophy in several aspects.[20] The protein product of the defective gene is present in skeletal muscle in Becker dystrophy but abnormal in molecular weight. In Duchenne dystrophy the protein is absent or scanty but of normal molecular weight. The principal difference between the two conditions is the slow progression of Becker dystrophy. However, unlike often mild or subclinical skeletal muscle involvement, the associated cardiomyopathy is common and tends to be progressive. Cardiac manifestation is characterised by early right ventricular involvement.[20] Subsequent or isolated left ventricular impairment may result in dilated cardiomyopathy. In some patients, life-threatening ventricular arrhythmias have been described.[21] However, there is very limited information about the clinical usefulness of risk stratification techniques in this condition. So far, heart rate variability analysis has been found to detect sympathetic predominance in a group of patients with Becker muscular dystrophy.[22] This finding corresponded to a higher occurrence of ventricular ectopic beats.

Emery–Dreifuss muscular dystrophy

This is a rare, X-linked disease characterised by a distinct pattern of muscle contractures and weakness with slow

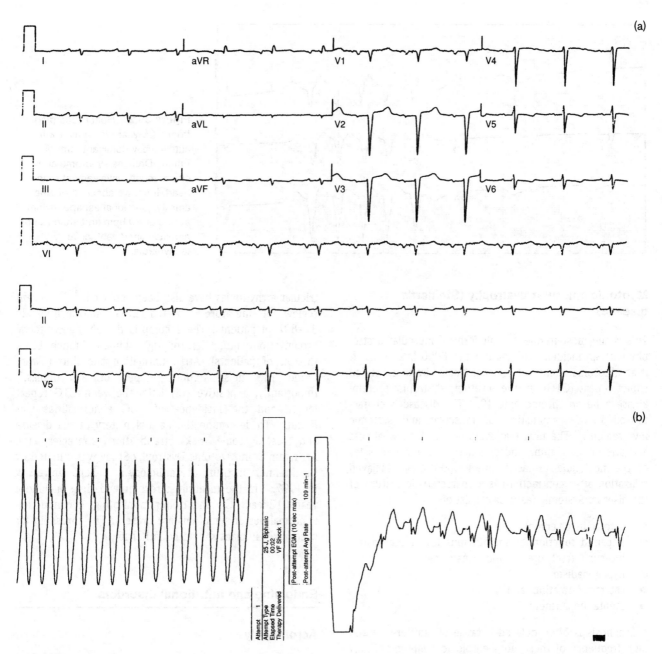

Figure 36.1 (a). An example of 12-lead ECG from a 45-year-old patient with documented AL amyloidosis and cardiac involvement. Note remarkably low voltage in the limb leads and QS pattern in right precordial leads. (b). Print-out from the memory of an ICD in the same patient showing termination of very rapid clinical ventricular tachycardia by 25 J biphasic shock.

progression, and predominant atrial arrhythmias. Exceptionally, the transmission may be autosomally dominant.[23] A defect in emerin, a specific protein, present in the nuclear membranes of cardiac and skeletal muscle, is the cause of the syndrome.[24] Importantly, even carrier females may have typical cardiac involvement that consists of permanent paralysis of the atria (atrial standstill).[25,26] This condition presents as a complete absence of P waves and lack of response to atrial stimulation (Fig. 36.2). Prior

to a complete atrial standstill, patchy involvement may support atrial macro-re-entrant tachycardias. A worrisome occurrence in these patients is unexpected sudden death.[27] As there is some evidence that early implantation of a cardiac pacemaker is likely to prolong lifespan,[28] sudden death appears to be, at least in a proportion of patients, due to bradyarrhythmias. Some affected individuals may also present with abnormalities in infranodal conduction, and/or ventricular tachycardia.[25,26]

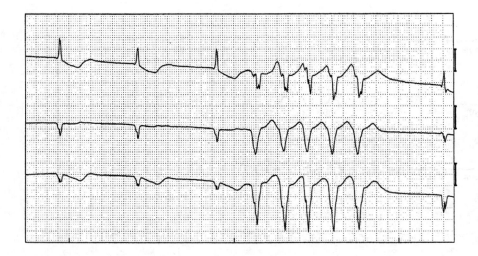

Figure 36.2 Holter recording from a 26-year-old woman with autosomally dominant form of Emery–Dreifuss syndrome and characteristic involvement of the heart. It shows absence of atrial activity, junctional escape rhythm at rate of 40 bpm and short run of non-sustained ventricular tachycardia.

Myotonic muscular dystrophy (Steinert's disease)

This is the most frequent adult form of muscular dystrophy with an incidence of about 1 per 8000 live births. It is an autosomal dominant disorder caused by an expanded triplet repeat $(CTG)_n$ in the myotonic dystrophy protein-kinase gene on chromosome 19.[29] The disease is characterised by a combination of muscular and systemic involvement.[30] The muscular symptoms include weakness and atrophy, beginning and dominating in flexor muscles of the neck and in facial muscles. Myotonia (delayed relaxation after contraction) is a characteristic feature of the disease. Systemic features consist of:

- cardiac involvement
- impaired function of smooth muscles in the gastro-intestinal tract, uterus, and urinary tract
- hypogonadism
- cataract formation, and
- mental impairment.

Diagnosis is often delayed because of indifference and high frequency of these non-neurologic symptoms. Many patients thus are initially under the care of other specialists who are not familiar with the disorder. The detection of CTG expansion as from blood assay confirms disease. Correct diagnosis is essential for genetic counselling, and detection of silent cardiac complications with a risk of sudden death.

Clinically significant heart disease consists predominantly of conduction defects. Although the majority of patients are asymptomatic, syncope, palpitations, or dyspnoea may sometimes even precede neurological symptoms. Sudden cardiac death appears to be responsible for up to one-third of deaths in this condition.[31] Most often, complete atrioventricular block is believed to be the cause, although some cases of sudden death owing to ven-

tricular arrhythmias have also been reported.[32,33] A recent review of literature reported ECG abnormalities in 37–80% of patients. These comprised mainly PR interval prolongation and/or left or right bundle branch block (5–25% of patients). Atrial fibrillation and flutter were found the most frequent types of arrhythmias.[34] Importantly, a positive correlation between CTG repeat length and the incidence of ECG abnormalities was found.[35] To determine the natural history of the disease and assess some risk stratification strategies, the Arrhythmias in Myotonic Dystrophy Study was initiated by the Krannert Institute of Cardiology at Indiana University in 1997.[36] In the meantime, recommendations include a yearly 12-lead ECG and Holter monitoring, if conduction abnormalities or symptoms are present. The threshold for pacemaker implant should be rather low.

Endocrine and nutritional disorders

Acromegaly

Acromegaly is notoriously associated with an increased cardiac mortality and morbidity. Affected patients have a limited life expectancy with about 80% of cases dying before the age of 60, predominantly of cardiac causes.[37] However, it is not clear whether this is a consequence of increased incidence of arterial hypertension or ischaemic heart disease, or a result of specific myocardial involvement.[38,39] In one case-controlled study, both prevalence and complexity of ventricular arrhythmias on Holter monitoring were significantly higher in acromegalic patients compared with controls.[37] More importantly, severity of these arrhythmias correlated with left ventricular mass and clinical activity score but not with plasma growth hormone levels. As none of the patients died during the short observational period, information about the risk of sudden death is not available.

Phaeochromocytoma

This is an uncommon tumour associated with overproduction of catecholamines. The most common symptoms are headache, palpitation, and sweating, combined with paroxysmal or persistent arterial hypertension.[40] Affected patients may occasionally present with atrial or ventricular arrhythmias associated with ECG changes consistent with those in myocardial ischaemia.[41] Life-threatening ventricular arrhythmias were even described after myocardial infarction in the presence of phaeochromocytoma.[42] Therefore, this diagnosis should be suspected in any patient with recurrent arrhythmias associated with hypertension.

Hyperthyroidism

This is the clinical state resulting from the excess production of tri-iodothyronine, thyroxine, or both. Most commonly, it is the result of diffuse toxic goitre or nodular toxic goitre. Hyperproduction of thyroidal hormones is thought to result from circulating IgG autoantibodies that bind to the thyrotropin receptor, in the thyroid gland in the former case. Apart from multiple systemic signs of hypermetabolism, the heart is one of the most responsive organs in thyroid disease. In addition to the direct myocardial effect, thyroid hormones interact with the sympathetic nervous system by altering responsiveness to sympathetic stimulation and thus mimicking adrenergic hyperfunction.[43] Sinus tachycardia occurs in over 40% of patients, and 15–25% of them have persistent atrial fibrillation.[44] Importantly, even subclinical hyperthyroidism may manifest predominantly by atrial fibrillation.[45] Hyperthyroidism appears to account for 15% of newly diagnosed cases of atrial fibrillation,[46] and approximately the same proportion of patients with thyrotoxic atrial fibrillation can develop thromboembolism.[47] Ventricular arrhythmias, when present, often indicate the presence of underlying heart disease.[48]

Hypothyroidism

Hypothyroidism results from reduced secretion of thyroidal hormones, predominantly as a consequence of destruction of the gland, usually by the inflammatory process. Manifestations are variable and related to the degree and duration of the disease.[49] The classic findings of cardiac involvement in myxoedema comprise cardiac enlargement, sinus bradycardia, hypotension, pericardial effusion, and evidence of congestive heart failure. ECG changes also include prolongation of the QT interval and changes associated with pericardial effusion.[50] Occasionally, life-threatening ventricular arrhythmias may appear.[51]

Obesity

The association of obesity and sudden death has been known since ancient times. However, the mechanism of sudden death in obesity is still not completely understood. Although even relatively mild obesity is a risk factor for dying suddenly, morbid obesity (defined as a body mass index $\geq 39.0 \, kg/m^2$, i.e. approximately 80–100% above desirable bodyweight) was found to be associated with about 40 times higher risk.[52] Few autopsy studies addressed the issue of sudden death in morbid obesity.[53,54] Findings suggested the presence of specific dilated cardiomyopathy, characterised by cardiomegaly with predominant left ventricular dilatation (eccentric hypertrophy) and myocyte hypertrophy without interstitial fibrosis. Of 22 cases of sudden death in one study, 14 were linked to cardiomyopathy.[54] In this respect, previous studies have shown that morbid obesity with documented left ventricular hypertrophy is associated with an increased propensity for ventricular ectopy.[55] A prolonged QT interval was found on preoperative ECG recordings in 76% of cases of cardiac arrest in surgical patients with morbid obesity.[56] The fact that the majority of these events occurred immediately after surgery may suggest that malignant arrhythmias are triggered by autonomic imbalances or postoperative shifts in electrolytes and fluids. This view appears to be supported by a known association of starvation diets for weight reduction in obese people and sudden death from ventricular arrhythmias.[57] Another study stressed the findings of significant involvement of the conduction system in young obese patients who died suddenly.[58] Risk of sudden death may be also increased in severely obese subjects with a history of heavy snoring and daytime sleepiness indicative of obstructive sleep apnoea syndrome.[59]

Anorexia nervosa

This is becoming the most frequent condition of malnutrition in industrialised countries that affects approximately 1% of female population between 15–25 years.[60] Its incidence is much lower in males and older age groups. Importantly, anorexia nervosa is associated with increased mortality, particularly of sudden death.[61] Mortality rates vary among reports, ranging between 5 and 20%. The most realistic estimate of total mortality rate is 5.9%, based on recent meta-analyses. As a certain proportion of these deaths occurs suddenly without apparent cause at postmortem examination, arrhythmic aetiology has been suggested.[62] In this respect, several studies evaluated potential links to arrhythmogenesis. In one of them, the QT interval on the 12-lead ECG was found significantly longer in 41 patients with anorexia nervosa as compared to control subjects.[63] The fact that there was a tendency towards normalisation of the QT interval after re-feeding may suggest that it can be used as a marker of increased arrhythmic risk. There are also some limited data about cardiac autonomic control in anorexia nervosa. Heart rate variability analysis documented significant increase in parasympathetic modulation of heart rate in these patients.[64] However, its relationship to risk of sudden death is unknown.

Metabolic disturbances

Chronic renal failure/haemodialysis

Cardiovascular disease is a common cause of death in haemodialysed patients with end-stage renal disease,[65] accounting for 40–60% of an estimated 7–10% annual mortality.[66,67] Up to 30% of them experience sudden death, suggesting that arrhythmia is the terminal event.[66,68] However, studies on cardiac arrhythmias during haemodialysis have brought conflicting results: some describe a high incidence of ventricular arrhythmias whilst others are not able to confirm this observation.[67,69] A more recent study documented a 51% incidence of arrhythmias.[70] Whilst infrequent supraventricular and ventricular beats were detected at all stages of the study period, complex arrhythmias were observed primarily during haemodialysis. This finding, that strongly suggests a direct cause–effect relationship, is consistent with other studies, which documented complex ventricular arrhythmias with an incidence of 39–66%.[71,72]

Many pathogenetic factors have been investigated; however, conclusive data are not available. It appears that an increased number of ventricular ectopics and their complexity during haemodialysis are associated with electrolyte changes[66] and/or rapid correction of metabolic acidosis.[71] In this respect, a lower occurrence of arrhythmias was found with higher potassium concentration in the dialysate.[73] However, other studies did not confirm any differences in plasma electrolyte values during haemodialysis between patients with or without arrhythmias.[71,74] Interestingly, haemodialysed patients with frequent ventricular ectopy were found to have lower intra-erythrocyte potassium content as compared with patients without arrhythmias, despite similar plasma electrolyte values.[75] The fact that depletion of potassium in erythrocytes reflects some degree of depletion of potassium in cardiomyocytes could explain lower transmembrane potentials in the heart and hyperexcitability.

Regarding the relationship of increased frequency of ventricular arrhythmias in haemodialysed patients to mortality, an Italian multicentre study of 127 subjects identified only age and the presence of ischaemic heart disease as independent predictors of mortality over a 4-year period of follow-up.[76] Overall mortality in the study reached 14% at 2 years and 28% at 4 years with 16 deaths from cardiovascular causes and 20 from other causes. One-quarter of cardiovascular deaths occurred suddenly. Similar data were confirmed by other authors, even for peritoneal dialysis.[77] To exclude the effect of higher age and ischaemic heart disease, a study from Brazil assessed predictors of mortality by studying relatively young haemodialysis patients with a low prevalence of comorbid conditions:[78] 5-year total mortality reached 30% and cardiovascular mortality 17%. Interestingly, age over 44 years and low serum creatinine levels were the only predictors of mortality. The latter parameter is thought to indicate poor nutritional status.

Several studies have attempted to use various risk stratification techniques to assess determinants of repetitive ventricular arrhythmias in patients receiving haemodialysis. In this respect, no association has been found between arrhythmias and the presence of late potentials or depressed heart rate variability.[79] The only predictors of complex ventricular ectopy were male sex, age, and left-ventricular motion abnormalities. This is consistent with the results of another study in which the presence of late potentials in haemodialysed patients corresponded with underlying coronary heart disease and left ventricular dysfunction.[80]

Thus, in view of the above data, it appears that, although some form of ventricular ectopy is a frequent finding in chronic renal failure, especially during haemodialysis, it is rather age, nutritional status, and the presence of associated coronary heart disease that determine cardiac mortality.

Electrolyte abnormalities

Abnormalities are often found in individuals following resuscitation from a cardiac arrest.[81] Hypokalaemia, one of the most significant abnormalities, may be either a secondary phenomenon owing to catecholamine-induced shift of the potassium into the cells, or a primary abnormality. Low extracellular potassium leads to hyperpolarisation of the resting membrane potential, shortening the plateau phase and increase in pacemaker activity in Purkinje cells.

Hypomagnesaemia has been shown to promote drug-induced torsade de pointes arrhythmias.[82] Importantly, both electrolyte abnormalities are associated with the use of diuretics[83] and other drugs. The pro-arrhythmogenic effect of increased intracellular calcium concentration reflects oscillatory release of calcium from the sarcoplasmic reticulum and resulting after-depolarisations.[81] Increased intracellular calcium is believed to play a role in catecholamine-induced ventricular tachycardias, reperfusion arrhythmias, and arrhythmias associated with digitalis intoxication.

Acute cerebral disorders accompanied by cardiovascular abnormalities

An association between acute cerebral events and cardiac arrhythmias has been recognised for nearly a century. It is estimated that approximately 90% of subjects with acute cerebral accidents (most notably spontaneous cerebral or subarachnoid haemorrhage or acute cerebral trauma) exhibit some ECG abnormalities, which consist mainly of impaired repolarisation and/or disturbances of cardiac rhythm.[84,85] Repolarisation abnormalities may be quite prominent and closely resemble electrocardiographic ischaemic changes with abnormal ST segments, symmetrical T wave inversions, and prolongation of the QT interval.[86] The underlying mechanism for these changes seems to be the "catecholamine storm" associated with an acute cerebral event. Catecholamines are held responsible for detectable myocardial damage (e.g. increased release of cardiospecific enzymes or left ventricular wall motion abnormalities) and may contribute to the genesis of malignant arrhythmias.[87] The possibility of catecholamine-induced myocardial damage should be taken into consideration when potential donors are being evaluated for heart transplantation, as the major sources of these organs are victims of accidents with serious cerebral injury.

Earlier case-reports have shown that subarachnoid haemorrhage may be one of the causes of acquired long QT syndrome presenting with polymorphic ventricular tachycardia of torsade de pointes type.[88] More recently, this association has been questioned.[89] A comprehensive review of literature by Machado *et al.*[90] revealed that, contrary to popular belief, a cause and effect relationship between subarachnoid haemorrhage and torsade de pointes cannot be convincingly demonstrated. In 20 reported cases over the period of 15 years, it was impossible to exclude at least one alternative explanation for ventricular arrhythmia such as congenital long QT syndrome, drug-induced torsade de pointes, hypokalaemia or hypomagnesaemia. In six cases (30%), potentially contributory factors were clearly identified with hypokalaemia being the principal one. The higher occurrence of documented hypokalaemia in the setting of subarachnoid haemorrhage might be a consequence of a hyperadrenergic state, namely of a cellular effect of catecholamines on potassium transport. Therefore, it appears that there is little scientific evidence to support the view that subarachnoid haemorrhage *per se* (i.e. in the absence of other predisposing factors) could cause torsade de pointes.

Drug-induced cardiac arrhythmias

The association of abnormalities of ventricular repolarisation, syncopal episodes from polymorphic ventricular tachycardia, and treatment with the antiarrhythmic agent quinidine was recognised for the first time in the 1960s.[91] The distinctive polymorphic nature of the ventricular tachycardia was later termed in French as "torsade de pointes" (twisting of the points) (Fig. 36.3). Since these original descriptions, many causes of the so-called acquired long QT syndrome have been identified. The most common cause for torsade de pointes is administration of drugs that prolong ventricular repolarisation and, thus, the QT interval (Box 36.1). Apart from antiarrhythmic drugs, this includes also a wide spectrum of drugs that are not thought to have important cardiovascular effects.[92] As already discussed above, other causes for torsade de pointes include severe hypokalaemia or hypomagnesaemia. Other causes, such as hypocalcaemia or acute cerebral injury, are very rare or questionable.

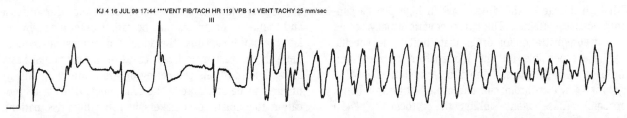

KJ 4 16 JUL 98 17:44 ***VENT FIB/TACH HR 119 VPB 14 VENT TACHY 25 mm/sec
III

Figure 36.3 ECG strip from a 72-year-old woman with a rare, amiodarone-induced torsade de pointes. Note isolated ventricular ectopics that encroach upon the end of the prolonged QT interval and a run of torsade de pointes triggered by the third ectopic beat.

Box 36.1 Drugs most commonly associated with torsade de pointes

- Antiarrhythmics
    - quinidine
    - disopyramide
    - procainamide
    - sotalol
    - ibutilide
    - (amiodarone)
    - other
- Calcium channel blockers
    - bepridil
    - lidoflazine
- Non-antiarrhythmic drugs
    - Antibiotics
        - erythromycin and other macrolides
        - pentamidine
        - co-trimoxazole
        - chloroquine
    - Antihistamines
        - terfenadine
        - astemizole
    - Drugs acting on CNS
        - phenothiazines (thioridazine, haloperidol)
        - tricyclic antidepressants
    - Miscellaneous
        - terolidine
        - cisapride
        - probucol
        - ketanserin

From the pathophysiological point of view, drugs appear to influence identical ion channels that are affected in congenital long QT syndromes.[93] In this condition, different mutations of genes encoding ion channels lead to QT interval prolongation. In the majority of cases, a defect in potassium channels results in reduction of the amplitude of outward currents. One of these is called I_{Kr} and is also blocked by many drugs that cause torsade de pointes. Similarly, hypokalaemia is capable of producing the same effect by decreasing I_{Kr}. This explains the similar clinical features of the congenital and acquired long QT syndromes.

Torsade de pointes associated with administration of the "non-cardiac" drugs appears to occur in conjunction with high dosage of the drug or when high plasma concentrations are attained. The latter scenario usually occurs with co-administration of drugs that inhibit the specific enzymes responsible for the biotransformation to non-cardioactive metabolites.[92] Inhibitors implicated include erythromycin, clarithromycin, and azole antifungals (ketoconazole). These agents inhibit the cytochrome P450 enzyme system resulting in increased concentrations of the "non-cardiac" drug. Another possibility is accumulation of the drug owing to impaired renal secretion.[94]

Patients have now been reported in whom rare mutations of genes encoding current channels exist but appear to be silent until the patient is challenged with a drug prolonging action potential.[95]

Successful prevention of drug-induced ventricular arrhythmias requires an increased awareness of the phenomenon of drug-induced torsade de pointes. An analysis of the available data has led to a delineation of some predictors for this potentially life-threatening arrhythmia.[93] The QT interval should be measured and should not exceed 520 ms when the patient receives a QT-prolonging drug. In the presence of bundle branch block the QT interval may be longer. QT interval may also be longer in patients receiving amiodarone; however, here the risk of torsade de pointes is substantially lower compared with other drugs. QT interval is longer in women than in men and this most probably makes women more susceptible to torsade de pointes. Such a notion is supported by reports of a 2–3 fold higher incidence of the arrhythmia among women compared with men, irrespective of the aetiology (i.e. acquired or congenital long QT syndrome). Another predisposing factors for development of torsade de pointes appears to be hypokalaemia and hypomagnesaemia. The presence of underlying cardiac disease may also increase the incidence of torsade de pointes. Last but not least, bradycardia is another factor that increases risk of torsade de pointes. The greatest problem is to predict arrhythmia in the absence of high doses or plasma concentrations. In this respect, development of a novel technique for quantification of repolarisation and its dynamicity from ECG recordings might be of significant help.

Conclusions

It is apparent that ventricular arrhythmias are quite frequent in various non-cardiac diseases, both with direct or indirect involvement of the heart. Some conditions are too rare to evaluate strategies focused on risk stratification and prophylaxis of sudden death. In other conditions, the nature of the disease and resulting metabolic and/or hormonal changes make assessment of risk difficult as the cause of sudden death is multifactorial. In addition, some diseases are known to accelerate ischaemic heart disease and then, the prognosis may be rather determined by the latter condition. Thus, therapeutic decisions need to be done in the vast majority of cases on an individual basis, as randomised trials comparing different interventions are unlikely to be attempted. The same holds true for an indication to implant pacemakers in some high-risk patients presenting with bradyarrhythmias. Nevertheless, increased awareness about the topic should promote further research in this interdisciplinary field.

References

1. Shammas RL, Movahed A. Sarcoidosis of the heart. *Clin Cardiol* 1993;**16**:462–72.
2. Veinot JP, Johnston B. Cardiac sarcoidosis – an occult cause of sudden death: a case report and literature review. *J Forens Sci* 1998;**43**:715–17.
3. Sekiguchi M, Yazaki Y, Isobe M, Hiroe M. Cardiac sarcoidosis: diagnostic, prognostic, and therapeutic considerations. *Cardiovasc Drugs Ther* 1996;**10**:495–510.
4. Stein E, Jackler I, Stimmel B, Stein W, Siltzbach LE. Asymptomatic electrocardiographic alterations in sarcoidosis. *Am Heart J* 1973;**86**:474–7.
5. Winters SL, Cohen M, Greenberg S *et al.* Sustained ventricular tachycardia associated with sarcoidosis: assessment of the underlying cardiac anatomy and the prospective utility of programmed ventricular stimulation, drug therapy and an implantable antitachycardia device. *J Am Coll Cardiol* 1991;**18**:937–43.
6. Paz HL, McCormick DJ, Kutalek S, Patchevsky A. The automated implantable cardiac defibrillator. Prophylaxis in cardiac sarcoidosis. *Chest* 1994;**106**:1603–7.
7. McCarthy RE, Kasper EK. A review of the amyloidoses that infiltrate the heart. *Clin Cardiol* 1998;**21**:547–52.
8. Parthenakis FI, Vardas PE, Ralidis L, Dritsas A, Nihoyannopoulos P. QT interval in cardiac amyloidosis. *Clin Cardiol* 1996;**19**:51–4.
9. Falk RH, Rubinow A, Cohen AS. Cardiac arrhythmias in systemic amyloidosis: correlation with echocardiographic abnormalities. *J Am Coll Cardiol* 1984;**3**:107–13.
10. Dubrey SW, Bilazarian S, LaValley M, Reisinger J, Skinner M, Falk RH. Signal-averaged electrocardiography in patients with AL (primary) amyloidosis. *Am Heart J* 1997;**134**:994–1001.
11. Reisinger J, Dubrey SW, LaValley M, Skinner M, Falk RH. Electrophysiologic abnormalities in AL (primary) amyloidosis with cardiac involvement. *J Am Coll Cardiol* 1997;**30**:1046–51.
12. Stamato A, Cahill J, Goodwin M, Winters G. Cardiac amyloidosis causing ventricular tachycardia. Diagnosis made by endomyocardial biopsy. *Chest* 1989;**96**:1431–3.
13. Arahata R, Ishii H, Hayashi YK. Congenital muscular dystrophies. *Curr Opin Neurol* 1995;**8**:385–90.
14. Perloff JK, Roberts WC, de Leon AC, Jr, O' Doherty D. The distinctive electrocardiogram of Duchenne's progressive muscular dystrophy. *Am J Med* 1967;**42**:179–88.
15. Nigro G, Comi LI, Politano L, Rain RJI. The incidence and evolution of cardiomyopathy in Duchenne muscular dystrophy. *Int J Cardiol* 1990;**26**:271–7.
16. Chenard AA, Becane HM, Tertrain F, de Kermadec JM, Weiss YA. Ventricular arrhythmia in Duchenne muscular dystrophy: prevalence, significance and prognosis. *Neuromusc Disorders* 1993;**3**:201–6.
17. Yanagisawa A, Miyagawa M, Yotsukura M *et al.* The prevalence and prognostic significance of arrhythmias in Duchenne type muscular dystrophy. *Am Heart J* 1992;**124**:1244–50.
18. Yotsukura M, Ishizuka T, Shimada T, Ishikawa K. Late potentials in progressive muscular dystrophy of the Duchenne type. *Am Heart J* 1991;**121**:1137–42.
19. Kubo M, Matsuoka S, Hayabuchi Y, Akita H, Matsuka Y, Kuroda Y. Abnormal signal-averaged electrocardiogram in patients with Duchenne muscular dystrophy: comparison of time and frequency domain analyses from the signal-averaged electrocardiogram. *Clin Cardiol* 1993;**16**:723–8.
20. Hoffman EP, Fishbeck KH, Brown RH *et al.* Characterization of dystrophin in muscle-biopsy specimens from patients with Duchenne's or Becker's muscular dystrophy. *New Engl J Med* 1988;**318**:1363–8.
21. Melacini P, Fanin M, Danieli GA *et al.* Cardiac involvement in Becker's dystrophy. *J Am Coll Cardiol* 1993;**22**:1927–34.
22. Ducceschi V, Nigro G, Sarubbi B *et al.* Autonomic nervous system imbalance and left ventricular systolic dysfunction as potential candidates for arrhythmogenesis in Becker muscular dystrophy. *Int J Cardiol* 1997;**59**:275–9.
23. Voit T, Krogmann H, Lenard G. Emery–Dreifuss muscular dystrophy: disease spectrum and differential diagnosis. *Neuropediatrics* 1988;**19**:62–71.
24. Bione S, Maestrini E, Rivella S *et al.* Identification of a novel X-linked gene responsible for Emery–Dreifuss muscular dystrophy. *Nature Genet* 1994;**9**:323–7.
25. Bialer MG, McDaniel NL, Kelly TE. Progression of cardiac disease in Emery–Dreifuss muscular dystrophy. *Clin Cardiol* 1991;**14**:411–16.
26. Rakovec P, Zidar J, Šinkovec M, Zupan I, Brecelj A. Cardiac involvement in Emery–Dreifuss muscular dystrophy: role of a diagnostic pacemaker. *PACE* 1995;**18**:1721–4.
27. Wyse DG, Nath FC, Brownell AK. Benign X-linked (Emery–Dreifuss) muscular dystrophy is not benign. *PACE* 1987;**10**:533–7.
28. Marshall TM, Huckell VF. Atrial paralysis in a patient with Emery–Dreifuss muscular dystrophy. *PACE* 1992;**15**:135–40.
29. Harley HG, Rundle SA, Reardon W *et al.* Unstable DNA sequence in myotonic dystrophy. *Lancet* 1992;**339**:1125–8.
30. Harper PS. *Myotonic dystrophy*. 2nd edn. Philadelphia: WB Saunders Co., 1989.
31. Hiromasa S, Ikeda T, Kubota K *et al.* Myotonic dystrophy: ambulatory electrocardiogram, electrophysiologic study, and echocardiographic evaluation. *Am Heart J* 1987;**113**:1482–8.
32. Grigg LE, Chan W, Mond HG, Vohra JK, Downey WF. Ventricular tachycardia and sudden death in myotonic dystrophy: clinical, electrophysiologic and pathologic features. *J Am Coll Cardiol* 1985;**6**:254–6.
33. Hiromasa S, Ikeda T, Kubota K *et al.* Ventricular tachycardia and sudden death in myotonic dystrophy. *Am Heart J* 1988;**115**:914–15.
34. Phillips MF, Harper PS. Cardiac disease in myotonic dystrophy. *Cardiovasc Res* 1997;**33**:13–22.
35. Melacini P, Villanova C, Menegazzo E *et al.* Correlation between cardiac involvement and CTG trinucleotide repeat length in myotonic dystrophy. *J Am Coll Cardiol* 1995;**25**:239–45.
36. Groh WJ. The problem of arrhythmias in myotonic dystrophy: A United States perspective. Satellite symposium "Pacing in myotonic dystrophy: benefits in this unrecog-

nized population". *XIth World Symposium on Cardiac Pacing and Electrophysiology*, Berlin, June 29, 1999.

37. Kahaly G, Olshausen KV, Kahaly-Mohr S et al. Arrhythmias profile in acromegaly. *Eur Heart J* 1992;**13**:51–6.

38. McGuffin WL, Sherman BM, Roth J et al. Acromegaly and cardiovascular disorders. A prospective study. *Ann Intern Med* 1974;**81**:11–18.

39. Rodrigues EA, Caruana MP, Lahiri A, Nabarro JD, Jacobs HS, Raftery EB. Subclinical cardiac dysfunction in acromegaly: evidence for a specific disease of heart muscle. *Br Heart J* 1989;**62**:185–94.

40. Ross EJ, Griffith DNW. The clinical presentation of phaeochromocytoma. *Q J Med* 1989;**71**:485–96.

41. Haas GJ, Tzagournis M, Boudolas H. Pheochromocytoma catecholamine-mediated electrocardiographic changes mimicking ischemia. *Am Heart J* 1988;**116**:1363–5.

42. McNeill AJ, Adgey AAJ, Wilson C. Recurrent ventricular arrhythmias complicating myocardial infarction in the presence of phaeochromocytoma. *Br Heart J* 1992;**67**:97–8.

43. Levey GS, Klein I. Catecholamine-thyroid hormone interactions and the cardiovascular manifestations of hyperthyroidism. *Am J Med* 1990;**88**:642–6.

44. Wolf PA, Abott RD, Kannel WB. Atrial fibrillation: A major contributor to stroke in the elderly: The Framingham Study. *Arch Intern Med* 1987;**147**:1561–4.

45. Sawin CT, Geller A, Wolf PA et al. Low serum thyrotropin concentrations as a risk factor for atrial fibrillation in older persons. *New Engl J Med* 1994;**331**:1249–52.

46. Furszyfer J, Kurland LT, McConahey WM, Elveback LR. Graves' disease in Olmstead County, Minnesota, 1935 through 1967. *Mayo Clin Proc* 1970;**45**:636–44.

47. Presti CF, Hart RG. Thyrotoxicosis, atrial fibrillation, and embolism, revisited. *Am Heart J* 1989;**117**:976–7.

48. Ladenson PW. Thyrotoxicosis and the heart: something old and something new. *J Clin Endocrinol Metab* 1993;**77**:332–3.

49. Gavin LA. The diagnostic dilemmas of hyperthyroxinemia and hypothyroxinemia. *Adv Intern Med* 1988;**33**:185–203.

50. Tajiri J, Morita M, Higashi K, Fuji H, Nakamura N, Sato T. The cause of low voltage QRS complex in primary hypothyroidism. Pericardial effusion or thyroid hormone deficiency? *Jap Heart J* 1985;**26**:539–47.

51. Kumar A, Bhandari AK, Rahimtoola SH. Torsade de pointes and marked QT prolongation in association with hypothyroidism. *Ann Intern Med* 1987;**106**:712–13.

52. Sjostrom LV. Mortality of severely obese subjects. *Am J Clin Nutr* 1992;**55** (Suppl. 2):516S–23S.

53. Alexander JK. The cardiomyopathy of obesity. *Progr Cardiovasc Dis* 1985;**27**:325–34.

54. Duflou J, Virmani R, Rabin I et al. Sudden death as a result of heart disease in morbid obesity. *Am Heart J* 1995;**130**:306–13.

55. Messerli FH, Nunez BD, Ventura HO, Snyder DW. Overweight and sudden death: increased ventricular ectopy in cardiomyopathy of obesity. *Arch Intern Med* 1987;**147**:1725–8.

56. Drenick EJ, Fisler JS. Sudden cardiac arrest in morbidly obese surgical patients unexplained after autopsy. *Am J Surg* 1988;**155**:720–6.

57. Fisler JS. Cardiac effects of starvation and semistarvation diets: safety and mechanisms of action. *Am J Clin Nutr* 1992;**56**:230S–4S.

58. Bharati S, Lev M. Cardiac conduction system involvement in sudden death of obese young people. *Am Heart J* 1995;**129**:273–81.

59. Rossner S, Lagerstrand L, Persson HE, Sachs C. The sleep apnoea syndrome in obesity: risk of sudden death. *J Int Med* 1991;**230**:135–41.

60. Garner DM. Pathogenesis of anorexia nervosa. *Lancet* 1993;**341**:1631–5.

61. Neumarker KJ. Mortality and sudden death in anorexia nervosa. *Int J Eating Disorders* 1997;**21**:205–12.

62. Isner JM, Roberts WC, Heymsfield SB, Yager J. Anorexia nervosa and sudden death. *Ann Intern Med* 1985;**102**:49–52.

63. Cooke RA, Chambers JB, Singh R et al. QT interval in anorexia nervosa. *Br Heart J* 1994;**72**:69–73.

64. Petreita M, Bonaduce D, Scalfi L et al. Heart rate variability as a measure of autonomic nervous system function in anorexia nervosa. *Clin Cardiol* 1997;**20**:219–24.

65. Bradley JR, Evans DB, Calne RY. Long-term survival in haemodialysis patients. *Lancet* 1987;**i**:295–6.

66. Gruppo Emodialisi e Patologie Cardiovascolari. Multicenter, cross-sectional study of ventricular arrhythmias in chronically haemodialysed patients. *Lancet* 1988;**2**:305–8.

67. Kimura K, Tabei K, Asano Y, Hosoda S. Cardiac arrhythmias in hemodialysis patients: a study of incidence and contributory factors. *Nephron* 1989;**53**:201–7.

68. Chazan JA. Sudden death in patients with chronic renal failure on hemodialysis. *Dial Transplant* 1987;**16**:447–8.

69. Chhabra SC, Sandha GS, Wander GS. Incidence of cardiac arrhythmias in chronic renal failure, especially during hemodialysis. *Nephron* 1991;**57**:500–1.

70. Shapira OM, Bar-Khayim Y. ECG changes and cardiac arrhythmias in chronic renal failure patients on hemodialysis. *J Electrocardiol* 1992;**25**:273–9.

71. Ramirez G, Brueggemeyer CD, Newton JL. Cardiac arrhythmias on hemodilaysis in chronic renal failure patients. *Nephron* 1984;**36**:212–18.

72. Abe S, Yoshizawa M, Nakanishi A et al. Electrocardiographic abnormalities in patients receiving hemodialysis. *Am Heart J* 1996;**131**:1137–44.

73. Morrison G, Michelson EL, Brown S, Morganroth J. Mechanism and prevention of cardiac arrhythmias in chronic hemodialysis patients. *Kidney Int* 1980;**17**:811–19.

74. Quereda C, Orte L, Martesan R, Ortuno J. Ventricular ectopic activity in hemodialysis. *Nephron* 1986;**42**:181–2.

75. Rombola G, Colussi G, DeFerrari ME, Frontini A, Minetti L. Cardiac arrhythmias and electrolyte changes during haemodialysis. *Nephrol Dial Transplant* 1992;**7**:318–22.

76. Sforzini S, Latini R, Mingardi G et al. Ventricular arrhythmias and four-year mortality in haemodialysis patients. *Lancet* 1992;**339**:212–14.

77. Gokal R, Jakubowsky C, King J et al. Outcome in patients on continuous ambulatory peritoneal dialysis and haemodialysis: 4-year analysis of a prospective multicentre study. *Lancet* 1987;**ii**:1105–9.

78. De Lima JJG, Sesso R, Abensur H et al. Predictors of mor-

tality in long-term haemodialysis patients with a low prevalence of comorbid conditions. *Nephrol Dial Transplant* 1995;**10**:1708–13.

79. Tamura K, Tsuji H, Nishiue T *et al.* Determinants of ventricular arrhythmias in hemodialysis patients. *Am J Nephrol* 1998;**18**:280–4.

80. Morales MA, Gremigni C, Dattolo P *et al.* Signal-averaged ECG abnormalities in haemodialysis patients. Role of dialysis. *Nephrol Dial Transplant* 1998;**13**:668–73.

81. Gettes LS. Electrolyte abnormalities underlying lethal ventricular arrhythmias. *Circulation* 1992;**85**(Suppl. I):I70-6.

82. Eisenberg MJ. Magnesium deficiency and sudden death. *Am Heart J* 1992;**124**:544–9.

83. Hoes AW, Grobbe DE, Peet TM, Lubsen J. Do non-potassium-sparing diuretics increase the risk of sudden cardiac death in hypertensive patients? Recent evidence. *Drugs* 1994;**47**:711–33.

84. Tobias SL, Bookatz BJ, Diamond TH. Myocardial damage and electrocardiographic changes in acute cerebrovascular hemorrhage: A report of three cases and review. *Heart Lung* 1987;**16**:521–6.

85. Mikolich JR, Jacobs WC, Fletcher GF. Cardiac arrhythmias in patients with acute cerebrovascular accidents. *JAMA* 1981;**246**:1314–17.

86. Samuels MA. Electrocardiographic manifestations of neurologic disease. *Semin Neurol* 1984;**4**:453–9.

87. Dimant J, Grob D. Electrocardiographic changes and myocardial damage in patients with acute cerebrovascular accidents. *Stroke* 1977;**8**:448–55.

88. Jackman WM, Friday KJ, Anderson JL *et al.* The long QT syndromes: a critical review, new clinical observations and a unifying hypothesis. *Progr Cardiovasc Dis* 1988;**31**:115–72.

89. Surawicz B, Knoebel S. Long QT: good, bad or indifferent. *J Am Coll Cardiol* 1984;**4**:398–413.

90. Machado C, Baga JJ, Kawasaki R, Reinoehl J, Steinman RT, Lehman MH. Torsade de pointes as a complication of subarachnoid hemorrhage. A critical reappraisal. *J Electrocardiol* 1997;**30**:31–7.

91. Selzer A, Wray HW. Quinidine syncope, paroxysmal ventricular fibrillations occurring during treatment of chronic atrial arrhythmias. *Circulation* 1964;**30**:17–27.

92. Doig JC. Drug-induced cardiac arrhythmias: Incidence, prevention and management. *Drug Safety* 1997;**17**:265–75.

93. Roden DM. A practical approach to torsade de pointes. *Clin Cardiol* 1997;**20**:285–90.

94. Bährle S, Schöls W. Torsade de pointes in haemodialysis patients. *Nephrol Dial Transplant* 1996;**11**:944–6.

95. Napolitano C, Priori SG, Schwartz PJ *et al.* Identification of a long QT syndrome molecular defect in drug-induced torsades de pointes. *Circulation* 1997;**96**:1–211.

Part IV

Antiarrhythmic trials

37 Antiarrhythmic device trials

Arthur J Moss

The implantable cardioverter defibrillator (ICD) was introduced into clinical medicine by Dr Michel Mirowski in 1980.[1] Several randomised ICD trials were initiated in the early 1990s to evaluate the safety and efficacy of the ICD to reduce mortality as part of primary and secondary prevention strategies. Three major ICD trials were reported in the 1-year period between 1996 and 1997,[2–4] and each of these studies used a different approach to identify patients at high risk for malignant ventricular arrhythmias. The findings from these studies substantiated the role of ICDs as the therapy of first choice for specific high-risk subgroups. During the same time frame, several major antiarrhythmic drug trials with amiodarone and sotalol were reported in similar groups of patients at increased risk for sudden cardiac death, and the antiarrhythmic drugs were no better than placebo, and possibly worse. The recent studies have identified the ICD as appropriate therapy to improve survival and prevent sudden arrhythmic cardiac death in appropriately selected high-risk patients.

Device trials

General comments

ICD trials are unblinded by the nature of the operative intervention. In order to minimise selection bias in ICD trials, randomisation of patients to ICD versus no ICD is essential. Sudden arrhythmic death is not a satisfactory end-point, since the interpretation of the mechanism of the terminal event is often uncertain and the assignment of the cause of death can be difficult. In the early 1990s, two small randomised studies indicated that amiodarone suppressed complex ventricular ectopy and was associated with improved survival when compared with placebo.[5,6] When randomised ICD trials were initiated in the 1990s, the ICD was compared against amiodarone. Subsequently, three large-scale, randomised, double-blind, placebo-controlled amiodarone trials revealed that survival was similar in the amiodarone- and placebo-treated patients.[7–9]

When an ICD trial is being designed, the projected sample size is based on an anticipated reduction in the mortality rate among ICD-treated patients as compared with patients with non-ICD therapy, with a two-sided significance level ≤5% to minimise a false-positive finding and a power of 80% or greater to minimise a false-negative finding. The magnitude of the estimated reduction in mortality with ICD therapy is based on the hypothesised mortality in the non-device group, the estimated proportion of the mortality from ventricular tachyarrhythmia, and the anticipated efficacy of the ICD in preventing arrhythmic mortality. An independent data and safety monitoring committee should review the results of the trial at regular intervals throughout the study, and this committee should be given the responsibility to recommend termination of the trial for reasons of safety, efficacy, or no difference between the two treatment groups. All analyses and potential covariates should be specified in advance of the trial's completion, and the primary analysis should follow the intention-to-treat principle.

Primary prevention trials

Multicenter automatic defibrillator implantation trial (MADIT)

MADIT was designed as a prophylactic primary prevention trial to determine if implantation of an ICD in patients with coronary heart disease, left ventricular dysfunction, and asymptomatic non-sustained ventricular tachycardia would result in improved survival when compared to conventional therapy.[2] To ensure a population at high risk for ventricular fibrillation, eligible patients had to have a documented prior myocardial infarction, an ejection fraction ≤35%, and inducible, sustained, non-suppressible ventricular tachycardia at electrophysiological study. The end-point of the trial was total mortality during a 5-year follow-up period. The eligibility and exclusion criteria for MADIT are presented in Box 37.1. Patients were excluded if there was an indication for coronary revascularisation. A total of 196 patients were randomly assigned to receive either an

Box 37.1   MADIT eligibility and exclusion criteria*

- Eligibility criteria
  - male or female aged 25–80 years
  - one or more prior myocardial infarctions
  - documented episode of non-sustained ventricular tachycardia (run of 3–30 ventricular ectopic beats at a rate >120 bpm) within 3 months before enrolment
  - ejection fraction ≤35%
  - New York Heart Association Class I–III
  - inducible, non-suppressible ventricular tachycardia at electrophysiological study
- Exclusion criteria
  - aborted cardiac arrest at any time in the past
  - history of sustained ventricular tachycardia unrelated to an acute myocardial infarction
  - enzyme positive myocardial infarction in the past 3 weeks
  - coronary artery bypass graft surgery within the past 8 weeks or coronary angioplasty within the past 12 weeks
  - indication for coronary revascularisation
  - major co-morbidity with a reduced likelihood of survival for the duration of the trial
  - cardiogenic shock, symptomatic hypotension, or New York Heart Association Class IV
  - participation in other clinical trials
  - patients unwilling to sign a consent form for participation in MADIT

*Modified from Moss AJ et al.[2]

ICD or conventional medical therapy. The trial used a triangular, two-sided sequential design with preset stopping boundaries for benefit, no difference, or harm from the ICD compared with conventional therapy.[2] The first patient was enrolled in December 1990, and the trial was stopped in March 1996 on advice of the Data Safety Monitoring Board.

The pertinent baseline characteristics of the 196 enrolled patients are presented in Table 37.1. The two groups were clinically similar. The MADIT-defined patients had severe chronic coronary disease with one-third of the patients having had two or more prior myocardial infarctions, one-half having received prior treatment for congestive heart failure, and almost one-quarter having had prior coronary artery bypass-graft surgery. It should be emphasised that the length of the qualifying run of non-sustained ventricular tachycardia averaged 9–10 beats. There was an imbalance in the cardiac medications used 1 month after enrolment, with the non-ICD group having a higher use of amiodarone and a lower use beta-blockers than the ICD group.

The distribution of deaths, the cause of death, and the suspected mechanism of cardiac death by treatment assignment are presented in Table 37.2. There was more than a 2.5-fold higher rate of deaths in the non-ICD than the ICD group, with considerably more deaths classified as arrhythmic deaths in the former than the latter group. The Kaplan–Meier life-table survival curves for the two treatment groups are shown in Fig. 37.1. The two survival

Table 37.1   Baseline characteristics of MADIT by treatment group*

Characteristic	Treatment group	
	Conventional (No. = 101)	Defibrillator (No. = 95)
Age (years)	64 ± 9	62 ± 9
Male sex (%)	92	92
Cardiac history (%)		
two or more prior myocardial infarctions	29	34
treatment for ventricular arrhythmias	35	42
NYHA Class II–III	67	63
treatment for congestive heart failure	51	52
treatment for hypertension	35	48
insulin-dependent diabetes	5	7
coronary bypass surgery	44	46
implanted pacemaker	7	2
Cardiac findings at enrolment (%)		
blood urea nitrogen >25 mg/dl	21	22
left bundle branch block	8	7
mean ejection fraction	25 ± 7	25 ± 7
Qualifying non-sustained ventricular tachycardia		
number of consecutive beats	9 ± 10	10 ± 9

Plus–minus values are mean ±SD.
*Modified from Moss AJ et al.[2]

Table 37.2 Distribution of deaths in MADIT by treatment group*

Cause	Conventional (N = 101)	Defibrillator (N = 95)
All causes		
cardiac	27	11
non-cardiac	6	4
unknown	6	0
Total	39	15
Cardiac cause		
primary arrhythmia	13	3
non-arrhythmia	13	7
uncertain	1	1

*Modified from Moss AJ *et al. N Engl J Med* 1996;**335**:1933–40.

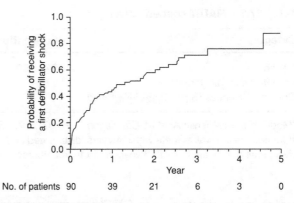

Figure 37.2 Probability of first ICD shock over time in MADIT. Reproduced with permission from Moss *et al. N Engl J Med* 1996;**335**:1933–40. Copyright ©1996 Massachusetts Medical Society. All rights reserved.)

curves separate early and remain well separated throughout the 5-year trial, with significantly improved survival for patients randomised to ICD therapy ($P = 0.009$). The cumulative time to first shock is presented in Fig. 37.2. Forty percent of the patients with an ICD had a shock discharge within 1 year after device implantation, 60% within 2 years, and 90% within 5 years. This rate of shock discharge is in good alignment with the improved survival in the ICD groups as shown in Fig. 37.1.

The hazard ratio comparing the risk of death per unit time in the ICD group with that in the non-ICD group was 0.46 (95% CI, 0.26–0.82; $P = 0.009$), i.e. there was a 54% reduction in death during any follow-up time interval in

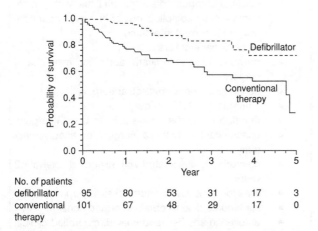

No. of patients
defibrillator	95	80	53	31	17	3
conventional therapy	101	67	48	29	17	0

Figure 37.1 Kaplan–Meier survival by treatment group in MADIT. The survival difference between the treatment groups was significant ($P = 0.009$). (Reproduced with permission from Moss *et al. N Engl J Med* 1996;**335**:1933–40. Copyright ©1996 Massachusetts Medical Society. All rights reserved.)

patients randomised to ICD versus non-ICD therapy. Additional analyses revealed that the beneficial effects of ICD therapy were similar in patients implanted with transthoracic and transvenous leads, and in several relevant subgroups.[2]

MADIT was associated with an imbalance in amiodarone and beta-blocker therapy between the two treatment groups. Amiodarone was used in almost 75% of the patients randomised to non-ICD therapy and in only 2% of patients in the ICD group. If amiodarone increased mortality, then it could have contributed to a beneficial ICD hazard ratio. However, all available randomised trials with amiodarone in similar high-risk populations show either no difference between amiodarone and placebo therapy, or a mild beneficial effect with amiodarone. It is unlikely that amiodarone contributed to the observed beneficial results with ICD therapy.

Beta-blockers were used in 26% of the ICD-treated patients and in 8% of the conventionally treated patients. The Cox proportional hazard model was used to evaluate the effect of beta-blocker use on the observed benefit with ICD therapy.[10] The benefit achieved with ICD therapy remained significant ($P = 0.02$) after adjustment for beta-blocker use. Although the beta-blocker imbalance in the two treatment arms could have had some minor effect on the results, it is unlikely that this imbalance contributed significantly to the observed beneficial findings with ICD therapy in this patient population.

A prospective cost-effectiveness analysis was carried out as part of MADIT, and the results were recently published.[11] The average survival for the defibrillator group over a 4-year period was 3.66 years compared with 2.80 years for conventionally treated patients. Accumulated average net costs were $97 560 in the ICD group compared with $75 980 in the non-ICD group. The resulting incremental cost-effectiveness ratio of $27 000 per life-year saved (Table 37.3) compares favourably with other

Table 37.3 MADIT cost effectiveness*

Category	Conventional	Defibrillator	Difference	95% CI†
Net costs‡	$75 980	$97 506	$21 580	$100–43 100
Expected survival (years)	2.66	3.46	0.8	0.41–1.22
Cost effectiveness ($ per year-of-life saved)			$27 000**	$200–68 200

*Modified from Mushlin AI *et al. Circulation* 1998;**97**:2129–35.
†Confidence interval. ‡Costs within 4 years, discounted at 3% per annum. **Ratio of net costs ($21 580) divided by expected survival for all device implants (0.8 years for both transthoracic and transvenous implants).

cardiac interventions such as CABG surgery. Sensitivity analyses showed that this cost-effectiveness would be reduced to approximately $22 800 per life-year saved if transvenous systems were used, as is currently the case.

MADIT was the first device trial showing that prophylactic ICD therapy saves lives and is cost-effective in patients with coronary heart disease at high risk for malignant ventricular arrhythmias.

Coronary artery bypass graft – ICD study (CABG-Patch)

The primary hypothesis of CABG-Patch was that the prophylactic implantation of an ICD at the time of CABG surgery in patients with symptomatic chronic coronary disease, left ventricular dysfunction, and a positive signal-averaged ECG would improve survival.[3] Patients were screened for entry into CABG-Patch after they were scheduled for operative coronary revascularisation for treatment of symptomatic ischaemic heart disease and obstructive coronary disease identified by coronary angiography. The end-point of the trial was total mortality. Enrolment in CABG-Patch began in January 1993, and the trial was stopped on advice of the Data and Safety Monitoring Board on April 2, 1997, because of no difference in mortality between the ICD and non-ICD groups, with a negligible chance that a difference would ever be found if the trial continued.[3]

The eligibility and exclusion criteria for CABG-Patch are presented in Box 37.2. Electrophysiological eligibility required only one abnormality on a signal-averaged ECG, i.e. either the duration of the filtered QRS ≥114 ms; root-mean-square voltage in the terminal 40 ms of the QRS <20 μV; or duration of the terminal 40 ms of the QRS at <40 μV, >38 ms. At the time CABG-Patch was started, a positive signal-averaged ECG was thought to be a good identifier of patients at high risk for sudden death, but subsequent studies failed to substantiate the usefulness of this technique in risk stratification for sudden cardiac death. As the investigators of CABG-Patch pointed out in the primary publication,[3] the signal-averaged ECG was used as a potential marker for high risk at enrolment because of the short time between hospital admission and surgery. In retrospect, this may have been the fatal flaw in the CABG-Patch trial.

The pertinent baseline characteristics of the 900 enrolled patients are presented in Table 37.4. The ICD and non-ICD treatment groups were clinically similar. The CABG-Patch patients had severe coronary heart disease with more than one-half of the patients having three-vessel coronary disease, almost a third having two or more

---

Box 37.2 CABG-patch eligibility and exclusion criteria*

- Eligibility criteria
  - male or female age <80 years of age
  - scheduled for coronary bypass graft surgery
  - ejection fraction ≤35%
  - positive signal-averaged electrocardiogram
- Exclusion criteria
  - history of sustained VT, VF, or cardiac arrest with inducible VT
  - renal dysfunction
  - insulin-dependent diabetes mellitus with significant vascular complications or history of poor control and recurrent infections
  - unipolar pacemakers
  - previous or concomitant aortic or mitral valve surgery
  - concomitant cerebrovascular surgery
  - emergency CABG surgery
  - thrombolysis in the 7 days prior to CABG surgery
  - concomitant arrhythmia surgery or aneurysmectomy
  - co-morbidity associated with expected survival <2 years
  - lives too far away to return for follow-up visits
  - inadequate time to obtain informed consent
  - enrolled in another randomised, controlled clinical trial
  - physician, surgeon, or patient refusal

Abbreviations: CABG = coronary bypass graft; VF = ventricular fibrillation; VT = ventricular tachycardia.
*Modified from Bigger JT *et al. N Engl J Med* 1997;**337**:1569–75.

Table 37.4 Baseline characteristics of CABG-patch by treatment group*

| | Treatment group | |
	Control (N = 454)	Defibrillator (N = 446)
Characteristic		
Age (years)	64 ± 9	63 ± 9
Male sex (%)	82	87
Cardiac history (%)		
two or more prior myocardial infarctions	33	30
treatment for ventricular arrhythmias	7	7
NYHA Class II–III	74	71
treatment for congestive heart failure	47	49
treatment for hypertension	52	54
diabetes treated with insulin	20	17
coronary bypass surgery	10	12
implanted pacemaker	2	2
Cardiac findings at enrolment (%)		
left bundle branch block	12	10
mean ejection fraction	27 ± 6	27 ± 6
Finding on coronary angiography (%)		
one-vessel disease	9	8
two-vessel disease	36	36
three-vessel disease	55	55

Plus–minus values are mean ±SD.
*Modified from Bigger JT *et al. N Engl J Med* 1997;**337**:1569–75.

prior myocardial infarctions, one-half having received treatment for congestive heart failure, but only one-tenth having had prior CABG surgery. The average EF was 27%. At 3 months after enrolment, the use of cardiac drugs, including antiarrhythmic agents and beta-blockers, was similar in the two treatment groups.

During an average follow-up of 32 months, the number of deaths in the two groups was very similar, and the Kaplan–Meier cumulative mortality curves showed no meaningful difference in the ICD and non-ICD treated patients (Fig. 37.3). The hazard ratio from Cox regression analysis was 1.07 (95% CI, 0.81–1.42), a value indicating that the ICD did not save lives in this population. In a follow-up publication, it was shown that ICD therapy reduced arrhythmic death by 45% without significant effect on non-arrhythmic deaths.[12]

The investigators concluded that, because 71% of the deaths were non-arrhythmic, total mortality was not significantly reduced. Other explanations for the absence of a survival benefit with ICD therapy in CABG-Patch have been given. Patients enrolled in CABG-Patch were selected from a pool of patients with symptomatic coronary disease who underwent coronary revascularisation surgery, an intervention known to reduce myocardial ischaemia and the risk of ischaemia-mediated malignant ventricular arrhythmias. Although the overall clinical characteristics of the CAGB-Patch and MADIT populations

were similar (Table 37.1 and 37.4), the MADIT patients had more extensive coronary disease with a 4-fold greater frequency of prior bypass surgery at enrolment than the CABG-Patch patients. Many of the MADIT patients probably had further progression of their coronary and bypass

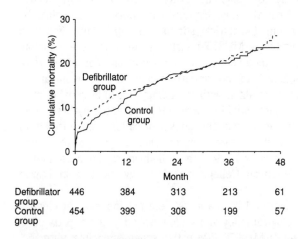

Defibrillator group	446	384	313	213	61
Control group	454	399	308	199	57

Figure 37.3 Kaplan–Meier survival by treatment group in CABG-Patch. The survival difference between the treatment groups was not significant (*P* = 0.64). (Reproduced with permission from Bigger JT *et al. N Engl J Med* 1997;**337**: 1569–75. Copyright ©1997 Massachusetts Medical Society. All rights reserved.)

grafts in the years between the prior CABG surgery and enrolment. Furthermore, patients with an indication for coronary revascularisation were excluded from MADIT. In contrast, patients enrolled in CABG-Patch, by definition, had symptomatic indication for coronary revascularisation.

Current evidence suggests that a positive signal-averaged ECG is only a non-specific marker for mortality, and does not identify patients at risk for arrhythmic death. CABG-Patch eligibility required only one of three criteria for an abnormal signal-averaged ECG, and the use of two of three criteria may be more sensitive for identifying high-risk, arrhythmia-prone patients. Furthermore, a positive signal-averaged ECG is not the arrhythmic risk equivalent of overt non-sustained ventricular tachycardia and a positive electrophysiological study, an eligibility requirement in MADIT. An additional explanation for the trial results may relate to the lower actuarial 2-year mortality in CABG-Patch (18%) compared with the non-ICD-treated patients in MADIT (32%). Once again, the relatively low mortality rate in CABG-Patch probably reflects the beneficial results from revascularisation.

Patients defined by the CABG-Patch criteria do not achieve long-term benefit from implantation of an ICD at the time of CABG surgery.

Multicenter unsustained tachycardia trial (MUSTT)

MUSTT was designed to test the hypothesis that electrophysiologically-guided antiarrhythmic therapy will reduce the risk of arrhythmic death or cardiac arrest in coronary patients with unsustained ventricular tachycardia and left ventricular dysfunction (ejection fraction ≤40%). Patients who met the eligibility criteria were offered an electrophysiological study. Patients who were not inducible by programmed electrical stimulation were simply followed as part of the MUSTT registry. Those who were inducible into sustained ventricular tachycardia and consented were randomised to no antiarrhythmic therapy (comparison group) or to antiarrhythmic therapy guided by serial electrophysiological studies. If an effective antiarrhythmic drug was not identified, this subset of patients was offered an ICD. MUSTT started in October 1991 and the study ended in early 1999 with preliminary results presented at the American College of Cardiology meeting in March 1999.

A total of 1396 patients were not inducible at electrophysiological study and were enrolled in the registry component of MUSTT; 704 patients were inducible, with 353 patients randomised to no antiarrhythmic therapy and 351 patients to electrophysiologically-guided antiarrhythmic treatment. In half of the later group, an effective antiarrhythmic drug was not identified and an ICD was implanted. The 5-year survival rate was approximately 75%

in those who received an ICD, 55% in those receiving electrophysiolgically-guided antiarrhythmic therapy, and 50% in those randomised to no therapy. The survival benefit with ICD therapy was quite striking, and the overall findings were remarkably similar to the results of MADIT.

Secondary prevention trials

Antiarrhythmics versus implantable defibrillator trial (AVID)

AVID was a secondary prevention trial and was designed to determine if ICD therapy in patients resuscitated after near-fatal ventricular fibrillation or those with symptomatic, sustained ventricular tachycardia with haemodynamic compromise would result in improved survival when compared to antiarrhythmic therapy with amiodarone or sotalol.[4] The ICD had already been approved by the FDA for use in such high-risk patients with aborted or threatened cardiac arrest, but no prior randomised prospective trial had been performed in this patient group. AVID was designed to evaluate treatment strategies using several different ICD devices and two different antiarrhythmic drugs. The trial used a traditional fixed-sample-size design. The eligibility and exclusion criteria for AVID are presented in (Box 37.3). One thousand and sixteen patients were randomly assigned to receive ICD or one of two Class III antiarrhythmic drugs. The first patient was enrolled in June 1993, and the trial was terminated on April 7, 1997 on recommendation of the Data and Safety Monitoring Board when analysis revealed a significant reduction in mortality in the ICD group compared to the patients randomised to antiarrhythmic drug therapy.

The pertinent baseline characteristics of the enrolled patients are presented in Table 37.5. The two treatment groups were similar; 45% had ventricular fibrillation as the index arrhythmia, and 55% had ventricular tachycardia. The AVID-defined patient had an average EF of 32%, with over 80% having a history of coronary artery disease, two-thirds having had a prior myocardial infarction, and slightly less than half with a history of congestive heart failure. During hospitalisation for the index arrhythmia, 11% of the patients underwent coronary revascularisation. Over 95% of the patients randomised to the antiarrhythmic drug group received amiodarone, with good compliance in taking amiodarone during the course of the trial (87% still receiving amiodarone at 1 year, and 85% at 2 years). The mean daily dose of amiodarone progressively decreased during follow-up, from 389 ± 112 mg at 3 months to 256 ± 95 mg at 3 years. As in the MADIT study, beta-blockers were used more frequently ($P < 0.001$) in the ICD group than in the antiarrhythmic drug group, 42% versus 17% at initial hospital discharge, and

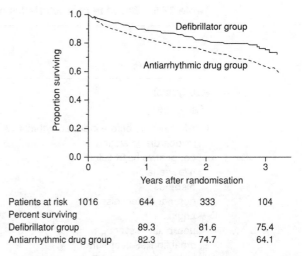

Figure 37.4 Kaplan–Meier survival by treatment group in AVID. The survival difference between the treatment groups was significant (*P* <0.02). (Reproduced with permission from The AVID Investigators. *N Engl J Med* 1997;**337**: 1576–83. Copyright ©1997 Massachusetts Medical Society. All rights reserved.)

Patients at risk	1016	644	333	104
Percent surviving				
Defibrillator group		89.3	81.6	75.4
Antiarrhythmic drug group		82.3	74.7	64.1

this imbalance persisted throughout the course of the trial.

During a mean follow-up of 18 months, the mortality in the ICD group was 16% versus 24% in the antiarrhythmic drug group. The Kaplan–Meier life-table survival curves for the two treatment groups are shown in Fig. 37.4. The average unadjusted length of additional life associated with ICD therapy was 2.7 months at 3 years. Activation of the ICD, either antitachycardia pacing or shock, was considerably more frequent if the index arrhythmia was ventricular tachycardia than ventricular fibrillation. Approximately 20% of patients crossed over to or had the other therapy added by 24 months. The Cox proportional-hazards regression model was used to adjust for baseline differences in several relevant clinical factors and for imbalance in beta-blocker use. The benefit achieved with ICD therapy in improving survival was essentially unchanged from the unadjusted raw data. The hazard ratios for various subgroups are presented in Fig. 37.5. It is interesting that patients with ejection fractions ≤35% achieved more bene-

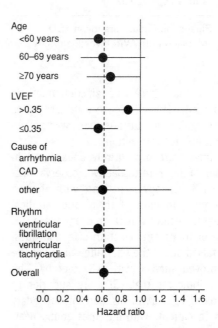

Figure 37.5 Hazard ratios and 95% confidence limits (horizontal lines) for death from any cause in prespecified AVID subgroups. The dotted line represents the results for the entire study (hazard ratio 0.62). LVEF = left ventricular ejection fraction; CAD = coronary artery disease. (Reproduced with permission from The AVID Investigators. *N Engl J Med* 1997;**337**:1576–83. Copyright ©1997 Massachusetts Medical Society. All rights reserved.)

Table 37.5   Baseline characteristics of AVID by treatment group*

Characteristic	Treatment group Antiarrhythmic drug (N = 509)	Defibrillator (N = 507)
Age (years)	65 ± 10	65 ± 11
Male sex (%)	86	87
Cardiac history before index arrhythmia (%)		
myocardial infarction	67	67
congestive heart failure	47	46
hypertension	56	55
diabetes	24	25
coronary artery disease	81	81
angina	50	48
unexplained syncope	10	11
atrial fibrillation or flutter	26	21
ventricular tachycardia	15	14
ventricular fibrillation	5	5
Index arrhythmia (%)		
sustained ventricular tachycardia	55	55
ventricular fibrillation	45	45
Cardiac findings at enrolment (%)		
angina	34	36
congestive heart failure	60	55
bundle branch block	25	23
corrected QT interval (msec)	445 ± 39	441 ± 40
mean ejection fraction	40 ± 13	32 ± 13

Plus−minus values are mean ±SD.
*Modified from AVID Investigators. *N Engl J Med* 1997;**337**:1576–83.

fit (hazard ratio <0.6) than those with ejection fractions >35% (hazard ratio >0.8). This difference in hazard ratios was not statistically significant and thus there was no significant ICD-ejection fraction interaction.

These AVID findings were not entirely unexpected in view of a spectrum of prior retrospective, observational experiences of the ICD therapy in patients with aborted cardiac arrest. However, in most of these prior studies, the groups of patients receiving ICD or drugs were not equivalent because of treatment selection bias, and questions were always raised about the scientific validity of the observation of improved survival with ICD therapy. The AVID study clearly indicates that ICDs are superior to amiodarone in prolonging survival as part of secondary prevention therapy in patients with life-threatening, near-fatal ventricular arrhythmias.

Cardiac arrest study Hamburg (CASH)

CASH was designed as a four-arm study to evaluate ICD, propafenone, amiodarone, and metoprolol therapy in cardiac arrest survivors. A combined end-point was used that included total mortality, aborted cardiac arrest, or docu-

mented ventricular tachycardia. The propafenone arm of the trial was stopped early because of increased cardiac events with this therapy. The preliminary results of the other three arms of the trial (N = 229) were reported in March 1998, with improved survival with ICD when compared with patients randomised to either amiodarone or metoprolol therapy ($P = 0.094$, two-sided). CASH was severely underpowered to detect significant differences in survival among the antiarrhythmic therapies. Nevertheless, there was a meaningful trend with ICD-treated patients having a lower mortality than patients treated with conventional antiarrhythmic drug therapy.

Canadian implantable defibrillator study (CIDS)

The design of CIDS was similar to AVID and involved a comparison of ICD versus amiodarone in patients with prior cardiac arrest, haemodynamically unstable ventricular tachycardia, or unexplained syncope. The primary outcome event was arrhythmic death and any death occurring within 30 days of initiation of either ICD or amiodarone therapy. Approximately 600 patients were enrolled, and ICD therapy was associated with improved survival when compared to amiodarone ($P = 0.072$, two sided). CIDS enrolled about one-half as many patients as AVID, with similar overall results but a less significant P-value due to the smaller sample size.

Comparison of antiarrhythmic device trials

The primary and secondary device trials were designed to evaluate the efficacy of ICD therapy in reducing mortality in high-risk cardiac patients. MADIT, CABG-Patch, and MUSTT focused on primary prevention of sudden arrhythmic death and used non-invasive (SAECG in CABG-Patch) or invasive (EPS in MADIT and MUSTT) testing to identify such high-risk patients. In MADIT and MUSTT, the eligibility requirements were quite stringent and involved patients with documented coronary disease who had advance mechanical and electrical dysfunction. In CABG-Patch, the eligibility requirements were less stringent, ambient ventricular arrhythmias were not required, and ICD implantation was an "add on" to surgical revascularisation, which is known to reduce the arrhythmic risk potential in patients with obstructive coronary disease. AVID, CASH, and CIDS were designed as secondary prevention trials and used documented spontaneous life-threatening arrhythmias as the identifier of high risk.

The six device studies were designed in the early 1990s, and they were the first set of prospective randomised device trials ever performed. The initiation of each trial should be viewed in the light of the clinical knowledge and experience that was available at that time. MADIT, CABG-Patch, and MUSTT started when only first-generation (shock-only) transthoracic defibrillators were approved for ICD therapy, and this certainly influenced trial design (stringent non-invasive and invasive criteria for entry into MADIT and MUSTT and concurrent ICD implantation at the time of thoracotomy during surgical revascularisation in CABG-Patch). By the time AVID started in 1993, second and third generation ICD devices were available, and the transvenous approach was approved. During the past 5 years, the structure and func-

tion of ICD devices have continued to improve with reduced size and increased therapeutic capability. During this same time, the limited usefulness of antiarrhythmic drug therapy in improving survival has become evident. A summary comparison of the six randomised trials that were designed to prevent sudden cardiac death and reduce mortality is presented in Fig. 37.6.

Recently initiated device trials

The current MADIT II, sudden cardiac death-heart failure trial (SCD-HeFT), and defibrillator implantation in non-ischaemic cardiomyopathy treatment evaluation (DEFINITE) trials are designed to test new hypotheses with the latest device technology (Table 37.6). All three studies are secondary prevention trials involving patients with more

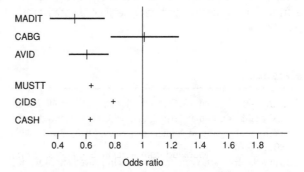

Figure 37.6 Results of six randomised trials to reduce mortality by ICD therapy. The solid vertical line represents equal effectiveness of the ICD vs. non-ICD therapies, with the odds of dying equivalent (odds ratio 1.0). In the upper three reported studies (MADIT, CABG-Patch, and AVID), the short vertical lines are the point estimates of the odds ratios, with the horizontal lines a rough indication of the 95% confidence intervals. In the lower three studies (MUSTT, CIDS, and CASH), the + sign indicates the point estimate of the odds ratios for each study from the preliminary results presented at cardiology meeting in 1998 and 1999; confidence intervals are not available. See text for further details.

Table 37.6   Recently initiated ICD trials

Study	Comparison therapy	Population	Size	End point
MADIT II	Conventional therapy	CAD and EF ≤30%	1200	Total mortality
SCD-HeFT	Placebo or amiodarone	EF ≤35%	2400	Total mortality
DEFINITE	Conventional therapy	CM and EF ≤35%	440	Total mortality

Abbreviations: CAD = coronary artery disease; DEFINITE = Defibrillator Implantation in Non-Ischaemic Cardiomyopathy Treatment Evaluation; EF = ejection fraction; MADIT II = Multicenter Automatic Defibrillator Trial II; SCD-HeFT = Sudden Cardiac Death-Heart Failure Trial.

advanced left ventricular failure than the earlier reported trials. The results from these studies are anticipated within the first few years of the 21st century.

Conclusion

The reported device trials have substantiated the safety and efficacy of ICD therapy in high-risk cardiac patients with electrical vulnerability. The newly initiated studies are focusing on patients with more advanced left ventricular dysfunction, a substrate with high potential for generating malignant ventricular arrhythmias. Overt and induced ventricular arrhythmias are not part of the eligibility criteria of any of the ongoing studies. Recently, left ventricular free wall pacing has been demonstrated to improve left ventricular function in patients with heart failure and intraventricular conduction disturbance. In the future, electrical therapy for treatment of mechanical and electrical cardiac dysfunction may be incorporated into a single device.

References

1. Mirowski M, Reid PR, Mower MM *et al.* Termination of malignant ventricular arrhythmias with an implanted automatic defibrillator in human beings. *N Engl J Med* 1980; **303**:322–4.

2. Moss AJ, Hall WJ, Cannom DS *et al.* Improved survival with an implanted defibrillator in patients with coronary disease at high risk for ventricular arrhythmia. *N Engl J Med* 1996; **335**:1933–40.

3. Bigger JT Jr, for the Coronary Artery Bypass Graft (CABG) Patch Trial Investigators. Prophylactic use of implanted cardiac defibrillators in patients at high risk for ventricular arrhythmias after coronary artery bypass graft surgery. *N Engl J Med* 1997;**337**:1569–75.

4. The antiarrhythmics versus implantable defibrillators (AVID) investigators. A comparison of antiarrhythmic drug therapy with implantable defibrillators in patients resuscitated from near-fatal ventricular arrhythmias. *N Engl J Med* 1997;**337**:1576–83.

5. Ceremuzynski L, Kleczar E, Krzeminska-Pakula M *et al.* Effect of amiodarone on mortality after myocardial infarction: a double-blind, placebo-controlled, pilot study. *J Am Coll Cardiol* 1992;**20**:1056–62.

6. Doval HC, Nul DR, Grancelli HO *et al.* Randomized trial of low-dose amiodarone in severe congestive heart failure. *Lancet* 1994;**344**:493–8.

7. Singh SN, Fletcher RD, Fisher SG *et al.* Amiodarone in patients with congestive heart failure and asymptomatic ventricular arrhythmia. *N Engl J Med* 1995;**333**:77–82.

8. Julian DG, Camm AJ, Frangin G *et al.* Randomized trial of effect of amiodarone on mortality in patients with left-ventricular dysfunction after recent myocardial infarction: EMIAT. *Lancet* 1997;**349**:667–74.

9. Cairns JA, Connolly SJ, Roberts R *et al.* Randomized trial of outcome after myocardial infarction in patients with frequent or repetitive ventricular premature depolarisations: CAMIAT. *Lancet* 1997;**349**:675–82.

10. Moss AJ. Background, outcome, and clinical implications of the multicenter automatic defibrillator implantation trial (MADIT). *Am J Cardiol* 1997;**80**(5B):28F–32F.

11. Mushlin AI, Hall WJ, Zwanziger J *et al.* The multicenter automatic defibrillator implantation trial: results from the cost-effectiveness analysis. *Circulation* 1998;**97**:2129–35.

12. Bigger JT Jr, Whang W, Rottman JN *et al.* Mechanisms of death in the CABG Patch Trial: a randomized trial of implantable cardiac defibrillator prophylaxis in patients at high risk of death after coronary artery bypass graft surgery. *Circulation* 1999;**99**:1416–21.

38 Recent antiarrhythmic drug trials

Michiel J Janse

The suppression of ventricular arrhythmias

In 1993, Teo, Yusuf, and Furberg published an overview of 138 trials on antiarrhythmic drugs against ventricular arrhythmias involving a total of 98 000 patients.[1] For the 51 trials on sodium-channel blocking drugs (Class I agents), 571 patients in the control groups died (out of 11 517 patients) versus 660 in the treated groups (11 712 patients) The odds ratio was 1.14, the 95% CI 1.01–1.28, and the *P* value 0.03.

In the 55 trials on beta-adrenergic blockers (Class II agents), in which a total of 43 268 patients were enrolled, the beneficial effects of these drugs were clearly demonstrated: odds ratio 0.81, CI 0.75–0.87, *P* value 0.00011.

The 24 trials on calcium-entry blockers, in which 20 342 patients participated, gave indifferent results: odds ratio 1.04, CI 0.95–1.14, *P* value 0.41.

The only antiarrhythmic drug, apart from beta-blockers, that showed any promise was amiodarone. Although the number of patients studied at that time was small, totalling 1557, the odds ratio in favour of amiodarone was 0.71, with a CI of 0.51–0.97, and a *P* value of 0.03. The endpoint of all trials mentioned here was all-cause mortality.

As summarised in Box 38.1, the conclusion was that class I agents increased mortality, class II drugs provided benefit, class IV compounds were unpromising, and amiodarone was promising.

Since sodium-channel blockers are effective in suppressing ventricular arrhythmias, but actually increase mortality, whereas beta-blockers are not particularly effective in suppressing arrhythmias but are effective in preventing sudden death, it was suggested that "decreasing heart rate and reducing sympathetic activity may be a more promising approach to the prevention of sudden death than suppression of ambient arrhythmias recorded on Holter monitoring."[1] Indeed, as shown by Kjekshus, those beta-blockers that produced the greatest reduction in sinus rhythm were the most effective in preventing sudden death in patients with myocardial infarction.[2] Another reason why beta-blockers were effective in reducing mortality in the acute phase of myocardial infarction is that they reduce the incidence of cardiac rupture.[3] Two

very recent trials, in which the effects of beta-blockers were tested in patients with congestive heart failure,[4,5] showed that bisoprol and metoprolol not only significantly reduced all-cause mortality, but also the incidence of sudden death. In the largest of these two trials,[5] in which 3991 patients were enrolled, 79 cases of sudden death occurred in the group treated with metoprolol versus 132 in the placebo group (odds ratio 0.59, CI 0.45–0.78, *P* = 0.0002). There is no doubt that the only class of drugs offering significant protection against sudden death in high-risk patients are the beta-blockers.

Because of the disappointing results of trials involving sodium-channel blocking drugs, and of the neutral effects of calcium antagonists, the antiarrhythmic drug trials of the past decade concentrated on on amiodarone and other drugs that prolong repolarisation (class III agents). At the time these trials were designed, i.e. around 1990, it was believed that prolonging repolarisation, and thus the refractory period, would prevent or abolish re-entrant arrhythmias by prolonging the wavelength (the product of

---

Box 38.1 Summary of data on suppression of ventricular arrhythmias

- 138 antiarrhythmic drug trials on 98 000 patients
- Na-channel blocking drugs (51 trials):
  - 11 712 patients in the treated group; 660 deaths
  - 11 713 patients in the control group; 571 deaths
  - Odds ratio 1.14; 95% CI 1.01–1.28; *P* = 0.03
- Beta-adrenergic receptor blocking drugs (55 trials):
  - 26 973 patients in the treated group; 1464 deaths
  - 26 974 patients in the control group; 1727 deaths
  - Odds ratio 0.81; 95% CI 0.75–0.87; *P* = 0.00001
- Ca-channel antagonists (24 trials):
  - 10 154 patients in the treated group; 982 deaths
  - 10 155 patients in the control group; 949 deaths
  - Odds ratio 1.04; 95% CI 0.95–1.14; *P* = 0.41
- Amiodarone (8 trials):
  - 778 patients in the treated group; 77 deaths
  - 779 patients in the control group; 101 deaths
  - Odds ratio 0.71; 95% CI 0.51–0.97; *P* = 0.03

Data derived from Teo *et al.*[1]

---

conduction velocity and refractory period). In retrospect, one may wonder why imitating the congenital long QT syndrome by action potential prolonging drugs would be expected to be antiarrhythmic.

The pro-arrhythmic effects of drugs that prolong the action potential will be described in a separate section.

The amiodarone trials

Only three of 13 randomised controlled trials of amiodarone showed a significant reduction of all-cause mortality in the treated group (for overview see Table 38.1). The BASIS study[6] included 312 patients with a recent myocardial infarction and complex ventricular arrhythmias (Lown class 3 or 4b) who were randomised into three groups: placebo (control), Holter-guided antiarrhythmic treatment, and amiodarone. Mortality in the amiodarone group was significantly lower than in the control group (1-year mortality of 5.3% versus 14.3%). The Argentine pilot study of sudden death and amiodarone (EPAMSA)[7] recruited 127 patients with asymptomatic arrhythmias and a left ventricular ejection fraction lower than 35%. Mortality in the placebo group was almost three times higher than in the amiodarone group. The larger GESICA study[8] included 516 patients with advanced heart failure and a left ventricular ejection fraction equal to or lower than 35%. There was a risk reduction for total mortality of 28% (CI 0.54–0.95). Although these results were promising, all three studies suffered from having enrolled only a small number of patients. The role of amiodarone as preventive therapy for patients with left ventricular dysfunction

became unclear because of the results of the CHF-STAT study.[9] In this trial, 674 patients were included on the basis of two entry criteria: documented history of congestive heart failure and at least 10 ventricular premature beats per hour.

Amiodarone had no significant effect on all-cause mortality during 45 months of follow-up. However, amiodarone tended to reduce total mortality in patients with ischaemic cardiomyopathy ($P = 0.07$), and reduced the incidence of ventricular arrhythmias.

The two largest amiodarone trials are the European Myocardial Infarct Amiodarone Trial (EMIAT) and the Canadian Amiodarone Myocardial Infarction Arrhythmia Trial (CAMIAT),[10,11] enrolling 1486 and 1202 patients respectively. Although both trials recruited patients with a recent myocardial infarction, both the entry criteria and the primary end-points were different. EMIAT is the only amiodarone trial in which presence of arrhythmias was not an entry criterion. Eligible patients were those aged 18–75 years, who had a left ventricular ejection fraction of 40% or less, as determined with multiple-gated nuclear angiography between 5 and 28 days after onset of myocardial infarction. The reasoning behind this was that even at the time the trial was designed (1989) it was already clear that suppression of arrhythmias did not prevent sudden death and that left ventricular dysfunction was the most powerful predictor of sudden death.[12,13] EMIAT's primary end-point was all-cause mortality, and it was powered to detect a 35% reduction in total mortality. In CAMIAT, post-myocardial infarction patients were recruited who had 10 or more ventricular premature beats per hour, or at least one run of ventricular tachycardia, and its primary end-point was arrhythmic death.

Table 38.1 Results of 13 amiodarone trials*

Study	Reference	Number of patients		1 year all-cause mortality	
		Control	Amiodarone	Control	Amiodarone
EMIAT	10	743	743	8.1	8.2
CAMIAT	11	596	606	6.4	5.2
CHF-STAT	9	338	336	18.1	17.0
PAT	19	308	305	11.6	7.2
GESICA	8	256	260	40.4	28.3
SSSD	20	123	115	3.0	1.3
BASIS	6	114	98	14.3	5.3
Hockings	21	100	100	5.9	10.3
EPAMSA	7	49	57	30.2	10.5
Nicklas	22	52	49	17.7	25.1
GEMICA (6 months)	23	38	33	10.7	12.7
CAMIAT pilot	24	29	48	13.7	6.2
Hamer	25	15	19	26.4	21.4

*Data derived from Amiodarone Trials Meta-Analysis.[15]

CAMIAT patients were at lower risk than EMIAT patients (1-year placebo mortality of 6.4% versus 8.2%). Neither trial showed a significant reduction of all-cause mortality, but both reported on a substantial reduction in arrhythmic death and resuscitated cardiac arrest (risk reduction in EMIAT was 35%, in CAMIAT 48.8%). An accompanying Editorial highlighted the difficulties in defining arrhythmic death, and, more importantly, in diagnosing it.[14] Nevertheless, since in both studies the evaluation committees were blinded as to whether the patient was on placebo or amiodarone, one might assume that the uncertainties in diagnosing arrhythmic death were equally divided among the two groups. A meta-analysis of all amiodarone trials, involving 6500 patients, arrived at the conclusion that prophylactic amiodarone reduces the rate of arrhythmic/sudden death in high-risk patients with a recent infarct or congestive heart failure, resulting in an overall reduction of 13% in total mortality (Table 38.1).[15] Clearly, both EMIAT and CAMIAT were insufficiently powered to detect such a reduction in total mortality. The impact of the meta-analysis remains unclear; patient populations in the various studies are different, and confirmation of the results of this meta-analysis will not be performed, in view of the very large number of patients needed to conduct a prospective randomised trial. From a practical point of view, it may be noted that amiodarone therapy was discontinued in 41% of patients, because of adverse side effects, including thyroid disorders (in the vast majority only "biochemical" and not "clinical"), neuropathy, lung infiltration, bradycardia, and liver dysfunction.

Subsequent post hoc analysis of EMIAT and CAMIAT noted a positive interaction between beta-adrenergic blocking agents and amiodarone.[16,17] The concluding remarks of the last paper were: "For the clinician treating a patient after myocardial infarction or any patient with significant arrhythmia in whom treatment with amiodarone is planned, the results of this analysis is clear. Amiodarone does not replace a beta-blocker. Beta-blocker therapy should be continued if possible."[17] The reasons for the amiodarone–beta-blocker interaction are not clear. One might speculate that in patients with suboptimal beta-blockade, amiodarone may offer a more complete adrenergic blockade. Also, because of the direct effects of amiodarone on the sinus node,[18] the extra reduction in sinus rate may be beneficial.[16]

Trials with other drugs that prolong repolarisation

Following the disappointing results with sodium channel blocking agents, interest was renewed in drugs that prolong repolarisation, and special hopes were focused on so-called pure class III drugs. The potassium channel blocker *d*-sotalol, with minimal beta-blocking activity unlike sotalol,

was evaluated in the Survival With Oral *d*-Sotalol (SWORD) trial.[26] The patients were similar to those of EMIAT (left ventricular ejection fraction lower than 40%, in patients with both a recent (6–42 days) and a remote (more than 42 days) infarct), and recruitment of 6400 patients was planned. After inclusion of 3121 patients, the trial was prematurely terminated because 78 patients out of 1549 assigned to *d*-sotalol died (5.0%) versus 48 (3.1%) in the placebo group. Presumed arrhythmic death (odds ratio 1.77; CI 1.15–2.74; $P = 0.001$) accounted for the increased mortality. Although the reported incidence of torsade de pointes was low (0.2%) the authors wrote: "We believe that the higher risk of death with *d*-sotalol in women than in men suggests that the arrhythmia that caused the adverse effect was torsade de pointes."[26]

Another potassium channel blocker, dofetilide, was tested in the DIAMOND trial.[27] In postinfarction patients, the drug was well tolerated but had no significant effect on total mortality.

The overall experience of antiarrhythmic drug trials in the past decade clearly raises the question whether pro-arrhythmic effects of antiarrhythmic drugs may not offset potential benefits related to arrhythmia suppression. This has also become evident from the analysis of studies on antiarrhythmic drugs used to treat supraventricular arrhythmias. Thus, a meta-analysis of six trials, involving 808 patients, on quinidine therapy for atrial fibrillation[28] clearly showed that, although quinidine was more effective in maintaining sinus rhythm following cardioversion than no antiarrhythmic therapy, it was associated with increased mortality (all-cause mortality for the quinidine treated patients was 2.9%, versus 0.8% in the placebo group; $P < 0.05$). In a randomised trial comparing warfarin, aspirin, and placebo for the prevention of stroke or systemic emboli in patients with atrial fibrillation, it was noted that, in patients receiving antiarrhythmic therapy, cardiac mortality was increased 2.5 fold ($P = 0.006$, CI 1.3–4.9) and arrhythmic death 2.6 fold.[29] The authors wrote: "Although antiarrhythmic therapy was not randomly determined, the data suggest that in patients with atrial fibrillation and a history of congestive heart failure the risk may outweigh the potential benefit of maintaining sinus rhythm."[29]

At the end of this decade, the optimism of the early 1990s regarding drugs with class III effects has been replaced by concern of pro-arrhythmic effects of both cardiac and non-cardiac drugs that prolong the action potential.

Pro-arrhythmic effects of antiarrhythmic drugs

Sodium channel blockers

The electrophysiogical mechanisms for pro-arrhythmia have recently been reviewed by Nattel.[30] Following the

CAST study,[31] suggesting pro-arrhythmic effects of sodium channel blockers in patients with myocardial infarction, a number of experimental studies showed that flecainide caused preferential slowing of conduction, and conduction block, in the epicardial layers overlying the infarct, thereby facilitating re-entry.[32–34]

During the first 10 minutes of acute ischaemia, sodium channel blockers may both be antiarrhythmic and pro-arrhythmic: lidocaine specifically depresses excitability of ischaemic myocytes. When this leads to complete inexcitability of the ischaemic zone, no re-entrant circuits can be set up, and the drug is actually antifibrillatory;[35] when ischaemia is less severe, areas with well-maintained conduction may be converted to zones of unidirectional block and the drug may promote re-entry.[36]

Very little is known about pro-arrhythmic effects of sodium channel blockers in hearts without ischaemia, infarction, or structural abnormalities.

Drugs that prolong the action potential

Prolongation of the action potential of ventricular myocytes, which causes prolongation of the QT interval in the electrocardiogram, is brought about by a reduction of outward currents, or to an enhancement of inward currents during the plateau phase of the action potential, or to both. The reduction in net outward current may lead to the development of early after depolarisations, which occur preferentially in M cells and Purkinje cells, due to reactivation of the *L*-type calcium current and/or activation of the sodium–calcium exchange current during the plateau phase.[37–39]

Action potential and QT prolongation *per se*, even when leading to early after-depolarisations, need not to be arrhythmogenic. Only when accompanied by a marked increase in dispersion of repolarisation (and thus in refractoriness) can an early after-depolarisation-induced premature beat trigger re-entry and torsade de pointes.[40–43]

The development of early after-depolarisations and torsade de pointes occurs mostly with drugs, both antiarrhythmic drugs and non-cardiac drugs, that block the rapid component of the delayed rectifyer, I_{kr}. However, not all drugs that block I_{kr} have the same arrhythmogenic potential. For example, the estimated incidence of torsade de pointes for cisapride is 1 out of 120 000 patients treated,[44] while for sotalol the incidence is between 2 and 2.4%.[45,46] The exact reasons for the different effects of I_{kr} blockers is unknown, but there are many factors that modulate the effect of drugs that block I_{kr}. These include the following:

● *Bradycardia*: low heart rates prolong the action potential.

● *Hypokalaemia and hypomagnaesemia*: at low extracellular K concentrations I_{kr} blockade by quinidine and dofetilide is enhanced.[47]

● *Hypertrophy and heart failure*: in these conditions, the action potential is prolonged and further reduction of I_{kr} may result in excessive action potential prolongation.[48]

● *Gender*: torsade de pointes occurs more frequently in women,[49] and female rabbits have less I_{kr} than male rabbits.[50]

● *Metabolic factors*: certain drugs, such as cisapride and terfenadine, are metabolised by the P450 isoenzyme CYP3A4. When drugs that inhibit CYP3A4 (erythromycin and other macrolide antibiotics, ketoconazole and other azole antifungals, mibefradil) are co-administered, plasma levels of the parent drug may rise considerably, thus leading to further lengthening of the action potential.

● *Sympathetic activity*: I_{kr} block combined with beta-adrenergic stimulation increases transmural dispersion of repolarisation because of "a large augmentation of I_{ks} in epicardial and endocardial cells but not in M cells where I_{ks} is intrinsically weak".[51] This favours re-entry.

● *Formes frustes of the congenital long QT syndrome*: although as yet there are insufficient data to support this, non- symptomatic carriers of mutated genes for sodium or potassium channels may be more susceptible for drugs that prolong the action potential.

● *Multiple actions of drugs that block I_{kr}*: The best example is amiodarone, which in addition to blocking I_{kr} also blocks sodium and calcium currents and has beta-adrenergic effects. Despite the fact that it prolongs the QT interval, amiodarone is associated with a very low incidence of torsade de pointes.[52] This may be due to its blocking effects of the sodium and calcium currents (thus suppressing early after-depolarisations) and to the fact that it does not increase, or actually decrease, transmural dispersion of repolarisation (thus preventing re-entry).[40,53]

From the above it is evident that many factors may interact with drugs that prolong the action potential duration, and that in ordinary practice it is extremely difficult to predict whether or not such a drug may exhibit a pro-arrhythmic effect. The results of the clinical trials thus far suggest that "pure class III drugs" may be more pro-arrhythmic than antiarrhythmic, whereas drugs with multiple actions such as amiodarone may in certain patients be beneficial, and are at least not dangerous. The positive interaction of beta-blockers and amiodarone needs to be proven prospectively. Thus far, the only drugs that have been proved to offer protection against sudden death in high-risk patients are the beta-adrenergic blocking agents.

References

1. Teo KK, Yusuf S, Furberg CD. Effects of prophylactic antiarrhythmic drug therapy in acute myocardial infarction: an overview of results of randomised controlled clinical trials. *JAMA* 1993;**270**:1589–95.

2. Kjekshus JK. Importance of heart rate in determining beta-blocker efficacy in acute and long-term acute myocardial infarction intervention trials. *Am J Cardiol* 1986;**57**:43F–49F.

3. ISIS-1 Collaborative Group. Mechanisms for the early mortality reduction produced by beta-blockade started early in acute myocardial infarction. *Lancet* 1988;1:921–3.

4. CIBIS-II Investigators. The Cardiac Insufficiency Bisoprolol Study II (CIBIS-II): a randomised trial. *Lancet* 1999;**353**:9–13.

5. MERIT-HF Study Group. Effect of metoprolol CR/XL in chronic heart failure: Metoprolol CR/XL Randomised Intervention Trial in Congestive Heart Failure (MERIT-HF). *Lancet* 1999;**353**:2001–7.

6. Burkart F, Pfisterer M, Kiowski W, Follath F, Burckhardt D. Effect of antiarrhythmic therapy on mortality in survivors of myocardial infarction with asymptomatic complex ventricular arrhythmias: Basel Antiarrhythmic Study of Infarct Survival (BASIS). *J Am Coll Cardiol* 1990;**16**:1711–18.

7. Garguichevich JJ, Ramos JL, Gambarte A *et al.* for the Argentine Pilot Study of Sudden Death and Amiodarone Investigators. Effect of amiodarone therapy on mortality in patients with left ventricular dysfunction and asymptomatic complex ventricular arrhythmias: Argentine pilot study of sudden death and amiodarone. *Am Heart J* 1995;**130**:494–500.

8. Doval HC, Nul DR, Grancelli HO, Perrone SV, Bortman GR, Curiel R, for Grupo de Estudio de la Sobrevida en la Insuficiencia Cardiaca en Argentina (GESICA). Randomised trial of low-dose amiodarone in severe congestive heart failure. *Lancet* 1994;**344**:493–8.

9. Singh SN, Fletcher RD, Fisher SG *et al.* for the Survival Trial in Congestive Heart Failure. Amiodarone in patients with congestive heart failure and asymptomatic ventricular arrhythmias. *New Engl J Med* 1995;**333**:77–82.

10. Julian DG, Camm AJ, Frangin G, Janse MJ, Munoz A, Schwartz PJ, Simon P for the EMIAT Investigators. Randomised trial of effect of amiodarone on mortality in patients with left-ventricular dysfunction after recent myocardial infarction: EMIAT. *Lancet* 1997;**349**:667–74.

11. Cairns JA, Conolly SJ, Roberst RS, Gent M and the CAMIAT Investigators. Randomised trial of outcome after myocardial infarction in patients with frequent or repetitive premature depolarisations. *Lancet* 1997;**349**:675–82.

12. Bigger JT Jr, Flaiss JL, Kleiger J *et al.* The relationship among ventricular arrhythmias, left ventricular dysfunction, and mortality two years after myocardial infarction. *Circulation* 1984;**69**:250–8.

13. Pitt B. Sudden cardiac death: role of left ventricular dysfunction. *NY Acad Sci* 1982;**382**:218–28.

14. Gottlieb SS. Dead is dead – artificial definitions are no substitute. *Lancet* 1997;**349**:662–3.

15. Amiodarone Trials Meta-Analysis Investigators. Effect of prophylactic amiodarone on mortality after acute myocardial infarction and in congestive heart failure: meta-analysis of individual data from 6500 patients in randomised trials. *Lancet* 1997;**350**:1417–24.

16. Janse MJ, Malik M, Camm AJ, Julian DG, Frangin GA, Schwartz PJ on behalf of the EMIAT investigators. Identification of post acute myocardial infarction patients with potential benefit from prophylactic treatment of amiodarone. A substudy of EMIAT. *Eur Heart J* 1998;**19**:85–95.

17. Boutitie F, Boissel J-P, Connolly S *et al.* and the EMIAT and CAMIAT Investigators. Amiodarone interaction with beta-blockers. Analysis of the merged EMIAT and CAMIAT databases. *Circulation* 1999;**99**:2268–75.

18. Kodama I, Kamiya K, Toyama J. Cellular electropharmacology of amiodarone. *Cardiovasc Res* 1997;**35**:13–29.

19. Ceremuzynski L, Kleczar E, Krzeminska-Pakula M *et al.* Effect of amiodarone on mortality after myocardial infarction: a double blind, placebo-controlled, pilot study. *J Am Coll Cardiol* 1992;**20**:1056–62.

20. Navarro-Lopez F, Cosin J, Marrugat J, Guindo J, Bayes de Luna A for the SSSD Investigators. Comparison of the effects of amiodarone versus metropolol on the frequency of ventricular arrhythmias and on mortality after acute myocardial infarction. *Am J Cardiol* 1993;**72**:1243–8.

21. Hockings BEF, George T, Mahrous F, Taylor RR, Hajar HA. Effectiveness of amiodarone on ventricular arrhythmias during and after myocardial infarction. *Am J Cardiol* 1987;**60**:967–70.

22. Nicklas JM, McKenna WJ, Stewart RA *et al.* Prospective, double-blind, placebo-controlled trial of low dose amiodarone in patients with severe heart failure and asympomatic frequent ventricular ectopy. *Am Heart J* 1991;**122**:1016–21.

23. Elizari M, Martinez JM, Belztitic C *et al.* Mortality following early administration of amiodarone in acute myocardial infarction: results of the GEMICA trial. *Circulation* 1996;**94**(Suppl. 1):90.

24. Cairns JA, Connolly SJ, Gent M, Roberts R. Post myocardial infarction mortality in patients with ventricular premature depolarizations. *Circulation* 1991;**84**:550–7.

25. Hamer AWF, Arkles B, Johns JA. Beneficial effects of low dose amiodarone in patients with congestive cardiac failure: a placebo-controlled trial. *J Am Coll Cardiol* 1989;**14**:1768–74.

26. Waldo AL, Camm AJ, de Ruyter H *et al.* for the SWORD investigators. Effects of d-sotalol on mortality in patients with left ventricular dysfunction after recent and remote myocardial infarction. *Lancet* 1996;**348**:7–12.

27. Danish Investigators of Arrhythmias and Mortality On Dofetilide (DIAMOND). Presented at The American Heart Association meeting in Orlando, Florida, November 1997.

28. Coplen SE, Antman EM, Berlin JA, Hewitt P, Chalmers FC. Efficacy and safety of quinidine therapy for maintenance of sinus rhythm after cardioversion. A meta-analysis of randomized control trials. *Circulation* 1990;**82**:1106–16.

29. Flaker GC, Blackshear JL, McBride R, Kronmal RA, Halperin JL, Hart RG. Antiarrhythmic drug therapy and cardiac mortality in atrial fibrillation. The stroke prevention in atrial fibrillation investigators. *J Am Coll Cardiol* 1992;**20**:527–32.

30. Nattel S. Experimental evidence for pro-arrythmic mechanisms of antiarrhythmic drugs. *Cardiovasc Res* 1998;**37**:567–77.

31. The Cardiac Arrhythmia Suppression Trial (CAST) Investigators. Preliminary report:effect of encainide and flecainide on mortality in a randomized trial of arrhythmia suppression after myocardial infarction. *New Engl J Med* 1989;**321**:406–12.

32. Ranger S, Nattel S. Determinants and mechanisms of flecainide-induced promotion of ventricular tachycardia in anesthetized dogs. *Circulation* 1995;**92**:1300–11.

33. Restivo M, Yin H, Caref EB *et al*. Reentrant arrhythmias in the subacute infarction period. The pro-arrhythmic effect of flecainide acetate on functional reentrant circuits. *Circulation* 1995;**91**:1236–46.

34. Coromilas J, Saltman AE, Waldecker B, Dillon SM, Wit AL. Electrophysiological effects of flecainide on anisotropic conduction and reentry in infarcted canine hearts. *Circulation* 1995;**91**:2245–63.

35. Cardinal R, Janse MJ, Van Eeden I *et al*. The effect of lidocaine on intracellular and extracellular potentials, activation, and ventricular arrhythmias during acute regional ischemia in the isolated porcine heart. *Circ Res* 1981;**49**:792–806.

36. Carson DL, Cardinal R, Savard P. *et al*. Relationship between an arrhythmogenic action of lidocaine and its effects on excitation patterns in acutely ischemic porcine myocardium. *J Cardiovasc Pharmacol* 1986;**8**:126–36.

37. Antzelevitch C, Sicouri S. Clinical relevance of cardiac arrhythmias generated by after-depolarizations. Role of M cells in the generation of U waves, triggered activity and torsade de pointes. *J Am Coll Cardiol* 1994;**23**:259–77.

38. Viswanathan PC, Rudy Y. Pause induced early after-depolarization in the long QT syndrome: a simulation study. *Cardiovasc Res* 1999;**42**:530–42.

39. Carlsson C, Abrahamsson C, Anderson B, Duker G, Schiller-Lindhardt G. Pro-arrhythmic effects of class III agent almokalant: importance of infusion rate, QT dispersion and early after-depolarizations. *Cardiovasc Res* 1993;**27**:2186–93.

40. Haverkamp W, Shenassa M, Borggrefe M, Breithardt G. Torsade de pointes. In: DP Zipes, J Jalife eds. *Cardiac electrophysiology, from cell to bedside*. 2nd edn. Philadelphia: WB Saunders Co., 1995, pp. 849–85.

41. El Sherif N, Caref FB, Yin H, Restivo M. The electrophysiological mechanism of ventricular arrhythmias in the long QT syndrome. Tridimensional mapping of activation and recovery patterns. *Circ Res* 1996;**79**:474–92.

42. Surawicz B. Electrophysiological substrate for torsade de pointes: dispersion of refractoriness or early after-depolarizations. *J Am Coll Cardiol* 1989;**14**:172–84.

43. Verduyn SC, Vos MA, Van der Zande J, Van der hulst FF, Wellens HJJ. Role of interventricular dispersion of repolarization in acquired torsade de pointes arrhythmias: reversal by magnesium. *Cardiovasc Res* 1997;**34**:453–63.

44. Vitola J, Vukanovic J, Roden DM. Cisapride-induced torsade de pointes. *J Cardiovasc Electrophysiol* 1998;**9**:1109–13.

45. Soyka LF, Wirz C, Spangenberg RB. Clinical safety profile of sotalol in patients with arrhythmias. *Am J Cardiol* 1990;**65**:74A–81A.

46. McNeill DJ, Davies RO, Deitchman D. Clinical safety profile of sotalol in the treatment of arrhythmias. *Am J Cardiol* 1993;**72**:44A–50A.

47. Yang T, Roden DM. Extracellular potassium modulation of drug block of I_{kr}. *Circulation* 1996;**93**:407–11.

48. Vermeulen JT, McGuire MA, Opthof T *et al*. Triggered activity and automaticity in ventricular trabeculae of failing human and rabbit hearts. *Cardiovasc Res* 1994;**28**:1547–54.

49. Lehmann MH, Hardy S, Archibald D, Quart B, McNeill DJ. Sex difference in risk of torsade de pointes with d,l-sotalol. *Circulation* 1996;**94**:2535–41.

50. Liu X-K, Katchman A Drici M-D *et al*. Gender differences in cycle-length dependent QT and potassium currents in rabbits. *J Pharm Exp Ther* 1998;**285**:672–9.

51. Shimizu W, Antzelevitch C. Cellular basis for the ECG features of the LQT1 form of the long-QT syndrome. Effects of beta-adrenergic agonists and antagonists and sodium channel blockers on transmural dispersion of repolarization and torsade de pointes. *Circulation* 1998;**98**:2314–22.

52. Singh BN. Amiodarone: pharmacological, electrophysiological, and clinical profile of an unusual antiarrhythmic compound. In: Singh BN, Wellens HJJ, Hiraoka M, eds. *Electropharmacological control of cardiac arrhythmias*. Mount Kisco, NY: Futura Publishing Company, Inc., 1994, pp. 497–522.

53. Sicouri S, Moro S, Litovski SH, Elizari M, Antzelevitch C. Chronic amiodarone reduced transmural dispersion of repolarization in the canine heart. *J Cardiovasc Electrophysiol* 1997;**8**:1269–79.

Index